Study Guide
for
# Medical-Surgical Nursing
Assessment and Manage...
Clinical Problems

## First Canadian Edition

**Sharon Mantik Lewis, RN, PhD, FAAN**
Professor, Schools of Nursing and Medicine
Castella Distinguished Professor of Nursing
University of Texas Health Science Center
Clinical Nurse Scientist
Geriatric Research, Education, and Clinical Center
South Texas Veterans Health Care System
San Antonio, Texas

**Margaret M. Heitkemper, RN, PhD, FAAN**
Professor, Biobehavioral Nursing and Health
Systems
School of Nursing
Adjunct Professor, Division of Gastroenterology
School of Medicine
University of Washington
Seattle, Washington

**Shannon Ruff Dirksen, RN, PhD**
Associate Professor, College of Nursing
Arizona State University
Tempe, Arizona

**Sandra Goldsworthy,
RN, BScN, MSc, CCN(C)**
Professor, Faculty of Nursing
Durham College/
University of Ontario Institute of Technology
Oshawa, Ontario

**Maureen A. Barry, RN, BScN, MScN**
Senior Lecturer, Faculty of Nursing
University of Toronto
Toronto, Ontario

Prepared by

**Patricia Graber O'Brien, RNCS, MSN, MA**
Instructor, College of Nursing
University of New Mexico
Clinical Resource Coordinator
Lovelace Scientific Resources
Albuquerque, New Mexico

**Sandra Goldsworthy, RN, BScN, MSc, CCN(C)**

**Maureen A. Barry, RN, BScN, MScN**

MOSBY

ELSEVIER

---

**Notice**

Nursing is an ever-changing field. Standard safety precautions must be followed, but as new research and clinical experience broaden our knowledge, changes in treatment and drug therapy may become necessary or appropriate. Readers are advised to check the most current product information provided by the manufacturer of each drug to be administered to verify the recommended dose, the method and duration of administration, and contraindications. It is the responsibility of the licensed prescriber, relying on experience and knowledge of the patient, to determine dosages and the best treatment for each individual patient. Neither the publisher nor the editor assumes any liability for any injury and/or damage to persons or property arising from this publication.

---

**Library and Archives Canada Cataloguing in Publication**

Lewis, Sharon Mantik
Study guide for medical-surgical nursing in Canada / Sharon
Lewis, Margaret Heitkemper, Shannon Dirksen; Sandra Goldsworthy,
Maureen Barry, editors. — 1st ed.

Supplement to: Medical-surgical nursing in Canada.
ISBN 0-7796-9968-8 (pbk.)

1. Surgical nursing—Textbooks. I. Heitkemper, Margaret M.
(Margaret McLean) II. Dirksen, Shannon Ruff III. Goldsworthy,
Sandra, 1961- IV. Barry, Maureen, 1951- V. Title.
RT41.L49 2006 Suppl.      617'.0231           C2006-902199-6


*Publisher:* John Horne
*Managing Developmental Editor:* Martina van de Velde
*Developmental Editor:* Dawn du Quesnay
*Managing Production Editor:* Lise Dupont
*Copy Editor:* Gilda Mekler
*Cover Design:* Kim Denando
*Typesetting and Assembly:* Wordbench
*Printing and Binding:* Transcontinental


Elsevier Canada
905 King Street West, Fourth Floor, Toronto, ON, Canada M6K 3G9
Phone: 1-866-896-3331
Fax: 1-866-359-9534

Printed in Canada
1 2 3 4 5   11 10 09 08 07

# Contents

**Worksheets**

1. Using your jurisdictional regulatory body's definition of nursing, identify which of the following activities are the domain of nursing.

_____ a. Writing an order for intake and output for a client who is vomiting

_____ b. Explaining the risks associated with the planned surgical procedure when a preoperative client asks

_____ c. Teaching a post-operative client relaxation and meditation techniques to manage pain

_____ d. Preventing pneumonia in an immobile client by ordering frequent turning, coughing, and deep breathing

_____ e. Determining and administering fluid replacement therapy needed for a client with serious burns

_____ f. Assessing the abdomen of an immobile client for bowel motility

2. In the following situation, identify five human responses to actual or potential health problems that are identified nursing diagnoses (see list of nursing diagnoses on inside back cover).

A 36-year-old woman is admitted to the hospital for a breast biopsy and possible mastectomy. The client tells the nurse she has known about the mass in her breast for about eight months but had not seen her doctor because she was afraid it might be cancer. She paces the room, telling the nurse she has a four-year-old son she wants to be able to care for and that she does not know what to expect if surgery is done. The following morning she undergoes a right modified radical mastectomy after a frozen section reveals cancer. Post-operatively, she experiences much incisional pain and swelling and limited movement of her right arm. She glances at the surgical site once when the dressings are changed and comments how awful she looks. When the doctor informs her that four of the lymph nodes were positive for cancer and she will have to undergo chemotherapy and radiation, she begins to cry. She says she had been worried that she would not be attractive to her husband, but now she just needs to focus on being able to live.

a.

b.

c.

d.

e.

3. The nurse knows that the use of evidence-based nursing practice

   a. is the same thing as research utilization.
   b. does not consider the individual client's preferences.
   c. improves the quality of client care and client outcomes.
   d. provides clinical practice guidelines that eliminate the need to make decisions about client care.

4. Classification of nursing interventions and outcomes is a process designed to

   a. standardize nursing care for clients with specific nursing diagnoses.
   b. identify client problems that are the specific domain of nursing practice.
   c. develop a standardized language for nursing planning, implementation, and evaluation.
   d. eliminate the need for nurses to identify individualized outcomes and interventions for clients.

5. Identify the three nursing languages that specifically relate to the steps of the nursing process.

   a.

   b.

   c.

6. Match the phases of the nursing process with the descriptions (answers may be used more than once).

   _____  a. Analysis of data                          1. Assessment

   _____  b. Priority setting                          2. Diagnosis

   _____  c. Nursing interventions                     3. Planning

   _____  d. Data collection                           4. Implementation

   _____  e. Identifying client strengths              5. Evaluation

   _____  f. Measuring client achievement of goals

   _____  g. Setting goals

   _____  h. Identifying health problems

   _____  i. Modifying the plan of care

   _____  j. Documenting care provided

7. A 62-year-old client hospitalized with heart failure has been receiving large doses of diuretics. The nurse notes that the client has increasing weakness, flabby muscles, increased irritability, and a weak, rapid pulse. The nurse notifies the physician regarding these findings, and asks the doctor if the client's potassium level should be checked. The physician orders a laboratory test for serum electrolytes. The results indicate hypokalemia, and the nurse calls the physician to report the results. The physician orders potassium supplements, daily serum electrolyte levels, and a high-potassium diet. The nurse administers the medication and discusses the dietary order and the client's status with the dietitian. The dietitian sees the client and does initial teaching regarding dietary intake of potassium. The nurse helps the client choose high potassium foods from the daily menu and evaluates the client's ability to make correct choices. The nurse also monitors the client's response to the potassium supplements with the daily lab results and physical assessment findings.

What are the independent, collaborative, and dependent functions that the nurse performed in this situation?

a.  Independent

b.  Collaborative

c.  Dependent

8. The following is a list of two-part nursing diagnoses. Identify whether each statement is correctly (C) or incorrectly (I) written. If it is incorrectly written, explain what is incorrect.

_____ a. Need for activity related to social isolation

_____ b. Inability to turn related to traction

_____ c. Dyspnea related to activity intolerance

_____ d. Body image disturbance related to loss of breast

_____ e. Pain related to surgery

_____ f. Ineffective individual coping related to inadequate support system

_____ g. Constipation related to bowel obstruction

_____ h. Cardiac monitoring related to cardiac arrhythmias

9. For the following problems, write "ND" in front of those that are nursing diagnoses and "CP" in front of those that are collaborative problems.

   _____  a. Infection related to immunosuppression

   _____  b. Ineffective airway clearance related to excessive mucus

   _____  c. Constipation related to irregular defecation habits

   _____  d. Deficient fluid volume related to NPO status

   _____  e. Fatigue related to sleep deprivation

   _____  f. Excess fluid volume related to high sodium intake

   _____  g. Imbalanced nutrition: less than body requirements related to anorexia

   _____  h. Risk for cardiac arrhythmias related to potassium deficiency

   _____  i. Stress urinary incontinence related to weak pelvic floor muscles

   _____  j. Hypoxia related to chronic obstructive pulmonary disease

10. Read all of the data for the case history below and write a three-part nursing diagnosis statement that clearly describes the problem.

    A 52-year-old client has been on prolonged bed rest following a fractured pelvis. When he begins ambulation, he develops the following signs and symptoms: shortness of breath on exertion; inability to carry out usual activities of daily living because of weakness and fatigue; pulse remains elevated after activity for more than five minutes.

11. Identify four guidelines that may be used in setting priorities of intervention for nursing diagnoses.

    a.


    b.


    c.


    d.


12. Describe how planned nursing interventions would differ between these two nursing diagnoses: (a) imbalanced nutrition: less than body requirements related to anorexia and (b) imbalanced nutrition: less than body requirements related to difficulty in swallowing.

13. Identify the expected client outcomes that are correctly (C) written, and identify what criteria are not met in those outcomes that are incorrectly (I) written.

_____ a. The client will recognize the importance of taking the medications as prescribed.

_____ b. The client lists the supplies needed to change the dressing by discharge.

_____ c. The client maintains a low-sodium diet.

_____ d. The client's activity tolerance will be increased by discharge.

_____ e. The client will ambulate with a walker from the room to the nurse's station three times a day without assistance.

14. For the nursing diagnoses and client outcomes listed below, write a specific nursing order indicated to help the client reach the outcome.

a. Nursing Diagnosis: Risk for impaired skin integrity related to immobility
   Client Outcome: Client will demonstrate skin integrity free of pressure ulcers

b. Nursing Diagnosis: Constipation related to inadequate fluid and fibre intake
   Client Outcome: Client will have daily soft bowel movements in one week

15. A client with a seizure disorder is admitted to the hospital following a sustained seizure. When the client tells the nurse that she has not taken her medication regularly, the nurse makes a nursing diagnosis of ineffective therapeutic regimen management related to lack of knowledge regarding medication regimen, and identifies an expected client outcome of "Takes prescribed medication as directed."

When the nurse tries to teach the client about the medication regimen, the client tells the nurse that she knows about the medications but she does not always have the money to refill the prescriptions. Where was the mistake made in the nursing process with this client?

How would the nurse revise the care plan based on this evaluation?

16. Identify four advantages of computerized documentation, especially when nursing languages are integrated in the computer programming.

a.

b.

c.

d.

# CHAPTER 2    CULTURALLY COMPETENT CARE

1. Match the following terms with their descriptions.

_____ a. Culture
1. Identification with a group whose members share a common social and cultural heritage passed through generations

_____ b. Values
2. Modification of one's culture as a result of contact with another culture

_____ c. Subculture
3. Forcing one's own cultural beliefs and practices on others without regard for their culture

_____ d. Acculturation
4. Principles and standards that serve as bases for beliefs, attitudes, and behaviours

_____ e. Assimilation
5. The knowledge, values, beliefs, laws, and customs of members of a society

_____ f. Ethnicity
6. Divisions of humankind sharing common ancestry and physical characteristics

_____ g. Race
7. Large groups of people who have shared characteristics that are not common to all members of the culture

_____ h. Ethnocentricity
8. The assumption that all members of a culture or ethnic group share the same values and beliefs

_____ i. Cultural imposition
9. Loss of one's cultural identity in the process of adaptation to the dominant culture

_____ j. Stereotyping
10. The belief that one's own values, beliefs, and behaviours are the only right and natural way

2. List the four basic characteristics of culture.

a.

b.

c.

d.

3. Identify the specific process of acquiring cultural competence reflected in the following examples.

   a.   Asking the client what caused the illness and what treatment would be appropriate.

   _____

   b.   Identifying one's own biases toward people of another culture.

   _____

   c.   Working directly with persons from different cultures over a period of time.

   _____

   d.   Creating a safe environment in which collection of relevant cultural data can be obtained during the health history and physical examination.

   _____

4. During the physical examination of a client from Southeast Asia, the nurse notes a number of round red bruises on the client's chest, back, and abdomen. The best response to this finding by the nurse is to ask the client,

   a.   "What has caused all these bruises you have on your body?"
   b.   "Has someone been hitting you or abusing you in some way?"
   c.   "Have you used any traditional treatments for your condition?"
   d.   "Did these bruises appear when you became ill with this condition?"

5. Identify one example of how each of the following cultural factors may affect the nursing care of a client of a different culture.

   a.   Time orientation        _____

   b.   Economic factors       _____

   c.   Nutrition              _____

   d.   Personal space         _____

   e.   Beliefs and values     _____

6. A hospitalized Aboriginal client tells the nurse that later in the day a healer from his nation is coming to perform a healing ceremony to return his world to balance. The nurse recognizes that

   a.   the client does not adhere to an organized, formal religion.
   b.   the client's spiritual needs may be met by traditional rituals.
   c.   the client may be putting his health in jeopardy by relying on rituals.
   d.   traditional Aboriginal medicine cannot alter the progression of the client's physical illness.

7. When the nurse takes a surgical consent form to an Asian woman for a signature after the surgeon has provided the information about the recommended surgery, the client refuses to sign the consent form. The best response by the nurse is

   a.   "Didn't you understand what the doctor told you about the surgery?"
   b.   "Are there others that you want to talk with before making this decision?"
   c.   "You are the only one who can sign this consent. It is your decision to make."
   d.   "I'll have to call the surgeon and have your surgery cancelled until you can make a decision."

8. A male nurse would be providing culturally competent care by requesting that a female nurse provide nursing care for a(n)

   a.   Arabic male.
   b.   Arabic female.
   c.   Hispanic female.
   d.   Black male.

9. A disease that occurs more frequently and has higher mortality rates in non-white populations is

   _____.

10. Identify at least six classes of drugs that are known to produce different responses in people of different ethnic groups.

   a.

   b.

   c.

   d.

   e.

   f.

11. In a Hispanic client who claims to have *susto*, the nurse would expect assessment findings to include

   a.   abdominal pain and cramping.
   b.   anxiety, insomnia, anorexia, and social isolation.
   c.   nightmares, weakness, and a sense of suffocation.
   d.   headaches, stomach problems, and loss of consciousness.

12. During the care of culturally diverse clients, the nurse must be aware that knowledge of cultural beliefs and behaviours may inadvertently lead to

   a.   stereotyping clients of one culture.
   b.   the tendency to develop ethnocentricity.
   c.   unconsciously imposing one's own culture on others.
   d.   confusing the values and beliefs of one culture with another.

13. Using the information presented in the textbook, identify the cultural characteristics that the nurse might find in the following areas during assessment of an Aboriginal client and a traditional Hispanic client.

| | **Aboriginal Client** | **Traditional Hispanic Client** |
| --- | --- | --- |
| **Communication** | | |
| **Illness factors** | | |
| **Culture-bound syndromes** | | |

# CHAPTER 3  HEALTH HISTORY AND PHYSICAL EXAMINATION

1. A newly admitted client has a medical history in his record file. Is it necessary for the nurse to complete a nursing history of the client? Why or why not?

2. While being admitted to the nursing unit from the emergency department, a client tells the nurse she is short of breath and has pain in her chest when she breathes. Her respiratory rate is 28 per minute, and she is coughing up yellow sputum. Her skin is hot and moist, and her temperature is 39°C (102.2°F). She says that coughing makes her head hurt and she aches all over. Identify the subjective and objective assessment findings in this client.

   **Subjective**                                              **Objective**

3. Give an example of a sensitive way to ask a client the following questions.

   a. Is a client on antihypertensive medication having a side effect of impotence?

   b. Has a client with a history of alcoholism had recent alcohol intake?

   c. Who are the sexual contacts of a client with gonorrhea?

   d. What complementary and alternative therapies are used by the client?

4. The nurse prepares to interview a client for a nursing history but finds the client in obvious pain. The best action by the nurse at this time is to

   a. delay the interview until the client is pain free.
   b. administer pain medication before initiating the interview.
   c. gather as much information as quickly as possible by using closed questions that require brief answers.
   d. ask only those questions pertinent to the specific problem and complete the interview when the client is more comfortable.

5. During an interview the client tells the nurse, "I am so tired and wrung-out I don't know what to do." The nurse's best action at this time is to

   a. arrange another time with the client to complete the interview.
   b. stop the interview and leave the client alone to sleep.
   c. question the client further about the characteristics of the symptoms.
   d. reassure the client that the symptoms will improve when treatment has time to be effective.

6. Rewrite each question asked by the nurse so that it is an open-ended question designed to gather information about the client's functional health patterns.

   a. Are you having any pain?

   b. Do you have a good relationship with your wife?

   c. How long have you been ill?

   d. Do you exercise regularly?

7. The following data are obtained from a client during a nursing history. Organize these data according to Gordon's functional health patterns. Patterns may be used more than once, and some data may apply to more than one pattern.

_____ a. 78-year-old woman

_____ b. Married, 3 grown children live out of town

_____ c. Cares for invalid husband in home with help of daily housekeeper

_____ d. Vision corrected with glasses; hearing normal

_____ e. Ht. 178 cm (5 ft 10 in); wt. 78 kg (172 lb)

_____ f. VS: T 99.2, HR 82, RR 32, BP 142/88

_____ g. 5-year history of adult-onset asthma; smokes 2–3 cigarettes a day

_____ h. Coughing, wheezing, with stated SOB

_____ i. Moderate, light-yellow sputum

_____ j. Says she now has no energy to care for husband

_____ k. Awakens 3–4 times a night and has to use bronchodilator inhaler

_____ l. Uses a laxative twice a week for bowel function; no urinary problems

_____ m. Feels her health is good for her age

_____ n. Allergic to codeine and aspirin

_____ o. Has esophageal reflux and eats bland foods

_____ p. Can usually handle stress of caring for husband, but if she becomes overwhelmed, asthma becomes worse

_____ q. Has been menopausal for 26 years; no sexual activity

_____ r. Takes medications for asthma, hypertension, hypothyroidism, and uses diazepam (Valium) prn for anxiety

_____ s. Goes out to lunch with friends weekly

_____ t. Says she misses going to church with husband but watches religious services with him on TV

1. Demographic data

2. Important health information

3. Health-perception–health-management pattern

4. Nutrition-metabolic pattern

5. Elimination pattern

6. Activity–exercise pattern

7. Sleep–rest pattern

8. Cognitive–perceptual pattern

9. Self-perception–self concept pattern

10. Role–relationship pattern

11. Sexuality–reproductive pattern

12. Coping–stress tolerance pattern

13. Value–belief pattern

8. An example of a negative finding during a physical examination is

    a. chest pain that does not radiate to the arm.
    b. elevated blood pressure in a client with hypertension.
    c. pupils that are equal and react to light and accommodation.
    d. clear and full lung sounds in a client with chronic bronchitis.

9. A screening physical examination is used by the nurse when examining a client who

    a. is being evaluated during routine health maintenance.
    b. is being seen two weeks following treatment of a peptic ulcer.
    c. has generalized weakness and fatigue without specific pain.
    d. wants to know the effectiveness of a prescribed hypertension medication.

10. Match the following data with the assessment technique used to obtain the information.

    _____  a. Blood flow through arteries            1. Inspection

    _____  b. Enlargement of the liver               2. Palpation

    _____  c. Tympany of the abdomen                 3. Percussion

    _____  d. Pain at a joint                        4. Auscultation

    _____  e. Cyanosis of the lips

    _____  f. Hyperactive peristalsis

11. The sequence of examination techniques that should be used when assessing the client's abdomen is

    a.  inspection, palpation, auscultation, percussion.
    b.  auscultation, inspection, percussion, palpation.
    c.  palpation, percussion, auscultation, inspection.
    d.  inspection, auscultation, percussion, palpation.

12. When performing a physical examination, it is most important that the nurse

    a. uses a head-to-toe approach to avoid missing an important area.
    b. uses the same systematic, efficient sequence for all examinations.
    c. follows a sequence that is least revealing and embarrassing for the client.
    d. allows time to collect the nursing history data while performing the examination.

13. Crossword Puzzle

**Across**

6. What clients do when they come for a physical examination
7. Reddened eardrum may indicate this
8. Upper chamber of the heart
10. Abnormal finding on examination of the skin
12. May be found on nasal examination
14. Rises in midline on "ahhh"
17. Laterally means to the _____
19. Referring to the eyes
20. Normal thyroid finding
21. Direction to a client to take a deep breath
22. Abnormal findings on abdominal palpation

**Down**

1. Prefix related to skeletal system
2. Where a pulse is palpated
3. Mouths or openings (var.)
4. Cancer that is localized is termed _____
5. Indicated by decreased hemoglobin and hematocrit
9. Dull sound heard on percussion
11. A mixed-up STAT
12. A drooping eyelid
13. Client's responses to a joke
15. Blue legs may indicate a _____ obstruction
16. Small or scant
18. Inspected reddened skin; edema massive (abbreviation)

# CHAPTER 4    CLIENT AND FAMILY TEACHING

1. In each of the nursing situations described below, identify the specific goal of client education:

   a. Teaching a new mother how to breast-feed

   b. Discussing recommended lifestyle changes with a client with newly diagnosed heart disease

   c. Counselling a client with a breast biopsy that is positive for cancer

   d. Demonstrating condom application to sexually active teenagers

2. In the following examples, indicate what principle(s) of adult education is (are) being used by the nurse in teaching clients.

   a. The nurse explains why it is important for a client with Parkinson's disease to walk with wide placement of the feet.

      _____

   b. The nurse asks a client what is most important to her to learn about managing a new colostomy.

      _____

   c. The nurse teaches a client how to reduce the risks for stroke after the client has had a transient ischemic attack, warning of carotid artery disease.

      _____

   d. The nurse provides a variety of printed materials and Internet resources for a client with impaired kidney function to use to learn about the disorder.

      _____

   e. When caring for a client with newly diagnosed asthma, the nurse explains that asthma is a disorder the client can control and allows the client to decide when teaching should be done and who else should be included.

      _____

   f. The nurse arranges for a client diagnosed with diabetes mellitus to perform self-monitoring of blood glucose and insulin administration in the nurse's presence.

      _____

   g. During preoperative teaching of a client scheduled for a total hip replacement, the nurse compares the post-operative care with that of the client's prior back surgery.

      _____

3. When using the Transtheoretical Model of Health Behaviour Change during client teaching, the nurse identifies that the client who states, "I walked regularly for about a year to help prevent osteoporosis, but recently I haven't been motivated to continue," is in the stage of

   a.  action.
   b.  preparation.
   c.  termination.
   d.  maintenance.

4. Translate the following medical terms or diagnoses into phrases that a client with little or no medical knowledge would be able to understand.

   a.  Acute myocardial infarction

   b.  Intravenous pyelogram

   c.  Diabetic retinopathy

5. An empathetic approach to client teaching is demonstrated when the nurse

   a.  assesses the client's needs before developing the teaching plan.
   b.  provides positive non-verbal messages that promote communication.
   c.  reads and reviews educational materials before distributing them to clients and families.
   d.  can overcome the personal frustration felt when clients are discharged before teaching is complete.

6. The nurse includes the needs of the family and significant others in planning client teaching because

   a.  family support of the client greatly affects the client's sense of well-being.
   b.  family members will be responsible for continued care of the client after discharge.
   c.  the client and family often have conflicting views of the illness and treatment options.
   d.  family members need to learn about the client's problems and need to know what to expect.

7. To promote the client's self-efficacy during the teaching-learning process, the nurse should

   a.  emphasize the relevancy of the teaching to the client's life.
   b.  begin with concepts and tasks that are easily learned to promote success.
   c.  provide stimulating learning activities that encourage motivation to learn.
   d.  encourage the client to learn independently without instruction from others.

8. Identify what teaching interventions are indicated when the following characteristics are found during assessment of a client for the purposes of developing a teaching plan.

    a. Impaired hearing

    b. Client refuses to see a need for a change in health behaviours

    c. Drowsiness caused by use of tranquilizers

    d. Presence of pain

    e. Severe anxiety about self-administering injections

    f. Lack of self-efficacy

    g. Decreased concentration because of cerebral injury

    h. Fatigue and weakness at early discharge from hospital

    i. Reading ability at national average

    j. Visual learning style

9. Upon assessment of a client's learning needs, the nurse determines that a client taking potassium-wasting diuretics does not know what foods are high in potassium. An appropriate nursing diagnosis for this client is

    a. risk for cardiac arrhythmias related to low potassium intake.
    b. deficient knowledge related to lack of recall of high-potassium foods.
    c. imbalanced nutrition: less than body requirements related to lack of intake of potassium-rich foods.
    d. deficient knowledge related to lack of interest regarding dietary requirements when taking diuretics.

10. Write a complete learning objective for the client taking potassium-wasting diuretics who does not know what foods are high in potassium.

11. Teaching strategies to meet learning objectives should be determined by the

    a. nurse.
    b. client.
    c. physician.
    d. nurse, client, and client's family.

12. Match the following descriptions or characteristics with the appropriate teaching strategy (answers may be used more than once).

_____ a. May require client to practise between teaching sessions

_____ b. Used to rehearse behaviours or feelings

_____ c. Participants are passive learners

_____ d. Most efficient in terms of time

_____ e. Useful when clients have previous experience with subject

_____ f. Allows for questions and exchange of ideas following content presentation

_____ g. Should be supplementary to the nurse's planned teaching sessions

_____ h. Useful when it is difficult to reach desired objectives of the session

_____ i. Requires clients to learn to identify reliable information

_____ j. Best strategy for teaching motor skills or procedures

_____ k. Nurse must have competency in the technology

_____ l. Requires maturity and confidence of participants

_____ m. May be used in combination with almost any other teaching strategy

_____ k. Offers extensive sources of information

1. Lecture

2. Lecture/discussion

3. Discussion

4. Peer teaching in support groups

5. Demonstration/return demonstration

6. Role play

7. Internet

8. Printed materials

13. When selecting audiovisual and written materials as teaching strategies, it is important for the nurse to

   a. provide the client with these materials before the planned learning experience.
   b. ensure that the materials include all the information the client will need to learn.
   c. review the materials before use for accuracy and appropriateness to learning objectives.
   d. assess the client's auditory and visual ability because these functions are necessary for these strategies to be effective.

14. A drug handbook provides the following information about the drug atorvastatin (Lipitor).

   • Action: Inhibits HMG-CoA reductase enzyme, which reduces cholesterol synthesis
   • Uses: As an adjunct in primary hypercholesterolemia (types Ia, Ib)
   • Side effects: Liver dysfunction, dyspepsia, flatus, pancreatitis, rash, pruritus, alopecia, lens opacities, myalgia, and headache
   • Precautions: Past liver disease, alcoholism, hypotension, severe acute infections, uncontrolled seizure disorders, severe metabolic disorders, trauma, and electrolyte imbalances
   • Interactions: Increased effects of warfarin, digoxin, oral contraceptives; increased myalgia with cyclosporine, gemfibrozil, niacin, erythromycin; decreased effects of atorvastatin with colestipol, antacids, bile acid sequestrants, propranolol; increased effects of atorvastatin with erythromycin, itraconazole

   Rewrite the above information as teaching material for a client with an average adult reading level.

15. Identify what short-term evaluation technique is appropriate to evaluate whether the client has met the following learning objectives.

   a. The client will demonstrate to the nurse the preparation and administration of a subcutaneous insulin injection to himself with correct technique.

   b. The client will identify five symptoms of digitalis toxicity.

   c. The client will select the foods highest in potassium for each meal from the hospital menu with 80% accuracy.

   d. The client will ambulate unassisted with the walker 30 m (100 feet) three times a day.

16. The best example of documentation of client teaching regarding wound care is

   a. "The client was instructed about care of wound and dressing changes."
   b. "The client demonstrated correct technique of wound care following instruction."
   c. "The client and family verbalize that they understand the purposes of wound care."
   d. "Written instructions regarding wound care and dressing changes were given to the client."

# CHAPTER 5  OLDER ADULTS

1. Identify two common social conceptions or myths about aging or the aged that illustrate the concept of ageism.

   a.

   b.

2. A 73-year-old man scheduled for surgery tells the nurse that if things do not go well during surgery, he has lived a full life and has no regrets. The nurse recognizes that this statement is consistent with

   a.  achievement of the developmental task of ego-integrity described by Erikson.
   b.  unsuccessful achievement of earlier developmental tasks described by Havighurst.
   c.  the wisdom and judgement that maintains self-esteem in Peck's theory of development.
   d.  the changes and redirected growth toward personal goals characteristic of Levinson's late adulthood transition.

3. Match the developmental theorists with their concepts (theorists may be used more than once).

   _____  a. Addresses only middle-adult and older adult tasks        1. Erikson

   _____  b. Family-oriented tasks                                     2. Peck

   _____  c. Individual life structure                                 3. Levinson

   _____  d. Experiences dictate self-adjustment                       4. Havighurst

   _____  e. Body transcendence vs. body preoccupation

   _____  f. Transitions vs. stability

   _____  g. Ego-integrity vs. despair

4. A characteristic common to all adult developmental models is that

   a.  acceptance of dying is the most important task of adulthood.
   b.  development is a continuous process throughout the lifespan.
   c.  the ultimate goal of adult development is to leave a genetic legacy.
   d.  chronological age is the most important factor in understanding adult behaviour.

5. Match the following characteristics with their related biological theory of aging.

_____    a. Inherent cellular biological clock that limits
cellular division

_____    b. Increased cellular rigidity related to
abnormal joining of metabolites

_____    c. Spontaneous mutation of body cells,
eventually causing organ failure

_____    d. Active self-destruction of normal cells
by immune system

_____    e. Altered DNA and protein synthesis
from oxidative process

_____    f. Loss of DNA enzymes resulting in limited
cell division

_____    g. Loss of response of nervous and glandular
tissue

_____    h. Gradual loss of genetic regulatory mechanisms resulting in mutational cells

1. Somatic mutation theory

2. Intrinsic mutagenesis theory

3. Free radical theory

4. Cross-link theory

5. Neuroendocrine theory

6. Programmed theory of cell death

7. Immunological theory

8. Telomere–telomerase theory

6. For each of the nursing diagnoses listed, identify at least two normal expected physiological changes related to aging that could be etiological factors of the diagnosis.

   a. Imbalanced nutrition: less than body requirements

     Change:

     Change:

   b. Activity intolerance

     Change:

     Change:

   c. Risk for injury

     Change:

     Change:

   d. Urge urinary incontinence

     Change:

     Change:

   e. Ineffective airway clearance

     Change:

     Change:

   f. Risk for impaired skin integrity

     Change:

     Change:

   g. Ineffective tissue perfusion: peripheral

     Change:

     Change:

   h. Constipation

     Change:

     Change:

7. The nurse identifies the presence of age-associated memory impairment in the older adult who says,

    a. "I just can't seem to remember the name of my new granddaughter."
    b. "I make out lists to help me remember what I need to do, but I can't seem to use them."
    c. "I forget movie stars' names more often now, but I can remember them later after the conversation is over."
    d. "I forgot that I went to the grocery store this morning and didn't realize it until I went again this afternoon."

8. Indicate what the acronym SCALES stands for in assessment of nutrition indicators in frail older adults.

    a. S

    b. C

    c. A

    d. L

    e. E

    f. S

9. When assessing the older adult's health status, the nurse finds a decline in the client's functional health status. This change often occurs as a result of the client

    a. manifesting symptoms of delirium.
    b. suffering from asymptomatic pathology.
    c. adjusting for disease symptoms by restricting activities.
    d. treating one symptom with a medication that causes detrimental side effects.

10. Identify one task required for daily living with chronic illness that would specifically apply to the following common chronic conditions present in the older adult.

    a. Diabetes mellitus
    b. Visual impairment
    c. Heart disease
    d. Hearing impairment
    e. Alzheimer's disease
    f. Arthritis
    g. Orthopedic impairment

11. When working with older clients who identify with a specific ethnic group, the nurse recognizes that health-care problems may occur because these clients often

    a. live with extended families that isolate the client.
    b. live in rural areas where services are not readily available.
    c. eat ethnic foods that do not provide all the essential nutrients.
    d. have less income to spend for medications and healthcare services.

12. An 88-year-old woman is brought to the health clinic for the first time by her 64-year-old daughter. During the initial comprehensive nursing assessment of the client, the nurse should

    a. ask the daughter whether the client has any urgent needs or problems.
    b. obtain a health history using a functional health pattern and assess ADLs and mental status.
    c. interview the client and daughter together so that pertinent information can be confirmed.
    d. refer the client for an interdisciplinary comprehensive geriatric assessment because she will have multiple needs at her age.

13. A mental status assessment of the older adult is especially important in determining

    a. potential for independent living.
    b. eligibility for federal health programs.
    c. if the person should be classified as frail.
    d. service and placement needs of the individual.

14. The nurse promotes learning activity when teaching older adult clients by providing

    a. written instructions instead of verbal explanations.
    b. information that relates to the client's actual experience.
    c. a review of basic concepts, because long-term memory is impaired.
    d. numerous repetitive presentations to promote memory retention.

15. One of the most frequent consequences of unscheduled surgery in the older adult is

    a. post-operative infection.
    b. acute confusional state.
    c. fluid and electrolyte imbalances.
    d. anaesthesia-induced arrhythmias.

16. An important nursing measure in the rehabilitation of the geriatric client to prevent loss of function from inactivity and immobility is

    a. performance of active and passive ROM exercises.
    b. using assistive devices such as walkers and canes.
    c. teaching good nutrition to prevent loss of muscle mass.
    d. performance of risk appraisals and assessments related to immobility.

17. A 78-year-old man is admitted to the orthopedic unit from the emergency department with a hip fracture. During the admission process the client does not complain of pain in the hip. The nurse should

    a. offer the client pain medication.
    b. ask the client to keep a pain diary.
    c. recognize that older adults' perception of pain is impaired.
    d. assume that the client is handling his pain in his own way.

18. An older adult client has hypertension and congestive heart failure and is treated with enalapril (Vasotec) and digoxin (Lanoxin). The pharmacodynamic and pharmacokinetic properties of these drugs include the following.

|  | **enalapril** | **digoxin** |
|---|---|---|
| Dynamics: | blocks conversion of angiotensin I to active angiotensin II, causing systemic vasodilation | increases intramedullary calcium, increasing cardiac muscle contraction; parasympathetic stimulation causing decreased heart rate |
| Kinetics: | | |
|    Absorption: | oral absorption 60% | oral absorption 60%–80% |
|    Distribution: | 20%–30% plasma protein-bound | 20%–30% plasma protein-bound |
|    Metabolism: | 60% converted by liver to active enalapril | small % metabolized by liver and GI flora |
|    Excretion: | 60% excreted by kidneys, rest in feces | most excreted unchanged by kidneys |
|    Half-life | 11 hours | 36 hours |

    a. What physiological changes in the older adult affect the absorption, metabolism, and excretion of enalapril?

    b. Describe the additional effect digoxin may have on the older adult also taking enalapril.

    c. What nursing interventions should the nurse plan to monitor for the potential side effects related to administration of these drugs?

19. In view of the fact that most older adults take at least six prescription drugs, what are four nursing interventions that can specifically help prevent problems caused by multiple drug use in older clients?

    a.

    b.

    c.

    d.

20. An 80-year-old woman is brought to the emergency department by her daughter, who says her mother has refused to eat for six days. The mother says she stays in her room all of the time because the family is mean to her when she eats or watches TV with them. She says her daughter only brings her one meal a day and that meal is cold leftovers from the family's meals days before. The daughter says her mother is too demanding and she just cannot cope with caring for her 24 hours a day.

   a. What types of elder abuse may be present in this situation?

   b. What might be an appropriate nursing diagnosis for the daughter?

   c. What resources can the nurse suggest to the daughter?

21. An 82-year-old client with multiple health problems is hospitalized with a fractured hip. Following the client's initial acute phase of care for the hip fracture, he is discharged from the hospital setting to live with his daughter and son-in-law in their home.

   a. The daughter asks the nurse discharging her father from the hospital what elements of her father's possible follow-up care at home may not be covered by medicare. Based on the nurse's knowledge of the potential course of rehabilitation following a hip fracture, what would be the nures's response to the daughter's question?

   b. What community-based service might be appropriate to allow the family members to continue in their jobs?

22. What are three common factors known to precipitate nursing home placement?

   a.

   b.

   c.

# CHAPTER 6    COMMUNITY-BASED NURSING AND HOME CARE

1. Settings in which a community health nurse (CHN) might practise include

   a. a school classroom
   b. a public health unit
   c. a home care provider organization
   d. the hospital
   e. a family physician's office
   f. all but d

2. A community health nurse's position title might be

   a. home health nurse
   b. public health nurse
   c. street nurse
   d. parish nurse
   e. all of the above

3. What historical milestones and trends influenced the birth of public health nursing?

4. The philosophy upon which CHNs base their practice is

   a. Benner's theory of novice to expert
   b. Jean Watson's theory of human caring
   c. primary health care
   d. Parse's theory of human becoming

5. What are the six principles of primary health care?

   a.

   b.

   c.

   d.

   e.

   f.

6. Identify five factors that have influenced the shift of client care from the hospital to the community.

   a.

   b.

   c.

   d.

   e.

7. A case manager is responsible for

    a. acting as advisor, advocate, and mentor.
    b. containing costs.
    c. coordinating and facilitating care.
    d. providing home health care to clients following hospitalization for acute illnesses.
    e. all of the above.

8. Match the following types of community health nurse with their defining characteristics:

    _____ a. public health nurse

    _____ b. home health nurse

    _____ c. community health centre/outreach nurse

    _____ d. outpost or rural nurse

    _____ e. parish nurse

    _____ f. occupational health nurse

    1. Promotes, maintains and restores health and prevents illness/injury

    2. Integrates a faith-based approach to care

    3. Often the only healthcare professional in the community

    4. provides primary health care and health promotion programs

    5. Initiates, manages, and evaluates the resources needed to promote the client's well-being and function

    6. Prevents disease and promotes healthy behaviours

9. The client care setting in which nurses are most likely to be required to adapt to a variety of circumstances and make independent decisions is

    a. outpost or rural nursing.
    b. family practice nursing.
    c. home health nursing.
    d. community health centre nursing.
    e. c and d.
    f. a and c.

10. Using the following three main functions of home care, identify the function that would be the most appropriate in each of the described client situations.

    maintenance and preventive function
    long-term care substitution function
    acute-care substitution function

    a. An ambulatory client with Alzheimer's disease is living with his wife in their home of 30 years.
       _____

    b. An elderly client with renal failure who lives alone in his home requires nightly visits from the nurse for monitoring and to set up the dialysis night cycler machine. _____

    c. A client requires wound care and support following a mastectomy. _____

    d. A client with diabetes with a wound infection at an above-the-knee amputation site requires IV antibiotics and frequent complex dressings for a short time. _____

    e. A mother and father are caring for their five-year-old child with cerebral palsy who requires tube feedings and total assistance with activities of daily living. _____

    f. A woman with advanced multiple sclerosis is being cared for by her family and needs physiotherapy and occupational therapy to maximize her mobility. _____

11. In Canada, home care services are free of charge

    a. always.
    b. if the frequency of care and length of stay fall within guidelines.
    c. in every province and territory.
    d. in some provinces and territories.
    e. a and c.
    f. b and c.
    g. a and d.

12. Hospice palliative care

    a. is outside the scope of practice for the home health nurse.
    b. is a philosophy that applies only to those with cancer.
    c. applies to hospital nursing only.
    d. is a specialty practice integral to home health nursing practice.

13. A 72-year-old man who has had two strokes is cared for by his wife and daughter in his home. The client is becoming weaker and is almost bedridden. The wife and daughter are becoming exhausted from the care he requires, but the client insists that his family care for him at home. What are two nursing diagnoses that might relate to this family situation?

    a.

    b.

14. In the home, the nurse is the _____

15. List five competencies required by home health nurses.

    1.

    2.

    3.

    4.

    5.

16. Standards of practice for Canadian Community Health Nurses were developed in order to

    1.

    2.

    3.

17. In Canada, how is community health nursing recognized as a specialty practice?



18. Nursing-sensitive outcomes are important because _____.

19. Examples of nursing-sensitive outcomes include

    a. pain, nausea, fatigue, and dyspnea
    b. client satisfaction
    c. nurses' work-life satisfaction
    d. all of the above

1. Match each description in the left column with its NCCAM classification (in the right column) and with its specific type of therapy (also in the right column).

### Descriptions

_____ _____ a. Use of hands to direct energy fields

_____ _____ b. Nutrition integrated with lifestyle and environment to promote health

_____ _____ c. Movement re-education to promote balanced, graceful movement

_____ _____ d. Manipulation of energy channels with fine needles

_____ _____ e. Involves assessment of client's sense of purpose and meaning of life and transcendence beyond context reality

_____ _____ f. Emphasizes inherent healing ability of body combined with natural therapies

_____ _____ g. Exercise system to manipulate internal energetic movement

_____ _____ h. Considers disease as an imbalance of life force and basic metabolic condition

_____ _____ i. Involves altering the length and tone of myofascial tissue to realign the body

_____ _____ j. Spinal and soft tissue manipulation

_____ _____ k. Use of plants or plant parts for specific effects

_____ _____ l. System of exercise involving movement integrated with breathing and visualization

_____ _____ m. Self-directed practice of focusing, centring, and relaxing

_____ _____ n. Uses the principle of "like cures like" with small doses of prepared extracts

### NCCAM Classification

1. Alternative medical systems

2. Mind–body interventions

3. Biologically based therapies

4. Manipulative and body-based methods

5. Energy therapies

### Specific Therapies

6. Acupuncture

7. Ayurveda

8. Alexander technique

9. Tai chi

10. Chiropractic therapy

11. Naturopathy

12. Therapeutic touch

13. Phytotherapy

14. Homeopathy

15. Meditation

16. Qigong

17. Spirituality

18. Macrobiotic diet

19. Rolfing

2. Indicate whether the following statements are true or false.

_____  a. The increase in the use of CAM therapies is due primarily to a growing distrust of allopathic medicine by the public.

_____  b. A limitation of the use of CAM therapies is the refusal of insurance companies to reimburse the cost of such therapies.

_____  c. Research and education in CAM therapies are supported by the National Centre for Complementary and Alternative Medicine of the National Institutes of Health.

_____  d. Practices that are considered complementary and alternative in one culture or time might be considered conventional in another place or time.

3. Complementary and alternative therapies are advocated by many nurses because these therapies

   a. promote self-care and self-determination by clients.
   b. are congruent with a view of humans as holistic beings.
   c. are less expensive for clients than conventional therapies.
   d. cause few adverse effects while achieving positive outcomes.

4. Traditional Chinese medicine holds that disease occurs when

   a. yin and yang become imbalanced, altering the flow of Qi.
   b. acupoints in Qi channels become obstructed, preventing the release of Qi.
   c. the body's natural healing abilities are impaired by obstruction of fluid channels.
   d. the elements of earth, metal, water, wood, and fire are restricted from interacting with each other.

5. Acupuncture is used to

   a. relieve pain by causing counterirritation in another area of the body.
   b. re-establish the flow of Qi through meridians to simulate the body's self-healing mechanism.
   c. create an inflammatory response at an acupoint, increasing blood circulation and healing energy.
   d. stimulate the electrical activity of the central nervous system, promoting movement of vital energy through the body.

6. The most common complications of acupuncture are those related to

   a. cardiac arrhythmias.
   b. infection transmission.
   c. post-treatment drowsiness.
   d. bleeding from needle sites.

7. Identify three interventions that are frequently used by nurses to help the client use the mind to affect bodily function.

   a.

   b.

   c.

8. The primary goal of biofeedback is to

   a. measure the physiological responses to stress.
   b. demonstrate the effect of stress reduction therapies on physiological function.
   c. teach the client to voluntarily control physiological processes that are usually involuntary.
   d. increase the client's awareness of autonomic nervous system responses to thoughts and feelings.

9. A complementary and alternative therapy shown to be effective in treatment of a client with chemotherapy-related nausea and vomiting is

   a. rolfing.
   b. acupuncture.
   c. aromatherapy.
   d. electromagnetic therapy.

10. Therapeutic touch is contraindicated in clients

   a. who are pregnant.
   b. who are immunosuppressed.
   c. who are receiving cancer chemotherapy.
   d. with critical or unstable conditions.

11. A client tells the nurse that she uses regular chiropractic therapy for treatment of dysmenorrhea. The nurse recognizes that chiropractic therapy

   a. is contraindicated for pain of visceral origin.
   b. is effective only for musculoskeletal abnormalities.
   c. involves the prescription of mild anti-inflammatory drugs for the menstrual pain.
   d. uses manipulation to correct spinal alterations that cause organ dysfunction and pain.

12. When discussing herbal therapy with a client, the nurse should advise the client that

   a. herbal remedies may interact with prescription medications.
   b. herbs rarely cause harm or side effects because they are natural plants.
   c. there are no known contraindications or conditions for which herbal therapy cannot be used.
   d. most herbal preparations have been clinically tested for safety and efficacy before marketing.

13. While the nurse is obtaining a health history for a client, the client tells the nurse that he uses a number of herbs to maintain his health. The most important thing the nurse can do to address the client's use of these products is to

   a. ask the client what effects the various products have.
   b. have a working knowledge of commonly used herbs and dietary supplements.
   c. reassure the client that the products can continue to be used with conventional therapies.
   d. warn the client that there is limited research concerning the therapeutic and harmful effects of herbal products.

14. Crossword Puzzle: Have You Met Herb?

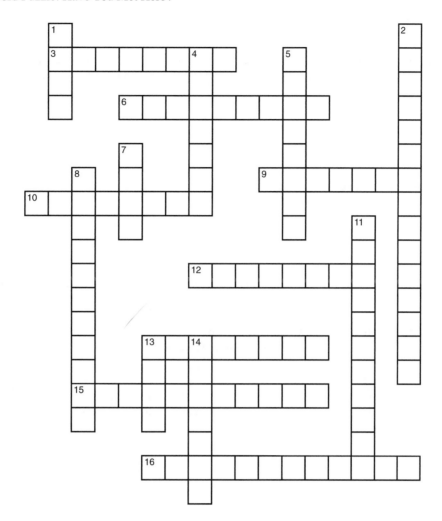

**Across**

3. Used for menstrual disorders because of its antispasmodic effects
6. Antibacterial and anti-inflammatory effects that are contraindicated in those with immunosuppression
9. You saw this one before, but it also increases serum cortisol and ability to respond to stress
10. Increases microcirculation in the eyes and used for eye problems
12. Another anti-inflammatory herb that inhibits prostaglandins and histamine
13. You saw this one before, but it also increases the risk for cancer while balancing the effects of estrogen
15. A commonly used herb for depression and anxiety
16. Promotes brain blood flow and memory

**Down**

1. As a skeletal muscle relaxant useful for fibromyalgia
2. Affects metabolism of fatty acids and useful in wound healing
4. Safe when used externally for wound healing
5. Sedative and anti-anxiety effects may interact with CNS depressants
7. Converted to androgens and should not be used in those with reproductive cancers
8. Often used for its estrogen effects by perimenopausal women
11. Slows prostate cell multiplication and used for benign prostatic hyperplasia
13. Common agent used for burns and wound healing
14. Used for its ability to increase endurance and stamina

# CHAPTER 8    STRESS

1. Below are common statements associated with the concept of stress. Indicate whether the term *stress* is used as a stimulus (S), response (R), or transaction (T), and identify the stress theorist(s) associated with the use of the term.

   _____ a. "I am so stressed out." _____

   _____ b. "She is under a lot of stress right now." _____

   _____ c. "What methods do you use to cope with stress?" _____

   _____ d. "This job causes too much stress." _____

   _____ e. "I always get sick at Christmas—it must be stress." _____

2. The stage of the general adaptation syndrome (GAS) in which the nurse would expect to observe the fewest signs and symptoms is the _____.

3. A client who is critically ill briefly shows an increase in pulse, respirations, and blood pressure and becomes more alert, followed by a return of previous vital signs and level of consciousness. The nurse identifies the client as being in which stage of GAS? _____.

4. Complete a personal inventory of your life events with the Social Readjustment Rating Scale in the textbook. What does your score indicate regarding your risk of developing a major illness?

5. Continuing research in the Stress as a Stimulus theory has shown that the factor that has a closer relationship with somatic illness than the life-event scale is

   a. threat demands.
   b. daily-hassle score.
   c. sense of coherence.
   d. challenge demands.

6. The nurse assesses that a client with a newly diagnosed chronic illness has a strong sense of coherence. The nurse anticipates that the client will probably

   a. be able to handle stress without help from healthcare professionals.
   b. require much emotional and psychological support to cope with the stress.
   c. ask for much information regarding the illness, its treatment, course, and expected outcome.
   d. go through a formal process of deciding what coping mechanisms and resources are available to manage the stress.

7. A 46-year-old client is told by his doctor that he has adult-onset diabetes and will require treatment and life-long changes in his lifestyle. The client is very distressed, but asks for information about the illness, visits the local office of the Canadian Diabetes Association, and elicits help and suggestions from his family in planning lifestyle changes.

Using the Stress as a Transaction theory, identify the following elements in the above situation.

a. Stimulus

b. Primary appraisal outcome

c. Type of demand

d. Secondary appraisal

8. Using the word and phrase list on the next page, fill in the boxes below with the numbers of the words or phrases that illustrate the physiological response to stress.

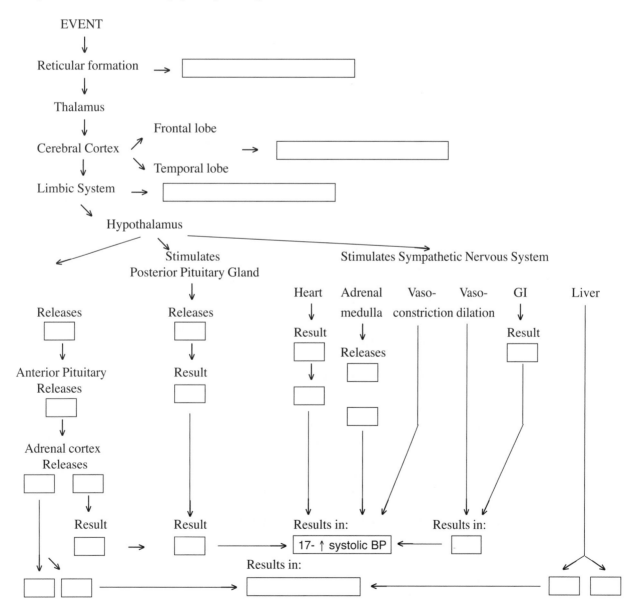

**Word and Phrase List**

1. Interpretation of event, fear
2. ↑ ADH
3. Cortisol
4. ↑ blood volume
5. ↑ HR and stroke volume
6. ↑ water retention
7. Wakefulness and alertness
8. ↑ sympathetic response
9. Behaviour change, ↑ pain perception
10. ↑ cardiac output
11. Corticotropin releasing hormone
12. Aldosterone
13. ACTH
14. ↑ gluconeogenesis
15. ↑ epinephrine and norepinephrine
16. ↓ digestion
17. ↑ systolic blood pressure
18. ↓ inflammatory response
19. Glycogenolysis
20. ↑ blood to vital organs and large muscles
21. ↑ blood glucose
22. ↑ Na and $H_2O$ reabsorption

9. From the diagram above and the physiological responses that are noted, identify eight objective clinical manifestations that the nurse might expect, and three or four subjective findings.

a. _____        g. _____

b. _____        h. _____

c. _____        i. _____

d. _____        j. _____

e. _____        k. _____

f. _____        l. _____

10. Place a check mark in front of each of the following findings or observations that illustrates the relationship between the immune system and stress.

_____ a. A client with moderate-to-severe post-operative pain experiences slow wound healing.

_____ b. A diabetic client experiences wide variations in blood glucose levels when he has an upper respiratory infection.

_____ c. After surgery to remove a malignant tumour, reducing the client's pain and stress may maintain tumour cell surveillance and destruction.

_____ d. The corticosteroids released during the stress response could prevent exacerbations of immune-based diseases such as multiple sclerosis and rheumatoid arthritis.

_____ e. A client with numerous daily hassles and with high scores on the Social Readjustment Rating Scale develops a urinary tract infection.

_____ f. Clients with metastatic breast cancer who attend a support group have a longer survival rate than clients who do not receive psychological support.

_____ g. A client who uses laughter to relieve pain and stress slows the progression of a rheumatoid condition.

11. While caring for a client with Alzheimer's disease and her husband, the nurse finds that the client's husband has progressively increased blood pressure and morning edema of the hands and feet. One explanation for this allostatic load is that

    a. allostasis is impaired during a time of stress.
    b. the husband does not perceive the care of his wife as stressful.
    c. allostatic responses to stress do not terminate when stress is chronic.
    d. chronic diseases always become more pronounced in stressful situations.

12. A client has recently had a myocardial infarction. Identify two specific problem-focused coping efforts and two specific emotion-focused coping efforts the nurse could encourage him to use to adapt to the physical and emotional stress of his illness.

    **Problem-Focused**                              **Emotion-Focused**

    a. _____        c. _____

    b. _____        d. _____

13. Identify the three major areas to be assessed in a client with stress, and describe techniques that would be appropriately used by the nurse to evaluate these areas.

    **Areas**                                        **Techniques**

    a.

    b.

    c.

14. A 42-year-old client with rheumatoid arthritis is withdrawn, pulls the bedcovers over her head, and does not initiate conversation with her husband or other visitors. Upon questioning, the client tells the nurse that she must either withdraw or cry all the time, that she just cannot cope with the chronic nature of the disease. An appropriate nursing diagnosis for the client is

    a. ineffective denial related to inability to cope.
    b. ineffective coping related to disruption of emotional bonds.
    c. ineffective coping related to inadequate psychological resources.
    d. impaired adjustment related to unwillingness to modify lifestyle to accommodate chronic illness.

15. List the nine factors that can increase resistance to stress in all individuals.

a.

b.

c.

d.

e.

f.

g.

h.

i.

## CASE STUDY

### STRESS

**Client Profile**

Ms. J., a 26-year-old unmarried secretary, is admitted to the hospital with right lower quadrant pain; 10 to 12 watery, blood-streaked stools in the past 24 hours; and a low-grade fever. She has a seven-year history of inflammatory bowel disease.

**Subjective Data**

Client relates the following:
• Has been hospitalized four times in the past year
• Not currently working because of the illness and has no income
• Has a boyfriend who has lived with her for two years
• Does not want her boyfriend to visit because she thinks he has enough of his own problems
• Has been in bed the past week because of weakness, nausea, and malaise and has been crying and depressed

**Objective Data**

Height: 168 cm (5 ft 6 in)
Weight: 47.3 kg (104 lb)
Hemoglobin: 105 g/L (10.5 g/dL)
Hematocrit: 0.30 (30%)
Temperature: 37.8°C (100°F)

## Critical Thinking Questions

1. What physiological and psychological stressors can be identified or anticipated in Ms. J.'s situation? Describe the possible effects of these stressors on the course of her illness.

2. What factors identified in Ms. J.'s nursing assessment may affect her current adaptation to stress?

3. What physiological changes would be expected in Ms. J. as she begins to respond to prescribed treatment?

4. Describe an approach that the nurse could use to assess Ms. J.'s perception of her situation. Include several specific questions to be asked by the nurse.

5. What specific nursing interventions can be implemented with Ms. J. to enhance her adaptation to stress?

6. Based on the assessment data provided, write one or more nursing diagnoses. Are there any collaborative problems?

# CHAPTER 9    PAIN

1. The practice by nurses of routinely administering the smallest prescribed opioid analgesic dose when a range of doses is prescribed

   a. protects the client from addiction and toxic effects of the drug.
   b. prevents hastening or causing a client's death from respiratory dysfunction.
   c. contributes to unnecessary suffering and physical and psychosocial dysfunction.
   d. indicates that the nurse understands the adage "start low and go slow" in administering analgesics.

2. *Pain* has been defined as "whatever the person experiencing the pain says it is, existing whenever the client says it does." The definition is problematic when caring for a client who has

   a. been placed on a ventilator.
   b. a history of opioid addiction.
   c. decreased cognitive function.
   d. pain resulting from severe trauma.
   e. all of the above.

3. List and briefly describe the five components of pain.

   a.


   b.


   c.


   d.


   e.


4. Match the following afferent nerve fibres with their characteristics (answers may be used more than once).

   _____    a. Transmit nociceptive signals at the fastest rate          1. A-alpha fibres

   _____    b. Rapid transmission of soft touch to the skin             2. A-beta fibres

   _____    c. The smallest peripheral nerve fibres                     3. A-delta fibres

   _____    d. Slowly transmit nociceptive signals                      4. C fibres

   _____    e. Myelinated fibre with rapid transmission of vibration
              and pressure from muscles

   _____    f. Myelinated fibre transmitting sharp, pointed stimulation

   _____    g. Non-myelinated fibre with slow transmission of dull,
              burning sensations

   _____    h. The smallest peripheral nerve fibres

5. Why is the size, myelinization, and conduction velocity of peripheral nerve fibres of significance in pain management?

6. During transmission of an action potential along a primary afferent nociceptor (PAN) to the dorsal root of the spinal cord,

   a. nothing can stop the action potential along an intact nerve until it reaches the spinal cord.
   b. the transmission may be interrupted by activation of large fibres (A beta) by massage, ice, and trans-electrical nerve stimulation, as well as drugs such as local anaesthetics and anticonvulsants.
   c. the fibre produces neurotransmitters that may activate nearby nerve fibres to transmit pain impulses.
   d. the action potential must cross several synapses, points at which the impulse may be blocked by drugs.

7. The development of referred pain during dorsal horn processing of nociceptive impulses is believed to occur when these impulses

   a. stimulate excitatory projection cells that send the impulse to the brain on the opposite side of the body.
   b. cause neural remodelling, increasing the number and excitability of areas activated by peripheral input.
   c. stimulate inhibitory wide dynamic range neurons in the dorsal horn.
   d. mix with impulses from A-beta fibres, causing perception of pain in the body part innervated by the A-beta fibre.

8. While caring for an unconscious client, the nurse knows that

   a. perception of pain will not occur.
   b. any noxious stimulus should be treated as potentially painful.
   c. if pain is perceived, the client will have a behavioural response.
   d. all nociceptive stimuli that are transmitted to the brain result in the perception of pain.

9. During pain modulation,

   a. opioid receptors in the brain are blocked to prevent the perception of nociceptive input.
   b. transmission of nociceptive stimuli is inhibited by inhibitory neurotransmitters released by afferent nerve fibres.
   c. descending fibres may release norepinephrine, serotonin, and enkephalins that prevent pain transmission to the brain.
   d. endorphins released from the cell during tissue damage occupy receptors on the PANs preventing transduction of pain.

10. When teaching a client with rheumatoid arthritis to avoid and/or pace repetitive motions such as knitting, the nurse is addressing the

    a. sensory component of pain.
    b. affective component of pain.
    c. cognitive component of pain.
    d. behavioural component of pain.

11. A client with trigeminal neuralgia has neuropathic pain. In helping the client manage the pain, the nurse recognizes that this type of pain

    a. is not as severe as nociceptive pain.
    b. is often described as aching and throbbing in nature.
    c. is chronic in nature and will require long-term treatment.
    d. involves treatment that includes the use of adjuvant analgesics.

12. List the sensory components of pain that should always be assessed in the client with pain, and give an example of a tool that is helpful in measuring these factors.

    | **Component** | **Tool** |
    | --- | --- |
    | a. | |
    | b. | |
    | c. | |
    | d. | |

13. List the eight basic principles that should guide the treatment of all pain.

    a.

    b.

    c.

    d.

    e.

    f.

    g.

    h.

14. A client with bowel cancer has continuous, poorly localized abdominal pain. The nurse teaches the client to use pain medications

    a. on a round-the-clock schedule.
    b. as often as necessary to keep the pain controlled.
    c. by alternating two different types of drugs to prevent tolerance.
    d. when the pain cannot be controlled with distraction or relaxation.

15. A client with chronic cancer-related pain has started using MS Contin for pain control and has developed the common side effects of the drug. The nurse reassures the client that tolerance will develop to most of these effects but that continued treatment will most likely be required for the

    a. sedation.
    b. dizziness.
    c. constipation.
    d. nausea and vomiting.

16. The use of a continuous infusion of an analgesic with patient-controlled-analgesia (PCA) prevents what disadvantage of PCA?

17. Match each step of the pain process (in the right column) with the measures or drugs (in the left column) that may be effective in controlling pain during that step.

    _____  a. NMDA antagonist drugs              1. Transduction

    _____  b. Massage                            2. Transmission along PAN

    _____  c. NSAIDs                             3. Dorsal horn processing

    _____  d. Local anaesthetics                 4. Modulation

    _____  e. TENS

    _____  f. Tricyclic antidepressants

    _____  g. Corticosteroids

    _____  h. Epidural opiates

    _____  i. Antiseizure medications

    _____  j. preoperative teaching

18. Mrs. S. has been on morphine 30 mg po q2h for three weeks following abdominal surgery complicated by multiple peritoneal abscesses. Her pain is now resolving and her morphine can be decreased. Her pain management should now include

    a. immediate discontinuation of her morphine
    b. reduction of her morphine dose by 50% over approximately one week
    c. teaching about becoming addicted to morphine
    d. substitution of morphine with TENS

19. A client with multiple injuries resulting from an automobile accident tells the nurse that he has "bad" pain but that he can "tough it out" and does not require pain medications. To encourage the client's participation in pharmacological pain management, the nurse explains that

    a. clients have a responsibility to keep the nurse informed about their pain.
    b. unrelieved pain has many harmful effects on the body that can impair recovery.
    c. using pain medications rarely leads to addiction when they are used for a pain problem.
    d. non-pharmacological therapies can be used to relieve his pain since he is afraid to use pain medications.

# CASE STUDY

## PAIN

### Client Profile

Mr. D., a 62-year-old postal worker, is being evaluated for a change in his pain therapy for chronic malignant pain from metastatic cancer.

### Subjective Data

- Desires 0 pain but will accept 3–4 on a 0–10 scale
- Has been taking two Percocet tablets q4h while awake but his pain is now usually at 4–5 with the medication
- Reports his pain varies over 24 hours from 5–10
- Always awakens in the morning with pain at 10 with nervousness and nausea and a runny nose
- When the pain becomes severe, he stays in bed and concentrates on blocking the pain by emptying his mind
- States he is worried that his increased pain means his disease is becoming worse
- States he is afraid to take additional doses or other opioids because he is afraid of addiction

### Objective Data

- Height: 183 cm (6 ft 0 in); Weight: 68 kg (150 lb)
- Rigid posturing, slow gait

### Critical Thinking Questions

1. What additional assessment data should the nurse obtain from Mr. D. before making any decisions about his problem?

2. What data from the nursing assessment are characteristic of the affective, behavioural, and cognitive dimensions of the pain experience?

3. Based on Mr. D.'s lack of pain control with his current dosage of opioid and his symptoms upon arising in the morning, what changes are indicated in his medication regimen?

4. What information would the nurse include in a teaching plan for Mr. D. to titrate his analgesic dose effectively?

5. How could the nurse best help Mr. D. overcome his fear of addiction to opioid drugs?

6. What additional pain therapies could the nurse plan to help Mr. D. manage his pain?

7. Based on the assessment data provided, write one or more nursing diagnoses. Are there any collaborative problems?

# CHAPTER 10    END-OF-LIFE CARE

1. The primary goal of end-of-life care is

   a. comfort and care that promote a dignified death.
   b. protecting the terminally ill client from needless grieving.
   c. implementation of measures to sustain physiological functioning.
   d. enhancing the client's progression through all stages of grieving.

2. For each of the following systems, identify three physical manifestations that the nurse would expect to see in a client approaching death.

   **Respiratory**

   a.

   b.

   c.

   **Skin**

   a.

   b.

   c.

   **Gastrointestinal**

   a.

   b.

   c.

   **Musculoskeletal**

   a.

   b.

   c.

3. A terminally ill client is unresponsive and has Cheyne-Stokes respiration. The client's husband and two grown children are arguing at her bedside about where the client's funeral should be held. The nurse should

   a. ask the family members to leave the room if they are going to argue.
   b. take the family members aside and explain that the client may be able to hear them.
   c. tell the family members that this decision is premature, since the client has not yet died.
   d. remind the family that this should be the client's decision and to ask her if she regains consciousness.

4. A 20-year-old client with a massive head injury is on life support, including a ventilator to maintain respirations. What three criteria for brain death are necessary to discontinue life support?

   a.

   b.

   c.

5. A 62-year-old woman has been diagnosed with metastatic lung cancer and is told that with therapy she may live for 12 to 18 months. Within the first month after her diagnosis, she prepares photo albums for her adult children, organizing and labelling all the photos of her family she has accumulated over the years. The nurse recognizes that this activity illustrates the psychosocial response of

   a. life review.
   b. peacefulness.
   c. saying goodbye.
   d. anxiety about unfinished business.

6. A client with end-stage liver failure tells the nurse, "If I can just live to see my first grandchild that is expected in five months, then I can die happy." The nurse recognizes that the client is demonstrating

   a. Rando's phase of avoidance.
   b. Kübler-Ross's stage of bargaining.
   c. Martocchio's stage of shock and disbelief.
   d. Martocchio's stage of reorganization and restoration.

7. Match the following types of grief with their characteristics.

   _____ a. Anticipatory grief

   _____ b. Pathological grief

   _____ c. Conflicted grief

   _____ d. Adaptive grief

   _____ e. Absent grief

   _____ f. Dysfunctional grief

   1. Appearance of coping and carrying on as if nothing has happened
   2. Exaggerated feelings and behaviours that are disruptive to the person's lifestyle
   3. Grieving based on perception of potential loss
   4. Unresolved ambivalent feelings toward the deceased
   5. Helps in acceptance of the reality of death
   6. Chronic grief that does not decrease after the first year

8. A terminally ill man tells the nurse, "I have never believed there is a God or an afterlife, but now it is too terrible to imagine that I will cease to exist. Why was I here in the first place?" The nurse recognizes that the client

   a. is experiencing spiritual distress.
   b. most likely will not have a peaceful death.
   c. needs to be reassured that his feelings are normal.
   d. should be referred to a clergyman for a discussion of his beliefs.

9. Identify the legal document or other term described by each of the following.

    a. A lay term for statements that give instructions about future treatment if the person is unable to do so for

       self: _____

    b. A term used to describe a document designating the person or persons who should make healthcare deci-

       sions if a client cannot make informed decisions for self: _____

    c. A written physician's order instructing healthcare providers not to attempt CPR:

       _____

    d. A general term used to describe all documents that give instructions about future medical care and treat-

       ments: _____

10. A client is receiving care to manage symptoms of a life-threatening illness when the disease no longer responds to curative treatment. This type of care is known as

    a. terminal care.
    b. palliative care.
    c. maintenance care.

11. A client with advanced cancer is referred to a community hospice program. The nurse explains to the client and the family that the main goal of hospice care is to

    a. provide for more complete pain control.
    b. provide compassion and support for persons living with terminal illnesses.
    c. support advance directives related to "right to die."
    d. always deliver care at home, rather than relying on the technology of hospitals.

12. End-of-life nursing care involves

    a. constant assessment for changes in physiological functioning.
    b. administering large doses of analgesics to keep the client sedated.
    c. providing as little physical care as possible to prevent disturbing the client.
    d. encouraging the client and family members to verbalize their feelings of sadness, loss, and forgiveness.

## CASE STUDY

### END-OF-LIFE CARE

**Client Profile**

Mrs. J., a 42-year-old housewife, had unsuccessful treatment for cancer of the breast one year ago and now has metastases to the lung and vertebrae. She lives at home with her husband, a 15-year-old daughter, and a 12-year-old son. She has been referred to a palliative care team because of her deteriorating condition and increasing pain. Her husband is an accountant and tries to do as much of his work at home as possible so that he can help care for his wife. Their children have become withdrawn, choosing to spend as much time as possible at their friends' homes and in outside activities.

**Subjective Data**

- Mrs. J. reports that she stays in bed most of the time because it is too painful to stand or sit
- She reports her pain as an 8/10 while taking MS Contin 15 mg po q12h.
- She reports shortness of breath with almost any activity, such as getting up to go to the bathroom.
- Mrs. J. says she knows she is dying, but her greatest suffering results from her children not caring about her.
- She and her husband have not talked with the children about her dying.
- Her husband reports that he just does not know how to help his wife any more and that he feels guilty sometimes when he just wishes it were all over.

**Objective Data**

- Height: 157 cm (5 ft 2 in); Weight: 44 kg (97 lb)
- Skin intact
- Vital signs: T 37.2°C (99°F); HR 92; RR 30; BP 102/60

### Critical Thinking Questions

1. What additional assessment data should the nurse obtain from Mr. and Mrs. J. before making any decisions about the care of the family?

2. What types of grieving appear to be occurring in the family?

3. What physical care should the nurse include in a plan for Mrs. J. at this time?

4. What is the best way to facilitate healthy grieving in this family?

5. What resources of a palliative care team are available to assist this client and her family?

6. Based on the assessment data provided, write one or more nursing diagnoses.

# CHAPTER 11

1. Match the following terms with their definitions.

_____  a. Addiction

_____  b. Abuse

_____  c. Craving

_____  d. Physical dependence

_____  e. Tolerance

_____  f. Withdrawal

_____  g. Abstinence

_____  h. Detoxification

_____  i. Relapse

_____  j. Misuse

_____  k. Psychological
         dependence

1. Absence of a substance will cause withdrawal symptoms

2. Responses occurring after abrupt cessation of a substance

3. Return to drug use after a period of abstinence

4. Drug use for purposes other than that intended

5. Compulsive need to experience pleasure

6. Overuse and dependence on substance that negatively affects functioning

7. Refraining from substance use

8. Decreased effect of substance following repeated exposure

9. Overwhelming desire for substance after decreased use

10. Removal of the drug and its effects from the body

11. Compulsive, uncontrollable use of substances, with cessation causing severe physical and emotional reactions

2. The neurotransmitter that appears to have a dominant effect on the process of addiction is

   a. serotonin.
   b. dopamine.
   c. norepinephrine.
   d. gamma-aminobutyric acid (GABA).

3. A client is admitted to the emergency department with chest pain and cardiac arrhythmias related to cocaine use. The client's wife tells the nurse she did not suspect a problem because her husband generally functioned normally, even though she now realizes he was using cocaine. The nurse explains to the wife that when addiction occurs, tolerance causes the individual to

   a. use the drug to feel and function normally.
   b. maintain normal behaviour to prevent detection of addiction.
   c. experience different behaviour only when the substance is not available.
   d. need less drug for the desired effects, decreasing the signs of drug use.

4. In working with culturally diverse populations, the nurse recognizes that health problems related to addiction include high rates of

   a. AIDS in Hispanic women.
   b. hepatitis C in Asian populations.
   c. alcoholism in Aboriginal persons.
   d. marijuana use in women of all cultures.

5. List two major health problems commonly seen in the acute care setting related to the abuse of the following substances.

**Nicotine/tobacco**

a.

b.

**Cocaine and amphetamines**

a.

b.

**Alcohol**

a.

b.

**Cannabis**

a.

b.

6. Match the following commonly abused substances with the physiological effects associated with their use (answers may be used more than once).

_____ a. Increase in appetite

_____ b. Sexual arousal

_____ c. Depersonalization

_____ d. Tachycardia with hypertension

_____ e. Reddened eyes

_____ f. Constricted pupils

_____ g. Nasal damage

_____ h. Decreased respirations

_____ i. Altered perception

_____ j. Euphoria and sedation

1. Cocaine/amphetamines

2. Opioids

3. Cannabis

4. Hallucinogens

7. Use the words below to fill in the blanks in the following statements.

sedative-hypnotic(s)                    narcotic(s)
stimulant(s)                            hallucinogen(s)

a. Seizures may be a symptom of toxicity in _____ addiction and a symptom of withdrawal in

   _____ addiction.

b. Assessment findings of tremors, chills and sweating, and nausea and cramps are most likely to be found in

   the client with _____ withdrawal.

c. The client who abuses _____ is least likely to have withdrawal symptoms.

d. Suicidal thoughts and proneness to violence should be assessed in clients during withdrawal from

   _____.

e. The safest and most effective method to withdraw the client from large doses of _____ is

   with hospitalization and gradual reduction of the drug.

f. A client with severe central nervous system depression with slow and shallow breathing and coma will

   respond to treatment with naloxone (Narcan) in acute _____ toxicity, but not in acute

   _____ toxicity.

8. When the nurse is encouraging a woman who smokes 1½ packs of cigarettes a day to quit with the use of
   nicotine replacement therapy, the woman asks how the nicotine in a patch or gum is different from the nicotine she gets from cigarettes. The nurse explains that that nicotine replacements

   a. include a substance that eventually creates an aversion to nicotine.
   b. provide a non-carcinogenic nicotine, unlike the nicotine in cigarettes.
   c. prevent the weight gain that is of concern to women who stop smoking.
   d. eliminate the thousands of toxic chemicals that are inhaled with smoking.

9. Match the following drugs used for treatment of cocaine toxicity with their uses (answers may be used more
   than once).

   _____  a. Haloperidol (Haldol)           1. Tachycardia

   _____  b. IV lidocaine                    2. Hallucinations

   _____  c. IV diazepam (Valium)            3. Arrythmias

   _____  d. Propranolol (Inderal)           4. Seizures

   _____  e. Bretylium (Bretylol)

   _____  f. IV lorazepam (Ativan)

   _____  g. Procainamide (Pronestyl)

10. A client who is a heavy caffeine user has been NPO all day in preparation for a late afternoon surgery. The nurse recognizes that the client may be experiencing caffeine withdrawal when the client complains of

    a. a headache.
    b. nervousness.
    c. mild tremors.
    d. shortness of breath.

11. A client admits to the nurse that she used to take diazepam (Valium) 5 mg twice a day when she became nervous, but recently has been taking 10 mg of the drug several times a day to keep herself calm. The nurse identifies that the pattern of abuse in this client is most likely that of

    a. illegal, intermittent social use that leads to daily use and rapid tolerance.
    b. early prescription use of the drug with increasing dose and frequency without medical indication.
    c. a psychological dependence that results in anxiety but not physical symptoms if the drug is stopped.
    d. learned behaviour from parents who demonstrated substance abuse for solutions to problems.

12. The third day after an alcohol-dependent client was admitted to the hospital for pancreatitis, the nurse determines that the client is experiencing alcohol withdrawal. Identify the four characteristic signs of withdrawal on which the nurse bases this judgement.

    a.

    b.

    c.

    d.

13. The best approach by the nurse to assess a newly admitted client's use of addictive drugs is to ask the client,

    a. "How do you relieve your stress?"
    b. "You don't use any illegal drugs, do you?"
    c. "What alcohol or recreational drugs do you use?"
    d. "Do you have any addictions we should know about to prevent complications?"

14. A client who abuses a variety of depressants and narcotics minimizes the amount and frequency of substances used, as well as the specific agents taken, and tells the nurse that a recent overdose episode was a result of experimentation. An appropriate nursing diagnosis for the client is

    a. defensive coping.
    b. ineffective denial.
    c. ineffective coping.
    d. ineffective health maintenance.

15. To stop the behaviour that leads to the most preventable cause of death in Canada, the nurse should support programs that

    a. prohibit alcohol use in public places.
    b. prevent tobacco use in children and adolescents.
    c. motivate individuals to enter addiction treatment.
    d. recognize addictions as illnesses rather than crimes.

16. A young woman is brought to the emergency department by police who found her lying on a downtown side-walk. Initial assessment finds that she is unresponsive and has a weak pulse of 112, shallow respirations of 8 per minute, and cold, clammy skin. Identify the two drugs that would most likely be given immediately to this client, and explain why.

    a.

    b.

17. A client with a history of alcohol abuse is admitted to the hospital following an automobile accident. To plan care for the client, it is most important for the nurse to assess

    a. when the client last had alcohol intake.
    b. how much alcohol has recently been used.
    c. what type of alcohol has recently been ingested.
    d. the client's current blood alcohol concentration.

18. A client in alcohol withdrawal has a nursing diagnosis of risk for injury related to sensorimotor deficits, seizure activity, and confusion. An appropriate nursing intervention for the client is to

    a. provide a darkened, quiet environment free from external stimuli.
    b. force fluids to assist in diluting the alcohol concentration in the blood.
    c. use restraints as necessary to prevent the client from reacting violently to hallucinations.
    d. monitor vital signs frequently as an indicator of an extreme autonomic nervous system response.

19. What are four precautions indicated for the alcoholic client who is alcohol intoxicated and is undergoing emergency surgery?

    a.

    b.

    c.

    d.

20. During admission to the emergency department, a client with chronic alcoholism is intoxicated and very disoriented and confused. The nurse anticipates that the client's management will initially include administration of

    a. intravenous thiamine.
    b. $D_5$ in ½ NS at 100 mL/hr.
    c. intravenous benzodiazepines.
    d. intravenous haloperidol (Haldol).

21. The nurse uses motivational interviewing with a client dependent on alcohol who is hospitalized for gastritis. When the client says she does not really think her use of alcohol is a problem because she can control her drinking when she wants, it would be most appropriate for the nurse to

    a. help the client consider the positive and negative factors of drinking.
    b. refrain from talking about her alcohol use while the client is in denial.
    c. explain that the gastritis is evidence that alcohol is affecting her health.
    d. reassure the client that she can quit drinking when she finally decides she wants to.

22. When assessing an older client for substance abuse, the nurse recognizes that abuse problems in older persons are most often related to the use of alcohol with

    a. opiates.
    b. sedative-hypnotics.
    c. central nervous system stimulants.
    d. prescription and over-the-counter medications.

## CASE STUDY

### COCAINE TOXICITY

**Client Profile**

Mr. C. is a 34-year-old man admitted to the emergency department with chest pain, tachycardia, dizziness, nausea, and severe migraine-like headache.

**Subjective Data**

- Is extremely nervous and irritable
- Thinks he is having a heart attack
- Admits that he was at a party earlier in the evening drinking alcohol, smoking pot, and snorting cocaine
- Noted a change in personality, including irritability and restlessness
- Experienced an increased need for cocaine in the past few months

**Objective Data**

Physical examination
- Appears pale and diaphoretic
- Has tremors
- BP 210/110, HR 100, RR 30

### Critical Thinking Questions

1. What other information is needed to assess Mr. C.'s condition?

2. How should questions regarding these areas be addressed?

3. What other clues should the nurse be alert for in assessing Mr. C.'s drug use?

4. What emergency conditions must be carefully monitored?

5. What nursing interventions are appropriate?

6. What is the best way to approach Mr. C. to engage him in a treatment program?

7. Based on the assessment data presented, write one or more nursing diagnoses. Are there any collaborative problems?

# CHAPTER *12*

## INFLAMMATION, INFECTION, AND HEALING

1. Match the definitions of cell adaptation and maladaptation to sublethal injury to their types.

   _____ a. Decrease in size or number of cells          1. Hypertrophy

   _____ b. Increase in size of cells                     2. Hyperplasia

   _____ c. Transformation of one cell type to another    3. Atrophy

   _____ d. Change in size, shape, and appearance of cells   4. Metaplasia

   _____ e. Increase in number of cells                  5. Dysplasia

   _____ f. Cells in a more embryonic form               6. Anaplasia

2. A client has suffered a penetrating injury to the abdomen causing a bowel perforation. The injury was

   caused by a hot coil flying off a machine. In this situation, four causes of lethal cell injury are

   _____, _____, _____, and _____.

3. For each of the following types of tissues or organs, identify the specific phagocytic cells of the mononuclear phagocyte system that are present, and whether the cells are fixed or free.

   a. Liver

   b. Lung

   c. Central nervous system

   d. Blood

   e. Connective tissue

   f. Bone

   g. Lymph nodes

4. A client with an inflammatory disease has the following symptoms. Identify the primary chemical mediators involved in producing the symptom and the physiological change that causes the symptoms.

| **Chemical mediators** | **Physiological change** |
| --- | --- |

a. Fever

b. Redness

c. Edema

d. Leukocytosis

5. In a client with leukocytosis with a shift to the left, the nurse recognizes that

   a. monocytes are released into the blood in larger than normal amounts.
   b. the complement system has been activated to enhance phagocytosis.
   c. the response to cellular injury is not adequate to remove damaged tissue and promote healing.
   d. the demand for increased neutrophils causes the release of immature neutrophils from the bone marrow into the circulation.

6. Chemotaxis is a mechanism that

   a. causes the transformation of monocytes into macrophages.
   b. involves a pathway of chemical processes resulting in cellular lysis.
   c. attracts the accumulation of neutrophils and monocytes to an area of injury.
   d. slows the blood flow in a damaged area allowing migration of leukocytes into tissue.

7. A client with an inflammation has a high eosinophil count. The nurse recognizes that this indicates that

   a. humoral and cell-mediated immunity is being stimulated.
   b. the inflammatory response has been stimulated by infection.
   c. tissue damage has been caused by an allergen–antibody reaction.
   d. the inflammation has become chronic with persistent tissue damage.

8. The action of the complement system in inflammation has the effect of

   a. modifying the inflammatory response to prevent stimulation of pain.
   b. increasing body temperature, resulting in destruction of micro-organisms.
   c. producing prostaglandins and leukotrienes that increase blood flow, edema, and pain.
   d. increasing inflammatory responses of vascular permeability, chemotaxis, and phagocytosis.

9. Identify whether the following statements are true or false. If a statement is false, correct the bold word(s) to make the statement true.

_____ a. Non-steroidal anti-inflammatory drugs used for inflammation inhibit the **release of leukotrienes from cells**.

_____ b. The primary effect of most **leukotrienes** is formation of the slow-reacting substance of anaphylaxis (SRS-A) that causes bronchial constriction.

_____ c. **Prostaglandins** are responsible for the constitutional symptoms of inflammation such as malaise, fatigue, and anorexia.

_____ d. Complement factors $C3_a$, $C5_a$, and $C4_a$ bind to receptors on **basophils**, causing histamine release and anaphylactoid reactions.

_____ e. Interleukin-1 (IL-1) and tumour necrosis factor (TNF) are cytokines that are released from **bacterial cells** during phagocytosis.

10. During the healing phase of inflammation, regeneration of cells would be most likely to occur in

a. neurons.
b. lymph glands.
c. cardiac muscle.
d. skeletal muscle.

11. Place the following events that occur during healing by primary intention in sequential order from 1 to 10:

_____ a. Contraction of healing area by movement of myofibroblasts

_____ b. Fibrin clot serves as meshwork for capillary growth and epithelial cell migration

_____ c. Accumulation of inflammatory debris

_____ d. Epithelial cells migrate across wound surface

_____ e. Fibroblasts migrate to site and secrete collagen

_____ f. Blood clots form

_____ g. Enzymes from neutrophils digest fibrin

_____ h. Avascular, pale, mature scar present

_____ i. Budding capillaries result in pink, vascular friable wound

_____ j. Macrophages ingest and digest cellular debris and red blood cells

12. The main difference between healing by primary intention and healing by secondary intention is that

a. secondary healing requires surgical debridement for healing to occur.
b. primary healing involves suturing two layers of granulation tissue together.
c. the presence of more granulation tissue in secondary healing results in more scarring.
d. healing by secondary intention takes longer because more steps in the healing process are necessary.

13. Complications of healing that are related to scar formation include _____, _____,

    _____, _____, and _____.

14. The three antibiotic-resistant bacteria that are of most current concern are _____,

    _____, and _____. The one most important method for nurses to prevent the

    spread of antibiotic-resistant organisms is _____.

15. The most important instruction the nurse should provide to a client to prevent the development of antibiotic-resistant bacterial infections is to

    a. wash the hands after toileting and before eating.
    b. avoid crowds and contact with others with infections.
    c. take prescribed antibiotics at the frequency and for the duration directed.
    d. request antibiotic therapy when a cold or the flu does not resolve in two to three days.

16. A client's normal calorie requirement is 1800 calories per day. During an infection, the client's temperature averages 38.5°C (101.2°F). The increase in calories the nurse plans to provide the client is

    a. 100.
    b. 150.
    c. 300.
    d. 900.

17. Match the characteristics and management techniques of wounds with their types (answers may be used more than once).

    _____ a. Serosanguineous drainage          1. Closed wound

    _____ b. Adherent grey necrotic tissue      2. Red wound

    _____ c. Spray films                        3. Yellow wound

    _____ d. Creamy ivory to yellow-green exudate    4. Black wound

    _____ e. Autolytic debridement

    _____ f. Dry sterile dressing

    _____ g. Soft necrotic slough

    _____ h. Clean, moist granulating tissue

    _____ i. Negative pressure wound therapy

18. A basic principle of wound management for all open wounds is to

    a. protect new granulation and epithelial tissue.
    b. apply topical antimicrobials to prevent wound infection.
    c. remove wound exudate with frequent dressing changes.
    d. use occlusive dressings to prevent wound contamination.

19. During care of clients, the most important precaution for preventing transmission of infections is

    a. wearing face and eye protection during routine care of the client.
    b. wearing a gown to protect skin and clothing during client care activities likely to soil clothing.
    c. wearing non-sterile gloves when in contact with body fluids, excretions, and contaminated items.
    d. hand washing following touching fluids and secretions, after removal of gloves, and between client contacts.

20. The client who is at greatest risk for developing pressure ulcers is

    a. a 42-year-old obese woman with type 2 diabetes.
    b. a 78-year-old man who is confused and malnourished.
    c. a 65-year-old woman who has urge and stress incontinence.
    d. a 30-year-old man who is comatose following a head injury.

21. The most important nursing intervention for the prevention and treatment of pressure ulcers is

    a. using pressure-reduction devices.
    b. massaging pressure areas with lotion.
    c. repositioning the client a minimum of every two hours.
    d. using lift sheets and trapeze bars to facilitate client movement.

22. Match the stages of pressure ulcers with their characteristics.

    _____ a. Necrosis of subcutaneous tissue to fascia        1. Stage I

    _____ b. Skin loss with damage to muscle or bone          2. Stage II

    _____ c. Loss of epidermis or dermis                      3. Stage III

    _____ d. Closed, nonblanchable erythema                   4. Stage IV

## CASE STUDY

### INFLAMMATION

#### Client Profile

Kate G., a 23-year-old diabetic, is admitted to the hospital with cellulitis of her left lower leg. She had been applying heating pads to the leg for the last 48 hours, but the leg has become more painful and she has developed chilling.

#### Subjective Data

- Complains of pain and heaviness in her leg
- States she cannot bear weight on her leg and has been in bed for three days
- Lives alone and has not had anyone to help her with meals

#### Objective Data

Physical examination:
- Round, yellow-red, 2-cm diameter, 1-cm deep, open wound above the medial malleolus with moderate amount of thick yellow drainage
- Left leg red from knee to ankle
- Calf measurement on left 7.5 cm (3 in.) larger than right
- Temperature: 38.9°C (102°F)
- Height: 163 cm (5 ft 4 in); weight: 83.5 kg (184 lb)

Laboratory:
- WBC: $18.3 \times 10^9$/L ($18.3 \times 10^3$/µl); 80% neutrophils, 12% bands
- Wound culture: *Staphylococcus aureus*

## Critical Thinking Questions

1. What clinical manifestations of inflammation are present in Kate?

2. What type of exudate is draining from the open wound?

3. What is the significance of Kate's WBC count and differential?

4. What factors are present in this situation that could delay wound healing?

5. Kate's physician orders ASA to be given prn for a temperature above 39°C (102°F). How does the ASA act to interfere with the fever mechanism? Why is the ASA to be given only if the temperature is above 39°C? To prevent cycling of chills and diaphoresis, how should the nurse administer the ASA?

6. What type of wound dressing would promote healing of the open wound?

7. What precautions to prevent infection transmission are required in the care of Kate's wound?

8. Based on the assessment data provided, write one or more nursing diagnoses. Are there any collaborative problems?

1. Match the following genetic terms with their descriptions.

_____ a. Phenotype

_____ b. Locus

_____ c. Allele

_____ d. Chromosome

_____ e. Dominant allele

_____ f. Genotype

_____ g. Recessive allele

_____ h. Autosomes

_____ i. DNA

_____ j. RNA

_____ k. Gene

1. The 22 homologous pairs of chromosomes

2. Double-stranded molecule-forming gene; stores genetic information

3. Position of a gene on a chromosome

4. Gene that has no noticeable effect on the phenotype in a heterozygous individual

5. Structure in cell nucleus that carries genes

6. Basic unit of heredity; arranged on chromosome

7. One of two or more alternative forms of a gene on a particular locus

8. Gene that is expressed in the phenotype of a heterozygous individual

9. Genetic physical traits expressed by an individual

10. Actual genetic make-up of an individual

11. Single-stranded nucleic acid that transfers genetic information for protein synthesis

2. When a pair of chromosomes fails to completely separate during meiosis, it may result in

a. the formation of oncogenes.
b. the creation of new autosomal-recessive disorders.
c. chromosomal abnormalities such as Down syndrome.
d. a greater diversity in the genetic make-up of oocytes and sperm.

3. When the father has Huntington's chorea, the nurse uses Punnett squares to illustrate the inheritance patterns and the probability of transmission of the autosomal-dominant disease. Complete the Punnett squares below to illustrate this inheritance pattern, using "H" as the normal gene, and "h" as the gene for Huntington's chorea.

Mother

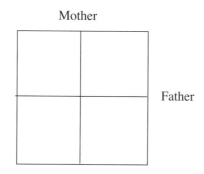

Father

There is a _____ % chance that offspring will be unaffected.

There is a _____ % chance that offspring will be carriers.

There is a _____ % chance that offspring will be affected.

4. The nurse uses Punnett squares to illustrate the inheritance patterns and the probability of transmission of phenylketonuria, an autosomal-recessive gene carried by the mother. Complete the Punnett squares below to illustrate this inheritance pattern, using "P" as the normal gene and "p" as the gene for phenylketonuria.

Mother

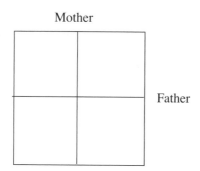

Father

There is a _____% chance that offspring will be unaffected.

There is a _____% chance that offspring will be carriers.

There is a _____% chance that offspring will be affected.

5. The use of a vector to carry genetic material into cells of the body is performed with

a. in vivo methods of gene therapy.
b. ex vivo methods of gene therapy.
c. both in vivo and ex vivo gene therapy.
d. physical transfection of the genetic material.

6. Match the descriptions of acquired specific immunity with their types of immunity (answers may be used more than once).

_____ a. Maternal immunoglobulins in neonate

_____ b. Contact with antigen through infection

_____ c. Immediate, lasting several weeks

_____ d. Longest lasting immunity

_____ e. Immunization with antigen

_____ f. Temporary for several months

_____ g. Boosters may be needed for extended protection

_____ h. Pooled gamma globulin

1. Active natural immunity

2. Active artificial immunity

3. Passive natural immunity

4. Passive artificial immunity

7. Complete the following statements.

a. The central organs of the lymphoid system are the _____ and the _____.

b. The primary cells involved in the immune response are _____, _____,

and _____.

c. The lymphoid organ primarily responsible for filtering foreign substances from the blood is the

_____.

d. Lymphocytes that differentiate into B lymphocytes are processed in the _____;

T lymphocytes are differentiated in the _____.

8. To stimulate an immune response, an antigen must be

a. captured, processed, and presented to a lymphocyte by a macrophage.
b. a foreign protein that has antigenic determinants different from the body.
c. circulated in the blood where it comes in contact with circulating lymphocytes.
d. combined with larger molecules that are capable of stimulating production of antibodies.

9. T lymphocytes that are involved in direct attack and destruction of foreign pathogens are

a. T cytotoxic cells.
b. natural killer cells.
c. T helper (CD4) cells.
d. T suppressor (CD8) cells.

10. Interferon is a cytokine that

a. directly attacks and destroys virus-infected cells.
b. augments the immune response by activating phagocytes.
c. induces production of antiviral proteins in cells that prevent viral replication.
d. is produced by virus-infected cells and prevents the transmission of the virus to adjacent cells.

11. The humoral immune response involves

    a. surveillance for malignant cell changes.
    b. production of antigen-specific immunoglobulins.
    c. direct attack of antigens by activated B lymphocytes.
    d. releasing cytokines responsible for destruction of antigens.

12. Activated B lymphocytes differentiate primarily into

    a. plasma cells that secrete antibodies.
    b. natural killer cells that destroy infected cells.
    c. memory B cells that retain a memory of the antigen.
    d. helper cells that in turn activate additional B lymphocytes.

13. Match the characteristics of the immunoglobulins with their types (answers may be used more than once).

    _____ a. Crosses placenta for fetal protection          1. IgA

    _____ b. Predominant in primary immune response          2. IgD

    _____ c. Predominant in secondary immune response        3. IgE

    _____ d. Responsible for allergic reactions              4. IgG

    _____ e. Assists in B lymphocyte differentiation         5. IgM

    _____ f. Protects body surfaces and mucous membranes

    _____ g. Antibodies against ABO blood antigens

    _____ h. Passed to neonate in colostrum

    _____ i. Assists in parasitic infections

14. Identify five important functions of cell-mediated immunity.

    a.

    b.

    c.

    d.

    e.

15. With advancing age, the immunological response that is increased is

    a. antibody responses.
    b. tumour surveillance.
    c. autoimmune responses.
    d. hypersensitivity responses.

16. Identify the types of hypersensitivity reactions from the following characteristics.

    1. Type I: anaphylactoid
    2. Type II: cytotoxic
    3. Type III: immune-complex mediated
    4. Type IV: delayed hypersensitivity

    _____ a. Cellular lysis or phagocytosis through complement activation following antigen–antibody binding on cell surfaces

    _____ b. Antigen links with specific IgE antibodies bound to mast cells or basophils releasing chemical mediators

    _____ c. T lymphocyte attack of antigens or release of lymphokines attract macrophages that cause tissue damage

    _____ d. Antigens combined with IgG and IgM too small to be removed by mononuclear phagocytic system deposit in tissue and cause fixation of complement

17. Match the following examples of hypersensitivity to their types (answers may be used more than once).

    _____ a. Transfusion reactions                    1. Type I

    _____ b. Asthma                                   2. Type II

    _____ c. Angioedema                               3. Type III

    _____ d. Transplant rejection                     4. Type IV

    _____ e. Rheumatoid arthritis

    _____ f. Allergic rhinitis

    _____ g. Tubercular caseous necrosis

    _____ h. Goodpasture's syndrome

    _____ i. Atopic dermatitis

    _____ j. Acute glomerular nephritis

    _____ k. Anaphylactic shock

    _____ l. Urticaria

    _____ m. Contact dermatitis

18. A client was given an IM injection of penicillin in the gluteus maximus and developed dyspnea and weakness within minutes following the injection.

    a. What are four additional assessment findings that would indicate that the client is having an anaphylactoid reaction?

       1)

       2)

3)

4)

b. Identify five nursing interventions to be taken to treat the client's problem.

1)

2)

3)

4)

5)

19. The rationale for treatment of atopic allergies with immunotherapy is that this therapy

a. decreases the levels of allergen-specific T helper cells.
b. decreases the level of IgE so that it does not react as readily with an allergen.
c. stimulates increased IgG to bind with allergen-reactive sites, preventing mast cell–bound IgE reactions.
d. gradually increases the amount of allergen in the body until it is no longer recognized as foreign and does not elicit an antibody reaction.

20. When administering immunotherapy to a client, the nurse must

a. give the injections at the same site each time.
b. give the injection in the upper arm near the shoulder.
c. observe the client for one hour following the injection.
d. have emergency equipment and drugs available for immediate use.

21. A nurse who develops contact dermatitis from wearing latex gloves

a. is demonstrating an allergy to natural latex proteins.
b. can use powder-free latex gloves to prevent the development of symptoms.
c. should use an oil-based hand cream when wearing gloves to prevent latex allergy.
d. has a type IV allergic reaction to chemicals used in the manufacture of latex gloves.

22. Although the cause of autoimmune disorders is unknown, the two factors believed to be present in most

conditions are _____ and _____.

23. Plasmapheresis is indicated in autoimmune disorders to

a. obtain plasma for analysis and evaluation of specific autoantibodies.
b. decrease high lymphocyte levels in the blood to prevent immune responses.
c. remove autoantibodies, antigen–antibody complexes, and inflammatory mediators of immune reactions.
d. add monocytes to the blood to promote removal of immune complexes by the mononuclear phagocyte system.

24. The human leukocyte antigen type appears to be closely related to

a. sex-linked genetic immunodeficiency disorders.
b. hereditary tendencies for immune or autoimmune disorders.
c. development of idiopathic environmental intolerances (IEI).
d. susceptibility to viral infection of the lymphoid organs and cells.

25. Explain what the term *histocompatibility complex* means, and identify which genes (of what chromosome) are involved in histocompatibility.

26. Currently, HLA typing can be used to

    a. determine paternity and predict risk for certain diseases.
    b. match tissue types for transplantation and determine paternity.
    c. establish racial background and predict risk for certain diseases.
    d. predict risk for certain diseases and match tissue types for transplantation.

27. The most common cause of secondary immunodeficiency disorders is _____.

28. The disorder in which viable T lymphocytes infused into an immunodeficient client destroy vulnerable host

    cells is _____.

29. A common combination of immunosuppressive agents used to prevent rejection of transplanted kidneys is

    a. cyclosporine, sirolimus, and muromonab-CD3.
    b. everolimus, mycophenolate mofetil, and sirolimus.
    c. tacrolimus, prednisone, and mycophenolate mofetil.
    d. prednisone, polyclonal antibodies, and cyclosporine.

## CASE STUDY

### ALLERGY

### Client Profile

Mr. W., age 54, has been diagnosed as having perennial allergic rhinitis. He is to undergo skin testing to identify specific allergens. His physician has prescribed oral antihistamines for control of his symptoms.

### Subjective Data

- Itching of eyes, nose, and throat
- Stuffy nose, head congestion

### Objective Data

Physical examination
- Clear nasal drainage
- Reddened eyes and lacrimation

**Critical Thinking Questions**

1. What immunoglobulins and chemical mediators are involved in Mr. W.'s allergic reaction?

2. Describe the procedure the nurse uses to perform the skin testing. What results indicate a positive response?

3. What precautions should be taken by the nurse during skin testing?

4. How do antihistamines act to relieve allergic symptoms? What information should the nurse include in teaching Mr. W. about using his antihistamines?

5. Skin testing indicates Mr. W. has an allergy to household dust. What information should the nurse include in teaching Mr. W. to control his exposure to this allergen?

6. Mr. W. is to begin immunotherapy. What precautions does the nurse use during the administration of the allergen extract?

7. Based on the assessment data provided, write one or more nursing diagnoses. Are there any collaborative problems?

# CHAPTER 14  HUMAN IMMUNODEFICIENCY VIRUS INFECTION

1. The most common method of transmission of HIV infection is

   a. sexual contact with an HIV-infected partner.
   b. sharing HIV-contaminated injection equipment.
   c. fetal exposure to infection from HIV-infected mother.
   d. transfusion of HIV-contaminated blood or blood products.

2. Underline the factors in the following situations in which the risk for HIV transmission is highest.

   a. Women compared with men during sexual intercourse

   b. Hollow-bore needle used for vascular access or used for IM injection

   c. Vaginal intercourse or anal intercourse

   d. Transfusion of whole blood or clotting factors

   e. First two to six months of infection or one year after infection

   f. Perinatal transmission from HIV-infected mothers taking antiretroviral therapy or HIV-infected mothers using no therapy

   g. A splash exposure of HIV-infected blood on skin with an open lesion or a needle-stick exposure to HIV-infected blood

3. Place the following events of HIV infection of a cell in sequence from 1 to 7.

   _____ a. Viral RNA is converted to single-strand viral DNA with assistance of reverse transcriptase

   _____ b. Viral DNA is spliced into cell genome using the enzyme integrase

   _____ c. gp 120 proteins on viral envelope combine with CD4 receptors of body cells

   _____ d. Cell replicates infected daughter cells and makes more HIV

   _____ e. Viral RNA and reverse transcriptase enzyme enter host cell

   _____ f. Long strands of viral RNA are cut in the presence of protease

   _____ g. Single-strand viral DNA replicates into double-stranded DNA

4. In the previous question, indicate what two events of HIV infection of a cell can be controlled with current drugs.

   a.


   b.

5. A primary reason that the normal immune response fails to contain HIV infection is that

   a. CD8⁺ T cells are stimulated, causing suppression of B lymphocyte activity.
   b. the virus inactivates B lymphocytes, preventing the production of HIV antibodies.
   c. activated CD4⁺ T cells drawn to HIV become infected and support viral replication.
   d. monocytes ingest infected cells, differentiate into macrophages, and shed viruses in body tissues.

6. List three methods by which HIV destroys CD4⁺ T cells.

   a.

   b.

   c.

7. Match the following characteristics with the corresponding stage of progression of HIV infection.

   _____ a. CD4⁺ T cells <600/μL                     1. Acute retroviral syndrome

   _____ b. Flu-like symptoms                          2. Early chronic infection

   _____ c. May last up to 10 years                    3. Intermediate chronic infection

   _____ d. HIV seroconversion                         4. AIDS or late chronic infection

   _____ e. Median length is two years

   _____ f. CD4⁺ T cell count usually normal

   _____ g. Lasts one to two weeks

   _____ h. Persistent fevers and night sweats

   _____ i. Reversal of CD4⁺ T cell to CD8⁺ T cell ratio

   _____ j. Oral hairy leukoplakia

8. A diagnosis of AIDS can be made in a client with HIV when there is

   a. a CD4⁺ T cell count of <500/μL.
   b. a WBC count <3 x 10⁹/L (3 x 10³/μL).
   c. development of oral candidiasis (thrush).
   d. onset of *Pneumocystis carinii* pneumonia.

9. Match the following characteristics with opportunistic diseases associated with AIDS.

_____ a. Hyperpigmented lesions of skin, lungs, and gastrointestinal tract

_____ b. Maculopapular, pruritic rash treated with acyclovir

_____ c. Common yeast infection involving mouth, esophagus, GI tract

_____ d. Viral infection affecting skin, eyes, and oral and esophageal mucosa

_____ e. May cause meningitis

_____ f. Diagnosed with lymph node biopsy

_____ g. Pneumonia with dry, non-productive cough

_____ h. Viral retinitis, stomatitis, esophagitis, gastritis, colitis

1. *Pneumocystis carinii* infection

2. Herpes simplex 1 infection

3. Kaposi's sarcoma

4. Cytomegalovirus infection

5. *Cryptococcus* infection

6. Varicella-zoster virus infection

7. Non-Hodgkin's lymphoma

8. *Candida albicans*

10. Opportunistic diseases develop in AIDS because these disorders are

   a. side effects of drug treatment of AIDS.
   b. sexually transmitted to individuals during exposure to HIV.
   c. characteristic in individuals with stimulated B and T lymphocytes.
   d. infections or tumours that occur when there is impaired immune function.

11. Identify whether the following statements are true or false. If a statement is false, correct the bold word(s) to make the statement true.

   _____ a. An individual with a positive result with the EIA is not considered HIV-antibody positive until confirmed with a repeat positive EIA and positive **Western blot or immunofluorescence assay (IFA) testing**.

   _____ b. **Polymerase chain reaction (PCR) tests** or **viral cultures** are done to confirm repeatedly positive ELISA testing for HIV antibodies.

   _____ c. The progression of HIV infection is monitored with the use of **Western blot** or **immunofluorescence assay (IFA)**.

   _____ d. An individual with HIV infection may have a **negative ELISA** for six months following infection.

   _____ e. **PCR and viral cultures** may be done to diagnose HIV infection in infants.

12. A newborn infant of a mother with HIV infection has a positive HIV antibody test. This indicates that the newborn

   a. has HIV infection.
   b. will require treatment for AIDS.
   c. will most likely develop AIDS within 15 months.
   d. has maternal HIV antibodies but may not have HIV infection.

13. Treatment with two nucleoside reverse transcriptase inhibitors (NRTIs) and a protease inhibitor (PI) is prescribed for a client with HIV infection who has a CD4+ T cell count of <400/µL. The client asks why three drugs are necessary for treatment. The nurse explains that the primary rationale for combination therapy is that

    a. cross-resistance between specific antiretroviral drugs is reduced when drugs are given in combination.
    b. combinations of antiretroviral drugs decrease the potential for development of antiretroviral-resistant HIV variants.
    c. side effects of the drugs are reduced when smaller doses of three different drugs are used rather than large doses of one drug.
    d. when CD4+ T cell counts are below 500/µL, a combination of drugs that have different actions is more effective in slowing HIV growth.

14. One of the most significant factors in determining when to start antiretroviral therapy in a client with HIV infection is

    a. whether the client has high levels of HIV antibodies.
    b. the confirmation that the client has contracted HIV infection.
    c. the client's readiness to commit to a complex, life-long, uncomfortable drug regimen.
    d. whether the client has a support system to help manage the costs and side effects of the drugs.

15. After teaching a client with HIV infection about using antiretroviral drugs, the nurse recognizes that further teaching is needed when the client says,

    a. "I should never skip doses of my medication, even if I develop side effects."
    b. "If my viral load becomes undetectable, I will no longer be able to transmit HIV to others."
    c. "I should not use any over-the-counter drugs without checking with my healthcare provider."
    d. "If I develop a constant headache that is not relieved with ASA or acetominophen, I should report it within 24 hours."

16. Prophylactic measures that are routinely used as early as possible in HIV infection to prevent opportunistic and debilitating secondary problems include administration of

    a. isoniazid (INH) to prevent tuberculosis.
    b. trimethoprim-sulphamethoxazole (TMP-SMX) for toxoplasmosis.
    c. vaccines for pneumococcal pneumonia, influenza, and hepatitis A and B.
    d. varicella zoster immune globulin (VZIG) to prevent chicken pox or shingles.

17. A client identified as HIV-antibody–positive one year ago manifests early HIV infection but does not want to start antiretroviral therapy at this time. An appropriate nursing intervention for the client at this stage of illness is to

    a. assist with end-of-life issues.
    b. provide care during acute exacerbations.
    c. provide physical care for chronic diseases.
    d. educate the client regarding immune enhancement.

18. Identify three methods to eliminate or reduce the risk for HIV transmission related to sexual intercourse and drug use.

**Sexual intercourse**

a.

b.

c.

**Drug use**

a.

b.

c.

19. A client with advanced AIDS has diarrhea and wasting syndrome. An appropriate nursing diagnosis for the client is

a. diarrhea related to opportunistic infection.
b. risk for fluid volume deficit related to diarrhea.
c. risk for infection related to immunosuppression.
d. risk for impaired skin integrity related to altered nutritional status and frequent stools.

20. A client with advanced AIDS has a nursing diagnosis of altered thought processes related to neurological changes. In planning care for the client, the nurse sets the highest priority on

a. providing a quiet, non-stressful environment to avoid overstimulation.
b. using memory cues such as calendars and clocks to promote orientation.
c. providing written instructions of directions to promote understanding and orientation.
d. maintaining a safe client environment.

## CASE STUDY

### HIV INFECTION

**Client Profile**

Doug K., a 28-year-old single man, had HIV antibody screening performed two weeks ago when he was seen at a health clinic for flu-like symptoms. At that time, he revealed that he had a history of multiple sexual partners. He has returned to the clinic for the results of his screening.

**Subjective Data**

- Vague symptoms of fatigue and headache
- Reports occasional night sweats

**Objective Data**

- Positive Western blot test
- Temperature: 37.8°C (100°F)
- Enlarged cervical and femoral lymph nodes

## Critical Thinking Questions

1. What specific post-test counselling activities should be performed by the nurse during Doug's visit?

2. Doug's CD4$^+$ T cell count is 650/μL. What stage of HIV infection is he most likely experiencing?

3. What additional diagnostic tests might be performed at this visit?

4. What prophylactic treatments should be used at this time to prevent the development of opportunistic diseases?

5. The physician encourages Doug to consider starting combination antiretroviral therapy. What can the nurse tell Doug about the expected effect of this therapy?

6. If Doug does not respond to treatment with an increased CD4$^+$ T cell count and a decreased viral load, what tests could be used to identify resistance to the antiretroviral agents?

7. Based on the assessment data presented, write one or more appropriate nursing diagnoses. Are there any collaborative problems?

# CHAPTER *15*   CANCER

1. When presenting a community education program related to cancer prevention, the nurse stresses that the leading cause of cancer death in both men and women is

   a. lung cancer.
   b. colorectal cancer.
   c. leukemias and lymphomas.
   d. cancer of the reproductive organs.

2. The defect in cellular proliferation that occurs in the development of cancer involves

   a. a rate of cell proliferation that is more rapid than that of normal body cells.
   b. shortened phases of cell life cycles with occasional skipping of $G_1$ or S phases.
   c. rearrangement of stem cell RNA that causes abnormal cellular protein synthesis.
   d. indiscriminate and continuous proliferation of cells with loss of contact inhibition.

3. The presence of carcinoembryonic antigens (CEAs) and alpha fetoprotein (AFP) on cell membranes is an indication that cells have

   a. shifted to more immature metabolic pathways and functions.
   b. spread from areas of original development to different body tissues.
   c. become more differentiated as a result of repression of embryonic functions.
   d. produced abnormal toxins or chemical that indicate abnormal cellular function.

4. The major difference between benign tumours and malignant tumours is that malignant tumours

   a. grow at a faster rate.
   b. are often encapsulated.
   c. invade and metastasize.
   d. cause death, while benign tumours do not.

5. Match the following malignancies with the carcinogenic factors associated with their initiation.

   _____ a. Skin cancer                     1. Alkylating agents

   _____ b. Acute myelogenous leukemia      2. Genetic susceptibility

   _____ c. Breast cancer                   3. Epstein-Barr virus

   _____ d. Cervical cancer                 4. Ultraviolet light

   _____ e. Burkitt's lymphoma              5. Ionizing radiation

   _____ f. Thyroid cancer                  6. Human papilloma virus

6. Identify whether the following statements are true or false. If a statement is false, correct the bold word(s) to make the statement true.

_____ a. **Initiation** is the stage of cancer development in which there is an irreversible alteration in the cell's DNA.

_____ b. Tobacco smoke is a complete carcinogen that is capable of both **initiation** and **promotion**.

_____ c. The promotion stage of cancer is characterized by the **irreversible** proliferation of altered, initiated cells.

_____ d. Obesity is an example of a **promoting factor**.

_____ e. The latent period of cancer is the same as **promotion**.

_____ f. Withdrawal of promoting factors will **reduce** the risk of cancer development.

_____ g. Metastasis of malignant cells to distant sites is promoted by the cell's production of **growth factor**.

_____ h. During cancer progression, metastatic cells become more **heterogeneous**, making treatment more difficult.

7. List three capabilities of tumour cells that facilitate spread of the tumour from the original site.

a.

b.

c.

8. Match the following terms with their descriptions.

_____ a. Mutations of proto-oncogenes that normally limit cell regulation

_____ b. Substance that promotes blood vessel development within tumours

_____ c. Tumour cell antigens that stimulate an immune response

_____ d. Capable of causing cellular alterations associated with cancer

_____ e. Antigens on tumour cells that reflect a return to embryonic cell differentiation

_____ f. Programmed cellular death

_____ g. Lesion with histological features of cancer except invasion

_____ h. Evasion of the immune system by cancer cells

1. Tumour-associated antigens

2. Immunological escape

3. Apoptosis

4. Oncofetal antigens

5. Oncogenes

6. Carcinoma in situ

7. Oncogenic

8. Tumour angiogenesis factor

9. Indicate the source and function of the following cytokines in immunological surveillance.

|  | **Source** | **Function** |
|---|---|---|
| a. Interleukin 1 (IL-1) | | |
| b. Interleukin 2 (IL-2) | | |
| c. Alpha-interferon | | |
| d. Gamma-interferon | | |
| e. Tumour necrosis factor | | |
| f. Colony-stimulating factors | | |

10. Compare a meningioma and a meningeal sarcoma according to the anatomical site classification system for tumours.

a. Tissue of origin:

b. Anatomical site:

c. Behaviour:

11. A client's tumour has been classified as grade II, $T_1N_1M_0$ carcinoma of the breast. What does this tell the nurse about the tissue of origin and the extent of the disease process?

a. Carcinoma:

b. Grade II:

c. $T_1N_1M_0$:

12. The nurse is counselling a group of individuals over the age of 50 about screening tests for cancer. What are six specific tests that should be performed by health professionals for the people in this group, and how frequently should each be performed?

a.

b.

c.

d.

e.

f.

13. The definitive method of diagnosing cancer is

    a. x-rays.
    b. biopsy.
    c. CT scan.
    d. presence of oncofetal antigens.

14. Match the surgical procedures with their primary purposes in cancer treatment (answers may be used more than once).

    _____ a. Colostomy to bypass bowel obstruction          1. Cure, control, or both

    _____ b. Bowel resection                                2. Supportive care

    _____ c. Mammoplasty                                    3. Palliation

    _____ d. Debulking procedure                            4. Rehabilitation

    _____ e. Insertion of suprapubic catheter

    _____ f. Cordotomy for pain control

    _____ g. Mastectomy

    _____ h. Insertion of feeding tube into stomach

15. Normal tissues that may manifest early, acute responses to radiation therapy include

    a. spleen and liver.
    b. kidney and nervous tissue.
    c. bone marrow and gastrointestinal mucosa.
    d. hollow organs such as the stomach and bladder.

16. The rationale for treatment of cancer with radiation includes the knowledge that

    a. radiation damages cellular DNA only in abnormal cells.
    b. malignant cells respond to the effects of radiation because they more frequently go through mitosis.
    c. damage to cells will occur only during M and $G_2$ phases of the cell cycle, necessitating a series of treatments.
    d. normal cells are able to repair radiation-induced damage to DNA and do not have permanent radiation damage.

17. When a client is undergoing brachytherapy, it is important for the nurse to recognize that

    a. the client will undergo simulation to identify and mark the field of treatment.
    b. the client is a source of radiation and personnel must wear film badges during care.
    c. the goal of this treatment is only palliative and the client should be aware of the expected outcome.
    d. computerized dosimetry is used to determine the maximum dose of radiation to the tumour within an acceptable dose to normal tissue.

18. A common side effect of radiation therapy that is not associated with the effect of radiation in the treatment field is

    a. fatigue.
    b. alopecia.
    c. skin reactions.
    d. bone marrow suppression.

19. Chemotherapy for the treatment of cancer would be most effective in

    a. a small tumour of the bone.
    b. a young tumour of the brain.
    c. a large tumour in a highly vascular area.
    d. malignant changes in hemopoietic cells.

20. Match the following descriptions of chemotherapeutic drugs with their classifications.

    _____   a. Cell cycle–specific drugs that mimic essential          1. Alkylating agents
                 cellular metabolites
                                                                        2. Antimetabolites
    _____   b. Cell cycle–non-specific drugs that break DNA
                 strands                                                3. Antitumour antibiotics

    _____   c. Cell cycle–specific drugs that cause mitotic            4. Plant alkaloids
                 arrest in metaphase
                                                                        5. Nitrosoureas
    _____   d. Bind with DNA to block RNA production

    _____   e. Cell cycle–non-specific drugs that block purine
                 synthesis

21. The nurse uses many precautions during intravenous administration of vesicant chemotherapeutic agents
    primarily to prevent

    a. septicemia.
    b. extravasation.
    c. catheter occlusion.
    d. anaphylactic shock.

22. Match the following malignancies with their associated routes of regional chemotherapeutic administration.

    _____   a. Bladder                                                 1. Intraperitoneal

    _____   b. Osteogenic sarcoma                                      2. Intra-arterial

    _____   c. Metastasis to the brain                                 3. Intravenous

    _____   d. Metastasis from a primary colorectal cancer             4. Intravesical

    _____   e. Leukemia                                                5. Intrathecal

23. A client is scheduled to have placement of a silastic right atrial catheter for administration of chemotherapy
    for breast cancer. When preparing the client for the catheter insertion, the nurse explains that this method of
    administration

    a. decreases the risk for extravasation at the infusion site.
    b. reduces the incidence of systemic side effects of the drug.
    c. does not become occluded as peripherally inserted catheters can.
    d. allows continuous infusion of the drug directly to the area of the tumour.

24. When teaching the client with cancer about chemotherapy, the nurse should

    a. avoid telling the client about possible side effects of the drugs to prevent anticipatory anxiety.
    b. explain that antiemetics, antidiarrheals, and analgesics will be provided as needed to control side effects.
    c. assure the client that the side effects from chemotherapy are merely uncomfortable, not life-threatening.
    d. inform the client that chemotherapy-related alopecia is usually permanent but can be managed with life-long use of wigs.

25. The late effects of chemotherapy and high-dose radiation may include

    a. third space syndrome.
    c. persistent myelosuppression.
    b. chronic nausea and vomiting.
    d. resistant secondary malignancies.

26. The primary use of biological therapy in cancer treatment is to

    a. prevent the fatigue associated with chemotherapy and high-dose radiation.
    b. enhance or supplement the effects of the host's immune responses to tumour cells.
    c. depress the immune system and circulating lymphocytes, as well as increasing a sense of well-being.
    d. protect normal rapidly reproducing cells of the gastrointestinal system from damage during chemotherapy.

27. A side effect common to all of the biological therapies is

    a. flu-like syndrome.
    b. bone marrow suppression.
    c. central nervous system deficits.
    d. nausea, vomiting, anorexia, and diarrhea.

28. To prevent the most frequent cause of death in clients undergoing radiation therapy and chemotherapy for treatment of cancer, the nurse implements measures to

    a. prevent infection.
    b. maintain nutrition.
    c. monitor kidney function.
    d. control vomiting and diarrhea.

29. An allogenic bone marrow transplant is considered as treatment for a client with acute myelogenous leukemia. The nurse explains that during this procedure

    a. there is no risk for graft-versus-host disease because the donated marrow is treated to remove cancer cells.
    b. bone marrow is obtained from a donor who has a human leukocyte antigen (HLA) match with the client.
    c. the client's bone marrow will be removed, treated, stored, and then reinfused after intensive chemotherapy.
    d. there is no need for post-transplant protective isolation because the stem cells are infused directly into the blood.

30. During initial chemotherapy a client with leukemia develops hyperkalemia and hyperuricemia. The nurse recognizes these symptoms as the oncological emergency of

    a. hypercalcemia.
    b. third space syndrome.
    c. tumour lysis syndrome.
    d. syndrome of inappropriate antidiuretic hormone (SIADH).

31. Identify five factors that will assist a client to cope positively with having cancer.

   a.

   b.

   c.

   d.

   e.

# CASE STUDY

## CANCER

### Client Profile

Mr. M. is a 45-year-old client who has recently been diagnosed with acute myelogenous leukemia. He began treatment with chemotherapy through a peripherally inserted central venous catheter five days ago.

### Subjective Data

- States he has almost continuous nausea, which becomes severe and causes vomiting following his dose of chemotherapy
- States he has no appetite
- Expresses no hope that the chemotherapy will have a positive effect

### Objective Data
- Temperature: 37.4°C (99.4°F)
- WBC: $3.2 \times 10^9$/L ($3.2 \times 10^3$/μL)
- Neutrophils: $0.5 \times 10^9$/L ($0.5 \times 10^3$/μL)
- Skin warm with decreased turgor

### Critical Thinking Questions

1. What factors may be responsible for Mr. M.'s decreased WBC and neutrophil count?

2. What assessment data indicate that Mr. M. may be experiencing an infection?

3. What additional assessment data should be collected from Mr. M. to determine the presence of an infection?

4. What factors may contribute to Mr. M.'s negative attitude toward the chemotherapy?

5. Identify nursing measures that could be instituted to help control his anorexia, nausea, and vomiting.

6. What should be included in the teaching plan for Mr. M. and his family to prevent infection?

7. Based on the assessment data presented, write one or more appropriate nursing diagnoses. Are there any collaborative problems?

1. Identify whether the following statements are true or false. If a statement is false, correct the bold word(s) to make the statement true.

   _____  a. A client with consistent dietary intake who loses 1 kg of weight in one day has lost **500** mL of fluid.

   _____  b. A man who weighs 90 kg has a total body water content of approximately **60 L**.

   _____  c. Major tissue damage that causes release of intracellular electrolytes into extracellular fluid will cause **hypernatremia**.

   _____  d. The primary difference in the electrolyte composition of intravascular fluid and interstitial fluid is the higher content of **protein** in plasma.

   _____  e. The different concentrations of sodium and potassium between interstitial fluid and intracellular fluid is maintained by the **sodium-potassium pump**.

   _____  f. A cell that is surrounded by a hypo-osmolar fluid will **shrink and die** as water moves **out of** the cell.

   _____  g. Third spacing refers to the abnormal movement of fluid into **interstitial spaces**.

   _____  h. The primary hypothalamic mechanism of water intake is **thirst**.

2. Match the following descriptions with the mechanisms of fluid and electrolyte movement.

   _____  a. Pressure exerted by proteins

   _____  b. ATP required

   _____  c. Flow of water from low solute concentration to high solute concentration

   _____  d. Force exerted by a fluid

   _____  e. Passive movement of molecules from a high concentration to lower concentration

   _____  f. Uses a carrier molecule

   _____  g. Force determined by osmolality of a fluid

   1. Facilitated diffusion

   2. Diffusion

   3. Osmotic pressure

   4. Oncotic pressure

   5. Active transport

   6. Osmosis

   7. Hydrostatic pressure

3. A client has a serum Na$^+$ of 147 mmol/L (147 mEq/L) and a blood glucose level of 7 mmol/L (126 mg/dL).

   The client's effective serum osmolality is _____ mOsm/kg. Is the client's serum osmolality

   increased, decreased, or normal? _____.

4. As fluid circulates through the capillaries, there is movement of fluid between the capillaries and the interstitium. In the following descriptions, match the direction of fluid movement and the location of the movement in the capillary.

   _____ a. Plasma hydrostatic pressure is less than plasma oncotic pressure

   _____ b. Interstitial hydrostatic pressure is lower than plasma hydrostatic pressure

   _____ c. Plasma hydrostatic pressure is less than interstitial hydrostatic pressure

   _____ d. Plasma hydrostatic pressure is higher than plasma oncotic pressure

1. Movement into capillary

2. Movement into interstitium

3. Occurs at arterial end

4. Occurs at venous end

5. Fill in the blanks *preceding* a–g below with 1, 2, 3, or 4 to indicate whether fluid shifts

   1) from vessels to interstitium
   2) from extracellular compartment to the cell
   3) from cell to extracellular compartment
   4) from interstitium to vessels

In each of the blanks *following* a–g, identify which mechanism of fluid movement is involved.

   _____ a. Low serum albumin _____

   _____ b. Hyponatremia _____

   _____ c. Administration of 10% glucose _____

   _____ d. Dehydration _____

   _____ e. Burns _____

   _____ f. Fluid overload _____

   _____ g. Application of elastic bandages _____

6. A woman has ham with gravy and green beans cooked with salt pork for dinner.

a. What could happen to the woman's serum osmolality as a result of this meal?

b. What fluid regulation mechanisms are stimulated by the intake of these foods?

7. Aldosterone is secreted by the adrenal cortex in response to

   a. excessive water intake.
   b. loss of serum potassium.
   c. loss of sodium and water.
   d. increased serum osmolality.

8. A major effect of aldosterone is increased

   a. water loss from kidney.
   b. reabsorption of sodium from the kidney.
   c. reabsorption of potassium from the kidney.
   d. permeability to water in the distal convoluted tubule and collecting duct.

9. A client at risk for hypernatremia is one who

   a. has a deficiency of aldosterone.
   b. has prolonged vomiting and diarrhea.
   c. receives excessive 5% dextrose solution intravenously.
   d. has impaired consciousness and decreased thirst sensitivity.

10. Manifestations of sodium imbalances are primarily manifested through altered

    a. kidney function.
    b. cardiovascular function.
    c. neuromuscular function.
    d. central nervous system function.

11. Match the electrolyte imbalances with their associated causes (answers may be used more than once).

   _____ a. Alcohol withdrawal                      1. Hypernatremia

   _____ b. Metabolic alkalosis                     2. Hyponatremia

   _____ c. Parathyroidectomy                       3. Hyperkalemia

   _____ d. Diabetes insipidus                      4. Hypokalemia

   _____ e. Fleet's enemas                          5. Hypercalcemia

   _____ f. Primary polydipsia                      6. Hypocalcemia

   _____ g. Milk of Magnesia use in renal failure   7. Hyperphosphatemia

   _____ h. Early burn stage                        8. Hypophosphatemia

   _____ i. Chronic alcoholism                      9. Hypermagnesemia

   _____ j. Vitamin D deficiency                   10. Hypomagnesemia

   _____ k. Osmotic diuresis

   _____ l. Prolonged immobilization

12. Several conditions will cause multiple imbalances of electrolytes. Identify three electrolyte imbalances that are caused by the following:

    a. Hyperaldosteronism

       1)

       2)

       3)

    b. Chronic renal failure

       1)

       2)

       3)

    c. Loop and thiazide diuretics

       1)

       2)

       3)

13. A client is taking diuretic drugs that cause sodium loss from the kidney. The fluid or electrolyte imbalance most likely to occur in this client is

    a. hyperkalemia.
    b. hyponatremia.
    c. hypocalcemia.
    d. isotonic fluid loss.

14. A common collaborative problem that is indicated for both hyperkalemia and hypokalemia is

    a. potential complication: seizures.
    b. potential complication: paralysis.
    c. potential complication: arrhythmias.
    d. potential complication: acute renal failure.

15. Hyperkalemia is frequently associated with

    a. hypoglycemia.
    b. metabolic acidosis.
    c. respiratory alkalosis.
    d. decreased urine potassium levels.

16. In a client with a positive Chvostek's sign, the nurse would anticipate the intravenous administration of

    a. calcitonin.
    b. vitamin D.
    c. loop diuretics.
    d. calcium gluconate.

17. A client with chronic renal failure has hyperphosphatemia. A commonly associated electrolyte imbalance is

    a. hypokalemia.
    b. hyponatremia.
    c. hypocalcemia.
    d. hypomagnesemia.

18. The normal pH range of the blood is _____ to _____. This reflects a ratio of base to acid of

    _____ to _____.

19. pH is a negative logarithm that is a measure of _____ in a solution.

20. Match the components of the buffer system with their characteristics (answers may be used more than once).

    _____  a. Neutralizes a strong base to a weak base and water        1. Carbonic acid–bicarbonate

    _____  b. Free acid radicals dissociate into $H^+$ and $CO_2$,       2. Phosphate buffer
              buffering excess base

                                                                         3. Hemoglobin buffer
    _____  c. Shifts chloride in and out of red blood cells in
              exchange for sodium bicarbonate, buffering both            4. Protein buffer
              acids and bases
                                                                         5. Cellular buffer
    _____  d. Resultant sodium biphosphate is eliminated by
              kidneys

    _____  e. Neutralizes HCl to yield carbonic acid and salt

    _____  f. Free basic radicals dissociate into ammonia and
              $OH^-$ that combines with $H^+$ to form water

    _____  g. Resultant $CO_2$ is eliminated by the lungs

    _____  h. Neutralizes a strong acid to yield sodium biphosphate,
              a weak acid, and salt

    _____  i. Shifts $H^+$ in and out of cell in exchange for other
              cations such as potassium and sodium

    _____  j. $H_2CO_3$ formed by neutralization dissociates into
              $H_2O$ and $CO_2$

21. A client who has a large amount of carbon dioxide in the blood has a

    a. large amount of carbonic acid and low hydrogen ion concentration.
    b. small amount of carbonic acid and low hydrogen ion concentration.
    c. large amount of carbonic acid and high hydrogen ion concentration.
    d. small amount of carbonic acid and high hydrogen ion concentration.

22. List the three ways that kidneys eliminate acids to maintain acid–base balance.

    a.

    b.

    c.

23. Match the acid-base imbalances with their mechanisms.

    _____ a. Increased base bicarbonate            1. Respiratory acidosis

    _____ b. Decreased carbonic acid ($H_2CO_3$)   2. Respiratory alkalosis

    _____ c. Increased carbonic acid ($H_2CO_3$)   3. Metabolic acidosis

    _____ d. Decreased base bicarbonate            4. Metabolic alkalosis

24. Identify the compensatory mechanism that occurs in each of the following.

    a.  Respiratory acidosis

    b.  Metabolic acidosis

    c.  Metabolic alkalosis

25. Match the acid–base imbalances with their common causes (answers may be used more than once).

    _____ a. Prolonged vomiting                    1. Respiratory acidosis

    _____ b. Renal failure                         2. Respiratory alkalosis

    _____ c. Response to anxiety, fear, and pain   3. Metabolic acidosis

    _____ d. Respiratory failure                   4. Metabolic alkalosis

    _____ e. Baking soda use as antacid

    _____ f. Severe shock

    _____ g. Diabetic ketosis

    _____ h. Mechanical overventilation

    _____ i. Sedative or narcotic overdose

26. A client with a pH of 7.29 has metabolic acidosis. A value that is useful in determining whether the cause of the acidosis is due to an acid gain or due to a bicarbonate loss is the

    a. $PaCO_2$.
    b. anion gap.
    c. serum $Na^+$ level.
    d. bicarbonate level.

27. Identify the acid–base imbalances represented by the following laboratory values.

a. pH           7.50
   $PaCO_2$     30 mm Hg
   $HCO_3^-$    24 mmol/L (24 mEq/L)

   Interpretation:

   _____

b. pH           7.2
   $PaCO_2$     25 mm Hg
   $HCO_3^-$    15 mmol/L (15 mEq/L)

   Interpretation:

   _____

c. pH           7.26
   $PaCO_2$     56 mm Hg
   $HCO_3^-$    24 mmol/L (24 mEq/L)

   Interpretation:

   _____

d. pH           7.62
   $PaCO_2$     48 mm Hg
   $HCO_3^-$    45 mmol/L (45 mEq/L)

   Interpretation:

   _____

e. pH           7.44
   $PaCO_2$     54 mm Hg
   $HCO_3^-$    36 mmol/L (36 mEq/L)

   Interpretation:

   _____

f. pH           7.35
   $PaCO_2$     60 mm Hg
   $HCO_3^-$    40 mmol/L (40 mEq/L)

   Interpretation:

   _____

28. An example of an intravenous solution that is used to provide free water and intracellular fluid hydration is

    a. lactated Ringer's.
    b. dextrose 5% in water.
    c. dextrose 10% in water.
    d. dextrose 5% in normal saline (0.9%).

29. An example of an intravenous solution that would be appropriate to treat an extracellular fluid volume deficit is

    a. $D_5W$.
    b. 3% saline.
    c. $D_5W$ in 1/2 NS (0.45%).
    d. lactated Ringer's solution.

# CASE STUDY

## FLUID AND ELECTROLYTE IMBALANCE

### Client Profile

Kathleen B., a 74-year-old woman who lives alone, is admitted to the hospital because of weakness and confusion. She has a history of chronic heart failure and chronic diuretic use.

### Objective Data

- Neurological: confusion, slow to respond to questioning, generalized weakness
- Cardiovascular: BP 90/62, HR 112 and irregular, peripheral pulses weak; ECG indicates sinus tachycardia
- Pulmonary: respirations 12 per minute and shallow
- Additional findings: decreased skin turgor; dry mucous membranes

### Significant Laboratory Results

- Serum electrolytes:
  | | | |
  |---|---|---|
  | $Na^+$ | 141 mmol/L (141 mEq/L) |
  | $K^+$ | 2.5 mmol/L (2.5 mEq/L) |
  | $Cl^-$ | 85 mmol/L (85 mEq/L) |
  | $HCO_3^-$ | 43 mmol/L (43 mEq/L) |
- BUN 15 mmol/L (42 mg/dL)
- Hct 0.49 (49%)
- Arterial blood gases:
  | | |
  |---|---|
  | pH | 7.52 |
  | $PaCO_2$ | 55 mm Hg |
  | $PaO_2$ | 88 mm Hg |
  | $HCO_3^-$ | 42 mmol/L (42 mEq/L) |

## Critical Thinking Questions

1. Evaluate Kathleen's fluid volume and electrolyte status. Which physical assessment findings support your analysis? Which laboratory results support your analysis? What is the most likely etiology of these imbalances?

2. Explain the reasons for Kathleen's ECG changes.

3. Analyze the arterial blood gas results. What is the etiology of the primary imbalance? Is the body compensating for this imbalance?

4. Why has Kathleen's advanced age placed her at risk for her fluid imbalance?

5. Discuss the role of aldosterone in the regulation of fluid and electrolyte balance. How will changes in aldosterone affect Kathleen's fluid and electrolyte imbalances?

6. Develop a plan of care for Kathleen while she is in the hospital. What daily assessments should be included in this plan of care?

7. Based on the assessment data presented, write one or more appropriate nursing diagnoses. Are there any collaborative problems?

1. Indicate the common purpose of surgery in the following procedures.

   a. Gastroscopy

   b. Rhinoplasty

   c. Tracheotomy

   d. Herniorrhaphy

   e. Cholecystectomy

2. A client is scheduled for a hemorrhoidectomy as a day surgery client. An advantage of ambulatory or same-day surgery is a decreased need for

   a. laboratory tests and perioperative medications.
   b. preoperative and post-operative teaching by the nurse.
   c. psychological support to alleviate fears of pain and discomfort.
   d. preoperative nursing assessment related to possible risks and complications.

3. A client who is being admitted for a hysterectomy to the surgical unit paces the floor, repeatedly saying, "I just want this to be over." To promote a positive surgical outcome for the client, the nurse should

   a. ask the client what her specific concerns are about the surgery.
   b. redirect the client's attention to the necessary preoperative preparations.
   c. reassure the client that the surgery will be over soon and she will be fine.
   d. tell the client she has no reason to be so anxious because she is having a common, safe surgery.

4. List six herbal products that the nurse should recognize as possibly increasing the risk for bleeding in a surgical client.

   a.

   b.

   c.

   d.

   e.

   f.

5. When the nurse asks a preoperative client about allergies, the client reports a history of seasonal environmental allergies and allergies to a variety of fruits. The nurse should

   a. note this information in the client's record as hayfever and food allergies.
   b. place an allergy alert wristband on the client identifying the specific allergies.
   c. ask the client to describe the nature and severity of any allergic responses experienced to these agents.
   d. notify the anaesthesiologist because the client may have an increased risk for allergies to anaesthetics.

6. During preoperative assessment of a client, the nurse obtains subjective data related to the client's functional health patterns. Identify one finding and a related surgical risk factor or need for nursing intervention for the following patterns.

|  | **Finding** | **Risk/Nursing Need** |
|---|---|---|
| a. Health perception–health management | | |
| b. Nutrition-metabolic | | |
| c. Elimination | | |
| d. Activity-exercise | | |
| e. Sleep-rest | | |
| f. Cognitive-perceptive | | |
| g. Self-perception–self-concept | | |
| h. Coping–stress tolerance | | |

7. During a preoperative systems review, the client reveals a history of renal disease. This finding suggests the need for preoperative diagnostic tests of

a. CBC.
b. ECG and chest x-ray.
c. ABGs and coagulation tests.
d. BUN, creatinine, and electrolytes.

8. During a preoperative physical examination, the nurse is alerted to the possibility of compromised respiratory function during or after surgery in the client with

a. obesity.
b. dehydration.
c. an enlarged liver.
d. decreased peripheral pulse volume.

9. Preoperative instruction that is appropriate for all clients includes

a. techniques of deep breathing and coughing.
b. descriptions of the planned surgical procedure.
c. physical procedures or preparation required before surgery.
d. the withholding of all oral fluids or food after midnight on the day of surgery.

10. When the nurse prepares to administer a preoperative medication to a client, the client tells the nurse that she really does not understand what the surgeon plans to do.

    a. What action should be taken by the nurse?

    b. What criterion of informed consent has not been met in this situation?

11. Preoperative checklists are used on the day of surgery to ensure that

    a. the client is correctly identified.
    b. clients' families have been informed where they may accompany and wait for clients.
    c. all preoperative orders and procedures have been carried out and records are complete.
    d. preoperative medications are the last procedure carried out before the client is transported to the operating room.

12. A client has the following preoperative medication order: morphine 10 mg with atropine 0.4 mg IM. The nurse informs the client that this injection will

    a. decrease nausea and vomiting during and after surgery.
    b. decrease oral and respiratory secretions, drying the mouth.
    c. decrease anxiety and produce amnesia of the preoperative period.
    d. induce sleep so the client will not be aware during transport to the operating room.

13. The nurse recognizes that extra time may be necessary when preparing an older adult for surgery because of

    a. ineffective coping.
    b. limited adaptation to stress.
    c. diminished vision and hearing.
    d. the need to include family members in preoperative activities.

# CASE STUDY

## PREOPERATIVE CLIENT

### Client Profile

Mr. Nathan J., a 49-year-old construction worker, is scheduled for a bronchoscopy. He initially sought medical care for hemoptysis and increasing fatigue. When the nurse asked him if he had any questions prior to surgery, he stated he was not certain if he should go ahead with the test because he feared a diagnosis of cancer.

### Subjective Data

- Has never been hospitalized
- Has had no medical problems except mild obesity
- Has a cigarette smoking history of 25 pack-years
- Is married with two children, ages 6 and 8; both children have cystic fibrosis
- Is fearful that his wife will not be able to manage without him

### Objective Data

- Diagnostic studies: Chest x-ray revealed mass in upper lobe of right lung
- Hematocrit: 0.31 (31%)

## Critical Thinking Questions

1. What factors in Nathan's background or personal situation may influence his emotional response and physical reactions to this surgery?

2. As Nathan will be an outpatient for this surgery, what preoperative teaching must be done to prepare him for surgery?

3. What risk factors for surgical and anaesthetic complications might you anticipate for Nathan? What potential interventions might minimize the risks?

4. Based on the assessment data provided, write one or more appropriate nursing diagnoses. Are there any collaborative problems?

1. The physical environment of a surgery suite is designed primarily to promote

   a. electrical safety.
   b. medical and surgical asepsis.
   c. comfort and privacy of the client.
   d. communication among members of the surgical team.

2. When transporting an in-patient to the surgical department, the nurse from another area of the hospital has access to

   a. the clean core.
   b. the holding area.
   c. corridors of the surgical suite.
   d. an unprepared operating room.

3. Match the surgical team members with their appropriate roles (answers may be used more than once).

   _____ a. Gowns and gloves self and other members of the surgical team

   _____ b. Admits client to the operating room

   _____ c. Responsible for maintenance of physiological homeostasis during surgery (MD)

   _____ d. Ensures all the necessary surgical instruments, sponges, and sutures are ready for the surgical procedure

   _____ e. Passes instruments to surgeon and assistants

   _____ f. Coordinates all activities in room with team members

   _____ g. Chooses surgical procedure and management of client

   _____ h. Prepares instrument table

   1. Circulating nurse

   2. Scrub nurse

   3. Surgeon

   4. Anaesthesiologist

4. Identify five examples of data collected during the perioperative nurse's assessment of the client that indicate special consideration of the client's needs during surgery.

    a.

    b.

    c.

    d.

    e.

5. During the admission of the client to the holding area or operating room before surgery, the perioperative nurse must

    a. identify the client with a formal identification process.
    b. verify the client's understanding of the risks of surgery.
    c. prepare the skin by scrubbing the surgical site with an antimicrobial agent.
    d. perform a preoperative assessment with a client history and physical examination.

6. The primary goal of the circulating nursing during preparation of the operating room, transferring and positioning the client, and assisting the anaesthesia team is

    a. avoiding any type of injury to the client.
    b. maintaining a clean environment for the client.
    c. providing for client comfort and sense of well-being.
    d. preventing breaks in aseptic technique by the sterile members of the team.

7. A break in sterile technique during surgery would occur when the scrub nurse touches

    a. the mask with gloved hands.
    b. gloved hands to the gown at chest level.
    c. the drape at the incision site with gloved hands.
    d. the lower arms to the instruments on the instrument tray.

8. During surgery, a client has a nursing diagnosis of risk for perioperative positioning injury. A common risk factor for this nursing diagnosis is

    a. skin lesions.
    b. break in sterile technique.
    c. musculoskeletal deformities.
    d. electrical or mechanical equipment failure.

9. At the end of the surgical procedure the perioperative nurse evaluates the client's response to the nursing care delivered during the perioperative period. Which of the following indicates that an outcome related to perioperative safety has been met?

    a. The client's right to privacy is maintained.
    b. The client's care is consistent with the perioperative plan of care.
    c. The client receives appropriate medication(s), safely administered during the perioperative period.
    d. The client's respiratory function is consistent with or improved from baseline levels established preoperatively.

10. The primary advantage of the use of midazolam (Versed) as an adjunct to general anaesthesia is its

    a. amnestic effect.
    b. analgesic effect.
    c. antiemetic effect.
    d. prolonged action.

11. Identify the rationale for the use of each of the following drugs during surgery and one nursing implication indicated in the care of the client immediately postoperatively related to the drug.

    | | **Use** | **Nursing Implication** |
    |---|---|---|
    | a. desflurane (Suprane) | | |
    | b. ketamine (Ketalar) | | |
    | c. fentanyl (Sublimaze) | | |
    | d. succinylcholine (Anectine) | | |

12. Match the methods of local anaesthetic administration with their descriptions.

    _____ a. Injection of anaesthetic agent directly into tissues         1. Nerve block

    _____ b. Injection of anaesthetic agent into space between             2. IV nerve block
              two vertebrae
                                                                           3. Spinal block
    _____ c. Injection of a specific nerve with an anaesthetic
              agent                                                        4. Epidural block

    _____ d. Injection of agent into subarachnoid space                   5. Local infiltration

    _____ e. Injection of agent into veins of extremity after limb
              exsanguinated

13. During epidural and spinal anaesthesia, the nurse should monitor the client for

    a. spinal headache.
    b. hypotension and bradycardia.
    c. loss of consciousness and seizures.
    d. downward extension of nervous block.

14. A preoperative client reveals that an uncle died during surgery because of a fever and cardiac arrest. The perioperative nurse alerts the surgical team, knowing that if the client is at risk for malignant hyperthermia

    a. the surgery will have to be cancelled.
    b. specific precautions can be taken to safely anaesthetize the client.
    c. dantrolene (Dantrium) must be given to prevent hyperthermia during surgery.
    d. the client should be placed on a cooling blanket during the surgical procedure.

1. In a PACU where fast tracking is used, the post-anaesthesia nurse

   a. initially admits all clients to phase I recovery areas.
   b. is responsible for determining outcome criteria for discharge from the unit.
   c. transfers clients to appropriate progressive care areas depending on the type of anaesthesia used.
   d. collaborates with a post-operative care team to establish standards for admission and progression of clients in recovery areas.

2. Upon admission of a client to the PACU, the nurse's priority assessment is the client's

   a. vital signs.
   b. surgical site.
   c. respiratory status.
   d. level of consciousness.

3. To provide care for a surgical client in the PACU, the nurse needs

   a. a copy of the written operative report.
   b. a verbal report from the circulating nurse.
   c. a verbal report from the anaesthesiologist.
   d. an explanation of the surgical procedure from the surgeon.

4. To prevent confusion during the client's recovery from anaesthesia, the nurse should begin orientation explanations when the client

   a. is awake.
   b. first arrives in the PACU.
   c. becomes agitated or frightened.
   d. is arousable and recognizes where he or she is.

5. Routine assessment of the client's cardiovascular function on admission to the PACU includes

   a. ECG monitoring.
   b. monitoring arterial blood gases.
   c. determining fluid and electrolyte status.
   d. direct arterial blood pressure monitoring.

6. Match the post-operative respiratory complications with their associated causes and mechanisms (answers may be used more than once).

   _____ a. Pain                              1. Airway obstruction

   _____ b. Tongue falling back               2. Hypoxemia

   _____ c. Medullary depression              3. Hypoventilation

   _____ d. Retained secretions

   _____ e. Inhalation of gastric contents

   _____ f. Atelectasis

   _____ g. Laryngospasm

   _____ h. Obesity

7. To prevent airway obstruction in the post-operative client who is unconscious or semiconscious, the nurse

    a. encourages deep breathing.
    b. elevates the head of the bed.
    c. administers oxygen per mask.
    d. positions the client in a side-lying position.

8. While assessing a client in the PACU, the nurse finds that the client's blood pressure is below the preoperative base line. An additional assessment finding that indicates the client has residual vasodilating effects of anaesthesia is

    a. an oxygen saturation of 88%.
    b. a urinary output greater than 30 mL/hr.
    c. a normal pulse with warm, dry, pink skin.
    d. a narrowing pulse pressure with normal pulse.

9. A client in the PACU has an elevated blood pressure and emergence delirium manifested by agitation and thrashing. The nurse should assess the client for

    a. hypoxemia.
    b. neurological injury.
    c. a distended bladder.
    d. cardiac arrhythmias.

10. The nurse applies warm blankets to a client who is shivering and has a body temperature of 35.6°C (96.0°F). The nurse would also anticipate the administration of

    a. oxygen.
    b. vasodilating drugs.
    c. anti-arrhythmic drugs.
    d. analgesics or sedatives.

11. List five criteria used to determine when clients are ready for discharge from the PACU.

    a.

    b.

    c.

    d.

    e.

12. Identify six nursing diagnoses or collaborative problems common in post-operative clients for which ambulation of the client is an appropriate intervention.

    a.

    b.

    c.

    d.

    e.

    f.

13. To promote effective coughing, deep breathing, and ambulation in the post-operative client, it is most important for the nurse to

    a. teach the client controlled breathing.
    b. explain the rationale for these activities.
    c. provide adequate and regular pain medication.
    d. use an incentive spirometer to motivate the client.

14. In the absence of post-operative vomiting, GI suctioning, and wound drainage, the physiological responses to the stress of surgery are most likely to cause

    a. diuresis.
    b. hyperkalemia.
    c. fluid overload.
    d. impaired blood coagulation.

15. Describe two independent nursing interventions in addition to ambulation that could be implemented to prevent or treat the following post-operative complications.

    a. Deep venous thrombosis

        1)

        2)

    b. Syncope

        1)

        2)

    c. Urinary retention

        1)

        2)

    d. Abdominal distension

        1)

        2)

    e. Wound infection

        1)

        2)

16. Match the following tubes and drains with their expected drainage (answers may be used more than once).

    _____   a. In-dwelling catheter                1. Wound drainage

    _____   b. Gastrostomy tube                    2. Urine

    _____   c. Hemovac                             3. Bile

    _____   d. Penrose drain                       4. Gastric contents

    _____   e. T-tube

    _____   f. Nasogastric tube

17. The nurse notes drainage on the surgical dressing when the client is transferred from the PACU to the clinical unit. The nurse should

    a. change the dressing and assess the wound.
    b. notify the surgeon of the drainage type and amount.
    c. note and record the type, amount, and colour of the drainage.
    d. observe the dressing every 15 minutes for an increase in drainage.

18. Thirty-six hours post-operatively a client has a temperature of 37.8°C (100°F). The nurse recognizes that this finding is most likely a result of

    a. dehydration.
    b. wound infection.
    c. lung congestion and atelectasis.
    d. the normal surgical stress response.

19. The physician has ordered morphine IV q2-4h prn for a client following major abdominal surgery. The nurse would plan to administer the morphine

    a. before all planned painful activities.
    b. every two to four hours during the first 48 hours.
    c. every four hours as the client requests the medication.
    d. after assessing the nature and intensity of the client's pain.

20. Instructions given to the post-operative client before discharge should include

    a. the need for follow-up care with home care nurses.
    b. directions for maintaining the routine postoperative diet.
    c. written information regarding self-care during recuperation.
    d. the necessity to restrict all activity until surgical healing is complete.

# CASE STUDY

## POST-OPERATIVE CLIENT

### Client Profile

Mrs. Beverly B., a 28-year-old schoolteacher, is admitted to the PACU following a cystoscopy for recurrent bladder infections and hematuria. The procedure was scheduled as outpatient surgery and was performed under intravenous sedation.

Physician Post-operative Orders
- Vital signs per routine
- D/C IV before discharge
- Client to void before discharge
- Cipro 500 mg PO q6h × 10 days
- Tylenol #3 1–2 tabs q3–4h prn pain
- Client to call office to schedule follow-up appointment

### Critical Thinking Questions

1. What nursing actions will be required to help Mrs. B. progress toward discharge?

2. What precautions will be required for Mrs. B. to ambulate after surgery?

3. What problems may interfere with discharging Mrs. B. to home in a timely manner?

4. How will the nurse determine that Mrs. B. is ready to be discharged home?

5. What are the unique needs of discharging a client home rather than to an in-patient unit?

6. Based on the data presented, write one or more appropriate nursing diagnoses. Are there any collaborative problems?

1. Use the following terms to fill in the labels in the illustration below.

**List of Terms**

Anterior chamber
Anterior compartment
Choroids
Ciliary body
Cornea
Iris
Lens

Optic nerve
Posterior chamber
Pupil
Retina
Sclera
Suspensory ligaments

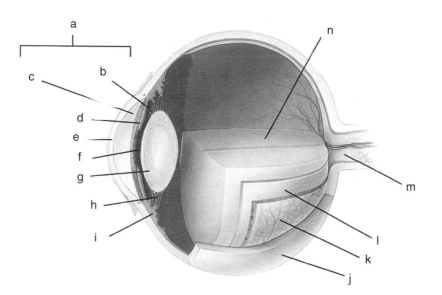

a. _____       h. _____

b. _____       i. _____

c. _____       j. _____

d. _____       k. _____

e. _____       l. _____

f. _____       m. _____

g. _____       n. _____

2. Word Search. Find the words that are described by the clues given below. The words may be located horizontally, vertically, or diagonally, and may be reversed.

```
Q  R  I  M  K  J  E  R  S  R  C  M  O  P
E  A  Q  U  E  O  U  S  H  U  M  O  R  R
A  V  I  T  R  E  O  U  S  H  U  M  O  R
D  I  O  R  O  H  C  D  L  I  I  P  O  M
W  T  H  U  M  T  O  U  M  E  R  O  U  S
E  C  E  R  T  R  E  D  L  I  P  U  P  O
A  N  T  C  O  R  N  E  A  T  C  N  U  P
Q  U  I  R  S  E  N  T  E  L  L  I  O  N
S  J  S  C  U  S  S  E  L  U  N  O  Z  T
E  N  I  T  B  O  P  T  I  C  D  I  S  C
N  O  R  A  M  I  L  T  A  R  E  L  C  S
O  C  I  L  I  A  R  Y  B  O  D  Y  E  T
C  A  N  A  L  O  F  S  C  H  L  E  M  M
S  P  C  S  C  R  E  L  O  T  M  L  E  T
```

**Clues**

a. Fibres holding the lens in place
b. Fills anterior cavity of the eye
c. Fills posterior cavity of the eye
d. Clear outer layer of anterior eyeball
e. Secretes aqueous humor
f. Photoreceptor cells stimulated in dim environments
g. Focuses light rays on retina
h. Needed for colour vision
i. Protective white outer layer of eyeball
j. Junction of the cornea and sclera
k. Transparent mucous membrane lining the eyelids
l. Drains tears from the surface of the eye into lacrimal canals
m. Point where optic nerve exits eyeball
n. Nourishes ciliary body, iris, and part of retina
o. Drainage path for aqueous humor
p. Coloured portion of eye
q. Opening in centre of iris

3. Identify whether the following statements are true or false. If a statement is false, correct the bold word(s) to make the statement true.

    _____ a. In an individual with **hyperopia** the image is focused in front of the retina and is corrected with a concave lens.

    _____ b. Presbyopia is a form of hyperopia that occurs as a result of loss of **lens elasticity**.

    _____ c. When the eyeball is too long or there is too much refracting power, the refractive error of **farsightedness** occurs.

    _____ d. Based on the visual pathway, a loss of perception in the left visual field results from a lesion in the **right** occipital lobe.

    _____ e. The cornea obtains oxygen from **tiny blood vessels in the bulbar conjunctiva**.

4. Match the following eye functions with the appropriate cranial nerve (answers may be used more than once).

    _____ a. Medial rectus muscle movement           1. CN II (optic)

    _____ b. Lateral rectus muscle movement           2. CN III (oculomotor)

    _____ c. Superior rectus muscle movement          3. CN IV (trochlear)

    _____ d. Inferior rectus muscle movement           4. CN V (trigeminal)

    _____ e. Inferior oblique muscle movement         5. CN VI (abducens)

    _____ f. Superior oblique muscle movement        6. CN VII (facial)

    _____ g. Eyelid movement

    _____ h. Corneal reflex

    _____ i. Pupil constriction

    _____ j. Pupil dilation

    _____ k. Visual acuity

5. Identify the causes of the following assessment findings of the eye that are associated with aging.

    a. Ectropium

    b. Pinguecula

    c. Arcus senilis

    d. "Floaters"

    e. Changes in colour perception

    f. Decreased pupil size

    g. Yellowish sclera

    h. Dry, irritated eyes

6. When obtaining health information from a client with cataracts, it is important for the nurse to ask about the use of

   a. corticosteroids.
   b. oral hypoglycemic agents.
   c. antihistamine/decongestants.
   d. beta-adrenergic blocking agents.

7. Identify one specific finding identified by the nurse during assessment of each of the client's functional health patterns that indicates a risk factor for visual problems or the response of the client to an eye problem.

   a. Health perception–health management

   b. Nutritional–metabolic

   c. Elimination

   d. Activity–exercise

   e. Sleep–rest

   f. Cognitive–perceptual

   g. Self-perception–self-concept

   h. Role–relationship

   i. Sexuality–reproductive

   j. Coping–stress tolerance

   k. Value–belief

8. Describe what is meant by the finding that the client has a visual acuity of OD: 20/40; OS: 20/50.

9. The nurse documents PERRLA following assessment of a client's eyes. One finding that supports these data is

   a. the slightly oval shape of the pupils.
   b. the presence of nystagmus on far lateral gaze.
   c. dilation of the pupil when a light is shined in the opposite eye.
   d. constriction of the pupils when an object is brought closer to the eyes.

10. Identify the assessment techniques used to obtain the following data.

   a. Peripheral vision field

   b. Extraocular muscle functions

   c. Near visual acuity

   d. Visual acuity

   e. Intraocular pressure

11. A yellow cast to the sclera is a normal assessment finding in

    a. infants.
    b. dark-skinned persons.
    c. persons with brown irises.
    d. inflammatory conditions of the eyes.

12. The presence of corneal abrasions or defects may be determined with the use of

    a. a tonometer.
    b. fluorescein dye.
    c. corneal reflex testing.
    d. corneal light reflex testing.

13. Match the following assessment abnormalities of the eye with their descriptions.

    _____    a. Scotoma                    1. Upper lid droop

    _____    b. Diplopia                   2. Irregularly shaped pupils

    _____    c. Exophthalmos               3. Blind spot

    _____    d. Chalazion                  4. Yellow conjunctival lesion

    _____    e. Ptosis                     5. Inflamed eyelid

    _____    f. Blepharospasm              6. Protrusion of eyeball

    _____    g. Pinguecula                 7. Double vision

    _____    h. Dyscoria                   8. Increased blink rate

14. The nurse explains to the client scheduled for a fluorescein angiography that the test involves

    a. anaesthetizing the cornea to attach a mirrored lens to examine the anterior chamber angle.
    b. application of eyedrops containing a dye that will localize arterial abnormalities in the retina.
    c. intravenous injection of a dye to evaluate blood flow through epithelial and retinal blood vessels.
    d. measurement of the electrical response of the retina to a flash of light using a contact lens electrode.

15. Match the structures of the ear with their functions.

_____ a. Semicircular canals

_____ b. Tympanic membrane

_____ c. Organ of Corti

_____ d. Cochlea

_____ e. Vestibular portion of CN VIII

_____ f. Acoustic portion of CN VIII

_____ g. External ear

_____ h. Ossicular chain

_____ i. Eustachian tube

1. Sets bones of middle ear in motion

2. Allows for equalization of pressure in middle ear

3. Receives sound waves and transmits to tympanic membrane

4. Converts mechanical sound waves into electro-chemical impulse

5. Organ of balance and equilibrium

6. Transmits sound stimuli to brain

7. Receptor organ of sound

8. Amplifies sound waves and transmits vibrations to inner ear

9. Transmits stimuli from semicircular canals to brain

16. Identify one change in the external, middle, and inner ear that can impair hearing in the older adult.

a. External ear

b. Middle ear

c. Inner ear

17. The nurse suspects a client has presbycusis when she complains of

a. ringing in the ears.
b. a sensation of fullness in the ears.
c. difficulty understanding the meaning of words.
d. a decrease in the ability to hear high-pitched sounds.

18. Describe the significance of the following questions asked of the client while obtaining subjective data during assessment of the auditory system.

    a. Do you have a history of childhood ear infections or ruptured eardrums?

    b. Do you use any over-the-counter or prescription medications on a regular basis?

    c. Have you ever been treated for a head injury?

    d. Is there a history of hearing loss in your parents?

    e. Have you been exposed to excessive noise levels in your work or recreational activities?

    f.   Has there been a change in your involvement in social activities?

19. Identify whether the following statements are true or false. If a statement is false, correct the bold word(s) to make the statement true.

_____ a. Examination of the external ear involves the techniques of **inspection and palpation**.

_____ b. To straighten the ear canal in an adult before insertion of the otoscope, the nurse grasps the auricle and pulls **downward and backward**.

_____ c. Major landmarks of the tympanic membrane are the **short process of the malleus, the handle of malleus, and the cone of light**.

_____ d. A normal finding upon physical assessment of the ear is the ability to hear a low whisper at **30 cm**.

_____ e. A client has a negative Rinne test of the left ear. The nurse would expect that with Weber testing the client would hear the tuning fork sound best in the **right** ear.

_____ f. The presence of a retracted eardrum on otoscopic examination is indicative of **negative pressure in the middle ear**.

_____ g. In **chronic otitis media**, the nurse would expect to find a lack of landmarks and a bulging eardrum on otoscopic examination.

20. Indicate whether conductive hearing loss (CHL) or sensorineural hearing loss (SHL) is associated with the following.

 \_\_\_\_\_ a. Positive Rinne test

 \_\_\_\_\_ b. Negative Rinne test

 \_\_\_\_\_ c. Weber lateralization to impaired ear

 \_\_\_\_\_ d. Weber lateralization to good ear

 \_\_\_\_\_ e. External or middle ear pathology

 \_\_\_\_\_ f. Inner ear or nerve pathway pathology

21. Results of an audiometry indicate that a client has a 10 dB hearing loss at 8000 Hz. The nurse recognizes that the client

 a. has only a mild hearing loss at high frequencies.
 b. will have problems in everyday communication situations.
 c. will have difficulty distinguishing high-pitched consonants.
 d. will need to use a hearing aid to amplify low-frequency sound.

22. Disease of the vestibular system of the ear is indicated with caloric testing when

 a. hearing is improved with irrigation of the external ear canal.
 b. no nystagmus is elicited with application of water in the external ear.
 c. the client experiences intolerable pain with irrigation of the external ear.
 d. irrigation of the external ear with water produces nystagmus opposite the side of instillation.

# CHAPTER 21  NURSING MANAGEMENT: VISUAL AND AUDITORY PROBLEMS

1. Match the refractive conditions with their characteristics (answers may be used more than once).

    _____ a. Corrected with cylinder lens

    _____ b. Absence of crystalline lens

    _____ c. Corrected with convex lens

    _____ d. Image focused behind retina

    _____ e. Abnormally long eyeball

    _____ f. Excessive light refraction

    _____ g. Corrected with concave lens

    _____ h. Unequal corneal curvature

    _____ i. No accommodation for distance vision with accommodation for near vision

    _____ j. Insufficient light refraction

    _____ k. Abnormally short eyeball

    _____ l. Image focused in front of retina

    1. Myopia

    2. Hyperopia

    3. Emmetropia

    4. Astigmatism

    5. Aphakia

2. To remove soft contact lenses from the eyes of an unconscious client, the nurse

    a. uses a small suction cup placed on the lenses.
    b. pinches the lens off the eye after sliding it off the cornea.
    c. lifts the lenses with a dry cotton ball that adheres to the lenses.
    d. tenses the lateral canthus while stimulating a blink reflex in the client.

3. The most common correction for aphakia is

    a. aphakic spectacles.
    b. aphakic contact lenses.
    c. photorefractive keratectomy.
    d. surgical implantation of intraocular lens.

4. A client tells the nurse on admission to the healthcare facility that he recently has been classified as legally blind. The nurse recognizes that the client

    a. has lost usable vision but has some light perception.
    b. will need time for grieving and adjusting to living with total blindness.
    c. will be dependent on others to ensure a safe environment for functioning.
    d. may be able to perform many tasks and activities with vision enhancement techniques.

5. Identify five nursing measures that should be implemented to increase a visually impaired client's safety and comfort.

   a.

   b.

   c.

   d.

   e.

6. A client is admitted to the emergency department with a wood splinter embedded in the right eye. An appropriate intervention by the nurse is to

   a. irrigate the eye with a large amount of sterile saline.
   b. carefully remove the splinter with a pair of sterile forceps.
   c. cover the eye with a dry sterile patch and a protective shield.
   d. apply light pressure on the closed eye to prevent bleeding or loss of aqueous humor.

7. Match the following extraocular disorders with their descriptions.

   _____  a. Acute bacterial conjunctivitis          1. Inflammation of the lid margin

   _____  b. Keratoconus                              2. Sty

   _____  c. Keratitis                                3. Blindness-causing keratoconjunctivitis

   _____  d. Epidemic keratoconjunctivitis            4. Pinkeye

   _____  e. Blepharitis                              5. Corneal degeneration

   _____  f. Trachoma                                 6. Spread by direct and sexual contact

   _____  g. Hordeolum                                7. Inflammation of the cornea

8. The nurse teaches all clients with conjunctival infections to use

   a. artificial tears to moisten and soothe the eyes.
   b. dark glasses to prevent discomfort of photophobia.
   c. warm moist compresses to the eyes to promote drainage and healing.
   d. frequent and thorough hand washing to avoid spreading the infection.

9. A client with early cataracts tells the nurse that he is afraid that cataract surgery may cause permanent visual damage. The nurse informs the client that

   a. progression of the cataracts can be prevented by avoidance of UV light and good dietary management.
   b. the cataracts will only become worse with time and they should be removed as early as possible to prevent blindness.
   c. cataract surgery is very safe and with the implantation of intraocular lenses the need for corrective lenses will be eliminated.
   d. vision enhancement techniques may improve vision until surgery becomes an acceptable option to maintain desired activities.

10. A 60-year-old client is being prepared for outpatient cataract surgery. When obtaining admission data from the client, the nurse would expect to find that the client has a history of

    a. a painless, sudden, severe loss of vision.
    b. blurred vision, coloured halos around lights, and eye pain.
    c. a gradual loss of vision with abnormal colour perception and glare.
    d. light flashes, floaters, and a "cobweb" in the field of vision with loss of central or peripheral vision.

11. A client with bilateral cataracts is scheduled for an extracapsular cataract extraction with an intraocular lens implantation of one eye. Preoperatively, the nurse should

    a. assess the visual acuity in the inoperative eye to plan the need for post-operative assistance.
    b. inform the client that the operative eye will need to be patched for three to four days post-operatively.
    c. assure the client that vision in the operative eye will be improved to near-normal on the first post-operative day.
    d. teach the client routine coughing and deep-breathing techniques to use post-operatively to prevent respiratory complications.

12. Complete the following sentences.

    a. Retinal tears leading to retinal detachment are most often caused by

    _____.

    b. The leakage of vitreous humor into the subretinal space, separating the sensory retina from the pigment

    epithelium, is termed a _____ retinal detachment.

    c. Treatments for retinal detachment that are used to create an inflammation and scarring between the retina

    and the choroid include _____ and _____.

    d. The surgical procedure that involves physical indentation of the globe to bring the pigmented epithelium,

    the choroid, and sclera in contact with a detached retina is known as _____.

13. Following a scleral buckling with a pneumatic retinopexy, the nurse plans post-operative care of the client based on the knowledge that

    a. specific positioning and activity restrictions are likely to be required for several days.
    b. the client is frequently hospitalized for seven to ten days on bed rest until healing is complete.
    c. clients experience little or no pain and development of pain indicates hemorrhage or infection.
    d. reattachment of the retina commonly fails and clients can be expected to grieve for loss of vision.

14. In caring for the client with age-related macular degeneration (ARMD), it is important for the nurse to

    a. teach the client how to correctly use topical eyedrops for treatment of ARMD.
    b. emphasize the use of vision enhancement techniques to improve what vision is present.
    c. encourage the client to undergo laser treatment to slow the deposit of extracellular debris.
    d. explain that nothing can be done to save the client's vision since there is no treatment for ARMD.

15. A client with wet ARMD is treated with photodynamic therapy. After the procedure the nurse instructs the client to

    a. maintain the head in an upright position for 24 hours.
    b. avoid blowing the nose or causing jerking movements of the head.
    c. completely cover all the skin to avoid a thermal burn from sunlight.
    d. expect to experience blind spots where the laser has caused retinal damage.

16. Visual impairment occurring with glaucoma results from

    a. ischemic pressure on the retina and optic nerve.
    b. clouding of aqueous humor in the anterior chamber.
    c. deposition of drusen and degeneration of the macula.
    d. loss of accommodation from paralysis of the ciliary body.

17. An important health promotion nursing intervention that is relevant to glaucoma is

    a. teaching individuals at risk for glaucoma about early signs and symptoms of the disease.
    b. preparing clients with glaucoma for lifestyle changes necessary to adapt to eventual blindness.
    c. promoting regular measurements of intraocular pressure for early detection and treatment of glaucoma.
    d. informing clients that glaucoma is curable if eye medications are administered before visual impairment has occurred.

18. Indicate whether the following characteristics of glaucoma are associated with primary open-angle glaucoma (POAG) or primary angle-closure glaucoma (PACG).

    _____  a. Resistance to aqueous outflow through trabecular meshwork

    _____  b. Treated with iridotomy/iridectomy

    _____  c. Administration of hypertonic oral and IV fluids

    _____  d. Caused by lens blocking pupillary opening

    _____  e. May be caused by increased production of aqueous humor

    _____  f. Causes sudden, severe eye pain associated with nausea and vomiting

    _____  g. Treated with beta-adrenergic blocking agents

    _____  h. Gradual loss of peripheral vision

    _____  i. Treated with trabeculoplasty/trabeculectomy

    _____  j. Causes loss of central vision with corneal edema

19. The physician has prescribed optic drops of betaxolol (Betoptic), dipivefrin (Propine), and carbachol (Isopto Carbachol) in addition to oral acetazolamide (Diamox) for treatment of a client with chronic open-angle glaucoma. What is the rationale for the use of each of these drugs in the treatment of glaucoma?

a. betaxolol

b. dipivefrin

c. carbachol

d. acetazolamide

20. Describe the method of removing and inserting an ocular prosthesis.

21. One of the nurse's roles in preservation of hearing includes
    a. advising clients to keep the ears clean of wax with cotton-tipped applicators.
    b. monitoring clients at risk for drug-induced ototoxicity for tinnitus and vertigo.
    c. promoting the use of ear protection in work and recreational activity with noise levels above 120 dB.
    d. advocating MMR (measles, mumps, rubella) immunization in susceptible women as soon as pregnancy is confirmed.

22. Number the following high-noise environments from the highest risk for ear injury to the lowest.

    _____    a. Noisy restaurant for 12 hours

    _____    b. Sitting in front of amplifiers at a rock band concert

    _____    c. Listening to music with stereo headphones for three hours

    _____    d. Guiding jet planes to and from airport gates

    _____    e. Heavy factory noise for eight hours

    _____    f. Using a chain saw continuously for two hours

23. A 74-year-old man has moderate presbycusis and heart disease. He takes one ASA a day as an antiplatelet agent and uses quinidine, furosemide (Lasix), and enalapril (Vasotec) for his heart condition. What risk factors are present for ototoxicity in this situation?

24. Nursing management of the client with external otitis includes

    a. irrigating the ear canal with body temperature saline several hours after instilling lubricating ear drops.
    b. inserting an ear wick into the external canal before each application of eardrops to disperse the medication.
    c. teaching the client to prevent further infections by instilling antibiotic drops into the ear canal before swimming.
    d. administering ear drops without touching the dropper to the auricle and positioning the ear upward for two minutes afterward.

25. Identify whether the following statements are true or false. If a statement is false, correct the bold word(s) to make the statement true.

    _____  a. Acute otitis media is most commonly treated with a **myringotomy** to resolve the increased pressure and inflammation in the middle ear.

    _____  b. In chronic otitis media, formation of an **acoustic neuroma** may destroy the structures of the middle ear or invade the dura of the brain.

    _____  c. A **tympanoplasty** may be used to insert an ossicular prosthesis and a tympanic membrane graft in clients with chronic otitis media.

    _____  d. The client who has had a myringotomy with placement of a ventilating tube should be instructed to **avoid getting water in the ear**.

    _____  e. **Acute** otitis media is an infection of the middle ear that frequently leads to mastoiditis and meningitis.

    _____  f. Impairment of the **eustachian tube** is most commonly associated with chronic otitis media with effusion.

    _____  g. Following middle ear surgery, the client should be positioned **flat in bed**.

26. The nurse teaches a client with chronic otitis media with effusion to equalize atmospheric pressure within the middle ear by

    a. using the Valsalva manoeuvre to force air into the middle ear.
    b. coughing or sneezing with the mouth open to prevent middle ear pressure.
    c. blowing the nose with both nostrils open to prevent eustachian tube collapse.
    d. keeping the head elevated and in straight alignment to decrease middle ear pressure.

27. While caring for a client with otosclerosis, the nurse would expect that the client has

    a. a strong family history of the disease.
    b. symptoms of sensorineural hearing loss.
    c. a positive Rinne test and lateralization to the good or better ear on Weber testing.
    d. an immediate and consistent improvement in hearing at the time of surgical treatment.

28. The nurse identifies a nursing diagnosis of risk for injury for a client following a stapedectomy based on the knowledge that

    a. nystagmus may result from perilymph disturbances caused by surgery.
    d. stimulation of the labyrinth during surgery may cause vertigo and loss of balance.
    c. blowing the nose or coughing may precipitate dislodgement of the tympanic graft.
    d. post-operative tinnitus may decrease the client's awareness of environmental hazards.

29. List the triad of symptoms that occur with Ménière's disease.

    a.

    b.

    c.

30. An appropriate nursing intervention for the client during an acute attack of Ménière's disease includes providing

    a. frequent positioning.
    b. a quiet, darkened room.
    c. a television for diversion.
    d. padded side rails on the bed.

31. The nurse counsels the client with an acoustic neuroma based on the knowledge that

    a. widespread metastasis usually occurs before symptoms of the tumour are noticed.
    b. facial nerve function will be sacrificed during surgical treatment to preserve hearing.
    c. treatment is usually delayed until hearing loss is significant since it is a benign tumour.
    d. early diagnosis and treatment of the tumour can preserve hearing and vestibular function.

32. Indicate whether the following characteristics of hearing loss are associated with conductive loss (C) or sensorineural loss (S).

    _____ a. Hears best in noisy environment

    _____ b. May be caused by impacted cerumen

    _____ c. Hearing aid is helpful

    _____ d. Speaks softly

    _____ e. Caused by noise trauma

    _____ f. Associated with otosclerosis

    _____ g. Presbycusis

    _____ h. Associated with Ménière's disease

    _____ i. Result of ototoxic drugs

    _____ j. Related to otitis media

33. When teaching a client to use a hearing aid, the nurse encourages the client to use the aid initially

    a. outdoors where sounds are distinct.
    b. at social functions where there are simultaneous conversations.
    c. in a quiet, controlled environment to experiment with tone and volume.
    d. in public areas such as malls or stores where others will not notice its use.

# CASE STUDY

## CHRONIC OPEN-ANGLE GLAUCOMA

### Client Profile

Mrs. G. is a 58-year-old Black woman seen in her ophthalmologist's office for a routine eye examination. Her last examination was five years ago.

### Subjective Data

- Has no current ocular complaints
- Has not kept annually scheduled examinations because her eyes have not bothered her
- Takes metoprolol tartrate (Lopressor) for hypertension
- Has a family history of glaucoma
- Uses over-the-counter diphenhydramine (Benadryl) for her seasonal allergies

### Objective Data

- Blood pressure: 130/78
- Heart rate: 72

### Ophthalmic Examination

- Visual acuity: OD 20/20, OS 20/20
- Intraocular pressure: OD 25, OS 28; by Tono-pen tonometry
- Direct and indirect ophthalmoscopy: small, scattered retinal hemorrhages, optic discs appear normal with no cupping
- Visual field perimetry: early glaucomatous changes, OU

### Collaborative Care

The physician prescribed betaxolol (Betoptic) 1 drop OU. The nurse instructed Mrs. G. on the reasons for the drug and how to do punctal occlusion.

## Critical Thinking Questions

1. Why should Mrs. G. have been seeing an ophthalmologist on a yearly basis even though she had no ocular complaints?

2. Explain why the nurse instructed Mrs. G. to use punctal occlusion when she uses the drops.

3. Why is it permissible for Mrs. G. to use her antihistamine? What would the nurse have told her if gonioscopy had revealed narrow angles?

4. Will this client be able to discontinue her eyedrops once her intraocular pressures are within the normal range? Explain your answer.

5. If topical therapy does not control Mrs. G.'s intraocular pressures, what should she be told about alternative therapies?

6. Describe the probable appearance of Mrs. G.'s optic discs in the future if her glaucoma is left untreated. What would her visual complaints be?

7. Based on the assessment data presented, write one or more appropriate nursing diagnoses. Are there any collaborative problems?

# CHAPTER 22 NURSING ASSESSMENT: INTEGUMENTARY SYSTEM

1. Use the following terms to fill in the labels in the illustration below.

**List of Terms**

Adipose tissue
Apocrine sweat gland
Arrector pili muscle
Blood vessels

Connective tissue
Dermis
Eccrine sweat gland
Epidermis

Hair follicle
Hair shaft
Melanocyte
Nerves

Sebaceous gland
Stratum corneum
Stratum germinativum
Subcutaneous tissue

From Jarvis C. (2004). *Student Laboratory Manual for Physical Examination and Health Assessment*, 4th ed. Philadelphia: Saunders.

a. _____

b. _____

c. _____

d. _____

e. _____

f. _____

g. _____

h. _____

i. _____

j. _____

k. _____

l. _____

m. _____

n. _____

o. _____

p. _____

2. Match the following skin structures and substances with their descriptions (answers may be used more than once).

| | |
|---|---|
| _____ a. Pigment-producing cells | 1. Epidermis |
| _____ b. Attaches skin to muscle and bone | 2. Dermis |
| _____ c. Site of vitamin D synthesis | 3. Subcutaneous tissue |
| _____ d. Specialized protective protein | 4. Keratinocytes |
| _____ e. Composed of collagen fibrils | 5. Melanocytes |
| _____ f. Produce collagen and elastin in dermis | 6. Keratin |
| _____ g. Form the basic cells of epidermis | 7. Papillary layer |
| _____ h. Form the stratum corneum | 8. Fibroblasts |
| _____ i. Dermal layer responsible for skin ridging | |
| _____ j. Location of skin glands and vessels | |
| _____ k. Location of skin-producing cells | |

3. Identify the causes of the following assessment findings of the skin associated with aging.

a. Wrinkling and skin laxity

b. Dryness

c. Easy bruising

d. Thick, ridged, brittle nails

4. When obtaining important health information from a client during assessment of the skin, it is important for the nurse to ask about

a. a history of freckles in childhood.
b. patterns of weight gain and loss.
c. communicable childhood illnesses.
d. skin problems related to the use of medications.

5.  Identify one specific finding identified by the nurse during assessment of each of the client's functional health patterns that would indicate a risk factor for skin problems or a client response to a skin problem.

    a.  Health perception–health management

    b.  Nutritional–metabolic

    c.  Elimination

    d.  Activity–exercise

    e.  Sleep–rest

    f.  Cognitive–perceptual

    g.  Self-perception–self-concept

    h.  Role–relationship

    i.  Sexuality–reproductive

    j.  Coping–stress tolerance

    k.  Value–belief

6.  When performing a physical assessment of the skin, the nurse

    a.  palpates the temperature of the skin with the fingertips.
    b.  assesses the degree of turgor by pinching the skin on the forearm.
    c.  inspects specific lesions before performing a general examination of the skin.
    d.  asks the client to completely undress so all areas of the skin may be inspected.

7.  The nurse observes that redness remains after palpation of a discoloured lesion on the client's leg. This finding is characteristic of

    a.  varicosities.
    b.  intradermal bleeding.
    c.  dilated blood vessels.
    d.  erythematous lesions.

8.  A woman calls the health clinic and describes a rash that she has over the abdomen and chest. She tells the nurse it has raised, fluid-filled, small blisters that are distinct.

    a.  Identify the type of primary skin lesion described by this client.

    b.  What is the distribution terminology for these lesions?

    c.  What additional information does the nurse need to record the critical components of these lesions?

9. Match the following skin lesions with their descriptions.

| | | |
|---|---|---|
| _____ a. Angioma | 1. Firm plaque caused by fluid in dermis |
| _____ b. Fissure | 2. A defined collection of free fluid up to 0.5 cm in diameter |
| _____ c. Macule | 3. Tiny purple spots resulting from tiny hemorrhage |
| _____ d. Papule | 4. A circumscribed, flat discoloration |
| _____ e. Plaque | 5. Linear loss of epidermis and dermis |
| _____ f. Scales | 6. Circumscribed collection of leukocytes and free fluid |
| _____ g. Wheal | 7. Elevated solid lesion up to 0.5 cm in diameter |
| _____ h. Ulcer | 8. Excess dead epidermal cells |
| _____ i. Vesicle | 9. Benign tumour of blood or lymph vessels |
| _____ j. Pustule | 10. Circumscribed, elevated solid lesion formed by confluence of papules |
| _____ k. Petechiae | 11. Irregular, crater-like loss of the epidermis and dermis |

10. The primary difference between an excoriation and an ulcer is that

   a. ulcers do not penetrate below the epidermal junction.
   b. excoriations involve only thinning of the epidermis and dermis.
   c. excoriations will form crusts or scabs whereas ulcers remain open.
   d. an excoriation heals without scarring since the dermis is not involved.

11. When assessing for changes in skin colour in Black persons, the nurse should assess the

   a. soles of the feet.
   b. palms of the hands.
   c. conjunctiva or sclera.
   d. nailbeds or oral mucosa.

12. A client has a plaque lesion on the dorsal forearm. The type of biopsy most likely to be used for diagnosis of the lesion is

   a. a punch biopsy.
   b. a shave biopsy.
   c. an incisional biopsy.
   d. an excisional biopsy.

13. The most common diagnostic test used to determine a causative agent of skin infections is

   a. a culture.
   b. the Tzanck test.
   c. immunofluorescent studies.
   d. potassium hydroxide slides.

14. Match the following assessment abnormalities with their descriptions.

_____ a. Intertrigo            1. Excavation of epidermis

_____ b. Hirsutism           2. Small, superficial dilated blood vessels

_____ c. Nevus              3. Loss of melanin

_____ d. Hematoma          4. Excessive scar tissue

_____ e. Excoriation         5. Abnormal hairiness in women

_____ f. Keloid             6. Thickening of skin

_____ g. Vitiligo            7. Mole

_____ h. Comedo            8. Swelling caused by bleeding

_____ i. Telangiectasia       9. Overlying skin surfaces

_____ j. Lichenification       10. Associated with acne vulgaris

1. Identify whether the following statements are true or false. If a statement is false, correct the bold word(s) to make the statement true.

_____ a. Exposure to **ultraviolet A (UVA) rays** is believed to be a major factor in the development of skin cancer.

_____ b. It is especially important for a client taking a **loop** diuretic to prevent sun exposure.

_____ c. In order to receive Canadian Dermatology Association approval, a sunscreen must contain an SPF of **at least 10**.

_____ d. The nurse should carefully question the client with urticaria about the use of **medications**.

_____ e. Dermatological symptoms of erythema, bullae, and seborrhea-like lesions are associated with deficiencies of **vitamin C**.

2. When teaching clients to prevent skin problems, the nurse stresses that the most important factor to avoid is overexposure to

a. sunlight.
b. radiation.
c. alkaline soaps.
d. over-the-counter skin preparations.

3. Match the following characteristics with the appropriate malignant skin conditions (answers may be used more than once).

_____ a. Skin cancer with highest mortality rate      1. Actinic keratosis

_____ b. Slow-growing tumour with rare metastasis      2. Dysplastic nevus syndrome

_____ c. Neoplastic growth of melanocytes      3. Basal cell carcinoma

_____ d. Precursor of squamous cell carcinoma      4. Squamous cell carcinoma

_____ e. Lesions keratitic and firm      5. Malignant melanoma

_____ f. Treated with topical 5-FU

_____ g. Frequently occurs on previously damaged skin

_____ h. Irregular colour and asymmetric shape

_____ i. Precursor of malignant melanoma

_____ j. Noduloulcerative type has "pearly" borders

4. Describe what is indicated by the ABCDs of malignant melanoma.

A:

B:

C:

D:

5. The nurse plans care for a client with a newly diagnosed malignant melanoma based on the knowledge that initial treatment most often involves

a. Mohs' surgery.
b. localized radiation.
c. wide surgical excision.
d. topical nitrogen mustard.

6. A client, a 78-year-old woman, has had chronic respiratory disease for 30 years. She weighs 96.4 kg (212 lb) and is 152.5 cm (5 ft 1 in.) tall. She has recently completed corticosteroid and antibiotic treatment for an exacerbation of her respiratory disease. Identify four specific predisposing factors for bacterial skin infection in this client.

a.

b.

c.

d.

7. Match the following skin conditions with the appropriate descriptions.

_____ a. Deep inflammation of subcutaneous tissue        1. Tinea

_____ b. Associated with poor hygiene        2. Herpes simplex 1

_____ c. White, patchy yeast infection        3. Acne

_____ d. Varicella infection of dermatome        4. Pediculosis

_____ e. Warty, irregular papules or plaques        5. Furuncle

_____ f. Papillomavirus infection        6. Candidiasis

_____ g. Head, body, or pubic lice        7. Cellulitis

_____ h. Excessive turnover of epithelial cells        8. Seborrheic keratosis

_____ i. Dermatophyte fungal infection        9. Lentigo

_____ j. Streptococcal infection of dermis        10. Impetigo

_____ k. Sebaceous gland inflammation        11. Herpes zoster

_____ l. Increase in normal melanocytes        12. Psoriasis

_____ m. Viral oral vesicles        13. Scabies

_____ n. Deep follicular staphylococcal infection        14. Warts

_____ o. Allergic reaction to mite eggs        15. Erysipelas

8. Three conditions of the skin that more commonly occur in immunosuppressed clients are

_____, _____, and _____.

9. The nurse should advise the client with urticaria to

a. apply topical benzene hexachloride.
b. avoid contact with the causative agent.
c. gradually expose the area to increasing amounts of sunlight.
d. use over-the-counter antihistamines routinely to prevent the condition.

10. A nurse caring for an ill-kempt client observes that the client has small red lesions flush with the skin on the head and body. The client complains of severe itching at the sites. The nurse should further assess the client for

a. nits on the shafts of his head hair.
b. a history of sexually transmitted infections.
c. the presence of ticks attached to the scalp.
d. the presence of burrows in the interdigital webs.

11. A client with a contact dermatitis is treated with calamine lotion. The nurse knows that the base for this topical preparation includes

    a. a suspension of oil and water to lubricate and prevent drying.
    b. an emulsion of oil and water used for lubrication and protection.
    c. insoluble powders suspended in water that leave a residual powder on the skin.
    d. a mixture of a powder and ointment that causes drying when moisture is absorbed.

12. A client with psoriasis is being treated with psoralen plus UVA light (PUVA) phototherapy. During the course of therapy, the nurse teaches the client to wear protective eyewear that blocks all UV rays

    a. continuously for six hours after taking the medication.
    b. until the pupils are able to constrict on exposure to light.
    c. for 12 hours following treatment to prevent retinal damage.
    d. for 24 hours following treatment when indoors near a bright window.

13. Identify one instruction the nurse should provide to a client receiving the following medications for dermatological problems.

    a. Topical antibiotics

    b. Topical corticosteroids

    c. Systemic antihistamines

    d. Topical fluorouracil

14. Match the surgical interventions with conditions they are used to treat.

    _____  a. Electrodesiccation/coagulation        1. Cutaneous malignancies

    _____  b. Excision                              2. Common and genital warts

    _____  c. Mohs' micrographic surgery            3. Small basal and squamous cell carcinomas

    _____  d. Curettage                             4. Telangiectasias

    _____  e. Cryosurgery                           5. Lesions involving the dermis

                                                    6. Seborrheic keratoses

15. The most appropriate dressings to use to promote comfort for a client with an inflamed, pruritic dermatitis are

    a. cool tap water dressings.
    b. cool acetic acid dressings.
    c. warm sterile saline dressings.
    d. warm potassium permanganate dressings.

16. An appropriate intervention to promote debridement and removal of scales and crusts of skin lesions is

    a. warm oatmeal baths.
    b. warm saline dressings.
    c. cool sodium bicarbonate baths.
    d. cool magnesium sulphate dressings.

17. Identify the rationale for using the following interventions to control pruritus.

    a. Cool environment

    b. Topical corticosteroids

    c. Decrease irritants

    d. Soaks and baths

18. A female client with chronic skin lesions of the face and arms tells the nurse that she cannot stand to look at herself in the mirror any more because of her appearance. Based on this information, the nurse identifies the nursing diagnosis of

    a. anxiety related to personal appearance.
    b. disturbed body image related to perception of unsightly lesions.
    c. social isolation related to decreased activities secondary to poor self-image.
    d. ineffective therapeutic regimen management related to lack of knowledge of cover-up techniques.

19. To prevent lichenification related to chronic skin problems, the nurse encourages the client to

    a. use measures to control itching.
    b. wear sterile gloves when touching the lesions.
    c. use careful hand washing and safe disposal of soiled dressings.
    d. use topical antibiotics with wet-to-dry dressings over the lesions.

20. A nursing intervention that is most helpful for a male client with the nursing diagnosis of anxiety related to personal appearance is to

    a. encourage the client to express feelings of anxiety.
    b. teach the client use of cosmetics and cover-up techniques.
    c. refer the client for counselling to help the client accept the situation.
    d. touch the client as appropriate to demonstrate acceptance of appearance.

21. The most common reason that elective cosmetic surgery is requested by clients is to

    a. improve self-image.
    b. remove deep acne scars.
    c. lighten the skin in pigmentation problems.
    d. prevent skin changes associated with aging.

22. Identify one cosmetic procedure indicated for each of the following problems.

    a. Redundant soft-tissue conditions

    b. Obesity with subcutaneous fat accumulation

    c. Hypertrophic scars and wrinkled skin

    d. Actinic and seborrheic keratoses

    e. Lentigines and freckles

23. A skin graft that is used to transfer skin and subcutaneous tissue to large areas of deep tissue destruction is a

    a. skin flap.
    b. free graft.
    c. soft-tissue extension.
    d. free graft with microscopic vascular anastomoses.

# CASE STUDY

## CELLULITIS

### Client Profile

Mr. J.B. cut his lower arm on a kitchen knife. At the time of the injury he did not seek medical attention. On the fourth day following the injury, he began to be concerned about the condition of the wound and the way he was feeling.

### Subjective Data

- States he has a fever and has had a general feeling of malaise
- Has pain in the area of the cut and the entire lower arm

### Objective Data

- 4-cm area around cut is hot, erythematous, and edematous
- Temperature: 38.2°C (100.8°F)

### Critical Thinking Questions

1. What care of the wound could J.B. have taken to have possibly prevented the occurrence of cellulitis in the wound?

2. What are the usual etiologies of this type of infection?

3. What would you tell J.B. about the usual treatment of cellulitis?

4. What could result if treatment is not initiated and maintained?

5. Based on the assessment data presented, write one or more appropriate nursing diagnoses. Are there any collaborative problems?

# CHAPTER 24  NURSING MANAGEMENT: BURNS

1. Match the following characteristics of burns with the types of burns (answers may be used more than once).

   _____ a. Risk for cardiac arrhythmias or arrest        1. Thermal

   _____ b. Hot cooking oil                                2. Chemical

   _____ c. Tissue adherence with protein hydrolysis       3. Smoke and inhalation

   _____ d. Causes coagulation necrosis                    4. Electrical

   _____ e. Can be caused by explosive flare

   _____ f. May cause carbon monoxide poisoning

   _____ g. Indicated by facial burns and hoarseness

2. Identify whether the following statements are true or false. If a statement is false, correct the bold word(s) to make the statement true.

   _____ a. Inhalation injury below the glottis may occur with **exposure to toxic fumes**.

   _____ b. **Acid substances** that cause chemical burns continue to cause tissue damage even after neutralized.

   _____ c. Lavage with large amounts of water is important to stop the burning process in **scald** injuries.

   _____ d. The visible skin injury seen with **an electrical burn** often does not represent the full extent of tissue damage.

   _____ e. Metabolic acidosis occurs immediately following an **acid chemical burn**.

3. Indicate the burn classification (minor, moderate uncomplicated, major) indicated in the following situations.

   _____ a. A 25-year-old with a 5% full-thickness burn of the left hand

   _____ b. A 45-year-old with smoke inhalation and superficial partial-thickness injury of the face

   _____ c. A 58-year-old with 20% deep partial-thickness burns of the legs

   _____ d. A 32-year-old who has been struck by lightning

   _____ e. A 19-year-old with a superficial partial-thickness sunburn of the legs, arms, and back

4. When assessing a client's full-thickness burn injury during the emergent phase, the nurse would expect to find

   a. leathery, dry, hard skin.
   b. red, fluid-filled vesicles.
   c. massive edema at the injury site.
   d. serous exudate on a shiny, dark-brown wound.

5. A client has the following mixed deep partial-thickness and full-thickness burn injuries: face, anterior neck, right anterior trunk, and anterior surfaces of the right arm and lower leg.

   a. According to the Lund-Browder chart, what is the extent of the client's burns? _____% TBSA

   b. According to the rule of nines chart, what is the extent of the client's burns? _____% TBSA

   c. Is it possible to determine the actual extent and depth of burn injury during the emergent phase of the burn? Why or why not?

   d. What would be the American Burn Association classification of this injury?

6. The initial intervention in the emergency management of a burn of any type is to

   a. establish and maintain an airway.
   b. assess for other associated injuries.
   c. establish an IV line with a large-gauge needle.
   d. remove the client from the burn source and stop the burning process.

7. Describe the criteria for each of the phases of burn injury and the approximate time frame of each phase.

   a. Emergent

   b. Acute

   c. Rehabilitation

8. During the early emergent phase of burn injury, the client's laboratory results would most likely include

   a. ↑ Hct, ↓ serum Na, ↑ serum K, ↓ urine Na.
   b. ↓ Hct, ↓ serum albumin, ↓ serum Na, ↑ serum K.
   c. ↓ Hct, ↑ serum Na, ↑ serum K, ↑ urine specific gravity.
   d. ↑ Hct, ↓ serum Na, ↓ serum K, ↓ urine specific gravity.

9. The initial cause of hypovolemia during the emergent phase of burn injury is

   a. increased capillary permeability.
   b. loss of sodium to the interstitium.
   c. decreased vascular oncotic pressure.
   d. fluid loss from denuded skin surfaces.

10. The response of the immune system to a burn injury includes

   a. decreased activity of neutrophils.
   b. an increase in T-helper lymphocytes.
   c. increased production of interleukin-1 and interleukin-2.
   d. becoming overwhelmed by micro-organisms entering denuded tissue.

11. One clinical manifestation that the nurse would expect to find during the emergent phase in a client with a full-thickness burn over the lower half of the body is

    a. fever.
    b. severe pain.
    c. intense thirst.
    d. unconsciousness.

12. A client has a 20% TBSA deep partial-thickness and full-thickness burn to the right anterior chest and entire right arm. It is most important that the nurse assess the client for

    a. presence of pain.
    b. swelling of the arm.
    c. formation of eschar.
    d. presence of pulses in the arms.

13. Nasotracheal or endotracheal intubation is instituted in burn clients who have

    a. electrical burns causing cardiac arrhythmias.
    b. thermal burn injuries to the face, neck, or airway.
    c. symptoms of hypoxia secondary to carbon monoxide poisoning.
    d. respiratory distress to inelastic eschar formation around the chest.

14. The physician orders IV mannitol (Osmitrol) and sodium bicarbonate to be given in addition to replacement fluids to a client in the emergent phase of burn injury. The nurse understands that the rationale for these drugs is to help prevent

    a. pulmonary edema.
    b. metabolic acidosis.
    c. hypovolemic shock.
    d. acute tubular necrosis.

15. A client is admitted to the emergency department at 1015 following a flame burn at 0930. The client has major 40% TBSA burns and weighs 60 kg (132 lb).

    a. According to the Parkland formula, the type of fluid prescribed for the client would be

       _____, and the total amount to be administered during the first 24 hours would be

       _____ mL.

    b. The schedule for the fluid administration would be _____ mL between _____ and _____ (time),

       _____ mL between _____ and _____ , and _____ mL between _____ and _____.

    c. Dextrose and water is given the second 24 hours at a rate determined by the _____.

    d. The three parameters used to determine the adequacy of the client's fluid replacement are

       _____, _____, and _____.

16. A client's deep partial-thickness burns are treated with the open method. The nurse plans to

    a. ensure that sterile water is used in the debridement tank.
    b. apply topical silver sulphadiazine (Silvadene) with clean gloves.
    c. use clean gloves to remove the dressings and wash the wounds.
    d. wear a cap, mask, gown, and gloves when caring for the client.

17. A client with deep partial-thickness burns over 45% of his trunk and legs is going for debridement in a hydrotherapy tank 48 hours post-burn. The drug of choice to control the client's pain during this activity is

    a. IV morphine.
    b. midazolam (Versed).
    c. IM meperidine (Demerol).
    d. long-acting oral morphine.

18. The nurse assesses absent bowel sounds and abdominal distension in a client 12 hours post-burn. The nurse notifies the physician and prepares to

    a. withhold all oral intake except water.
    b. insert a nasogastric tube for decompression.
    c. administer a histamine-2 blocking agent such as cimetidine (Tagamet).
    d. administer nutritional supplements through a feeding tube placed in the duodenum.

19. The nurse positions the client with ear, face, and neck burns

    a. prone.
    b. on the side.
    c. without pillows.
    d. with extra padding around the head.

20. Identify three factors that increase nutritional needs during the emergent and acute phases of burn injury.

    a.

    b.

    c.

21. At the end of the emergent phase and the initial acute phase of burn injury, a client has a serum sodium of 152 mmol/L (152 mEq/L) and a serum potassium of 2.8 mmol/L (2.8 mEq/L). The nurse recognizes that these imbalances could occur as a result of

    a. free oral water intake.
    b. prolonged hydrotherapy.
    c. mobilization of fluid and electrolytes at the acute phase.
    d. excessive fluid replacement with dextrose in water without potassium supplementation.

22. A burn client has a nursing diagnosis of impaired physical mobility related to a limited range of motion secondary to pain. An appropriate nursing intervention for this client is to

    a. have the client perform ROM exercises when pain is not present.
    b. teach the client the importance of exercise to prevent contractures.
    c. provide analgesic medications before physical activity and exercise.
    d. arrange for the physical therapist to encourage exercise during hydrotherapy.

23. The nurse suspects the possibility of sepsis in the burn client based on changes in

    a. vital signs.
    b. urinary output.
    c. gastrointestinal function.
    d. burn wound appearance.

24. Identify one major complication of burns that is believed to be stress related that may occur in each of the following systems during the acute burn phase.

    a.   Neurological

    b.   Gastrointestinal

    c.   Endocrine

25. Complete the following sentences.

    a. A permanent skin graft that may be available for the client with large body surface area burns who has

       limited skin for donor harvesting is _____.

    b. Early excision and grafting of burn wounds involves excising _____ down to clean viable tissue

       and applying _____.

    c. Blebs can be removed from skin grafts by _____ or _____.

26. To help a burn client who has developed an increasing dread of painful dressing changes, it would be most appropriate to ask the physician to prescribe

    a. midazolam (Versed) to be used with morphine before dressing changes.
    b. morphine in a dosage range so that more may be given before dressing changes.
    c. buprenorphine (Buprenex) to be administered with morphine before dressing changes.
    d. client-controlled analgesia so that the client may have control over analgesic administration.

27. During the rehabilitation phase of wound injury, the contour of scarring can be controlled with

    a. pressure garments.
    b. avoidance of sunlight.
    c. splinting joints in extension.
    d. application of emollient lotions.

# CASE STUDY

## BURN CLIENT IN REHABILITATION PHASE

### Client Profile

Kim is a 30-year-old woman who has been in the burn centre for one month. She sustained partial- and full-thickness burns to both hands and forearms while cooking with grease. She has undergone three surgeries to date for escharotomies and split-thickness skin grafting. Kim is married and has three young children at home. Her physicians feel she is nearly ready for discharge, but she has been tearful and non-compliant with therapy. Kim and her husband refuse to look at her hand grafts, which continue to require light dressings. She has not seen her children since admission.

### Critical Thinking Questions

1. When should discharge planning be initiated with Kim? Who should be involved in the planning and implementation of the educational process before discharge?

2. Describe the nutritional needs Kim will have after discharge and interventions to meet those needs.

3. Kim has been wearing hand and elbow splints at night while in the burn centre. What instructions will Kim need regarding her splinting and exercise routine at home?

4. Kim complains of tightness in her hands, which restricts her motion. She uses this excuse to avoid exercise and independent performance of her activities of daily living. What activities and education would be beneficial to address this?

5. Kim and her husband have been extremely upset and anxious regarding Kim's discharge. They are not actively participating in the discharge planning process. What interventions should the staff implement to assist the couple?

6. What are some of the feelings Kim and her family may experience following her return home? What can the nurse do to prepare the family?

7. What are the needs that must be addressed with Kim and her husband regarding dressing changes and graft care before discharge from the burn centre? Discuss how this should be managed.

8. Based on the assessment data presented, write one or more appropriate nursing diagnoses. Are there any collaborative problems?

# CHAPTER 25  NURSING ASSESSMENT: RESPIRATORY SYSTEM

1. Identify the structures in the following illustration.

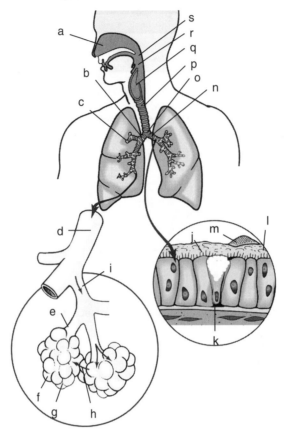

a. _____

b. _____

c. _____

d. _____

e. _____

f. _____

g. _____

h. _____

i. _____

j. _____

k. _____

l. _____

m. _____

n. _____

o. _____

p. _____

q. _____

r. _____

s. _____

2. Identify the structures and the landmarks of the chest wall in the following illustrations.

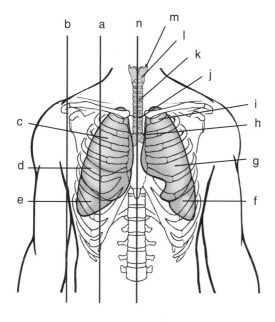

a. _____

b. _____

c. _____

d. _____

e. _____

f. _____

g. _____

h. _____

i. _____

j. _____

k. _____

l. _____

m. _____

n. _____

o. _____

p. _____

q. _____

r. _____

s. _____

t. _____

u. _____

3. Word Search: Find the words that are defined by the clues given below. The words may be located horizontally, vertically, or diagonally, and may be reversed.

```
E  D  T  N  A  T  C  A  F  R  U  S  T  A
S  E  M  P  Y  E  M  A  N  I  C  U  R  T
E  A  R  O  C  A  R  I  N  A  L  U  A  H
T  D  I  P  W  M  I  R  S  D  E  M  C  O
A  S  V  I  S  C  E  R  A  L  O  C  H  N
N  P  I  M  T  A  A  Y  P  S  I  M  E  G
I  A  S  O  I  L  A  L  M  L  G  B  A  O
B  C  T  H  O  R  A  C  I  C  C  A  G  E
R  E  F  E  S  T  L  A  R  Y  N  X  I  T
U  L  V  T  E  P  I  G  L  O  T  T  I  S
T  L  S  I  U  O  L  F  O  E  L  G  N  A
A  E  R  O  C  O  M  P  L  I  A  N  C  E
W  A  E  V  R  E  N  C  I  N  E  R  H  P
P  F  B  W  E  T  I  S  R  A  M  D  E  S
```

**Clues**

  a. Shapes and supports the chest wall
  b. Covers the larynx during swallowing
  c. Separates the larynx and the bronchi
  d. Point of bifurcation of trachea into bronchi
  e. 150 mL of air in this area not available for gas exchange
  f. Keeps the alveoli from collapsing
  g. Terminal structures of the respiratory tract
  h. Elasticity of the lungs and thorax
  i. Location of the vocal cords
  j. Warm and moisturize inhaled air
  k. Manubriosternal junction at level of carina
  l. Membrane lining the chest cavity
  m. Innervates the diaphragm
  n. Small hairs that move mucus up the respiratory tract
  o. The _____ pleura lines the lungs
  p. Collection of pus in thoracic cavity

4. Identify whether the following statements are true or false. If a statement is false, correct the bold word(s) to make the statement true.

_____ a. **Arterial oxygen tension (PaO$_2$)** is the amount of oxygen bound to hemoglobin in comparison with the amount of oxygen the hemoglobin can carry, and is expressed **in mm Hg**.

_____ b. **Arterial oxygen saturation (SaO$_2$)** is the amount of oxygen dissolved in plasma and is expressed **as a percentage**.

_____ c. If hemoglobin is **desaturated of oxygen**, more oxygen is released from the hemoglobin and dissolved in the blood to provide oxygen to the tissues.

_____ d. The oxygen–hemoglobin dissociation curve indicates that a client is adequately oxygenated when PaO$_2$ is above 60 mm Hg because hemoglobin saturation **remains above 90%**.

_____ e. A client has an oxyhemoglobin saturation of 90%. On the normal oxygen-hemoglobin dissociation curve with this saturation, he would have an arterial oxygen tension of about **90 mm Hg**.

5. In a client with a shift to the right in the oxygen–hemoglobin dissociation curve caused by an acidosis

a. low concentrations of oxygen are administered because more oxygen is delivered to the tissues.
b. high concentrations of oxygen are necessary because blood picks up less oxygen from the lungs.
c. low concentrations of oxygen are administered because blood picks up more oxygen from the lungs.
d. high concentrations of oxygen may be administered to compensate for decreased unloading of oxygen in tissues.

6. A client with an SaO$_2$ of 85% has a PaO$_2$ of 50 mm Hg. This indicates a

a. shift to the left in the oxygen–hemoglobin dissociation curve that could be caused by acidosis.
b. shift to the right in the oxygen–hemoglobin dissociation curve that could be caused by alkalosis.
c. shift to the left in the oxygen–hemoglobin dissociation curve that could be caused by hypothermia.
d. shift to the right in the oxygen–hemoglobin dissociation curve that could be caused by hyperthermia.

7. A 75-year-old client breathing room air has an analysis of arterial blood gases. Normal results the nurse would expect for the client include

a. pH 7.32; PaO$_2$ 90 mm Hg, PaCO$_2$ 50 mm Hg.
b. pH 7.40; PaO$_2$ 72 mm Hg, PaCO$_2$ 40 mm Hg.
c. pH 7.44; PaO$_2$ 84 mm Hg, PaCO$_2$ 33 mm Hg.
d. pH 7.51; PaO$_2$ 68 mm Hg, PaCO$_2$ 28 mm Hg.

8. Differences between normal arterial blood gas values and normal mixed venous blood gas values

a. indicate impaired cardiac output.
b. indicate that the client is hemodynamically unstable.
c. reflect the normal capillary oxygen–carbon dioxide exchange.
d. occur when the client has inadequate delivery of oxygen to the tissues.

9. A pulse oximetry monitor indicates that the client has a drop in SpO$_2$ from 95% to 85% over several hours. The first action the nurse should take is to

a. order stat ABGs to confirm the SpO$_2$ with a SaO$_2$.
b. notify the physician of the change in baseline PaO$_2$.
c. check the position of the probe on the finger or earlobe.
d. start oxygen administration by nasal cannula at 2 L/min.

10. Pulse oximetry may not be a reliable indicator of oxygen saturation in the client

     a. with a fever.
     b. who is anaesthetized.
     c. in hypovolemic shock.
     d. receiving oxygen therapy.

11. A client has an $SpO_2$ of 70%. What are four other assessments the nurse should consider in making a judgement about the adequacy of the client's oxygenation?

     a.

     b.

     c.

     d.

12. Criteria for the use of continuous oxygen therapy include

     a. $SpO_2$ of 95%; $PaO_2$ of 70 mm Hg.
     b. $SpO_2$ of 90%; $PaO_2$ of 60 mm Hg.
     c. $SpO_2$ of 88%; $PaO_2$ of 55 mm Hg.
     d. $SpO_2$ of 75%; $PaO_2$ less than 40 mm Hg.

13. An excess of carbon dioxide causes an increased respiratory rate and volume because

     a. $CO_2$ displaces oxygen on hemoglobin leading to a decreased $PaO_2$.
     b. $CO_2$ causes an increase in the amount of hydrogen ions available in the body.
     c. $CO_2$ combines with water to form carbonic acid, lowering the pH of cerebrospinal fluid.
     d. $CO_2$ directly stimulates chemoreceptors in the medulla to increase respiratory rate and volume.

14. The respiratory defence mechanism that is most impaired by smoking is

     a. filtration of air.
     b. the cough reflex.
     c. mucociliary clearance.
     d. reflex bronchoconstriction.

15. Identify two specific causes of the following age-related changes in the respiratory system.

     a. Decreased $PaO_2$

     b. Barrel-chest appearance

     c. Decreased secretion clearance

     d. Decreased resistance to infection

16. Identify one specific finding identified by the nurse during assessment of each of the client's functional health patterns that indicates a risk factor for respiratory problems or a client response to an actual respiratory problem.

   a. Health perception–health management

   b. Nutritional–metabolic

   c. Elimination

   d. Activity–exercise

   e. Sleep–rest

   f. Cognitive–perceptual

   g. Self-perception–self-concept

   h. Role–relationship

   i. Sexuality–reproductive

   j. Coping–stress tolerance

   k. Value–belief

17. Match the following abnormal assessment findings with the assessment technique used to detect them (answers may be used more than once).

   _____ a. Nasal polyps                   1. Inspection

   _____ b. Limited chest expansion         2. Palpation

   _____ c. Hyperresonance                  3. Percussion

   _____ d. Increased tactile fremitus      4. Auscultation

   _____ e. Finger clubbing

   _____ f. Tracheal deviation

   _____ g. Pleural friction rub

   _____ h. Wheeze

   _____ i. Use of accessory muscles

   _____ j. Barrel chest

18. To assess the client's chest expansion, the nurse places

   a. the thumbs at the midline of the chest.
   b. the palms of the hands against the chest wall.
   c. the index fingers on either side of the trachea.
   d. one hand on the lower anterior chest and one hand on the upper abdomen.

19. The nurse records the presence of an increased AP diameter of the chest when

    a. there is a prominent protrusion of the sternum.
    b. the width of the chest is equal to the depth of the chest.
    c. there is equal but diminished movement of the two sides of the chest.
    d. the client cannot fully expand the lungs because of kyphosis of the spine.

20. The presence of bronchovesicular breath sounds in the peripheral lung fields is described as

    a. rhonchi.
    b. crackles.
    c. adventitious sounds.
    d. abnormal lung sounds.

21. Match the descriptions or possible etiologies with the appropriate abnormal assessment findings.

    _____  a. Finger clubbing              1. Lung consolidation with fluid or exudate

    _____  b. Stridor                      2. Air trapping

    _____  c. Wheezes                      3. Atelectasis

    _____  d. Pleural friction rub         4. Interstitial filling with fluid

    _____  e. Increased tactile fremitus   5. Bronchoconstriction

    _____  f. Hyperresonance               6. Partial obstruction of trachea or larynx

    _____  g. Fine crackles                7. Chronic hypoxemia

    _____  h. Absent breath sounds         8. Pleurisy

22. A nurse has been exposed to tuberculosis during care of a client with TB and has TB skin testing performed. The nurse is considered uninfected if

    a. there is no redness or induration at the injection site.
    b. there is an induration of only 5 mm at the injection site.
    c. testing causes a 10-mm reddened flat area at the injection site.
    d. a negative skin test is followed by another negative skin test in three weeks.

23. A primary nursing responsibility after obtaining a blood specimen for ABGs is

    a. adding heparin to the blood specimen.
    b. applying pressure to the puncture site for two full minutes.
    c. taking the specimen immediately to the laboratory in an iced container.
    d. avoiding any changes in oxygen intervention for 20 minutes following the procedure.

24. When preparing a client for a pulmonary angiogram scan, the nurse

    a. assesses the client for iodine allergy.
    b. implements NPO orders for six to twelve hours before the test.
    c. ensures that informed consent has been obtained from the client.
    d. informs the client that radiation isolation for 24 hours after the test is necessary.

25. To prepare the client for a thoracentesis, the nurse positions the client

    a. side-lying with the affected side up.
    b. flat in bed with the arms extended out to the side.
    c. sitting upright with the elbows on an overbed table.
    d. in a semi-Fowler's position with the arms above the head.

26. The nurse observes the client for symptoms of a pneumothorax following a

    a. thoracentesis.
    b. ventilation-perfusion scan.
    c. bronchoscopic lung biopsy.
    d. positron emission tomography.

27. The physician orders a pulmonary angiogram for a client admitted with dyspnea and hemoptysis. The nurse recognizes that this test is most commonly used to diagnose

    a. tuberculosis.
    b. cancer of the lung.
    c. airway obstruction.
    d. pulmonary embolism.

28. Match the following pulmonary capacities and function tests with their descriptions.

    _____ a. VT              1. Amount of air exhaled in first second of forced vital capacity

    _____ b. RV              2. Maximum amount of air lungs can contain

    _____ c. TLC             3. Volume of air inhaled and exhaled with each breath

    _____ d. VC              4. Maximum amount of air that can be exhaled after maximum inhalation

    _____ e. FVC             5. Amount of air that can be quickly and forcefully exhaled after maximum
                                inspiration
    _____ f. PEFR
                             6. Maximum rate of airflow during forced expiration
    _____ g. $FEV_1$
                             7. Amount of air remaining in lungs after forced expiration

1. Identify whether the following statements are true or false. If a statement is false, correct the bold word(s) to make the statement true.

   _____ a. A major deviation in the nasal septum that causes obstruction of nasal airflow is usually corrected by a **rhinoplasty**.

   _____ b. In the client who has suffered a major frontal blow with a nasal fracture, the nurse should monitor for **leakage of cerebrospinal fluid**.

   _____ c. Preoperative teaching for the client planning an elective rhinoplasty for cosmetic effects includes informing the client to avoid **ASA-containing products** for two weeks before and immediately following the surgery.

   _____ d. **Perennial** rhinitis usually occurs as an allergic response when pollen counts are high in spring and fall.

   _____ e. Nasal polyps are a complication of long-term **allergic rhinitis**.

2. A client develops epistaxis upon removal of a nasogastric tube. The nurse should

   a. pinch the soft part of the nose.
   b. position the client on the side.
   c. apply an ice pack to the forehead.
   d. have the client hyperextend the neck.

3. When caring for a client hospitalized with posterior nasal packing for control of epistaxis, the nurse

   a. monitors for hypoxemia and hypercapnia.
   b. cleans the nares and applies petroleum jelly.
   c. expects the client to have a low-grade fever.
   d. administers non-steroidal anti-inflammatory drugs for pain.

4. The nurse teaches the client with allergic rhinitis that the most effective way to decrease allergic symptoms is to

   a. undergo weekly immunotherapy.
   b. identify and avoid triggers of the allergic reaction.
   c. use cromolyn nasal spray prophylactically year-round.
   d. use over-the-counter antihistamines and decongestants during an acute attack.

5. During assessment of the client with a viral upper respiratory infection, the nurse recognizes that antibiotics may be indicated based on the finding of

   a. fever.
   b. cough and sore throat.
   c. purulent nasal discharge.
   d. dyspnea and purulent sputum.

6. A 36-year-old client asks the nurse if an influenza vaccine is necessary every year. The best response by the nurse is

   a. "Only healthcare workers in contact with high-risk clients should be immunized each year."
   b. "Annual vaccination is not necessary because previous immunity will protect you for several years."
   c. "New antiviral drugs, such as zanamivir (Relenza), eliminate the need for vaccine except in the older adult."
   d. "You should get the vaccine if you have a chronic disease or want to reduce your chances of acquiring influenza."

7. A client uses echinacea and goldenseal herbal therapy when experiencing symptoms of a common cold. The nurse correctly explains that

   a. there is no proof that these agents have any effect on colds.
   b. these products work best when combined with antibiotic therapy.
   c. both products have limitations on the length of time they should be used as immunostimulants.
   d. zinc is a more effective agent to stimulate the immune system and relieve symptoms of a cold.

8. The nurse identifies a nursing diagnosis of altered health maintenance related to lack of knowledge of therapeutic regimen for a client with acute sinusitis who

   a. continues to take antibiotics for a week after symptoms are relieved.
   b. uses ASA or ASA-containing products to relieve headache and facial pain.
   c. uses over-the-counter antihistamines to relieve symptoms of congestion and drainage.
   d. reports a lack of improvement in symptoms after three days of taking broad-spectrum antibiotics.

9. A client with an acute pharyngitis is seen at the clinic with fever and severe throat pain that affects swallowing. On inspection the throat is reddened and edematous with patchy yellow exudates. The nurse anticipates that management will include

   a. treatment with antibiotics.
   b. treatment with antifungal agents.
   c. a throat culture or rapid strep antigen test.
   d. treatment with medication only if the pharyngitis does not resolve in three to four days.

10. A client's wife tells the nurse that she thinks her husband has sleep apnea because he snores very loudly. Additional information that should be collected by the nurse related to obstructive sleep apnea includes her husband's history of

    a. evening headaches.
    b. sleeping on a soft mattress.
    c. frequent awakening at night.
    d. frequent upper respiratory infections.

11. The physician prescribes nasal bilevel positive airway pressure (BiPAP) for the client with sleep apnea. To help the client tolerate this device, the nurse teaches the client

    a. to sleep with the head of the bed elevated.
    b. to use the device only on nights when insomnia occurs.
    c. to use nighttime sedatives to relax the tone of the upper airway.
    d. that although it is uncomfortable, it is very effective in relieving sleep apnea.

12. While the nurse is feeding a client, the client appears to choke on the food. List four symptoms that indicate to the nurse that the client has a partial airway obstruction.

    a.

    b.

    c.

    d.

13. An advantage of a tracheostomy over an endotracheal tube for long-term management of an upper airway obstruction is that a tracheostomy

    a. is safer to perform in an emergency.
    b. allows for more comfort and mobility.
    c. has a lower risk of tracheal pressure necrosis.
    d. is less likely to lead to lower respiratory tract infection.

14. Match the following descriptions with the types of tracheostomy tubes (answers may be used more than once).

    _____ a. Client can speak with attached air source with cuff inflated

    _____ b. Cuff pressure monitoring not required

    _____ c. Two tubings, one opening just above the cuff

    _____ d. Most likely to cause airway obstruction if exact steps are not followed to produce speech

    _____ e. Pilot tubing is not capped

    _____ f. Airflow around tube and through window allows speaking when cuff deflated and plug inserted

    _____ g. Cuff fills passively with air

    1. Speaking tracheostomy tube

    2. Fenestrated tracheostomy tube

    3. Tracheostomy tube with foam-filled cuff

15. If a tracheostomy tube has an inner cannula, it is designed to

    a. allow the client to speak.
    b. facilitate suctioning of secretions from the tube.
    c. promote cleaning of mucus from the inside of the tube.
    d. increase the volume of air that can be delivered by mechanical ventilation.

16. List three precautions used to prevent dislodgement of a tracheostomy tube the first several days after its placement.

    a.

    b.

    c.

17. Nursing care of the client with a cuffed tracheostomy tube in place includes

    a. changing the tube every three days.
    b. recording cuff pressure every eight hours.
    c. performing mouth care every 12 hours.
    d. assessing arterial blood gases every eight hours.

18. In the event that a tracheostomy tube becomes dislodged, the nurse should immediately

    a. notify the physician.
    b. attempt to replace the tube.
    c. place the client in high Fowler's position.
    d. ventilate the client with a manual resuscitation bag until the physician arrives.

19. To determine when the client with a tracheostomy tube can effectively swallow, the nurse deflates the cuff and

    a. checks for a gag reflex at the back of the tongue with a tongue blade.
    b. asks the client to drink 30 mL of milk and suctions the tube for coloured secretions.
    c. has the client swallow a small amount of water and observes for symptoms of respiratory distress.
    d. has the client drink a small amount of blue-coloured water, observing for coughing and coloured secretions.

20. During the nursing assessment of the client with cancer of the head and neck, the nurse would expect to find a history of

    a. long-term denture use.
    b. heavy tobacco and alcohol use.
    c. persistent swelling of the neck and face.
    d. chronic herpes simplex infections of the mouth and lips.

21. The management of early vocal cord malignancies usually includes

    a. radiation therapy that preserves the quality of the voice.
    b. a hemilaryngectomy that prevents the need for a tracheostomy.
    c. a radical neck dissection that removes possible sites of metastasis.
    d. a total laryngectomy to prevent development of second primary cancers.

22. During preoperative teaching for the client scheduled for a total laryngectomy, the nurse includes information related to

    a. the post-operative use of non-verbal communication techniques.
    b. techniques that will be used to alleviate a dry mouth and prevent stomatitis.
    c. the need for frequent, vigorous coughing in the first 24 hours post-operatively.
    d. self-help groups and community resources for clients with cancer of the larynx.

23. When assessing the client upon return to the surgical unit following a total laryngectomy and radical neck dissection, the nurse would expect to find

    a. a closed wound drainage system.
    b. a nasal endotracheal tube in place.
    c. a tracheostomy tube and mechanical ventilation.
    d. placement of a nasogastric tube with orders for tube feedings.

24. Following a supraglottic laryngectomy, the client is taught how to use the supraglottic swallow to minimize the risk of aspiration. In teaching the client about this technique, the nurse instructs the client to

    a. perform Valsalva manoeuvre immediately after swallowing.
    b. breathe between each Valsalva manoeuvre and cough sequence.
    c. cough after swallowing to remove food from the top of the vocal cords.
    d. practise swallowing thin, watery fluids before attempting to swallow solid foods.

25. Discharge teaching by the nurse for the client with a total laryngectomy includes

    a. how to use esophageal speech to communicate.
    b. how to use a mirror to suction the tracheostomy.
    c. the necessity of never covering the laryngectomy stoma.
    d. the need to use baths instead of showers for personal hygiene.

26. The most normal functioning method of speech restoration in the client with a total laryngectomy is

    a. a voice prosthesis.
    b. esophageal speech.
    c. an electrolarynx held to the neck.
    d. an electrolarynx placed in the mouth.

# CASE STUDY

## RHINOPLASTY

### Client Profile

Mr. N. is a 28-year-old married accountant who sustained a bilateral fracture of the nose in an automobile accident three days ago. He had a rhinoplasty to re-establish an adequate airway and improve cosmetic appearance.

### Subjective Data

- Upon return to his room following surgery, Mr. N. reports facial pain and mouth dryness
- Expresses concern about his "fat face" and appearance

### Objective Data

- Respirations 24 and shallow
- Nasal packing present in both nares
- Mustache dressing in place with a small amount of serosanguineous drainage
- Steri-Strips are applied to the skin under a plastic splint moulded to the nose
- Nose and upper cheeks are edematous

## Critical Thinking Questions

1. What assessments should the nurse make of Mr. N. in the immediate post-operative period?

2. What interventions should the nurse implement to increase Mr. N.'s comfort?

3. What information should the nurse provide to Mr. N. regarding his appearance?

4. Mr. N.'s nasal packing is removed in 24 hours and he is to be discharged. What pre-discharge teaching should the nurse perform?

5. Based on the assessment data presented, write one or more appropriate nursing diagnoses. Are there any collaborative problems?

1. A client has chronic bronchitis. To prevent the development of an acute exacerbation of chronic bronchitis (AECB), the nurse teaches the client to take provided antibiotics with the onset of

   a. rhinitis and headache.
   b. diffuse wheezing.
   c. fever and increased productive cough.
   d. chest pain with a non-productive cough.

2. List the three methods by which micro-organisms that cause pneumonia reach the lungs.

   a.

   b.

   c.

3. The classification of pneumonia as community-acquired pneumonia (CAP) or hospital-acquired pneumonia (HAP) is clinically useful because

   a. atypical pneumonia syndrome is more likely to occur in HAP.
   b. diagnostic testing does not have to be used to identify causative agents.
   c. causative agents can be predicted and empirical treatment is often effective.
   d. intravenous antibiotic therapy is necessary for HAP while oral therapy is adequate for CAP.

4. Match the following micro-organisms to the type of pneumonia they are most commonly associated with (answers may be used more than once).

   _____ a. *Pneumocystis carinii*          1. Community-acquired pneumonia

   _____ b. *Escherichia coli*              2. Hospital-acquired pneumonia

   _____ c. *Pseudomonas aeruginosa*        3. Opportunistic pneumonia

   _____ d. *Legionella pneumophila*

   _____ e. *Staphylococcus aureus*

   _____ f. *Streptococcus pneumoniae*

   _____ g. *Enterobacter*

   _____ h. *Klebsiella*

   _____ i. *Haemophilus influenzae*

   _____ j. Cytomegalovirus

   _____ k. *Mycoplasma pneumoniae*

5. Identify the pathophysiological stages of pneumococcal pneumonia.

    a. Massive dilation of capillaries with alveolar filling with organisms, neutrophils, and fibrin

    _____

    b. Exudate becomes lysed and processed by macrophages and normal lung tissue restored

    _____

    c. Outpouring of fluid into alveoli that supports micro-organism growth and spread

    _____

    d. Blood flow decreases and leukocytes and fibrin consolidate in affected lung tissue

    _____

6. When obtaining a health history from the client with suspected community-acquired pneumonia (CAP), the nurse expects the client to report

    a. an insidious onset.
    b. a dry, productive cough.
    c. a recent loss of consciousness.
    d. an abrupt onset of fever and chills.

7. Initial antibiotic treatment for pneumonia is usually based on

    a. the severity of symptoms.
    b. the presence of characteristic leukocytes.
    c. Gram stains and cultures of sputum specimens.
    d. history and physical examination and characteristic chest x-ray findings.

8. An example of a metastatic infection that occurs as a complication of pneumococcal pneumonia is

    a. pleurisy.
    b. empyema.
    c. meningitis.
    d. pleural effusion.

9. Complete the following sentences related to antibiotic treatment for pneumonia.

    a. The class of antibiotics most commonly used to treat an outpatient with CAP and no modifying factors is

    _____.

    b. The drug of choice for treatment of *Pneumocystis carinii* pneumonia is _____.

    c. An HAP client with a methicillin-resistant *Staphylococcus aureus* is usually treated with

    _____.

10. Identify five clinical situations in which hospitalized clients are at risk for aspiration pneumonia and one nursing intervention for each situation that is indicated to prevent pneumonia.

| Situation | Intervention |
| --- | --- |
| a. | |
| b. | |
| c. | |
| d. | |
| e. | |

11. A client with pneumonia has a nursing diagnosis of ineffective airway clearance related to pain, fatigue, and thick secretions. An appropriate nursing intervention for this diagnosis is to

    a. encourage fluid intake of at least 3 L/day.
    b. administer oxygen as prescribed to maintain optimal oxygenation.
    c. place the client in semi-Fowler's position to maximize lung expansion.
    d. teach the client to take three or four shallow breaths before coughing to minimize pain.

12. A client is admitted to the hospital with fever, chills, productive cough with rusty sputum, and pleuritic chest pain. Pneumococcal pneumonia is suspected. An appropriate nursing diagnosis for the client based on the systemic manifestations of pneumococcal pneumonia is

    a. diarrhea related to inflammatory process.
    b. hyperthermia related to acute infectious process.
    c. risk for injury related to disorientation and confusion.
    d. acute pain related to pleuritis and ineffective pain management.

13. The nurse advises a 75-year-old man that to prevent pneumonia, he should

    a. obtain the pneumococcal vaccine every five or six years.
    b. obtain the pneumococcal vaccine and an annual influenza vaccine.
    c. seek medical care and antibiotic therapy for all upper respiratory infections.
    d. obtain the pneumococcal vaccine if he is exposed to individuals with pneumonia.

14. Indicate whether the following statements about SARS are true or false:

    a. SARS is spread through contact with infected animals.

    b. Aminoglycosides are commonly used to treat SARS.

    c. Early symptoms of SARS include hyperthermia, cough, and dyspnea.

15. The resurgence in tuberculosis due to emergence of multidrug-resistant strains of *M. tuberculosis* is primarily the result of

    a. a lack of effective means to diagnose TB.
    b. poor compliance with drug therapy in clients with TB.
    c. the increased population of immunosuppressed individuals with AIDS.
    d. indiscriminate use of antitubercular drugs in treatment of other infections.

16. One of the characteristic pathophysiological responses to infection by the tubercular bacillus is

    a. metastases of osteocytes from the bone to the lung where they calcify lung tissue.
    b. necrotic abscesses formed from reactions of the tubercular bacilli with lymphocytes.
    c. deposition of antibody–antigen immune complexes in the alveoli of the affected lung.
    d. formation of epithelioid cell granulomas from activation of the cellular immune system.

17. A client diagnosed with Class 3 TB one week ago is admitted to the hospital with symptoms of chest pain and a possible myocardial infarction. The nurse knows that

    a. the client has a TB infection without clinical evidence of the disease.
    b. respiratory isolation may be required while the client is hospitalized.
    c. the client has a history of a previous episode of TB with no evidence of current disease.
    d. the client is suspected of having TB but a definite diagnosis is pending the results of diagnostic studies.

18. Usual initial clinical manifestations of TB include

    a. chest pain, hemoptysis, and weight loss.
    b. fatigue, low-grade fever, and night sweats.
    c. cough with purulent mucus and fever with chills.
    d. pleuritic pain, non-productive cough, and temperature elevation at night.

19. Circle the appropriate words from the choices in parentheses to complete the following sentences related to classifications and treatment protocols for TB.

    a. A healthcare provider who has cared for a client with TB has a 7-mm reaction to PPD skin testing. This individual has been (exposed to/infected with) TB.
    b. When a person who is taking corticosteroids for rheumatoid arthritis has a positive PPD skin test, treatment would include drugs for (clinical/latent) TB infection.
    c. A client who has HIV and clinical TB should receive combination drug therapy for a minimum of (nine/twelve) months and (six/nine) months beyond culture conversion.
    d. Latent TB infection is treated with (INH/combination) therapy.
    e. The minimum treatment period for a client with active TB infection is (six/nine) months.
    f. A diagnosis of TB is established with (chest x-ray/positive smear and culture).

20. Identify the recommended drug protocol for the *initial* treatment of clinically active TB.

21. A client with active TB does not have negative sputum cultures after six months of treatment because she says she cannot remember to take the medication all the time. The best action by the nurse is to

    a. schedule the client to come to the clinic every day to take the medication.
    b. have a client who has recovered from TB tell the client about his successful treatment.
    c. schedule more teaching sessions so the client will understand the risks of non-compliance.
    d. arrange for directly observed therapy by a responsible family member or a public health nurse.

22. A client receiving chemotherapy for breast cancer develops cryptococcosis and is treated with IV amphotericin B. The nurse monitors the client for side effects of the amphotericin B with the knowledge that this client is at risk for increased

    a. renal impairment.
    b. immunosuppression.
    c. nausea and vomiting.
    d. hypersensitivity reactions.

23. The nursing assessment of a client with bronchiectasis is most likely to reveal a history of

    a. chest trauma.
    b. childhood asthma.
    c. smoking or oral tobacco use.
    d. recurrent lower respiratory tract infections.

24. In planning care for the client with bronchiectasis, the nurse includes measures that will

    a. relieve or reduce pain.
    b. prevent paroxysmal coughing.
    c. prevent spread of the disease to others.
    d. promote drainage and removal of mucus.

25. The nurse uses protective measures with clients at risk for lung abscesses based on the knowledge that lung abscesses occur most frequently in clients with

    a. lung tumours.
    b. altered consciousness.
    c. altered immune response.
    d. pulmonary infarct infections.

26. The most important precaution in reducing the risk of most occupational lung diseases is

    a. maintaining smoke-free work environments for all employees.
    b. using masks and effective ventilation systems to reduce exposure to irritants.
    c. inspection and monitoring of workplaces by national occupational safety agencies.
    d. requiring periodic chest x-rays and pulmonary function tests for exposed employees.

27. During a health-promotion program, the nurse teaches the participants that the best way to prevent lung cancer is to

    a. stop smoking and avoid second-hand smoke.
    b. have an annual chest x-ray after the age of 50.
    c. wear masks when exposed to industrial carcinogens.
    d. seek medical care for a cough that persists for more than two to three weeks.

28. A client with cancer of the lung is diagnosed with paraneoplastic syndrome. The nurse recognizes that the lung malignancy most commonly related to this symptom

    a. can be successfully treated with radiation.
    b. metastasizes early and has the poorest prognosis.
    c. has a good prognosis if surgical resection is possible.
    d. is associated with lung scarring and chronic interstitial fibrosis.

29. A client with a lung mass found on chest x-ray is undergoing further testing. A definitive diagnosis of cancer of the lung may be made with

    a. CT scans.
    b. lung tomograms.
    c. pulmonary angiography.
    d. identification of malignant cells in sputum.

30. Match the following treatments for lung cancer with their descriptions.

    _____ a. Standard treatment for NSCLC

    _____ b. Dye activated by laser light that destroys cancer cells

    _____ c. Freezes bronchial tumours with use of bronchoscope radiation

    _____ d. Palliative treatment for airway collapse or compression therapy

    _____ e. Best procedure for cure of lung cancer

    _____ f. Palliative treatment by bronchoscope to remove obstructing bronchial tumours

    _____ g. Improves survival when combined with chemotherapy and surgery

    _____ h. Used with chemotherapy to overcome effect of blood–brain barrier

    1. Surgical therapy
    2. Radiation therapy
    3. Chemotherapy
    4. Prophylactic cranial radiation
    5. Bronchoscopic laser therapy
    6. Phototherapy
    7. Airway stenting
    8. Cryotherapy

31. In assisting a client to stop smoking, the nurse advises the client that the most successful programs for smoking cessation include

    a. hypnosis and acupuncture.
    b. self-help programs with group therapy.
    c. aversion therapy and individual psychotherapy.
    d. behaviour modification approach with nicotine replacement.

32. A client with advanced lung cancer refuses pain medication, saying, "I deserve everything this cancer can give me." The nurse's best response to the client is

    a. "Would you like to talk to a counsellor?"
    b. "Can you tell me what the pain means to you?"
    c. "Are you using the pain as a punishment for your past behaviour?"
    d. "Pain control will help you to deal more effectively with your feelings."

33. Complete the following statements.

    a. Collapse of the lung due to accumulation of air in the intrapleural space caused by a sucking chest wound

       is a(n) _____.

    b. Multiple fractured ribs causing paradoxic chest movement is known as _____.

    c. Collapse of the lung due to accumulation of blood in the intrapleural space is a(n)

       _____.

    d. Collapse of the lung due to accumulation of air in the intrapleural space caused by an injury to the lungs

       from closed rib fractures is known as a(n) _____.

    e. When air in the intrapleural space progressively increases intrathoracic pressure because it cannot escape

       during expiration, a(n) _____ occurs.

    f. Accumulation of lymphatic fluid in the pleural space due to a leak in the thoracic duct is known as

       _____.

    g. The usual treatment for a large pneumothorax or hemothorax of any cause is a(n) _____

       connected to _____.

34. Signs and symptoms that indicate to the nurse that a tension pneumothorax is developing in a client with chest trauma include

    a. dull percussion sounds on the injured side.
    b. severe respiratory distress and tracheal deviation.
    c. muffled and distant heart sounds with decreasing blood pressure.
    d. decreased movement and diminished breath sounds on the affected side.

35. Indicate the function of each of the chambers in a three-chamber water-seal pleural drainage system.

    a. First chamber

    b. Second chamber

    c. Third chamber

36. The nurse should check for leaks in the chest tube and water-seal system when

    a. there is constant bubbling of water in the suction-control chamber.
    b. there is continuous bubbling from the tube in the water-seal chamber.
    c. the water levels in the water-seal and suction-control chambers are decreased.
    d. fluid in the tubing in the water-seal chamber fluctuates with the client's breathing.

37. When caring for the client with a chest tube, the nurse questions the practice of

    a. looping the drainage tubing on the bed.
    b. clamping the chest tube momentarily to check for leaks.
    c. having the client cough and breathe deeply every two hours.
    d. stripping or milking a chest tube used to treat a pneumothorax.

38. Match the following chest surgeries with their descriptions.

    _____ a. Thoracotomy                 1. Removal of a small lesion

    _____ b. Lobectomy                   2. Removal of a lung

    _____ c. Wedge resection             3. Incision into the thorax

    _____ d. Segmental resection         4. Stripping of a fibrous membrane

    _____ e. Decortication               5. Removal of one lung lobe

    _____ f. Pneumonectomy               6. Removal of lung segment

39. Following a thoracotomy, the client has a nursing diagnosis of ineffective airway clearance related to inability to cough secondary to pain and positioning. The best nursing intervention for this client is to

    a. have the client drink 475 mL of water before attempting to breathe deeply.
    b. auscultate the lungs before and after deep-breathing and coughing regimens.
    c. place the client in the Trendelenburg position for 30 minutes before the coughing exercises.
    d. medicate the client with analgesics 20 to 30 minutes before assisting to cough and deep breathe.

40. Match the following restrictive lung conditions with the mechanisms that cause decreased vital capacity (VC) and decreased total lung capacity (TLC).

    _____ a. Pleural effusion            1. Central depression of respiratory rate and depth

    _____ b. Empyema                     2. Lung expansion restricted by fluid in pleural space

    _____ c. Pleurisy                    3. Paralysis of respiratory muscles

    _____ d. Atelectasis                 4. Excess fat restricts chest wall and diaphragmatic excursion

    _____ e. Idiopathic pulmonary fibrosis
                                         5. Inflammation of the pleura restricting lung movement
    _____ f. Kyphoscoliosis
                                         6. Lung expansion restricted by pus in intrapleural space
    _____ g. Narcotic and sedative overdose
                                         7. Presence of collapsed, airless alveoli
    _____ h. Muscular dystrophy
                                         8. Spinal angulation restricting ventilation
    _____ i. Pickwickian syndrome
                                         9. Excessive connective tissue in lungs

41. Match the following conditions with their related mechanisms of pulmonary hypertension.

_____ a. Chronic obstructive pulmonary disease (COPD)

_____ b. Pulmonary fibrosis

_____ c. Pulmonary embolism

_____ d. Neuromuscular disorders

1. Stiffening of pulmonary vasculature

2. Obstruction of pulmonary blood flow

3. Pulmonary capillary/alveolar damage

4. Local vasoconstriction and shunting

42. While caring for a client with primary pulmonary hypertension, the nurse observes that the client has exertional dyspnea and chest pain, in addition to fatigue. The nurse knows that these symptoms are related to

a. decreased left ventricular output.
b. right ventricular hypertrophy and dilation.
c. increased systemic arterial blood pressure.
d. development of alveolar interstitial edema.

43. The primary treatment for cor pulmonale is directed toward

a. controlling arrhythmias.
b. dilating the pulmonary arteries.
c. strengthening the cardiac muscle.
d. treating the underlying pulmonary condition.

44. Six days after a heart-lung transplant, a client develops a low-grade fever and a decreased $SpO_2$ with exercise. The nurse recognizes that this indicates

a. a normal response to extensive surgery.
b. a frequently fatal cytomegalovirus infection.
c. acute rejection that can be treated with corticosteroids.
d. obliterative bronchiolitis that plugs terminal bronchioles.

## CASE STUDY

### PULMONARY HYPERTENSION

### Client Profile

Ms. S. is a 46-year-old client who was diagnosed with primary pulmonary hypertension at the age of 42. At that time she presented to her primary care physician with a history of increasing fatigue and recent onset of swelling in her feet and ankles. A chest x-ray revealed severe cardiomegaly with pulmonary congestion. She underwent a right cardiac catheterization, which showed very high pulmonary artery pressures. Since then, she has been treated with several drugs, but her pulmonary hypertension has never been controlled and her peripheral edema has progressively worsened.

### Subjective Data

- Short of breath at rest and exercise intolerant to the extent that she had to quit her job
- Recently divorced from her husband
- Has two children, a daughter who is 10 years old and a son who is four years old

### Objective Data

- 3+ pitting edema from her feet to her knees
- Respirations: 28 at rest
- Heart rate: 92 and bounding

## Critical Thinking Questions

1. What drugs might Ms. S. have been given to treat her pulmonary hypertension?

2. Is Ms. S. a candidate for heart-lung transplantation or lung transplantation? Why or why not?

3. What transplantation procedure would be considered for Ms. S? What is the rationale?

4. What preoperative counselling would be necessary for Ms. S. to prepare for a transplantation procedure?

5. Based on the assessment data presented, write one or more appropriate nursing diagnoses. Are there any collaborative problems?

# CHAPTER 28 NURSING MANAGEMENT: OBSTRUCTIVE PULMONARY DISEASES

1. Obstructive pulmonary disease is characterized by

   a. destruction of lung tissue.
   b. decreased total lung capacity.
   c. obstruction or narrowing of airways.
   d. constant limitations in expiratory airflow.

2. Number in sequence the processes that occur in the early- and late-phase responses of asthma.

   _____ a. Onset of bronchial smooth muscle constriction, vascular permeability, and increased mucus secretion

   _____ b. Inflammation causing mucosal edema and obstruction of airways

   _____ c. Allergen or irritant cross-links IgE receptors on mast cells in bronchial basement membrane

   _____ d. Eosinophils and neutrophils infiltrate airway releasing mediators that cause further mast cell degranulation

   _____ e. Monocytes and lymphocytes infiltrate airways

   _____ f. Epithelial damage causes heightened airway reactivity that worsens symptoms of future attacks

   _____ g. Activated mast cells release histamine, leukotrienes, bradykinin, prostaglandins, and chemotactic factors

3. In assisting a client with asthma to identify specific asthma triggers, the nurse recognizes that

   a. food and drug allergies do not manifest in respiratory symptoms.
   b. exercise-induced asthma is seen only in individuals with sensitivity to cold air.
   c. asthma attacks are psychogenic in origin and can be controlled with relaxation techniques.
   d. viral upper respiratory infections are a common precipitating factor in acute asthma attacks.

4. On assessment the nurse determines that the client has severe obstruction and impending respiratory failure based on the findings of

   a. markedly diminished breath sounds with no wheezing.
   b. inspiratory and expiratory wheezing with an unproductive cough.
   c. use of accessory muscles of respiration and a feeling of suffocation.
   d. a respiratory rate of 34 breaths per minute and increased pulse and blood pressure.

5. Arterial blood gas results that would be expected in a client early in an acute asthma attack include

   a. pH 7.20, $PaCO_2$ 52 mm Hg, $PaO_2$ 60 mm Hg.
   b. pH 7.35, $PaCO_2$ 42 mm Hg, $PaO_2$ 74 mm Hg.
   c. pH 7.40, $PaCO_2$ 50 mm Hg, $PaO_2$ 80 mm Hg.
   d. pH 7.48, $PaCO_2$ 30 mm Hg, $PaO_2$ 78 mm Hg.

6. One indication for intubation and mechanical ventilation for the client in status asthmaticus is when

   a. $PaCO_2$ levels are at 60 mm Hg.
   b. $PaO_2$ levels decrease to 70 mm Hg.
   c. severe respiratory muscle fatigue occurs.
   d. the client has extreme anxiety and fear of suffocation.

7. Marked bronchoconstriction of the lungs in the client with asthma is indicated by

   a. $SaO_2$ of 85%.
   b. $FEV_1$ of 85% of predicted.
   c. PEFR of 100 to 150 L/min.
   d. chest x-ray showing a flattened diaphragm.

8. Match the following drugs, first with their use in promoting quick-relief of asthma symptoms or long-term control of symptoms and then with their primary mode of action (answers may be used more than once).

   **Use / Action**

   _____  _____    a. Salbutamol inhaler          1. Long-term control

   _____  _____    b. Oral prednisone             2. Quick-relief agent

   _____  _____    c. Fluticasone inhaler         3. Beta-adrenergic agonist

   _____  _____    d. Ipratropium bromide inhaler 4. Mast-cell stabilizer

   _____  _____    e. Oral theophylline           5. Leukotriene receptor agonist

   _____  _____    f. Cromolyn inhaler            6. Steroidal anti-inflammatory

   _____  _____    g. Budesonide inhaler          7. Methylxanthine agent

   _____  _____    h. Intravenous aminophylline   8. Anticholinergic

   _____  _____    i. Formoterol inhaler

   _____  _____    j. Terbutaline inhaler

9. Of the following instructions for clients about the use of asthma medications, check all those that are correct.

_____    a. When using your metered-dose inhaler, it is best to use it with a spacer.

_____    b. Salbutamol or terbutaline or cromolyn inhalers can be used before exercise or when anticipating exposure to allergens known to cause asthma.

_____    c. The mouth should be rinsed thoroughly after using the ipratropium (Atrovent) inhaler to prevent oral candidiasis.

_____    d. Salmeterol (Serevent) should not be used more than every 12 hours.

_____    e. When asthma symptoms are increasing, you should use your reliever (salbutamol) inhaler as often as every 20 minutes until the symptoms are relieved.

_____    f. The best way to use a metered-dose inhaler is to hold it about 4 cm (one to two inches) in front of your mouth before depressing the inhaler.

_____    g. You must use your budesonide (Pulmicort) inhaler every day as prescribed to prevent worsening of your asthma, even if you have no asthma symptoms.

_____    h. You should wait five minutes before taking a second puff of any inhaled medication.

_____    i. If you use a spacer with your inhaler, depress the inhaler before starting to inhale.

_____    j. You should take zafirlukast (Accolate) tablets on an empty stomach.

_____    k. To use your dry powder inhaler (DPI), empty your lungs of air, close your lips around the mouthpiece, and inhale quickly and deeply.

10. One of the best ways to decrease the client's sense of panic during an acute asthma attack is for the nurse to

   a. leave the client alone to rest in a quiet, calm environment.
   b. stay with the client and encourage slow, pursed-lip breathing.
   c. reassure the client that the attack can be controlled with treatment.
   d. let the client know his or her status is being closely monitored with frequent measurement of vital signs and $SpO_2$.

11. When a client with asthma is admitted to the emergency department for worsening asthma, the nurse anticipates that initial drug treatment will most likely include administration of

   a. inhaled fluticasone.
   b. inhaled salbutamol.
   c. intravenous aminophylline.
   d. intravenous hydrocortisone.

12. The nurse recognizes that additional teaching is needed when the client with asthma says,

    a. "I should exercise every day if my symptoms are controlled."
    b. "I should use cough drops to control my son's cough at night."
    c. "I should inform my spouse about my medications and how to get help if I have a severe asthma attack."
    d. "An asthma action plan will help in adjusting my therapy."

13. Match the following effects of smoking with the related components of cigarette smoke (answers may be used more than once).

    _____ a. Destruction of alveolar walls                                    1. Nicotine

    _____ b. Hyperplasia of bronchial cells                                   2. Carbon monoxide

    _____ c. Decreased ciliary action                                         3. Smoke gases

    _____ d. Increased mucus production by goblet cells                       4. Oxidants

    _____ e. Peripheral vasoconstriction and increased BP

    _____ f. Inactivation of the protease inhibitor alpha$_1$-antitrypsin

    _____ g. Decreased oxygen-carrying capacity

    _____ h. Stimulate neutrophil and macrophage release of proteases

    _____ i. Psychomotor impairment and impaired judgement

    _____ j. Increased oxygen need of heart

14. Use the given words to complete the following sentences (some words may be used more than once).

    alpha$_1$-antitrypsin (AAT)          collagen              elastin
    smoking                              infection             hereditary AAT deficiency
    inhaled irritants

    a. In the normal lung, the action of proteases and elastases released from macrophages and neutrophils is

       balanced by the presence of the protease inhibitor _____.

    b. In emphysema, three known factors that increase the release of proteases and elastases are

       _____, _____, and _____.

    c. The action of the proteases and elastases destroy _____ and _____ of the alveolar

       walls and the supporting structures of the lung.

    d. The action of the proteases and elastases is inhibited by _____.

    e. Two factors that are known to cause a decrease in AAT levels or activity are _____

       and _____.

    f. _____ is the one factor that both increases protease release and decreases AAT activity.

15. The effect of alveolar destruction in emphysema results in

    a. decreased lung compliance.
    b. air trapping in distal alveoli.
    c. dilation of small bronchioles.
    d. obstruction of airflow into alveoli.

16. Chronic inflammation of the bronchi characteristic of chronic bronchitis results in

    a. collapse of small bronchioles on expiration.
    b. permanent, abnormal dilation of the bronchi.
    c. hyperplasia of mucus-secreting cells and bronchial edema.
    d. destruction of the elastic and muscular structures of the bronchial wall.

17. Indicate whether the following clinical manifestations of COPD are most characteristic of emphysema (E), chronic bronchitis (CB), or both (B).

    _____ a. Barrel chest

    _____ b. Persistent cough

    _____ c. Flattened diaphragm

    _____ d. Early polycythemia

    _____ e. Decreased breath sounds

    _____ f. Cor pulmonale

    _____ g. Weight loss

    _____ h. Early onset

    _____ i. Finger clubbing

    _____ j. Early hypercapnia

    _____ k. Decreased diaphragmatic excursion

    _____ l. Copious mucus production

18. The pulmonary vasoconstriction leading to the development of cor pulmonale in the client with COPD results from

    a. increased viscosity of the blood.
    b. alveolar hypoxia and hypercapnia.
    c. long-term low-flow oxygen therapy.
    d. administration of high concentrations of oxygen.

19. Explain how the following findings on pulmonary function testing relate to the pathophysiological changes of COPD.

    a.  decreased $FEV_1$

    b.  decreased VC

    c.  increased RV

    d.  increased TLC

20. Arterial blood gas results that are characteristic of late stage COPD include

    a.  pH 7.26, $PaCO_2$ 58 mm Hg, $PaO_2$ 60 mm Hg, $HCO_3$ 30 mmol/L.
    b.  pH 7.30, $PaCO_2$ 45 mm Hg, $PaO_2$ 55 mm Hg, $HCO_3$ 18 mmol/L.
    a.  pH 7.40, $PaCO_2$ 40 mm Hg, $PaO_2$ 70 mm Hg, $HCO_3$ 25 mmol/L.
    a.  pH 7.52, $PaCO_2$ 30 mm Hg, $PaO_2$ 80 mm Hg, $HCO_3$ 35 mmol/L.

21. In addition to smoking cessation, treatment for COPD that is indicated to slow the progression of the disease includes

    a.  use of bronchodilating drugs.
    b.  use of inhaled corticosteroids.
    c.  lung volume reduction surgery.
    d.  prevention of respiratory tract infections.

22. Match the following characteristics with their methods of oxygen administration.

    _____  a.  Provides highest oxygen concentrations          1. Nasal cannula

    _____  b.  May cause aspiration of condensed fluid          2. Simple face mask

    _____  c.  Safest system to use in client with COPD         3. Partial rebreathing mask

    _____  d.  Most comfortable and causes least                4. Non-rebreathing mask
              restriction on activities
                                                                5. Venturi mask
    _____  e.  Provides 40–60% oxygen concentration
                                                                6. Tracheostomy collar
    _____  f.  Invasive placement of catheter into trachea
                                                                7. Transtracheal catheter
    _____  g.  Used to give oxygen quickly for short time

23. Identify whether the following statements are true or false. If a statement is false, correct the bold word(s) to make the statement true.

_____    a. A decrease in mental status and hypoventilation that occurs after oxygen administration is started may indicate **oxygen toxicity**.

_____    b. The risk for oxygen toxicity is high in the client receiving **more than 50% oxygen for more than 24 hours**.

_____    c. Absorption atelectasis occurs when high $FIO_2$ causes displacement of **carbon dioxide** from the alveoli.

_____    d. Clients at highest risk for $CO_2$ narcosis are those with chronic **high carbon dioxide** levels.

_____    e. Alterations in skin integrity with pressure ulcer formation during oxygen therapy is most likely to occur at the **top of the ears**.

24. A client is being discharged with plans for home oxygen therapy provided by a liquid oxygen reservoir with a refillable portable unit. In preparing the client to use the equipment, the nurse teaches the client that

   a. the portable tank filled from the reservoir will last about six to eight hours at 2 L/min.
   b. the unit concentrates oxygen from the air, providing a continuous oxygen supply.
   c. the unit should be kept out of the bedroom and extension tubing used at night because of the noise.
   d. weekly delivery of four or five large cylinders of oxygen will be necessary for a seven- to ten-day supply of oxygen.

25. A breathing technique the nurse should teach the client with COPD to promote exhalation is

   a. huff coughing.
   b. thoracic breathing.
   c. pursed-lip breathing.
   d. diaphragmatic breathing.

26. A dietary modification that helps meet the nutritional needs of clients with COPD is

   a. a high-carbohydrate, low-fat diet.
   b. avoiding foods that require a lot of chewing.
   c. preparing most foods of the diet to be eaten hot.
   d. drinking fluids with meals to promote digestion.

27. During an acute exacerbation of COPD, the client is severely short of breath and the nurse identifies a nursing diagnosis of ineffective breathing pattern related to obstruction of airflow and anxiety. The best action by the nurse is to

   a. prepare and administer inhaled corticosteroids.
   b. perform chest physiotherapy to promote removal of secretions.
   c. administer oxygen at 5 L/min until the shortness of breath is relieved.
   d. position the client upright with the elbows resting on the overbed table.

28. The husband of a client with COPD tells the nurse that they have not had any sexual activity since the client was diagnosed with COPD because she becomes too short of breath. The best response of the nurse is

a. "You need to discuss your feelings and needs with your wife so she knows what you expect of her."
b. "There are other ways to maintain intimacy besides sexual intercourse that will not make her short of breath."
c. "Would you like for me to talk to you and your wife about some modifications that can maintain sexual activity?"
d. "You should explore other ways to meet your sexual needs, since your wife is no longer capable of sexual activity."

29. In teaching the client with COPD about the need for physical exercise, the nurse informs the client that

a. all clients with COPD should be able to gradually increase walking to 20 minutes a day.
b. a bronchodilator inhaler should be used to relieve exercise-induced dyspnea immediately after the exercise.
c. shortness of breath is expected during exercise but should return to baseline within five minutes after the exercise.
d. monitoring the heart rate before and after exercise is the best way to determine how much exercise can be tolerated.

30. The pathophysiological mechanism of cystic fibrosis leading to obstructive lung disease is

a. fibrosis of mucous glands and destruction of bronchial walls.
b. destruction of lung parenchyma from inflammation and scarring.
c. production of abnormally thick, copious secretions from mucous glands.
d. increased serum levels of pancreatic enzymes that are deposited in the bronchial mucosa.

31. The primary treatment for cystic fibrosis is

a. heart-lung transplantation.
b. administration of prophylactic antibiotics.
c. administration of nebulized bronchodilators.
d. vigorous and consistent chest physiotherapy.

32. Meeting the developmental tasks of young adulthood becomes a major problem for young adults with cystic fibrosis primarily because

a. they have an expected shortened lifespan.
b. any children they have will develop cystic fibrosis.
c. they must also adapt to a newly diagnosed chronic disease.
d. their illness keeps them from becoming financially independent.

## CASE STUDY

### CHRONIC OBSTRUCTIVE PULMONARY DISEASE

#### Client Profile

Mr. D. has a history of emphysema and chronic bronchitis. He is a 73-year-old retired farmer who can no longer walk in his farm without extreme breathlessness. He is treated at the outpatient medicine clinic today for increasing shortness of breath, even at rest.

#### Subjective Data

- Reports that his sputum production has increased over the past week and the colour has changed to a greenish yellow
- Has more sputum in the morning that gradually reduces over the day
- Has been taking salbutamol MDI and beclomethasone MDI two puffs every six hours
- Takes no other medication at this time

#### Assessment Data

- Appears to be a frail older adult on observation
- Laboured breathing and use of accessory muscles of respiration
- Sitting in a tripod position and using pursed-lip breathing
- Chest assessment: crackles in left lower lobe and diffuse expiratory wheezing throughout his chest; left lower lobe dull to percussion
- Vital signs: BP normal; P 96; R 28; T 38.8°C (101.8°F)
- ABGs:    pH 7.36
          $PaO_2$ 55 mm Hg
          $PaCO_2$ 65 mm Hg

Treatment is initiated with an intravenous catheter and IV fluids at 50 mL/hr, nebulized salbutamol, sputum for culture and sensitivity, IV antibiotics, antipyretics, and oral corticosteroids.

### Critical Thinking Questions

1. Mr. D. is most likely experiencing an exacerbation of his COPD. What assessment data provided indicates the presence of pneumonia?

2. What are the nursing care priorities for Mr. D.?

3.  What are possible causes of Mr. D.'s exacerbation of COPD?

4.  What do his ABG values indicate?

5.  What is the home care plan for this client?

6.  Based on the assessment data presented, write one or more appropriate nursing diagnoses. Are there any collaborative problems?

1. Match the following characteristics with the appropriate blood cells (answers may be used more than once).

_____ a. May become tissue macrophages      1. Erythrocyte

_____ b. 30% of volume stored in spleen      2. Reticulocyte

_____ c. Primarily responsible for immune response      3. Neutrophil

_____ d. Make up 4–8% of WBCs      4. Basophil

_____ e. Production stimulated by hypoxia      5. Eosinophil

_____ f. Make up 0–2% of WBCs      6. Lymphocyte

_____ g. Immature cell is a band      7. Monocyte

_____ h. Increased in individuals with allergies      8. Platelet

_____ i. Responds first at injury site

_____ j. Make up 20–40% of WBCs

_____ k. Releases granules that increase allergic and inflammatory responses

_____ l. Arises from megakaryocyte

_____ m. Make up 50–70% of WBCs

_____ n. Increases indicate an increased rate of erythropoiesis

_____ o. Make up 2–4% of WBCs

_____ p. Also known as "segs"

2. Complete the following statements.

a. Granulocytic leukocytes include _____, _____, and

_____.

b. Red blood cell production is stimulated by the release of the hormone _____ from the

kidney.

c. Nutrients essential for red blood cell production include _____, _____, and

_____.

d. Obstruction of the lymph flow results in accumulation of lymph fluid known as _____.

e. Organs of the hematological system that have filtering functions include the _____,

_____, and _____.

3. Match the following processes with the appropriate response of normal blood coagulation (answers may be used more than once).

    \_\_\_\_\_  a. Thrombin converts fibrinogen to fibrin        1. Vascular response

    \_\_\_\_\_  b. Release of adenosine diphosphate            2. Platelet response

    \_\_\_\_\_  c. Release of tissue thromboplastin            3. Plasma clotting factors

    \_\_\_\_\_  d. Release of PF3, serotonin, and epinephrine

    \_\_\_\_\_  e. Vasoconstriction

    \_\_\_\_\_  f. Prothrombin converted to thrombin

    \_\_\_\_\_  g. Damaged vascular surface

    \_\_\_\_\_  h. Serum calcium activity as factor IV

    \_\_\_\_\_  i. Platelet clumping and plugging

4. Fibrinolysis involves the action of

   a. heparin.
   b. plasmin.
   c. fibrinogen.
   d. prothrombin.

5. The effects of fibrin split products (FSPs) include

   a. clot stabilization.
   b. increase in prothrombin.
   c. impaired platelet aggregation.
   d. decreased release of tissue thromboplastin.

6. In analyzing the results of an 83-year-old client's CBC, the nurse would expect to find as a normal age-related change a decrease in

   a. platelets.
   b. total WBC.
   c. hemoglobin.
   d. red blood cells.

7. A client's CBC indicates a pancytopenia. The nurse suspects that the client has an impairment of the

   a. liver.
   b. spleen.
   c. bone marrow.
   d. lymph system.

8. During the nursing assessment of a client with anemia, the nurse notes as significant the client's history of

   a. recurring infections.
   b. a partial gastrectomy.
   c. corticosteroid therapy.
   d. oral contraceptive use.

9. Identify one specific finding identified by the nurse during assessment of each of the client's functional health patterns that indicates a risk factor for hematological problems or a client response to an actual hematological problem.

    a. Health perception–health management

    b. Nutritional–metabolic

    c. Elimination

    d. Activity–exercise

    e. Sleep–rest

    f. Cognitive–perceptual

    g. Self-perception–self-concept

    h. Role–relationship

    i. Sexuality–reproductive

    j. Coping–stress tolerance

    k. Value–belief

10. Using light pressure with the index and middle fingers, the nurse cannot palpate any of the client's superficial lymph nodes. The nurse

    a. records this finding as normal.
    b. should reassess the lymph nodes using deeper pressure.
    c. asks the client if there is a history of any radiation therapy.
    d. notifies the physician that x-rays of the nodes will be necessary.

11. During physical assessment of a client with thrombocytopenia, the nurse would expect to find

    a. sternal tenderness.
    b. petechiae and purpura.
    c. jaundiced sclera and skin.
    d. tender, enlarged lymph nodes.

12. A client with a hematological disorder has a smooth, shiny red tongue. The nurse would expect the client's laboratory results to include

    a.  WBC 13.5 x $10^9$/L (13.5 x $10^3$/$\mu$L).
    b.  neutrophils 45%.
    c.  RBC 6.4 x $10^{12}$/L (6.4 x $10^6$/$\mu$L).
    d.  Hb 96 g/dL (9.6 g/dL).

13. A client is being treated with chemotherapeutic agents. The nurse revises the client's care plan based on the CBC results of

    a. Hct 0.38 (38%).
    b. MCV 85 fl.
    c. WBC 4 x $10^9$/L (4 x $10^3$/$\mu$L).
    d. platelets 80 x $10^9$/L (80 x $10^3$/$\mu$L).

14. Identify the type of condition that is indicated by the following laboratory study results.

    a.  Serum iron 7 µmol/L (40 µg/dL)

    b.  Erythrocyte sedimentation rate (ESR) 30 mm/hr

    c.  Increased band neutrophils

    d.  Activated partial thromboplastin time 60 sec

    e.  Indirect bilirubin 34 µmol/L (2.0 mg/dL)

    f.  Urine Bence Jones protein

15. If a client with blood type O Rh$^+$ is given AB Rh$^-$ blood, the nurse would expect

    a.  the client's Rh factor to react with the red blood cells of the donor blood.
    b.  no adverse reaction, since the client has no antibodies against the donor blood.
    c.  the anti-A and anti-B antibodies in the client's plasma to hemolyze the donor red cells.
    d.  the anti-A and anti-B antibodies in the donor plasma to hemolyze the client's red cells.

16. A client is undergoing a contrast computed tomography (CT) of the spleen. Before this test it is important for the nurse to ask the client about

    a.  iodine sensitivity.
    b.  prior blood transfusions.
    c.  phobia of confined spaces.
    d.  internal metal implants or appliances.

17. The most common site for a bone marrow aspiration in an adult is the

    a.  tibia.
    b.  scapula.
    c.  sternum.
    d.  iliac crest.

18. When preparing the client for a bone marrow examination, the nurse explains that

    a.  the procedure will be done under general anaesthesia because it is very painful.
    b.  the client will not have any pain after the area at the puncture site is anaesthetized.
    c.  the client will experience a brief, very sharp pain during aspiration of the bone marrow.
    d.  there will be no pain during the procedure but an ache will be present several days afterward.

19. A lymph node biopsy is most often performed to diagnose

    a.  leukemias.
    b.  hemorrhagic tendencies.
    c.  the cause of lymphedema.
    d.  neoplastic cells in the lymph nodes.

# CHAPTER *30* NURSING MANAGEMENT: HEMATOLOGICAL PROBLEMS

1. Match each of the anemic states with both etiological and morphological classification systems (answers may be used more than once).

   \_\_\_\_\_  \_\_\_\_\_  a. Acute trauma

   \_\_\_\_\_  \_\_\_\_\_  b. Malaria

   \_\_\_\_\_  \_\_\_\_\_  c. Anemia of gastritis

   \_\_\_\_\_  \_\_\_\_\_  d. Anemia of renal failure

   \_\_\_\_\_  \_\_\_\_\_  e. Aplastic anemia

   \_\_\_\_\_  \_\_\_\_\_  f. G6PD

   \_\_\_\_\_  \_\_\_\_\_  g. Iron-deficiency anemia

   \_\_\_\_\_  \_\_\_\_\_  h. Thalassemia

   \_\_\_\_\_  \_\_\_\_\_  i. Pernicious anemia

   \_\_\_\_\_  \_\_\_\_\_  j. Sickle cell anemia

   \_\_\_\_\_  \_\_\_\_\_  k. Anemia of leukemia

   \_\_\_\_\_  \_\_\_\_\_  l. Anemia associated with prosthetic heart valve

   **Etiological:**

   1. Decreased RBC production

   2. Blood loss

   3. Increased RBC destruction

   **Morphological:**

   4. Normocytic, normochromic

   5. Macrocytic, normochromic

   6. Microcytic, hypochromic

2. A client with a hemoglobin level of 78 g/L (7.8 g/dL) has cardiac palpitations, a heart rate of 102, and an increased reticulocyte count. At this severity of anemia, the nurse would also expect the client to manifest

   a. pallor.
   b. dyspnea.
   c. a smooth tongue.
   d. sensitivity to cold.

3. A 76-year-old woman has an Hb of 73 g/L (7.3 g/dL) and is experiencing ataxia and confusion. During assessment of the client, it is most important for the nurse to ask about

   a. food and drug intake.
   b. a family history of anemia.
   c. any exposure to chemical toxins.
   d. the presence of post-menopausal bleeding.

4. On physical assessment of the client with severe anemia, the nurse would expect to find

   a. nervousness and agitation.
   b. fever and tenting of the skin.
   c. systolic murmurs and tachycardia.
   d. bluish mucous membranes and reddened skin.

5. A nursing diagnosis that is appropriate for clients with moderate to severe anemia of any etiology is

    a. impaired skin integrity related to edema and pruritus.
    b. disturbed body image related to changes in appearance and body function.
    c. imbalanced nutrition: less than body requirements related to lack of knowledge of adequate nutrition.
    d. activity intolerance related to decreased hemoglobin and imbalance between oxygen supply and demand.

6. Match the following descriptions with their associated types of anemia (answers may be used more than once).

| | |
|---|---|
| \_\_\_\_\_ a. Chronic bone marrow hyperplasia | 1. Iron deficiency |
| \_\_\_\_\_ b. Hypoxia-induced change in RBCs | 2. Thalassemia |
| \_\_\_\_\_ c. Responds to treatment with erythropoietin | 3. Cobalamin deficiency |
| \_\_\_\_\_ d. Most common type of anemia | 4. Folic acid deficiency |
| \_\_\_\_\_ e. Related to RBC metabolism of glucose | 5. Anemia of chronic disease |
| \_\_\_\_\_ f. Megaloblastic cells without neurological involvement | 6. Aplastic anemia |
| \_\_\_\_\_ g. Autoimmune-related disease | 7. Sickle cell |
| \_\_\_\_\_ h. May occur with removal of the duodenum | 8. G6PD anemia |
| \_\_\_\_\_ i. May occur with removal of the stomach | |
| \_\_\_\_\_ j. Altered globin synthesis of hemoglobin | |
| \_\_\_\_\_ k. Lack of intrinsic factor | |
| \_\_\_\_\_ l. Associated with vascular occlusion and tissue infarction | |
| \_\_\_\_\_ m. Decrease in all blood cells | |
| \_\_\_\_\_ n. May be caused by adrenal hypofunction | |
| \_\_\_\_\_ o. Associated with chronic blood loss | |
| \_\_\_\_\_ p. Treatment causes chronic iron toxicity | |
| \_\_\_\_\_ q. Oral contraceptives a contributing factor | |

7. Explain the following laboratory findings in anemia.

   a. Reticulocyte counts are increased in chronic blood loss but decreased in cobalamin (vitamin $B_{12}$) deficiency.

   b. Bilirubin levels are increased in sickle cell anemia but are normal in acute blood loss.

   c. MCV is increased in folic acid deficiency but is decreased in iron-deficiency anemia.

8. To prevent a common side effect of oral iron supplements, the nurse teaches the client to

   a. take the iron preparations with meals.
   b. increase fluid and dietary fibre intake.
   c. report the presence of black stools to the physician.
   d. use enteric-coated preparations taken with orange juice.

9. To administer iron intramuscularly, the nurse should

   a. use a short, fine needle to avoid causing pain.
   b. massage the site after the injection to promote absorption.
   c. include 0.5 mL of air in the syringe to clear the iron from the needle.
   d. administer the injection in the vastus lateralis to prevent nerve damage.

10. The nurse evaluates that teaching for the client with iron-deficiency anemia has been effective when the client states,

    a. "I will need to take the iron supplements the rest of my life."
    b. "I will increase my dietary intake of milk and milk products."
    c. "I should increase my activity to increase my aerobic capacity."
    d. "I should take the iron for several months after my blood is normal."

11. In teaching the client with pernicious anemia about the disease, the nurse explains that it results from a lack of

    a. folic acid.
    b. intrinsic factor.
    c. extrinsic factor.
    d. cobalamin intake.

12. In addition to the general symptoms of anemia, the client with pernicious anemia also manifests

    a. neurological symptoms.
    b. coagulation deficiencies.
    c. cardiovascular disturbances.
    d. a decreased immunological response.

13. The nurse explains to the client with pernicious anemia that

    a. death can be prevented by cobalamin supplementation for the rest of the client's life.
    b. the symptoms of the disease can be completely reversed with cobalamin (vitamin B$_{12}$) therapy.
    c. bone marrow transplantation to change the defective marrow cells is an alternative therapy for pernicious anemia.
    d. dietary intake of foods high in cobalamin is the most inexpensive and convenient treatment of pernicious anemia.

14. Laboratory and diagnostic test findings the nurse would expect in an anemic client with chronic alcoholism include

    a. achlorhydria and macrocytic erythrocytes.
    b. decreased serum folate and increased MCHC.
    c. increased indirect bilirubin and increased reticulocytes.
    d. decreased total iron-binding capacity and increased MCH.

15. The strict vegetarian is at highest risk for the development of

    a. thalassemias.
    b. iron-deficiency anemia.
    c. folic acid–deficiency anemia.
    d. cobalamin-deficiency anemia.

16. A nursing diagnosis that is appropriate for the effects of the deficiency of all of the cells associated with aplastic anemia is

    a. risk for injury: falls.
    b. impaired physical mobility.
    c. risk for impaired skin integrity.
    d. risk for impaired oral mucous membrane.

17. Nursing interventions for the client with aplastic anemia are directed toward the prevention of the complications of

    a. fatigue and dyspnea.
    b. hemorrhage and infection.
    c. thromboemboli and gangrene.
    d. cardiac arrhythmias and heart failure.

18. Identify whether the following statements are true or false. If a statement is false, correct the bold word(s) to make the statement true.

    _____ a. The most reliable way to evaluate the effect and degree of blood loss in a client with hemorrhage is with **laboratory data**.

    _____ b. A client with acute blood loss that has normal vital signs at rest but has increased heart rate and postural hypotension with exercise has lost approximately **30%** of the total blood volume.

    _____ c. The anemia that follows acute blood loss is most frequently treated with **increased dietary iron intake**.

    _____ d. In addition to the general symptoms of anemia, the client with a hemolytic anemia also manifests **jaundice**.

    _____ e. A major concern in hemolytic anemias is maintenance of **liver** function.

    _____ f. An example of an intravascular extrinsic hemolytic anemia results from **blood transfusion reactions**.

19. The anemia of sickle cell disease is caused by

    a. intravascular hemolysis of sickled RBCs.
    b. accelerated breakdown of abnormal RBCs.
    c. autoimmune antibody destruction of RBCs.
    d. isoimmune antibody–antigen reactions with RBCs.

20. A client with sickle cell anemia asks the nurse why the sickling crisis does not stop when oxygen therapy is started. The nurse explains that

    a. sickling occurs in response to decreased blood viscosity, which is not affected by oxygen therapy.
    b. when red cells sickle, they occlude small vessels, which causes more local hypoxia and more sickling.
    c. the primary problem during a sickle cell crisis is destruction of the abnormal cells resulting in fewer RBCs to carry oxygen.
    d. oxygen therapy does not alter the shape of the abnormal erythrocytes but only allows for increased oxygen concentration in hemoglobin.

21. A nursing intervention that is indicated for the client during a sickle cell crisis is

    a. frequent ambulation.
    b. application of antiembolism hose.
    c. restriction of sodium and oral fluids.
    d. administration of large doses of continuous narcotic analgesics.

22. During discharge teaching with a client with newly diagnosed sickle cell disease, the nurse teaches the client to decrease the risk of a sickle cell crisis by

    a. limiting fluid intake.
    b. avoiding hot, humid weather.
    c. eliminating exercise from the lifestyle.
    d. seeking early medical intervention for upper respiratory infections.

23. Identify whether the following statements are true or false. If a statement is false, correct the bold word(s) to make the statement true.

    _____ a. Genetic counselling and family planning is indicated for couples when one of them has **thalassemia**.

    _____ b. Immune thrombocytopenic purpura is characterized by increased platelet destruction by the **spleen**.

    _____ c. Alterations in platelet function are assessed with the use of **prothrombin** times.

    _____ d. Thrombotic thrombocytopenic purpura is characterized by **decreased** platelets, **decreased** RBCs, and **decreased** agglutination function of platelets.

    _____ e. A classic clinical manifestation of thrombocytopenia that the nurse would expect to find on physical examination of the client is **ecchymosis**.

    _____ f. Clients with platelet deficiencies usually bleed from **superficial sites**, while those with diminished clotting factors experience **deep or internal** bleeding.

    _____ g. Treatment of **hemachromatosis** involves weekly phlebotomy for two to three years.

    _____ h. The nurse suspects heparin-induced thrombocytopenia and thrombosis syndrome when a client receiving heparin requires **decreased** heparin to maintain therapeutic activated thromboplastin times.

24. In planning the care of a client hospitalized with polycythemia vera, the nurse recognizes that a nursing intervention that is most likely to prevent organ damage or death is

   a. maintaining protective isolation.
   b. promoting leg exercises and ambulation.
   c. protecting the client from injury or falls.
   d. promoting hydration with a large fluid intake.

25. A client has a platelet count of $50 \times 10^9/L$ ($50 \times 10^3/\mu L$) and is diagnosed with immune thrombocytopenic purpura. The nurse would expect initial treatment to include

   a. splenectomy.
   b. corticosteroids.
   c. administration of platelets.
   d. immunosuppressive therapy.

26. During the care of the client with thrombocytopenia, the nurse

   a. takes frequent temperatures to assess for fever.
   b. maintains the client on strict bed rest to prevent injury.
   c. monitors the client for headaches, vertigo, or confusion.
   d. removes oral crusting and scabs with firm friction every two hours.

27. In analyzing the laboratory results of a client with classic hemophilia, the nurse would expect to find

   a. an absence of factor IX.
   b. a decreased platelet count.
   c. a prolonged bleeding time.
   d. a prolonged partial thromboplastin time.

28. Treatment of hemophilia most often includes periodic administration of

   a. whole blood.
   b. thromboplastin.
   c. factor concentrates.
   d. fresh frozen plasma.

29. A client with hemophilia is hospitalized with acute knee pain and swelling. Nursing interventions for the client include

   a. wrapping the knee with an elastic bandage.
   b. placing the client on bed rest and applying ice to the joint.
   c. gently performing ROM exercises to the knee to prevent adhesions.
   d. administering non-steroidal anti-inflammatory drugs as needed for pain.

30. Number in sequence the events that occur in disseminated intravascular coagulation (DIC).

_____  a. Activation of fibrinolytic system

_____  b. Uncompensated hemorrhage

_____  c. Widespread fibrin and platelet deposition in capillaries and arterioles

_____  d. Release of fibrin split products

_____  e. Fibrinogen converted to fibrin

_____  f. Inhibition of normal blood clotting

_____  g. Production of intravascular thrombin

_____  h. Depletion of platelets and coagulation factors

31. Early recognition of acute DIC by the nurse in a client includes

    a. providing appropriate care for managing the causative problem.
    b. a knowledge of signs and symptoms of microvascular thrombosis.
    c. administering necessary blood products and anticoagulants to susceptible clients.
    d. astute, ongoing assessment with awareness of risk for DIC in clients with predisposing conditions.

32. A client has a WBC of 2.3 x $10^9$/L (2.3 x $10^3$/μL) and a neutrophil percentage of 40%.

    a. Does the client have a leukopenia?


    b. What is the client's neutrophil count?


    c. Does the client have a neutropenia?


    d. What is the client's risk for developing a bacterial infection?


33. The most important method for identifying the presence of infection in a neutropenic client is

    a. frequent temperatures.
    b. routine blood and sputum cultures.
    c. assessing for redness and swelling.
    d. monitoring white blood cell counts.

34. The major method of preventing infection in the client with neutropenia is use of

    a. HEPA filtration rooms.
    b. prophylactic antibiotics.
    c. private, laminar airflow rooms.
    d. strict hand washing by all persons in contact with the client.

35. Myelodysplastic syndrome (MDS) differs from acute leukemias in that MDS

    a. has a slower disease progression.
    b. does not result in bone marrow failure.
    c. is a clonal disorder of hematopoietic cells.
    d. only affects the production and function of platelets and WBCs.

36. Match the following characteristics with their related types of leukemia (answers may be used more than once).

    _____    a. Neoplasm of activated B lymphocytes           1. AML

    _____    b. Mature-appearing, but functionally inactive   2. ALL
              lymphocytes
                                                               3. CML
    _____    c. 85% of acute leukemia in adults
                                                               4. CLL
    _____    d. Most common in children

    _____    e. Only cure is bone marrow transplant

    _____    f. Proliferation of immature lymphocytes in bone marrow

    _____    g. Increased incidence in atomic bomb survivors

    _____    h. Proliferation of precursors of granulocytes

    _____    i. Associated with Philadelphia chromosome

    _____    j. CNS manifestations common

    _____    k. Most common leukemia of adults

37. A client with acute myelogenous leukemia is to start chemotherapy. During the induction stage of chemotherapy, the nurse can expect the client to

    a. experience mild side effects of the drugs.
    b. experience additive bone marrow suppression.
    c. receive high-dose treatment daily for several months.
    d. regain energy and become more resistant to infection.

38. Lymphadenopathy, splenomegaly, and hepatomegaly are common clinical manifestations of leukemia that are due to

    a. the development of infection at these sites.
    b. increased compensatory production of blood cells by these organs.
    c. infiltration of the organs by increased numbers of WBCs in the blood.
    d. normal hypertrophy of the organs in an attempt to destroy abnormal cells.

39. A client with acute myelogenous leukemia is considering a bone marrow transplant and asks the nurse what is involved. The best response by the nurse is

    a. "Your bone marrow is destroyed by radiation and new bone marrow cells from a matched donor are injected into your bones."
    b. "A specimen of your bone marrow may be aspirated and treated to destroy any leukemic cells, and then reinfused when your disease becomes worse."
    c. "During chemotherapy and total body radiation to destroy all your blood cells, you are given transfusions of red cells and platelets to prevent complications."
    d. "All leukemic cells and bone marrow stem cells are eliminated with chemotherapy and total body radiation, and new bone marrow cells from a donor are infused."

40. Nursing diagnoses that are appropriate for the client with newly diagnosed chronic lymphocytic leukemia include

    a. pain and hopelessness.
    b. anxiety and risk for infection.
    c. self-care deficit and ineffective health maintenance.
    d. decisional conflict: treatment options and risk for injury.

41. Indicate whether the following characteristics are associated with Hodgkin's disease (HD), non-Hodgkin's lymphoma (NHL), or both (B).

    _____ a. Multiple histopathological classifications

    _____ b. Presence of Reed-Sternberg cells

    _____ c. Treated with radiation and chemotherapy

    _____ d. Affects all ages

    _____ e. Originates in lymph nodes in most clients

    _____ f. Often widely disseminated at time of diagnosis

    _____ g. Alcohol-induced pain at site of disease

    _____ h. Primary initial clinical manifestation is painless lymph node enlargement

    _____ i. Over 90% cure rate in stage I disease

    _____ j. Associated with Epstein-Barr virus

42. The nurse prepares to administer IV GM-CSF (Leukine) to a client with neutropenia resulting from chemotherapy for non-Hodgkin's lymphoma. The nurse explains to the client that this preparation

    a. can stimulate the production and function of neutrophils and monocytes.
    b. is a type of interferon that may inhibit DNA and protein synthesis in tumour cells.
    c. is a chemotherapeutic agent that is less toxic to the bone marrow than other chemotherapeutic agents.
    d. is a monoclonal antibody linked to a radioactive isotope that will directly deliver radiation to malignant cells.

43. Identify whether the following statements are true or false. If a statement is false, correct the bold word(s) to make the statement true.

_____ a. Staging of lymphomas is important to **predict prognosis**.

_____ b. Nursing management of the client undergoing treatment for Hodgkin's disease includes measures to prevent **infection**.

_____ c. Multiple myeloma is characterized by proliferation of malignant activated **T cells** that destroy the **kidneys**.

_____ d. Two important nursing interventions in the care of clients with multiple myeloma are increasing fluids to manage **hypercalcemia** and careful handling of the client to prevent **pathological fractures**.

44. When analyzing laboratory results of a client with multiple myeloma, the nurse would expect to find

a. lymphopenia and myeloma protein.
b. neutrophilic leukocytosis and anemia.
c. decreased serum creatinine and BUN.
d. hyperuricemia and increased immunoglobulinemia.

45. Following a splenectomy for treatment of immune thrombocytopenic purpura, the nurse would expect the client's laboratory results to reveal

a. decreased RBCs.
b. decreased WBCs.
c. increased platelets.
d. increased immunoglobulins.

46. While receiving a unit of packed red blood cells, the client develops chills and a temperature of 39°C (102.2°F). The nurse

a. notifies the physician and the blood bank.
b. stops the transfusion and removes the IV catheter.
c. adds a leukocyte reduction filter to the blood administration set.
d. recognizes this as a mild allergic transfusion reaction and slows the transfusion.

47. A client with thrombocytopenia with active bleeding is to receive a bag of five units of platelets prescribed. To administer the platelets, the nurse

a. uses standard IV tubing with external filler.
b. agitates the bag periodically during the transfusion.
c. takes vital signs before, during, and after the procedure.
d. refrigerates the second unit until the first unit has transfused.

48. Match the following characteristics with their related transfusion reactions (answers may be used more than once).

_____ a. May restart transfusion with antihistamine therapy in mild cases

_____ b. May be avoided by leukocyte reduction filters

_____ c. Acute renal failure may occur

_____ d. Destruction of donor RBCs

_____ e. Hypothermia common

_____ f. Leukocyte or plasma protein incompatibility

_____ g. ABO incompatibility

_____ h. Hypocalcemia and hyperkalemia

_____ i. Epinephrine used for severe reaction

_____ j. May occur in cardiac and renal insufficiency

1. Acute hemolytic reaction

2. Febrile reaction

3. Allergic reaction

4. Circulatory overload

5. Massive blood transfusion reaction

49. The signs of transfusion-related acute lung injury (TRALI), a serious and potentially fatal transfusion reaction, could be:

a. acute shortness of breath and oxygen desaturation during or within six hours of completion of a transfusion.
b. fever, productive cough, and lower lobe consolidation 48 hours after a transfusion.
c. elevated CVP and cardiogenic pulmonary edema 24 hours after completion of a transfusion.
d. cyanosis in the absence of chest x-ray changes 12 hours after completion of a transfusion.

# CASE STUDY

## DISSEMINATED INTRAVASCULAR COAGULATION

**Client Profile**

Mrs. G., a 35-year-old mother of two, is admitted in active labour to the labour and delivery department for delivery of her third child. She delivers a 4.1-kg (9-lb) boy following an unusually hard and prolonged labour.

**Objective Data**

- During her recovery period she continues to have heavy uterine bleeding and a boggy fundus.
- Her skin is pale and diaphoretic.
- BP 70/40; HR 150.
- Although the placenta appeared intact on examination, she is suspected of having retained placental fragments causing DIC.

## Critical Thinking Questions

1. What is the pathological mechanism that triggers DIC in this case?

2. What additional clinical findings would indicate the presence of DIC?

3. Describe the common laboratory findings that are indicative of DIC.

4. What therapeutic modalities are most appropriate for this client and why?

5. Based on the assessment data presented, write one or more appropriate nursing diagnoses. Are there any collaborative problems?

1. Using the list of terms below, identify the structures in the following illustration.

**List of Terms**

Chordae tendineae          Papillary muscle
Cusp                       Tricuspid valve
Mitral valve               Ventricular septum

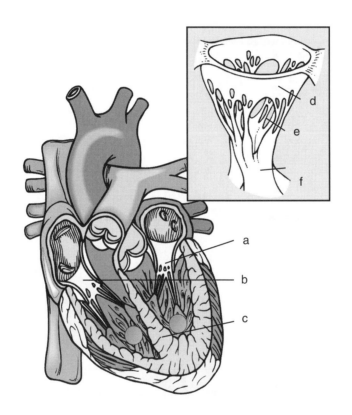

a. _____     d. _____

b. _____     e. _____

c. _____     f. _____

2. Identify the structures in the following illustrations by placing the correct term from the list below in the corresponding answer blank on the next page (some terms will be used more than once).

**List of Terms**

Anterior interventricular artery
Aorta
Aortic semilunar valve
Circumflex artery
Coronary sinus
Great cardiac vein
Left atrium
Left coronary artery
Left marginal artery
Left ventricle

Middle cardiac vein
Posterior interventricular artery
Posterior vein
Pulmonary trunk
Right atrium
Right coronary artery
Right marginal artery
Right ventricle
Small cardiac vein
Superior vena cava

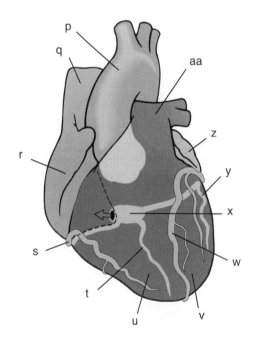

a. _____      o. _____

b. _____      p. _____

c. _____      q. _____

d. _____      r. _____

e. _____      s. _____

f. _____      t. _____

g. _____      u. _____

h. _____      v. _____

i. _____      w. _____

j. _____      x. _____

k. _____      y. _____

l. _____      z. _____

m. _____      aa. _____

n. _____

3. Complete the following statements.

a. The three main coronary arteries are the _____,

_____, and _____.

b. In most people, the _____ artery supplies the AV node.

c. Blood flow into the coronary arteries occurs primarily during the _____ phase of the cardiac cycle.

4. Number in sequence the path of the action potential along the conduction system of the heart.

_____ a. AV node

_____ b. Purkinje fibres

_____ c. Internodal pathways

_____ d. Bundle of His

_____ e. Ventricular cells

_____ f. SA node

_____ g. Right and left atrial cells

_____ h. Right and left bundle branches

5. Match the cardiac activity and time frames characteristic of the waveforms of the electrocardiogram (answers may be used more than once).

_____ a. Time of impulse spread from SA node to ventricles

_____ b. Repolarization of the ventricles

_____ c. 0.12 to 0.20 sec

_____ d. Depolarization from SA node throughout atria

_____ e. 0.16 sec

_____ f. Time of depolarization and repolarization of ventricles

_____ g. 0.06 to 0.10 sec

_____ h. Depolarization from AV node throughout ventricles

_____ i. 0.06 to 0.12 sec

1. P wave

2. P-R interval

3. QRS interval

4. T wave

5. Q-T interval

6. Indicate what factor of stroke volume (i.e., preload, afterload, or contractility) is primarily affected by the following situations, and whether cardiac output (CO) is increased or decreased by the factor.

a. Valsalva manoeuvre        _____        CO _____

b. Venous dilation        _____        CO _____

c. Hypertension        _____        CO _____

d. Administration of epinephrine        _____        CO _____

e. Obstruction of pulmonary artery        _____        CO _____

f. Hemorrhage        _____        CO _____

7. Match the effects of the autonomic nervous system stimulation with the receptors responsible for the effects (answers may be used more than once).

_____ a. Increased force of cardiac contraction

_____ b. Decreased rate of impulse conduction

_____ c. Vasoconstriction

_____ d. Increased heart rate

_____ e. Increased rate of impulse conduction

_____ f. Decreased heart rate

1. α-Adrenergic stimulation

2. β-Adrenergic stimulation

3. Parasympathetic stimulation

8. Complete the following statements.

   a. Since blood pressure is a factor of cardiac output (heart rate x stroke volume) x systemic vascular resistance, three effects of sympathetic nervous system stimulation responsible for increased blood pressure are _____, _____, and _____.

   b. The one effect of parasympathetic nervous system stimulation that is responsible for decreased blood pressure is _____.

   c. When a client who has been in bed for a prolonged time is assisted to a standing position, the client's heart rate increases by 20 beats per minute. The regulatory mechanism of the cardiovascular system that is responsible for this change is _____.

   d. A client has a BP of 136/76. The client's pulse pressure is _____, and the client's mean arterial pressure (MAP) is _____.

9. Identify the age-related physiological changes that occur in the older adult that result in the following.

   a.  Widened pulse pressure


   b.  Decreased cardiac reserve


   c.  Increased cardiac arrhythmias


   d.  Decreased response to sympathetic stimulation


   e.  Aortic systolic murmur


10. Information related to the client's past health and medication history that the nurse identifies as significant during assessment of the cardiovascular system is a history of

    a. metastatic cancer.
    b. calcium supplementation.
    c. frequent viral pharyngitis.
    d. use of recreational/abused drugs.

11. Identify one specific finding identified by the nurse during assessment of each of the client's functional health patterns that indicates a risk factor for cardiovascular disease or a client response to an actual cardiovascular problem.

    a.   Health perception–health management

    b.   Nutritional–metabolic

    c.   Elimination

    d.   Activity–exercise

    e.   Sleep–rest

    f.   Cognitive–perceptual

    g.   Self-perception–self-concept

    h.   Role–relationship

    i.   Sexuality–reproductive

    j.   Coping–stress tolerance

    k.   Value–belief

12. A normal positional blood pressure in lying, sitting, and standing positions is

    a.  106/70; 100/65; 90/62.
    b.  114/82; 110/76; 108/74.
    c.  120/82; 110/80; 100/78.
    d.  134/84; 130/80; 126/80.

13. When palpating the client's popliteal pulse, the nurse feels a vibration at the site. This finding is recorded as a

    a.  thready, weak pulse.
    b.  bruit at the artery site.
    c.  bounding pulse volume.
    d.  thrill of the popliteal artery.

14. Match the points that are inspected and palpated on the chest wall with their locations (answers may be used more than once).

_____ a. Pulmonic area

_____ b. PMI

_____ c. Erb's point

_____ d. Tricuspid area

_____ e. Precordium

_____ f. Angle of Louis

_____ g. Aortic area

_____ h. Apex of heart

_____ i. Mitral area

_____ j. Base of the heart

1. Second ICS left of sternum

2. Manubrium and sternal junction at level of second rib

3. Second ICS right of sternum

4. Third ICS left of sternum

5. Fifth ICS left of sternum

6. Fifth ICS at left mid-clavicular line

7. Located between apex and sternum

15. Indicate whether the following are characteristic of the first heart sound ($S_1$) or the second heart sound ($S_2$).

_____ a. Indicates the onset of diastole

_____ b. Associated with closure of tricuspid and mitral valves

_____ c. Is loudest at pulmonic and aortic areas

_____ d. Soft lubb sound

_____ e. Heard when carotid pulse felt

_____ f. Indicates beginning of systole

_____ g. Associated with closure of semilunar valves

_____ h. Sharp dupp sound

_____ i. Is loudest at tricuspid and mitral areas

16. Match the following abnormal assessment findings with their descriptions or significance.

    _____  a. Positive Homan's sign               1. Associated with increased right atrial pressure

    _____  b. Heave                                2. Flattening of angle of nail base and finger

    _____  c. Central cyanosis                     3. Decreased peripheral perfusion

    _____  d. $S_3$                                4. Lift of chest wall in precordial area

    _____  e. Cardiac murmurs                      5. Blue tinge around nose and ears

    _____  f. Finger clubbing                      6. Extra heart sound ending in late diastole

    _____  g. Jugular vein distension              7. Calf pain on dorsiflexion of foot

    _____  h. Delayed capillary filling time       8. Common with heart valve disorders

    _____  i. $S_4$                                9. Blue tinge around lips and conjunctiva

    _____  j. Peripheral cyanosis                  10. Extra heart sound ending in early diastole

17. A client is scheduled for a Cardiolite scan with stress testing. The nurse explains to the client that this test involves

    a. placement of electrodes inside the right heart chambers through a vein to directly record the electrical activity of the heart.
    b. exercising on a treadmill or stationary bicycle with continuous ECG monitoring to detect ischemic changes during exercise.
    c. the IV administration of a radioisotope of technetium-99 Sestimibi at the maximum heart rate during exercise to identify areas of cardiac damage.
    d. placement of a small transducer in four positions on the chest to record the direction and flow of blood through the heart by reflection of sound waves.

18. Evaluation of electrocardiographic responses to normal activity over a period of a day or two is performed with

    a. serial ECGs.
    b. Holter monitoring.
    c. electrophysiology studies.
    d. positron emission tomography.

19. Following a cardiac catheterization with coronary angiography, it is most important for the nurse to

    a. observe the catheter insertion site for swelling.
    b. assess for pain at the side of the catheter insertion.
    c. check the pulses distal to the catheter insertion site.
    d. monitor for symptoms of allergy to the constrast media.

20. A laboratory test that is a specific indicator of cardiac muscle damage is

    a. troponin I.
    b. apoproteins.
    c. lactic dehydrogenase (LDH)-3.
    d. serum aspartate aminotransferase (AST).

21. A female client has a total cholesterol level of 6 mmol/L (232 mg/dL) and an HDL of 1.68 mmol/L (65 mg/dL). A male client has a total cholesterol level of 210 and an HDL of 32. Based on these findings, the client with the highest cardiac risk is

    a. the male, because his HDL is lower.
    b. the female, because her HDL is higher.
    c. the female, because her cholesterol is higher.
    d. the male, because his cholesterol-to-HDL ratio is higher.

# CHAPTER 32 NURSING MANAGEMENT: HYPERTENSION

1. In the regulation of normal blood pressure, indicate whether the following mechanisms elevate blood pressure by increasing cardiac output (CO), increasing systemic vascular resistance (SVR), or increasing both (B), and identify how these mechanisms cause the increases indicated.

   _____ a. $\beta_1$-Adrenergic stimulation _____

   _____ b. $\alpha_1$-Adrenergic stimulation _____

   _____ c. $\alpha_2$-Adrenergic stimulation _____

   _____ d. Enothelin release _____

   _____ e. Angiotensin II _____

   _____ f. Aldosterone release _____

   _____ g. ADH release _____

2. A client is given an $\alpha_1$-adrenergic agonist and experiences a reflex bradycardia. What normal mechanism of blood pressure control is stimulated in this situation?

3. A client uses a mixed $\beta$-adrenergic blocking agent for treatment of migraine headaches. What effect may this drug have on blood pressure and why?

4. A client has blood pressures taken at an outpatient clinic. Blood pressure measurements that would indicate that the client has hypertension include

   a. an initial visit blood pressure of 156/96.
   b. two different visit blood pressures of 142/92 and 136/86.
   c. three different visit blood pressures of 144/94, 156/90, and 142/88.
   d. three different visit blood pressures of 158/94, 136/88, and 146/92.

5. The nurse recognizes that the client has stage 2 hypertension when the client's average blood pressure is

   a. 155/88 mm Hg.
   b. 172/92 mm Hg.
   c. 160/110 mm Hg.
   d. 182/106 mm Hg.

6. Identify four risk factors for primary hypertension that are not related to lifestyle behaviours.

   a.

   b.

   c.

   d.

7. Secondary hypertension is differentiated from primary hypertension in that secondary hypertension

   a. has a more gradual onset than primary hypertension.
   b. does not cause the target organ damage that occurs with primary hypertension.
   c. has a specific cause, such as renal disease, that often can be corrected by medicine or surgery.
   d. is caused by age-related changes in blood pressure regulatory mechanisms in those individuals over 65 years of age.

8. The client with stage 2 hypertension is likely to report

   a. no symptoms.
   b. cardiac palpitations.
   c. dyspnea on exertion.
   d. dizziness and vertigo.

9. Most organ damage that occurs from hypertension is related to

   a. increased fluid pressure exerted against organ tissue.
   b. atherosclerotic changes in vessels that supply the organs.
   c. erosion and thinning of blood vessels from constant pressure.
   d. increased hydrostatic pressure causing leakage of plasma into organ interstitial spaces.

10. The organ that is damaged most directly as a result of high systemic vascular resistance is the

   a. brain.
   b. heart.
   c. retina.
   d. kidney.

11. Identify the significance of the following laboratory results found in clients with hypertension.

   a. BUN 17.1 mmol/L (48 mg/dL); creatinine 380 μmol/L (4.3 mg/dL)

   b. Serum $K^+$ 3.1 mmol/L (3.1 mEq/L)

   c. FBS 10.2 mmol/L (183 mg/dL)

   d. Serum uric acid 547 μmol/L (9.2 mg/dL)

   e. Low-density lipoproteins (LDL) 4 mmol/L (154 mg/dL)

12. A 42-year-old male client has been diagnosed with essential hypertension with an average blood pressure of 162/92 on three consecutive clinic visits. What are four lifestyle modifications that may be indicated in the initial treatment of the client?

    a.

    b.

    c.

    d.

13. A client does not respond to treatment of stage 2 hypertension with lifestyle modifications within one year. Initial drug therapy that would be indicated for the client includes

    a. a thiazide diuretic.
    b. a β-adrenergic blocker and an ACE inhibitor.
    c. a loop diuretic and a direct-acting vasodilator.
    d. a calcium channel blocker and an α-adrenergic blocker.

14. Match the following primary effects in reducing blood pressure with the classifications of drugs used to treat hypertension.

    _____ a. Decrease extracellular fluid volume by decreasing Na+ and water reabsorption in loop of Henle and distal tubule

    _____ b. Decrease cardiac output by decreasing rate and strength of heart and decreasing renin secretion by kidney

    _____ c. Act directly on smooth muscle of arterioles to cause vasodilation

    _____ d. Cause vasodilation of arterioles by blocking movement of calcium into cells

    _____ e. Decrease Na+ and water reabsorption by blocking effect of aldosterone

    _____ f. Block peripheral α-adrenergic receptors to cause arteriole and venous dilation

    _____ g. Cause vasodilation by inhibiting sympathetic outflow from CNS

    _____ h. Interfere with enzyme conversion necessary for production of angiotensin II

    1. Central adrenergic antagonists
    2. Spironolactone
    3. ACE inhibitors
    4. Thiazide diuretics
    5. β-adrenergic blockers
    6. Calcium channel blockers
    7. α-adrenergic blockers
    8. Direct vasodilators

15. Teaching to include dietary sources of potassium is indicated for the hypertensive client taking

    a. enalapril (Vasotec).
    b. labetalol (Normodyne).
    c. spironolactone (Aldactone).
    d. hydrochlorothiazide (HydroDiuril).

16. A client with stage 3 hypertension taking hydrochlorothiazide (HydroDiuril) and lisinopril (Prinivil) has prazosin (Minipress) added to the medication regimen. It is most important for the nurse to teach the client to

    a. weigh every morning to monitor for fluid retention.
    b. change position slowly and avoid prolonged standing.
    c. use sugarless gum or candy to help relieve dry mouth.
    d. take the pulse daily to note any slowing of the heart rate.

17. A 38-year-old man is treated for hypertension with amiloride/hydrochlorothiazide (Maxide) and metaprolol (Lopressor). Four months after his last clinic visit, his blood pressure returns to pretreatment levels and he admits he has not been taking his medication regularly. The best response of the nurse is

    a. "Try to always take your medication when you carry out another daily routine so you do not forget to take it."
    b. "If you would exercise more and stop smoking, you probably would not need to be on medications for hypertension."
    c. "The drugs you are taking cause sexual dysfunction in many clients. Are you experiencing any problems in this area?"
    d. "You need to remember that hypertension can only be controlled with medication, not cured, and you must always take your medication."

18. When teaching a client for whom clonidine (Catapres) has been prescribed, the nurse stresses that

    a. the drug should never be stopped abruptly.
    b. the drug should be taken early in the day to prevent nocturia.
    c. the first dose should be taken when the client is in bed for the night.
    d. ASA will decrease the drug's effectiveness and acetaminophen should be substituted for ASA use.

19. The correct technique for blood pressure measurements includes

    a. always taking the blood pressure in both arms.
    b. releasing the pressure in the cuff at a rate of 1 mm Hg per second.
    c. inflating the cuff 10 mm Hg higher than the expected systolic pressure.
    d. taking additional readings if the first two readings differ more than 5 mm Hg.

20. A client's blood pressure has not responded consistently to the prescribed medications for hypertension. The first cause of this lack of responsiveness the nurse should explore is

    a. progressive target organ damage.
    b. the possibility of drug interactions.
    c. the client not adhering to therapy.
    d. the client's possible use of recreational drugs.

21. A client would be diagnosed with a hypertensive emergency when experiencing

    a. a systolic BP >200 mm Hg and a diastolic BP >120 mm Hg.
    b. a sudden rise in BP accompanied by neurological impairment.
    c. symptoms of a cerebrovascular accident (CVA) with an elevated BP.
    d. a severe elevation of the blood pressure that occurs over several days or weeks.

22. What drugs are used initially to treat a hypertensive crisis?

    a. labetalol (Normodyne) and diazoxide (Hyperstat).
    b. hydralazine (Apresoline) and captopril (Catapres).
    c. nitroglycerin (Tridil) and sodium nitroprusside (Nipride).
    d. intravenous enalaprilat (Vasotec) and minoxidil (Loniten).

23. During treatment of hypertensive emergencies with intravenous vasodilators, the initial goal of therapy is to

    a. lower the BP sufficiently to prevent target organ damage.
    b. decrease the BP to a normal level for the age of the client.
    c. decrease the mean arterial pressure 10–20% in the first one to two hours.
    d. reduce the systolic BP to 150 mm Hg and the diastolic BP to 90 mm Hg as quickly as possible.

24. A nursing responsibility in the management of the client with a hypertensive urgency often includes

    a. monitoring hourly urine output for drug effectiveness.
    b. providing for continuous ECG monitoring to detect side effects of the drugs.
    c. titrating intravenous drug dosages based on BP measurements every two to three minutes.
    d. instructing the client to follow up with a healthcare professional 24 hours after outpatient treatment.

## CASE STUDY

### ISOLATED SYSTOLIC HYPERTENSION

**Client Profile**

Mrs. J. is a 73-year-old white woman with no history of hypertension. She came to the doctor's office for a flu shot.

**Subjective Data**

- Says she has gained 9 kg (20 lb) over the past year since her husband died
- Has never smoked and uses no alcohol
- Only medication is one multivitamin per day
- Eats a lot of canned food
- Does not exercise

**Objective Data**

- Height 162.5 cm (64 in); weight 77 kg (170 lb)
- BP 170/82 mm Hg
- Physical examination shows no abnormalities
- Serum potassium 3.3 mmol/L (3.3 mEq/L)

The physician diagnosed isolated systolic hypertension (ISH) and prescribed lifestyle modifications.

## Critical Thinking Questions

1. What contributing factors to the development of ISH are present?

2. What additional risk factors are present?

3. What specific dietary changes would the nurse recommend for Mrs. J.?

4. What other teaching should be instituted by the nurse?

5. If drug therapy became necessary to treat Mrs. J.'s hypertension, what diuretic would be indicated on her laboratory results?

6. Based on the assessment data presented, write one or more appropriate nursing diagnoses. Are there any collaborative problems?

1. Identify the three stages of lesions that occur in the development of coronary artery disease and the ages at which the stages are present.

   **Stage**                                                **Age**

   a.

   b.

   c.

2. Identify whether the following statements are true or false. If a statement is false, correct the bold word(s) to make the statement true.

   _____ a. The leading theory of atherogenesis proposes that **aging** is the basic underlying cause of atherosclerosis.

   _____ b. Endothelial alteration may be caused by chemical irritants such as **hyperlipidemia** or by **hypertension**.

   _____ c. New findings indicate that certain **bacterial or viral infections** may damage the endothelium and contribute to the development of atherosclerosis.

   _____ d. During development of the raised fibrous plaque, arterial wall changes may be initiated by **carbon monoxide produced by smoking**.

   _____ e. Partial or total occlusion of the coronary artery occurs during the stage of **raised fibrous plaque**.

   _____ f. Collateral circulation in the coronary circulation is more likely to be present in the **young** client with **CAD**.

3. List the three most significant risk factors for atherosclerosis and indicate whether these risk factors are modifiable or unmodifiable.

   a.

   b.

   c.

4. While taking nursing histories of clients, the nurse identifies that the client with the highest risk for coronary artery disease is

   a. a black man, age 65, with obesity and a BP of 160/85.
   b. a white man, age 54, who is a smoker and has a stressful lifestyle.
   c. an Asian woman, age 45, with a cholesterol level of 6.21 mmol/L (240 mg/dL) and a BP of 130/75.
   d. a white woman, age 72, with a BP of 172/100 and who is physically inactive.

5. Match the following characteristics with their associated lipoproteins (answers may be used more than once).

   \_\_\_\_\_   a. Contains most of the triglycerides

   \_\_\_\_\_   b. Specific marker for cholesterol-depositing capacity of the blood

   \_\_\_\_\_   c. Contains the most cholesterol

   \_\_\_\_\_   d. The higher the level, the lower the risk for CAD

   \_\_\_\_\_   e. Carries lipids away from arteries to liver

   \_\_\_\_\_   f. Increases are associated with obesity

   \_\_\_\_\_   g. Increases with exercise

   \_\_\_\_\_   h. Genetically inherited lipoprotein that contributes to blood clot formation

   \_\_\_\_\_   i. High levels correlate most closely with CAD

   \_\_\_\_\_   j. Specific marker for cholesterol-clearing capacity of the blood

   \_\_\_\_\_   k. Has an affinity for arterial walls

1. HDL

2. LDL

3. VLDL

4. Apolipoprotein A-1

5. Apolipoprotein B

6. Lipoprotein (a)

6. Identify the desirable levels of the following serum lipoproteins.

   a. Total cholesterol _____

   b. Triglycerides _____

   c. LDL _____

   d. HDL in men _____

   e. HDL in women _____

7. The nurse is encouraging a sedentary client with major risks for CAD to perform physical exercise on a regular basis. In addition to decreasing the risk factor of physical inactivity, the nurse tells the client that exercise will also directly contribute to reducing the risk factors of

   a. hyperlipidemia and obesity.
   b. diabetes mellitus and hypertension.
   c. elevated serum lipids and stressful lifestyle.
   d. hypertension and elevated serum homocysteine.

8. Two risk factors for CAD that are considered to increase the workload of the heart and increase myocardial oxygen demand include

   a. hypertension and elevated serum lipids.
   b. cigarette smoking and diabetes mellitus.
   c. cigarette smoking and physical inactivity.
   d. type A behaviour pattern and hypertension.

9. During a routine health examination, a 48-year-old man is found to have a total cholesterol level of 5.8 mmol/L (224 mg/dL) and an LDL level of 3.6 mmol/L (140 mg/dL). The nurse teaches the client that a Step 1 dietary change should include

   a. use of skim or 1% milk.
   b. elimination of red meat from the diet.
   c. elimination of alcohol and use of simple sugars.
   d. avoidance of all egg yolks and food prepared with whole eggs.

10. A 62-year-old woman has hypertension and smokes one pack of cigarettes per day. She has no symptoms of CAD, but a recent LDL level is 3.98 mmol/L (154 mg/dl). Based on these findings, the nurse would expect that treatment for the client would include

    a. diet therapy only.
    b. drug therapy only.
    c. diet and drug therapies.
    d. exercise instruction only.

11. A client with CAD has a total cholesterol of 7.24 mmol/L (280 mg/dL), LDL of 3.62 mmol/L (140 mg/dL), and a triglyceride level of 3.84 mmol/L (340 mg/dL). The nurse recognizes that an antilipemic drug that would be indicated for the client is

    a. gemfibrozil (Lopid).
    b. lovastatin (Mevacor).
    c. nicotinic acid (niacin).
    d. cholestyramine (Questran).

12. Complete the following sentences.

    a. When myocardial ischemia is temporary and reversible, the condition is called

    _____.

    b. The three conditions that are included as manifestations of acute coronary syndrome are

    _____, _____, and _____.

    c. When myocardial cells die as a result of ischemia, the area of cellular necrosis is known as an

    _____.

13. Use the following terms to complete the statements:

   increased oxygen demand
   decreased oxygen supply

   a. Myocardial ischemia occurs as a result of two factors: _____ and

      _____.

   b. Any factor that increases cardiac workload causes _____.

   c. Narrowing of coronary arteries by atherosclerosis is the primary reason for _____.

   d. Chronic dilation of coronary arteries below an obstruction area results in _____.

   e. Low blood volume or a decreased hemoglobin leads to _____.

   f. Left ventricular hypertrophy caused by chronic hypertension leads to _____.

   g. Sympathetic nervous system stimulation by drugs, emotions, or exertion constricts blood vessels and

      increases heart rate, resulting in _____.

   h. In the client with atherosclerotic coronary arteries, anything that causes

      _____ may precipitate angina.

14. Angina pectoris, the pain, most likely occurs with myocardial ischemia as a result of

    a. death of myocardial tissue.
    b. arrhythmias caused by cellular irritability.
    c. lactic acid accumulation during anaerobic metabolism.
    d. elevated pressure in the ventricles and pulmonary vessels.

15. Tachycardia that is a response of the sympathetic nervous system to the pain of ischemia is detrimental because not only does it increase oxygen demand, but it

    a. decreases cardiac output.
    b. causes reflex hypotension.
    c. may lead to ventricular arrhythmias.
    d. impairs perfusion of the coronary arteries.

16. The client's cardiac catheterization report reveals a 95% blockage of the left anterior descending artery. The client is at greatest risk for an infarction of the

    a. lateral wall.
    b. inferior wall.
    c. anterior wall.
    d. posterior wall.

17. The point in the healing process of the myocardium following an infarct where early scar tissue results in an unstable heart wall is

    a. two to three days after MI.
    b. four to ten days after MI.
    c. 10 to 14 days after MI.
    d. six weeks after MI.

18. Match the following types of angina with their characteristics (answers may be used more than once).

    _____ a. Occurs only when the person is recumbent          1. Silent ischemia

    _____ b. Usually precipitated by exertion                  2. Prinzmetal's angina

    _____ c. Unpredictable and unrelieved by rest              3. Stable angina

    _____ d. Prevalent in persons with diabetes                4. Nocturnal angina

    _____ e. Characterized by progressive severity             5. Unstable angina

    _____ f. Occurs with same pattern of onset,                6. Angina decubitus
              duration, and intensity

    _____ g. Asymptomatic myocardial ischemia

    _____ h. Usually occurs in response to coronary artery spasm

    _____ i. Occurs only at night

    _____ j. May occur in the absence of coronary artery disease

19. As an acute coronary syndrome, unstable angina must be identified and treated because

    a. the pain may be severe and disabling.
    b. ECG changes and arrhythmias may occur during an attack.
    c. atherosclerotic plaque deterioration may cause complete thrombus of the vessel lumen.
    d. the spasm of a major coronary artery may cause total occlusion of the vessel with progression to MI.

20. The nurse suspects angina rather than myocardial infarction pain in the client who reports chest pain that

    a. is relieved by nitroglycerin.
    b. is a sensation of tightness or squeezing.
    c. does not radiate to the neck, back, or arms.
    d. is precipitated by physical or emotional exertion.

21. A client admitted to the hospital for evaluation of chest pain has normal cardiac enzyme values four hours after the onset of pain. A non-invasive diagnostic test that can differentiate angina from other types of chest pain is a(n)

    a. ECG.
    b. exercise stress test.
    c. coronary angiogram.
    d. transesophageal echocardiogram.

22. A 52-year-old man is admitted to the emergency department with severe chest pain. The nurse suspects an MI upon finding that the client

    a. has pale, cool, clammy skin.
    b. reports nausea and vomited once at home.
    c. is anxious and has a feeling of impending doom.
    d. has had no relief of the pain with rest or position change.

23. To detect and treat the most common complication of MI, the nurse

    a. measures hourly urine output.
    b. auscultates the chest for crackles.
    c. uses continuous cardiac monitoring.
    d. takes vital signs q2hr for the first eight hours.

24. Match the following complications of MI with the clinical manifestations that commonly indicate its occurrence.

    _____ a. Congestive heart failure

    _____ b. Cardiogenic shock

    _____ c. Papillary muscle dysfunction

    _____ d. Ventricular aneurysm

    _____ e. Pericarditis

    1. Intractable arrhythmias and CHF

    2. Systolic murmur at the cardiac apex radiation toward the axilla

    3. Persistent or intermittent pericardial friction rub

    4. Crackles in lungs and $S_3$ or $S_4$ heart sound

    5. Decreased cardiac output with falling BP

25. In the client with an acute MI, the nurse would expect diagnostic testing to reveal

    a. ECG changes at the onset of the pain.
    b. an enlarged heart with distended upper lobe veins.
    c. CK-MB enzyme elevations that peak 24 hours after the infarct.
    d. the appearance of troponin in the blood 48 hours after the infarct.

26. A second 12-lead ECG performed on a client four hours after the onset of chest pain reveals ST-segment elevation. The nurse recognizes that this finding indicates a

    a. transient ischemia typical of unstable angina.
    b. lack of permanent damage to myocardial cells.
    c. myocardial infarction associated with prolonged and complete coronary thrombosis.
    d. myocardial infarction associated with transient or incomplete coronary artery occlusion.

27. The following are effects of drugs used to prevent and treat angina. Identify the classes of the drugs that are used to promote these effects.

    a. Decrease preload

    b. Dilate coronary arteries

    c. Prevent thrombosis of plaques

    d. Decrease heart rate

    e. Decrease afterload

    f. Decrease myocardial contractility

28. When teaching the client with angina about taking nitroglycerin tablets, the nurse instructs the client

    a. to take the tablet with a large amount of water so it will dissolve right away.
    b. to lie or sit down and place one tablet under the tongue when chest pain occurs.
    c. that if one tablet does not relieve the pain in 15 minutes the client should go to the hospital.
    d. that if the tablet causes dizziness and a headache the medication should be stopped and the doctor notified.

29. A strategy used to prevent the development of tolerance to the effects of transdermal nitrates includes

    a. removing the patch during the night.
    b. changing the sites of the patch every day.
    c. using the patch only when chest pain occurs.
    d. applying the patch on an alternate-day schedule.

30. Match the following descriptions with the procedures used to treat CAD (answers may be used more than once).

    _____ a. Allows for dissolution of arterial plaques

    _____ b. Surgical construction of new vessels to carry blood beyond obstructed coronary artery

    _____ c. Requires anticoagulation following the procedure

    _____ d. Most common alternative to CABG

    _____ e. Structure applied to hold vessels open

    _____ f. Use limited to lesions in proximal and middle portion of vessel

    _____ g. Laser-created channels between left ventricular

    _____ h. Recommended for clients with poor response to treatment of unstable angina

    _____ i. Removal of plaque with a rotating cutter

    _____ j. Compression of artherosclerotic plaque with a balloon

    1. Percutaneous transluminal coronary angioplasty (PTCA)

    2. Stent placement

    3. Atherectomy

    4. Laser angioplasty

    5. Coronary artery bypass graft (CABG)

31. The nurse explains to the client who is to undergo a coronary artery bypass graft that the procedure may involve bypassing stenosed coronary arteries by

    a. using a synthetic graft as a conduit for blood flow from the aorta to a coronary artery distal to an obstruction.
    b. resecting a stenosed coronary artery and inserting a synthetic arterial tube graft to replace the diseased artery.
    c. removing the internal mammary artery and anastomosing it from the aorta to a coronary artery distal to a stenosis.
    d. anastomosing reversed segments of a saphenous vein from the aorta to the coronary artery distal to an obstruction.

32. A client with a previous CABG operation is scheduled for a coronary revascularization using the inferior epigastric artery. The nurse recognizes that this surgery has a higher mortality risk than the usual revascularization procedure primarily because

    a. arterial grafts have a higher rate of restenosis and occlusion than vein grafts.
    b. the need for a laparotomy to access the artery increases the length of the surgery.
    c. this artery does not provide as great a blood supply to the myocardium as other grafts.
    d. use of cardiopulmonary bypass is necessary during arterial graft procedures but not for vein grafts.

33. Collaborative care of the client with NSTEMI differs from that of a client with STEMI in that NSTEMI is more frequently treated with

    a. acute intensive drug therapy.
    b. reperfusion therapy with fibrinolytics.
    c. a coronary artery bypass graft (CABG).
    d. percutaneous coronary intervention (PCI).

34. Fibrinolytic therapy is initiated for a client with a STEMI. The nurse explains to the client that this treatment is performed to

    a. prevent the development of life-threatening arrhythmias.
    b. prevent the development of further clotting in the coronary arteries.
    c. assist ventricular contraction and promote coronary artery perfusion.
    d. dissolve the clot in the coronary artery and prevent further cellular death.

35. The nurse recognizes that fibrinolytic therapy for the treatment of an MI has not been successful when the client

    a. continues to have chest pain.
    b. develops major GI or GU bleeding during treatment.
    c. has a marked increase in CK enzyme levels within three hours of the therapy.
    d. develops premature ventricular contractions and ventricular tachycardia during treatment.

36. Match the following characteristics with the drugs used to treat myocardial infarction.

_____ a. Controls ventricular arrythmias

_____ b. Relieves pain by decreasing $O_2$ demand and increasing $O_2$ supply

_____ c. Helps prevent ventricular remodelling

_____ d. Relieves anxiety and cardiac workload

_____ e. Associated with decreased reinfarction and increased survival

_____ f. Minimizes bradycardia from vagal stimulation

1. Beta-adrenergic blockers

2. IV morphine

3. Stool softeners

4. IV amiodarone (Cordarone)

5. IV nitroglycerin

6. ACE inhibitors

37. Listed below are classes of drugs that may be used in a variety of situations and combinations to prevent or treat thrombus formation in the coronary arteries. Identify one specific use of each of the agents.

a. ASA

b. Glycoprotein (GP) IIB/IIIA inhibitors (abciximab, eptifibatide, tirofiban)

c. Direct thrombin inhibitors (bivalirudin, lepirudin, hirudin)

d. Adenosine diphosphate (ADP) receptor antagonists (ticlopidine, clopidogrel)

38. A client with an MI has a nursing diagnosis of anxiety related to possible lifestyle changes and perceived threat of death. The nurse determines that outcome criteria have been met when the client states,

a. "I'm just going to take this recovery one step at a time."
b. "I feel much better and am ready to get on with my life."
c. "How soon do you think I will be able to go back to work?"
d. "I know you are doing everything possible to save my life."

39. A client hospitalized for evaluation of unstable angina experiences severe chest pain and calls the nurse. List six interventions the nurse should implement in addressing the client's pain.

a.

b.

c.

d.

e.

f.

40. Indicate what emotional responses (denial, anger, etc.) to acute MI are indicated by the following statements by clients.

    a. "I don't think I can take care of myself at home yet."

    b. "What's going to happen if I have another heart attack?"

    c. "I'll never be able to enjoy life again."

    d. "I hope my wife is happy now after harping at me about my eating habits all these years."

    e. "Yes, I'm having a little chest pain. It's no big deal."

41. The nurse and client set a client outcome that at the time of discharge after an MI the client will be able to tolerate moderate-energy activities similar to

    a. golfing.
    b. walking at 8 km/hr (5 mph).
    c. cycling at 20 km/hr (13 mph).
    d. mowing the lawn using a push-mower.

42. When teaching the client who has had an MI about cardiac rehabilitation, the nurse recognizes that the phase of rehabilitation when a routine exercise program should be started is

    a. phase I.
    b. phase II.
    c. phase III.
    d. phase IV.

43. A 58-year-old client is in a cardiac rehabilitation program. The nurse teaches the client to stop exercising if

    a. the heart rate exceeds 150 beats/min.
    b. the client develops pain or dyspnea.
    c. the respiratory rate increases to 30 beats/min.
    d. the heart rate is 30 beats over the resting heart rate.

44. In counselling the client about sexual activity following an MI, the nurse

    a. should wait for the client to ask about resuming sexual activity.
    b. may discuss sexual activity while teaching about other physical activities.
    c. should have the client ask the physician when sexual activity can be resumed.
    d. should inform the client that impotence is a common long-term complication following MI.

45. The nurse advises the client who has had an MI that during sexual activity

    a. orogenital sex should be avoided.
    b. the client should use the superior position.
    c. foreplay may cause too great an increase in heart rate.
    d. prophylactic nitroglycerin may be used if angina occurs.

46. Sudden cardiac death in persons with CAD occurs most often as a result of

    a. an acute MI.
    b. heart trauma.
    c. cardiac arrhythmias.
    d. primary left ventricular outflow obstruction.

47. Clinical manifestations in the older adult that would alert the nurse to the possibility of acute MI include

    a. diaphoresis and nausea.
    b. back and abdominal pain.
    c. tachycardia and elevated BP.
    d. dyspnea and profound weakness.

48. When teaching an older adult with CAD how to manage the treatment program for angina, the nurse instructs the client

    a. to sit for three to five minutes before standing when getting out of bed.
    b. to exercise only twice a week to avoid unnecessary strain on the heart.
    c. that lifestyle changes are not as necessary as they would be in a younger person.
    d. that ASA therapy is contraindicated in older adults because of the risk for bleeding.

49. While teaching women about the risks and incidence of CAD, the nurse stresses that

    a. women have an increased incidence of sudden death compared with men.
    b. smoking is not as significant a risk factor for CAD in women as it is in men.
    c. estrogen replacement therapy in post-menopausal women decreases the risk for CAD.
    d. CAD is a leading cause of death in women, with a higher mortality rate following MI than men.

# CASE STUDY

## CORONARY ARTERY DISEASE

### Client Profile

Mrs. C., a 47-year-old Aboriginal woman, comes to the clinic with a burning sensation in her epigastric area extending into her sternum.

### Subjective Data

- Has had chest pain with activity that is relieved with rest for the past three months
- Has had type 2 diabetes mellitus since she was 35
- Has a 27 pack-year smoking history
- Is more than 30% over her ideal body weight
- Has no regular exercise program
- Expresses frustration with physical problems
- Is reluctant to get medical therapy because it will interfere with her life

### Objective Data

- Physical examination
    - Anxious, clutching fists
    - Appears overweight and withdrawn
- Diagnostic studies
    - Cholesterol 6.41mmol/L (248 mg/dL)
    - LDL 4.14 mmol/L (160 mg/dL)
    - Glucose 11.7 mmol/L (210 mg/dL)

### Collaborative Care

- Altace 10 mg tid
- Nitroglycerin 0.4 mg sublingual prn for chest pain
- Exercise treadmill testing

### Critical Thinking Questions

1. What are Mrs. C.'s risk factors for CAD?

2. What nursing measures should be instituted to help her decrease her risk factors?

3. What symptoms would lead you to suspect the pain may be angina?

4. What kind of ECG changes would indicate myocardial ischemia?

5. What is the rationale for the use of the Altace?

6. What information should the nurse provide for Mrs. C. before the treadmill testing?

7. Based on the assessment data presented, write one or more appropriate nursing diagnoses. Are there any collaborative problems?

1. Identify whether the following statements are true or false. If a statement is false, correct the bold word(s) to make the statement true.

    _____ a. **Systolic failure** is characterized by abnormal resistance to ventricular filling.

    _____ b. A primary risk factor for congestive heart failure is **coronary artery disease**.

    _____ c. A common cause of diastolic failure is **left ventricular hypertrophy**.

    _____ d. The mechanisms by which **hypervolemia** acts as a precipitating cause of heart failure include decreasing cardiac output and increasing the workload of oxygen requirements of the myocardium.

    _____ e. Systolic heart failure results in a **normal** left ventricular ejection fraction.

2. Describe the primary ways in which each of the following compensatory mechanisms of congestive heart failure increases cardiac output, and identify at least one effect of the mechanism that is detrimental to cardiac function.

    a. Cardiac dilation

        ↑ CO:

        Detrimental effect:

    b. Cardiac hypertrophy

        ↑ CO:

        Detrimental effect:

    c. Sympathetic nervous system stimulation

        ↑ CO:

        Detrimental effect:

    d. Neurohormonal response

        (1) Renin-angiotensin system

            ↑ CO:

            Detrimental effect:

        (2) Atrial natriuretic peptide (ANP) and brain natriuretic peptide (BNP)

            ↑ CO:

            Detrimental effect:

3. The following diagram illustrates the pathophysiology of left-sided heart failure that occurs from elevated systemic vascular resistance. Indicate the point in the process, by number, where the other causes of heart failure listed below the diagram (a–h) would most likely initiate the process.

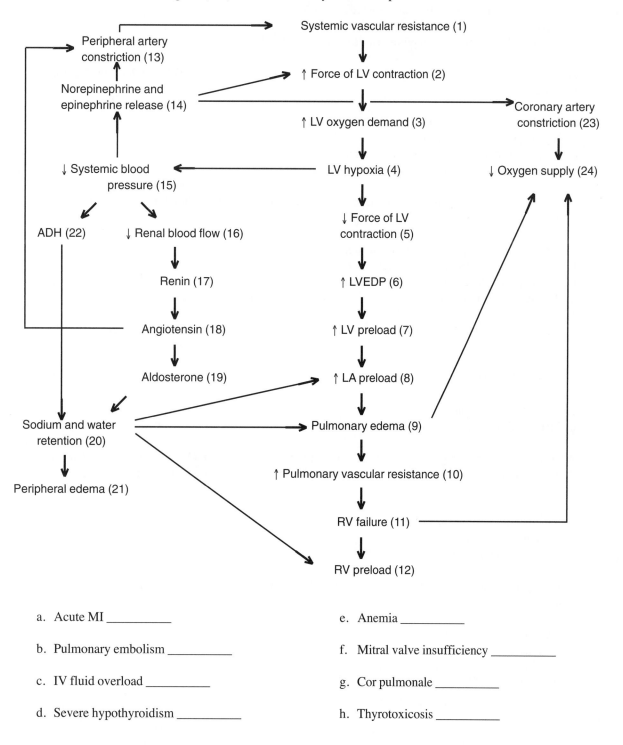

a. Acute MI _____

b. Pulmonary embolism _____

c. IV fluid overload _____

d. Severe hypothyroidism _____

e. Anemia _____

f. Mitral valve insufficiency _____

g. Cor pulmonale _____

h. Thyrotoxicosis _____

4. Using the diagram above, identify four points in the process, by number, where compensatory mechanisms

enter the process: _____, _____, _____, _____.

5. The pathophysiological mechanism that results in the pulmonary edema of left-sided heart failure is

   a. increased right ventricular preload.
   b. increased pulmonary hydrostatic pressure.
   c. impaired alveolar oxygen and carbon dioxide exchange.
   d. increased lymphatic flow of pulmonary extravascular fluid.

6. A physical assessment finding that the nurse would expect to be present in the client with acute left-sided heart failure is

   a. bubbling crackles and tachycardia.
   b. hepatosplenomegaly and tachypnea.
   c. peripheral edema and cool, diaphoretic skin.
   d. frothy blood-tinged sputum and distended jugular veins.

7. The nurse assesses the client with chronic biventricular congestive heart failure for paroxysmal nocturnal dyspnea by questioning the client regarding

   a. frequent awakening to void during the night.
   b. the presence of a dry, hacking cough when resting.
   c. difficulty breathing when lying flat in bed.
   d. the use of two or more pillows to help breathing during sleep.

8. An indication that the client with congestive heart failure is developing a complication of congestive heart failure is

   a. increased weight gain.
   b. development of ascites.
   c. restlessness and confusion.
   d. increased liver enzyme levels.

9. A client with chronic congestive heart failure has atrial fibrillation and an LV ejection fraction of 18%. To decrease the risk of complications from these conditions, the nurse anticipates the administration of

   a. diuretics.
   b. anticoagulants.
   c. β-adrenergic blockers.
   d. potassium supplements.

10. A diagnostic test that is most useful in assessing and monitoring the pulmonary effects of congestive heart failure is

   a. a chest x-ray.
   b. exercise stress testing.
   c. a cardiac catheterization.
   d. determination of blood urea nitrogen (BUN).

11. Using the diagram illustrated in question 4, indicate the point(s) in the process, by number, where the following treatment modalities are used to interrupt or reverse the pathophysiological process of congestive heart failure.

    a. Diuretics _____

    b. IV nitroglycerin _____

    c. IV nitroprusside _____

    d. Oxygen therapy _____

    e. ACE inhibitors _____

    f. Digitalis _____

    g. Milrinone (Primacor) _____

12. Match the following drugs used in the treatment of acute and chronic congestive heart failure with their therapeutic effects.

    _____ a. Spironolactone (Aldactone)

    _____ b. IV nitroglycerin

    _____ c. Digoxin (Lanoxin)

    _____ d. Furosemide (Lasix)

    _____ e. IV nitroprusside (Nipride)

    _____ f. Enalapril (Vasotec)

    _____ g. Dopamine (Intropin)

    _____ h. Milrinone (Primacor)

    _____ i. IV morphine

    _____ j. Carvedilol (Coreg)

    _____ k. Nesiritide (Natrecor)

    1. Improves cardiac contractions, decreases afterload, and increases cardiac output

    2. Dilates arterial and venous blood vessels in addition to relieving anxiety

    3. Recombinant form of a natriuretic peptide that decreases preload and afterload

    4. Primarily reduces preload and increases myocardial oxygen supply

    5. Directly blocks sympathetic nervous system's negative effects on the failing heart

    6. Potent vasodilator that decreases both preload and afterload, increasing cardiac contractility and output

    7. Decreases afterload by reducing levels of angiotensin II and aldosterone

    8. Primary effect is to decrease intravascular fluid volume, thus decreasing preload and improving left ventricular function

    9. Increases cardiac contractility but may increase ventricular irritability

    10. Increases cardiac contractility and output and slows heart rate

    11. Blocks action of aldosterone, decreasing intravascular volume by sodium excretion, but retains potassium

13. A client with chronic congestive heart failure is treated with hydrochlorothiazide, digoxin, and lisinopril (Prinivil). To prevent the risk of digitalis toxicity with these drugs, it is most important that the nurse monitor the client's

    a. heart rate.
    b. blood pressure.
    c. potassium levels.
    d. gastrointestinal function.

14. The physician prescribes spironolactone (Aldactone) for the client with chronic congestive heart failure. Diet modifications related to the use of this drug that the nurse includes in client teaching include

    a. decreasing both sodium and potassium intake.
    b. increasing calcium intake and decreasing sodium intake.
    c. decreasing sodium intake and increasing potassium intake.
    d. decreasing sodium intake and using salt substitutes for seasoning.

15. The nurse monitors the client receiving treatment for acute congestive heart failure with the knowledge that marked hypotension is most likely to occur with the intravenous administration of

    a. furosemide (Lasix).
    b. milrinone (Primacor).
    c. nitroglycerin.
    d. nitroprusside (Nipride).

16. A 2400-mg sodium diet is prescribed for a client with chronic congestive heart failure. The nurse recognizes that additional teaching is necessary when the client states,

    a. "I should limit my milk intake to two cups a day."
    b. "I can eat fresh fruits and vegetables without worrying about sodium content."
    c. "I can eat most foods as long as I do not add salt when cooking or at the table."
    d. "I need to read the labels on prepared foods and medicines for their sodium content."

17. List four heart conditions that may lead to congestive heart failure and what can be done to prevent the development of congestive heart failure in each condition.

    a.

    b.

    c.

    d.

18. The nurse determines that treatment of congestive heart failure has been successful when the client experiences

    a. weight loss and diuresis.
    b. warm skin and less fatigue.
    c. clear lung sounds and decreased heart rate.
    d. absence of chest pain and improved level of consciousness.

19. A client with CHF has tachypnea, severe dyspnea and an $SpO_2$ of 84%. The nurse identifies a nursing diagnosis of impaired gas exchange related to increased preload and mechanical failure. An appropriate nursing intervention for this diagnosis is

    a. assist the client to cough and breathe deeply q2h.
    b. assess intake and output q8h and weigh client daily.
    c. encourage alternate rest and activity periods to reduce cardiac workload.
    d. place the client in a high Fowler's position with the feet dangling over the bedside.

20. The nurse determines that additional discharge teaching is needed when the client with chronic congestive heart failure says,

    a. "I should hold my digitalis and call the doctor if I experience nausea and vomiting."
    b. "I will take my pulse every day and call the clinic if it is irregular or is less than 50."
    c. "I plan to organize my household tasks so I don't have to constantly go up and down the stairs."
    d. "I should weigh myself every morning and go on a diet if I gain more than two or three pounds in two days."

21. Indicate whether the following characteristics of cardiomyopathies are associated with dilated cardiomyopathy (D), hypertrophic cardiomyopathy (H), or restrictive cardiomyopathy (R).

    _____ a. The hyperdynamic systolic function creates a diastolic failure

    _____ b. Systemic embolization may occur because of stasis of blood in the ventricles

    _____ c. The most uncommon type of cardiomyopathy

    _____ d. Has a good prognosis with heart transplant

    _____ e. Autosomal-dominant genetic relationship

    _____ f. Differs from chronic congestive heart failure in that there is no ventricular hypertrophy

    _____ g. Echocardiogram reveals cardiomegaly with thin ventricular walls

    _____ h. Often results in syncope during increased activity due to obstructed aortic valve outflow

    _____ i. Often follows an infective myocarditis or exposure to toxins or drugs

    _____ j. Surgery to remove myocardial tissue may be indicated for symptoms refractory to treatment

    _____ k. Characterized by ventricular stiffness

    _____ l. Characterized by massive thickening of intraventricular septum and ventricular wall

22. When performing discharge teaching for the client with any type of cardiomyopathy, the nurse instructs the client to

    a. abstain from all alcohol intake.
    b. avoid strenuous activity and allow for periods of rest.
    c. restrict fluids to prevent volume overload and to decrease cardiac workload.
    d. plan for periodic returns to the healthcare facility for intermittent dobutamine (Dobutrex) or milrinone (Primacor) infusions.

23. The evaluation team for cardiac transplantation determines that the client who would most benefit from a new heart is

   a. a 24-year-old man with Down syndrome who has received excellent care from parents in their 60s.
   b. a 46-year-old single woman with a limited support system who has alcohol-induced cardiomyopathy.
   c. a 60-year-old man with inoperable coronary artery disease who has not been compliant with lifestyle changes and rehabilitation programs.
   d. a 52-year-old woman with end-stage coronary artery disease who has limited financial resources but is emotionally stable and has strong social support.

24. The nurse plans long-term goals for the client who has had a heart transplant with the knowledge that the most common cause of death in heart transplant clients is

   a. rejection.
   b. infection.
   c. heart failure.
   d. embolization.

## CASE STUDY

### DILATED CARDIOMYOPATHY

**Client Profile**

Mr. J. is a 43-year-old man who had an onset of flu with fever, pharyngitis, and malaise. Six days later he developed diffuse pericardial chest pain, jugular vein distension, dyspnea, and peripheral edema and was admitted to the hospital with a diagnosis of infectious myocarditis and possible dilated cardiomyopathy (CMP).

**Subjective Data**

- Has no history of cardiovascular disease
- Is very anxious and asks whether he is going to die
- Says his heart feels like it is "running away"
- Reports that he is so exhausted he cannot eat or drink by himself

**Objective Data**

- Height 175 cm (5 ft 10 in); weight 81.8 kg (180 lb)
- Vital signs: T 37.6°C (99. 6°F), HR 118 and irregular, RR 34, BP 90/58
- Cardiovascular: Distant $S_1$, $S_2$; $S_3$, $S_4$ present; PMI at sixth ICS and faint; all peripheral pulses are 1+; bilateral jugular vein distension, initial cardiac monitoring indicates a ventricular rate of 132 and atrial fibrillation
- Respiratory: Pulmonary crackles; decreased breath sounds right lower lobe; $SpO_2$ 82%
- Gastrointestinal: BS present; hepatomegaly 4 cm below costal margin

Laboratory work and diagnostic testing are scheduled.

## Critical Thinking Questions

1. What signs and symptoms of right and left heart failure is Mr. J. experiencing?

2. What difference in the ventricles is present in dilated cardiomyopathy as compared with congestive heart failure?

3. What diagnostic procedures and findings would help establish a diagnosis of dilated cardiomyopathy?

4. What nursing interventions are appropriate for Mr. J. at the time of his admission?

5. Drug therapy is started for Mr. J. to control his symptoms. What is the rationale for the administration of each of the following?

   a. digoxin (Lanoxin)

   b. furosemide (Lasix)

   c. milrinone (Primacor)

   d. enalapril (Vasotec)

   e. metoprolol (Lopressor)

6. Mr. J. does not respond well to treatment, and his condition deteriorates. Are there any alternative treatments for him?

7. Based on the assessment data presented, write one or more appropriate nursing diagnoses for Mr. J. Are there any collaborative problems?

# CHAPTER 35 NURSING MANAGEMENT: ARRHYTHMIAS

1. Identify whether the following statements are true or false. If a statement is false, correct the bold word(s) to make the statement true.

   _____ a. During **repolarization** of cardiac cells, sodium migrates rapidly into the cell, making the cell positive compared with the outside of the cell.

   _____ b. Depolarization of the cells in the ventricles produces the **T wave** on the ECG.

   _____ c. A client with a regular heart rate has four QRS complexes between every three-second marker on the ECG paper. The client's heart rate is **40 beats/min**.

   _____ d. The ECG pattern of a client with a regular heart rate reveals 20 small squares between each R-R interval. The client's heart rate is **75 beats/min**.

   _____ e. For cardiac monitor with a lead II, the **positive** electrode is placed on the upper right chest and the **negative** electrode is placed on the lower left chest.

   _____ f. Lead placement for $MCL_1$ monitoring is the positive electrode at the **fourth intercostal space at the right sternal border** and the negative electrode at the **left mid-clavicular line just below the clavicle**.

   _____ g. If the SA node fails to discharge an impulse, or discharges very slowly, a secondary pacemaker in the AV node is able to discharge at a rate of **30 to 40** times a minute.

   _____ h. **Re-entrant excitation** causing premature beats may occur when areas of the heart do not repolarize at the same rate because of depressed conduction.

   _____ i. An abnormal cardiac impulse that arises in the atria, ventricles, or AV junction that creates a premature beat is known as an **artifact**.

2. Match the following terms with their definitions.

   _____ a. Contractility

   _____ b. Conductivity

   _____ c. Excitability

   _____ d. Automaticity

   _____ e. Ectopic foci

   _____ f. Refractoriness

   1. Ability to spontaneously discharge an electrical impulse

   2. Abnormal electrical impulses

   3. Period in which heart tissue cannot be stimulated

   4. Ability to respond mechanically to an impulse

   5. Property of myocardial tissue that enables it to be depolarized by an impulse

   6. Ability to transmit an impulse along a membrane

3. The client's PR interval comprises six small boxes on the ECG graph. The nurse determines that this indicates

     a. a normal finding.
     b. a problem with ventricular depolarization.
     c. a disturbance in the repolarization of the atria.
     d. a problem with conduction from the SA node to the ventricular cells.

4. The nurse plans close monitoring for the client who has undergone electrophysiological testing because this test

     a. requires the use of dyes that irritate the myocardium.
     b. causes myocardial ischemia resulting in arrhythmias.
     c. induces arrhythmias that may require defibrillation to correct.
     d. involves the use anticoagulants to prevent thrombus and embolism.

5. Match the following arrhythmias with their descriptions.

     _____ a. Premature atrial contractions

     _____ b. Junctional escape rhythm

     _____ c. Sinus tachycardia

     _____ d. Asystole

     _____ e. Paroxysmal supraventricular tachycardia (PSVT)

     _____ f. First-degree AV block

     _____ g. Ventricular tachycardia

     _____ h. Sinus bradycardia

     _____ i. Atrial fibrillation

     _____ j. Premature ventricular contraction (PVC)

     _____ k. Type II AV block

     _____ l. Ventricular fibrillation

     _____ m. Third-degree AV block

1. Absence of ventricular activity
2. Wide, distorted QRS
3. Usual spontaneous onset and termination
4. Associated with bundle branch blocks
5. Chaotic ventricular rhythm
6. Normal rhythm pattern with rate < 60
7. Heart rate of 40 to 60 beats/min
8. May precipitate supraventricular tachycardia
9. Atria and ventricles dissociated
10. A run of PVCs
11. Prolonged PR interval
12. Chaotic P wave
13. Sinus rate >100

6. Complete the following statements.

   a. A client with an acute MI develops the following ECG pattern: atrial rate of 82 and regular; ventricular rate of 46 and regular; P wave and QRS complex are normal but there is no relationship between the P wave and the QRS complex. The nurse identifies the arrhythmia as _____, and the treatment indicated is _____.

   b. A common arrhythmia the nurse would expect to find in a client with hypoxemia and hypovolemia is _____.

   c. Vagal stimulation induced by carotid massage may be used to treat the arrhythmia of _____.

   d. An arrhythmia that is characterized by progressive lengthening of the PR interval until an atrial impulse is not conducted and a QRS complex is dropped is known as _____.

   e. PVCs that occur on the T wave of a preceding contraction are always treated because they may precipitate _____ or _____.

7. A client with heart disease has a sinus bradycardia of 48 beats/min. The nurse recognizes that the client is at greatest risk for

   a. asystole.
   b. heart block.
   c. sinus arrest.
   d. ectopic premature beats.

8. A client with an acute MI has a sinus tachycardia of 126 beats/min. The nurse recognizes that if this arrhythmia is not treated, the client is likely to experience

   a. hypertension.
   b. escape rhythms.
   c. ventricular tachycardia.
   d. an increase in infarct size.

9. A client with no history of heart disease has a rhythm strip that shows an occasional distorted P wave followed by normal AV and ventricular conduction. The nurse questions the client about

   a. the use of caffeine.
   b. the use of sedatives.
   c. any aerobic training.
   d. holding the breath during exertion.

10. A newly admitted client has the following rhythm pattern: heart rate 84 beats/min; regular rhythm; absent P wave; normal QRS complex. The nurse asks the client about the use of

    a. ASA.
    b. digoxin.
    c. caffeine.
    d. metoprolol (Lopressor).

11. A client's rhythm strip indicates a normal heart rate and rhythm with normal P wave and QRS complex, but the P-R interval is 0.26 seconds. The most appropriate action by the nurse is to

    a. continue to assess the client.
    b. administer atropine per protocol.
    c. prepare the client for synchronized cardioversion.
    d. prepare the client for placement of a temporary pacemaker.

12. In the client with an arrhythmia, the nurse identifies a nursing diagnosis of decreased cardiac output related to arrhythmias when the client experiences

    a. hypertension and bradycardia.
    b. chest pain and decreased mentation.
    c. abdominal distension and hepatomegaly.
    d. bounding pulses and a ventricular heave.

13. A client with an acute MI is having multifocal PVCs and ventricular couplets. He is alert and has a blood pressure of 118/78 with an irregular pulse of 86 beats/min. The most appropriate action by the nurse at this time is to

    a. continue to assess the client.
    b. be prepared to administer CPR.
    c. administer anti-arrhythmic drugs per protocol.
    d. ask the client to perform Valsalva manoeuvre.

14. Premature ventricular contractions are indicated by a rhythm pattern finding of

    a. a QRS complex of > 0.12 second followed by a P wave.
    b. continuous wide QRS complexes with a ventricular rate of 160 beats/min.
    c. sawtooth P waves with no measurable P-R interval and an irregular rhythm.
    d. P waves hidden in QRS complexes with a regular rhythm of 120 beats/min.

15. Following fibrinolytic therapy, the nurse monitors the client for the common reperfusion arrhythmias of

    a. sinus tachycardia and atrial fibrillation.
    b. supraventricular and ventricular tachycardia.
    c. premature atrial and ventricular contractions.
    d. premature ventricular contractions and ventricular tachycardia.

16. A client in the coronary care unit develops ventricular fibrillation. Within protocol guidelines, the first action the nurse should take is to

    a. initiate CPR.
    b. perform defibrillation.
    c. prepare for synchronized cardioversion.
    d. administer IV anti-arrhythmic drugs per protocol.

17. Cardiac defibrillation

    a. enhances repolarization and relaxation of ventricular myocardial cells.
    b. provides an electrical impulse that stimulates normal myocardial contractions.
    c. depolarizes the cells of the myocardium to allow the SA node to resume pacemaker function.
    d. delivers an electrical impulse to the heart at the time of ventricular contraction to convert the heart to a sinus rhythm.

18. Initial treatment of asystole and pulseless electrical activity is

    a. CPR.
    b. defibrillation.
    c. administration of atropine.
    d. administration of epinephrine.

19. The nurse's responsibilities in preparing to administer defibrillation include

    a. applying gel pads to the client's chest.
    b. setting the defibrillator to deliver 50 joules.
    c. setting the defibrillator to a synchronized mode.
    d. sedating the client with midazolam (Versed) before defibrillation.

20. While providing discharge instructions to the client who has had an implantable cardioverter-defibrillator (ICD) inserted, the nurse teaches the client that if she is alone when the ICD fires, she should

    a. lie down.
    b. call the physician.
    c. push the reset button on the pulse generator.
    d. immediately take her anti-arrhythmic medication.

21. A client with a sinus node dysfunction has a permanent pacemaker inserted. Before discharge, the nurse teaches the client to

    a. avoid cooking with microwave ovens.
    b. avoid high-voltage electrical generators.
    c. use mild analgesics to control the chest spasms caused by the pacing current.
    d. start lifting the arm above the shoulder right away to prevent a "frozen shoulder."

22. A client with a newly implanted pacemaker refuses to move his involved arm and shoulder and will not participate in his care. An appropriate nursing diagnosis for the client is

    a. decreased cardiac output related to arrhythmias.
    b. activity intolerance related to inadequate cardiac output.
    c. fear related to perceived vulnerability and reliance on pacemaker.
    d. impaired adjustment related to inability to modify lifestyle as needed.

23. The use of catheter ablation therapy to "burn" areas of the cardiac conduction system is indicated for treatment of

    a. sinus arrest.
    b. heart blocks.
    c. tachyarrhythmias.
    d. multifocal ectopic foci.

24. A 54-year-old client who has no structural heart disease has an episode of syncope. Upright tilt-table testing is performed to rule out neurocardiogenic syncope. The nurse explains to the client that if neurocardiogenic syncope is the problem, the client will experience

    a. palpitations and dizziness.
    b. tachyarrhythmias and chest pain.
    c. marked bradycardia and hypotension.
    d. no change in heart rate or blood pressure.

25. The nurse finds a client unresponsive in bed and determines that the client is in cardiopulmonary arrest. From the time of cardiac arrest until CPR is started, the maximum time that should elapse is

    a. 35 seconds.
    b. 60 seconds.
    c. three to four minutes.
    d. four to six minutes.

26. Listed below are the steps required in establishing one-person CPR by a health professional in the hospital system. Number the steps in sequence.

    _____ a. Call a code and ask for the crash cart

    _____ b. Determine cessation of breathing

    _____ c. Begin chest compressions

    _____ d. Open the airway

    _____ e. Determine unresponsiveness

    _____ f. Position the victim on back

    _____ g. Determine absence of pulse

    _____ h. Ventilate twice

27. After chest compressions are initiated in CPR, reassessment to determine if spontaneous breathing and circulation have returned should be done after

    a. two cycles of compressions and ventilations.
    b. four cycles of compressions and ventilations.
    c. eight cycles of compressions and ventilations.
    d. five minutes of compressions and ventilations.

28. The most significant factor in the positive outcome of a client with a cardiac arrest is

    a. absence of underlying heart disease.
    b. rapid institution of emergency services and procedures.
    c. performance of perfect technique in resuscitation procedures.
    d. maintenance of 50% of normal cardiac output during resuscitation efforts.

29. While the nurse is feeding a client who is sitting in a chair, the client chokes, cannot speak, and turns blue. The nurse should

    a. place the client on the floor and perform a finger-sweep manoeuvre to attempt to remove the obstruction.
    b. stand behind the chair, hug the client, and deliver abdominal thrusts with the fist of one hand held by the other hand.
    c. leave the client in the chair and attempt rescue breathing with mouth-to-mouth ventilation after hyperextending the head.
    d. move the client to the floor, kneel astride the client, and administer abdominal thrusts with the heel of one hand covered with the other hand.

30. Before administering drugs in cardiac emergencies as part of advanced cardiac life support (ACLS), it is important to first

    a. administer defibrillation.
    b. insert an endotracheal tube.
    c. check the client for the presence of a pulse.
    d. establish ECG monitoring and identify arrhythmias.

31. Identify the following cardiac rhythms using the systematic approach to assessing cardiac rhythms found in Table 35-7 in the textbook. All rhythm strips are six seconds.

    a.

    b.

    c.

d.

e.

f.

g.

h.

i.

j.

k.

l.

m.

n.

o.

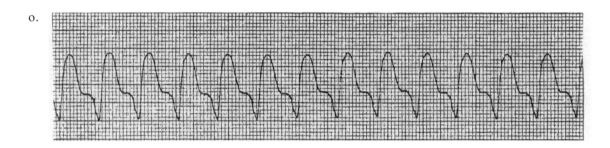

## CASE STUDY

### ARRHYTHMIA

### Client Profile

Mrs. S. is a 75-year-old woman admitted to the telemetry unit with a diagnosis of atrial fibrillation.

### Subjective Data

- Has a history of hypothyroidism and hypertension
- Has no history of atrial fibrillation
- Is taking levothyroxin (Synthroid) 0.05 mg PO qd and enalapril (Vasotec) 5 mg PO bid
- Complains of palpitations, dizziness, shortness of breath, and mild chest pressure

### Objective Data

- Physical examination
    Alert, anxious, elderly woman
    BP 100/70, HR 150/min, RR 32/min
    Lungs: bibasilar crackles
    Heart: $S_1$ and $S_2$, irregularly irregular
- Diagnostic study
    ECG: atrial fibrillation

### Collaborative Care

- Discontinue enalapril (Vasotec)
- Digoxin 0.25 mg PO qd
- Diltiazem (Cardizem) 60 mg PO q8h
- Warfarin (Coumadin) 5 mg PO qd

**Critical Thinking Questions**

1. What is the immediate goal of anti-arrhythmic drug therapy for Mrs. S.?

2. What non-pharmacological therapy may be used to treat the arrhythmia?

3. Explain the rationale for use of the medications ordered for Mrs. S.

4. Explain the pathophysiology of her symptoms on admission to the telemetry unit.

5. Describe the characteristics of her ECG wave form.

6. Based on the assessment data presented, write one or more appropriate nursing diagnoses. Are there any collaborative problems?

# CHAPTER 36    NURSING MANAGEMENT: INFLAMMATORY AND VALVULAR HEART DISEASES

1. A 20-year-old client has acute right-sided infective endocarditis. While obtaining a nursing history, the nurse recognizes as most significant the client's history of

   a. intravenous drug abuse.
   b. a recent urinary tract infection.
   c. a recent professional teeth cleaning.
   d. rheumatic fever without a heart murmur.

2. A client has an admitting diagnosis of acute left-sided infective endocarditis. The nurse explains to the client that this diagnosis is best confirmed with

   a. blood cultures.
   b. a complete blood count.
   c. a cardiac catheterization.
   d. a transesophageal echocardiogram.

3. Match the following manifestations of infective endocarditis with their descriptions.

   _____  a. Splinter hemorrhages          1. Hemorrhagic retinal lesions

   _____  b. Janeway's lesions             2. Painful red or purple lesions on
                                              fingers or toes
   _____  c. Osler's nodes
                                           3. Black longitudinal streaks in
   _____  d. Roth's spots                     nailbeds

   _____  e. Petechiae                     4. Small hemorrhages in conjunctiva,
                                              lips, and buccal mucosa

                                           5. Flat, red, painless spots on palms and soles of
                                              feet

4. A client with infective endocarditis of a prosthetic mitral valve develops a left hemiparesis and visual changes. The nurse expects that medical management of the client will include

   a. an embolectomy.
   b. surgical valve replacement.
   c. administration of anticoagulants.
   d. higher than usual antibiotic dosages.

5. A client with aortic valve endocarditis develops dyspnea, crackles in the lungs, and restlessness. The nurse suspects that the client is experiencing

   a. vegetative embolization to the coronary arteries.
   b. pulmonary embolization from valve vegetations.
   c. non-specific manifestations that accompany infectious diseases.
   d. valvular incompetence with possible infectious invasion of the myocardium.

250

6. A client hospitalized for one week with subacute infective endocarditis is afebrile and has no signs of heart damage, and discharge with outpatient antibiotic therapy is planned. During discharge planning with the client, it is most important for the nurse to

   a. plan how his needs will be met while he continues on bed rest.
   b. teach the client to avoid crowds and exposure to upper respiratory infections.
   c. encourage the use of diversional activities to relieve boredom and restlessness.
   d. assess the client's home environment in terms of family assistance and hospital access.

7. When teaching a client with endocarditis how to prevent recurrence of the infection, the nurse instructs the client to

   a. start on antibiotic therapy when exposed to persons with infections.
   b. take one ASA a day to prevent vegetative lesions from forming around the valves.
   c. obtain prophylactic antibiotic therapy before any invasive medical or dental procedures.
   d. always maintain continuous antibiotic therapy to prevent the development of any systemic infection.

8. A client is admitted to the hospital with a suspected acute pericarditis. To establish the presence of a pericardial friction rub, the nurse listens to the client's chest

   a. while timing the sound with the respiratory pattern.
   b. with the bell of the stethoscope at the apex of the heart.
   c. with the diaphragm of the stethoscope at the lower left sternal border of the chest.
   d. with the diaphragm of the stethoscope to auscultate a high-pitched continuous rumbling sound.

9. A client with acute pericarditis has markedly distended jugular veins, decreased blood pressure, tachycardia, tachypnea, and muffled heart sounds. The nurse recognizes that these symptoms occur when

   a. the pericardial space is obliterated with scar tissue and thickened pericardium.
   b. excess pericardial fluid compresses the heart and prevents adequate diastolic filling.
   c. the parietal and visceral pericardial membranes adhere to each other, preventing normal myocardial contraction.
   d. fibrin accumulation on the visceral pericardium infiltrates into the myocardium, creating generalized myocardial dysfunction.

10. Identify whether the following statements are true or false. If a statement is false, correct the bold word(s) to make the statement true.

   _____ a. To measure a pulsus paradoxus, the nurse determines the difference between the systolic pressure **at inspiration** and the systolic pressure **at expiration**.

   _____ b. A pulsus paradoxus of >10 mm Hg occurs with **cardiac tamponade**.

   _____ c. A pericardiocentesis is indicated for the client with pericarditis when there is a **pericardial effusion of any amount**.

   _____ d. Acute pericarditis may be diagnosed with **specific ECG changes that evolve over time.**

   _____ e. Treatment of chronic constrictive pericarditis may include a **pericardiectomy.**

11. A client with acute pericarditis has a nursing diagnosis of pain related to pericardial inflammation. An appropriate nursing intervention for the client is

   a. administering narcotics as prescribed on a round-the-clock schedule.
   b. promoting progressive relaxation exercises with the use of deep, slow breathing.
   c. positioning the client on the right side with the head of the bed elevated 15 degrees.
   d. positioning the client in Fowler's position with a padded overbed table for the client to lean on.

12. When obtaining a nursing history for a client with myocarditis, the nurse specifically questions the client about

   a. prior use of digoxin for treatment of cardiac problems.
   b. recent symptoms of a viral illness such as fever and malaise.
   c. a recent streptococcal infection requiring treatment with penicillin.
   d. a history of coronary artery disease with or without a myocardial infarction.

13. A 19-year-old client with rheumatic heart disease is admitted to the hospital with a recurrence of acute rheumatic fever. In planning care for the client, the nurse recognizes that an appropriate nursing diagnosis for the client is

   a. ineffective coping related to refusal to carry out health promotion activities.
   b. risk for infection related to recent exposure to group A β-hemolytic streptococci.
   c. impaired adjustment related to unsuccessful life style modifications, goal setting, and problem solving.
   d. ineffective management of therapeutic regimen related to lack of knowledge of or compliance with prophylactic antibiotic therapy.

14. The most important role of the nurse in preventing rheumatic fever is to

   a. teach clients with infective endocarditis to adhere to antibiotic prophylaxis.
   b. identify clients with valvular heart disease who are at risk for rheumatic fever.
   c. encourage the use of antibiotics for treatment of all infections involving a sore throat.
   d. promote the early diagnosis and immediate treatment of group A β-hemolytic streptococcal pharyngitis.

15. A client with rheumatic carditis asks the nurse if his heart is infected with streptococcal organisms. The best response of the nurse is

   a. "It is thought that antibodies produced in response to a streptococcal infection then attack normal body tissues."
   b. "Yes, it is a complication that may occur with any group A β-hemolytic streptococcal infection if it is not treated early."
   c. "The heart is not really infected, but toxins produced by streptococci infecting the throat can damage the heart and other tissues."
   d. "The relationship between streptococcal infections and rheumatic fever is not known, but penicillin is used in treatment just in case there is an infection."

16. The diagnosis of acute rheumatic fever is most strongly supported in the client with

   a. organic heart murmurs, fever, and elevated ESR.
   b. polyarthritis, chorea, and increased anti-streptolysin O titre.
   c. cardiac enlargement, polyarthritis, and erythema marginatum.
   d. positive C-reactive protein, elevated WBC, subcutaneous nodules.

17. Residual and chronic cardiac damage from acute rheumatic fever most often includes

   a. myocardial scarring.
   b. chronic constrictive pericarditis.
   c. blockade of the conduction system.
   d. scarring and contractures of the mitral valve.

18. Identify the rationale for the use of the following drugs in the treatment of acute rheumatic fever.

    a. Penicillin

    b. ASA

    c. Corticosteroids

19. To establish a balance of activity-rest to prevent hazards of immobility yet decrease cardiac workload in the client with acute rheumatic carditis, the nurse

    a. allows full ambulation as soon as acute symptoms have subsided.
    b. promotes bed rest until anti-inflammatory therapy has been discontinued.
    c. encourages non-strenuous activities as soon as antibiotic therapy is initiated.
    d. maintains the client on bed rest until symptoms of congestive heart failure are controlled.

20. The nurse teaches the adult client recovering from rheumatic heart disease that antibiotic prophylaxis

    a. is required for only five years in adults with rheumatic heart disease.
    b. promotes bed rest until anti-inflammatory therapy has been discontinued.
    c. encourages non-strenuous activities as soon as antibiotic therapy is initiated.
    d. is not required if good nutrition, adequate rest, and stringent hygiene are maintained.

21. Identify whether the following statements are true or false. If a statement is false, correct the bold word(s) to make the statement true.

    _____ a. Valvular stenosis leads to **backward flow** of blood and **dilation** of the preceding chamber.

    _____ b. **Valvular regurgitation** causes a pressure gradient difference across an open valve.

    _____ c. The heart valve most commonly affected by stenosis or regurgitation is the **tricuspid** valve.

    _____ d. One of the most common forms of valvular heart disease is **mitral stenosis**.

22. Number in sequence the pathophysiological processes of mitral valve stenosis.

    _____ a. Fluid moves into the pulmonary extravascular space and alveoli.

    _____ b. Pulmonary artery pressure increases.

    _____ c. During diastole, a pressure gradient difference occurs between the left atrium and the left ventricle.

    _____ d. The left atrium dilates and pulmonary vessels hypertrophy.

    _____ e. The right ventricle fails.

    _____ f. Adhesions and contractures of valve leaflets and chordae tendineae occur, narrowing the valve opening.

    _____ g. The right ventricle hypertrophies in response to pressure overload in the pulmonary vasculature.

    _____ h. Pressure increases in left atrium, pulmonary veins, and pulmonary capillaries.

23. Match the following characteristics with the related type of valvular disease (answers may be used more than once).

_____ a. Sudden onset of cardiovascular collapse

_____ b. May be caused by pulmonary hypertension

_____ c. Rapid development of pulmonary edema and cardiogenic shock

_____ d. Dyspnea is prominent symptom

_____ e. Loud pansystolic or holosystolic murmur

_____ f. Ballooning of valve into left atrium during ventricular systole

_____ g. Characteristic systolic crescendo-decrescendo murmur

_____ h. Corrigan's (water-hammer) pulses

_____ i. Angina and syncope result from decreased cardiac output

_____ j. Embolization may result from chronic atrial fibrillation

_____ k. Major symptoms related to elevated systemic venous pressures

_____ l. Rapid onset prevents left chamber dilation

_____ m. Brisk carotid pulses present

1. Mitral stenosis

2. Acute mitral regurgitation

3. Chronic mitral regurgitation

4. Mitral valve prolapse

5. Aortic stenosis

6. Acute aortic regurgitation

7. Chronic aortic regurgitation

8. Tricuspid valve disease

24. Drugs that the nurse would expect to be prescribed for most clients with valvular heart disease include

a. oral nitrates.
b. anticoagulants.
c. atrial anti-arrhythmics.
d. β-adrenergic blocking agents.

25. A client with symptomatic mitral valve prolapse has atrial and ventricular arrhythmias. In addition to monitoring for decreased cardiac output related to the arrhythmias, an appropriate nursing diagnosis related to the arrhythmias identified by the nurse is

a. ineffective breathing pattern related to hypervolemia.
b. risk for injury related to dizziness and light-headedness.
c. disturbed sleep pattern related to paroxysmal nocturnal dyspnea.
d. ineffective therapeutic regimen management related to lack of knowledge of prevention and treatment strategies.

26. A client is scheduled for a percutaneous transluminal balloon valvuloplasty. The nurse understands that this procedure is indicated for

    a. any client with aortic regurgitation.
    b. older clients with tricuspid valve stenosis.
    c. young adult clients with mild mitral valve stenosis.
    d. clients with valvular stenosis who are poor surgical risks.

27. A client is scheduled for an open surgical valvuloplasty of the mitral valve. In preparing the client for surgery, the nurse recognizes that

    a. cardiopulmonary bypass is not required with this procedure.
    b. valve repair is a palliative measure, while valve replacement is curative.
    c. the operative mortality rate is lower in valve repair than in valve replacement.
    d. clients with valve repair do not require post-operative anticoagulation as they do with valve replacement.

28. A mechanical prosthetic valve is most likely to be preferred over a biological valve for valve replacement in a

    a. 41-year-old man with peptic ulcer disease.
    b. 22-year-old woman who desires to have children.
    c. 35-year-old man with a history of seasonal asthma.
    d. 62-year-old woman with early Alzheimer's disease.

29. When performing discharge teaching for the client following a mechanical valve replacement, the nurse determines that further instruction is needed when the client says,

    a. "I may begin an exercise program to gradually increase my cardiac tolerance."
    b. "I will always need to have my blood checked once a month for its clotting function."
    c. "I should wear a Medic Alert bracelet to identify my valve and anticoagulant therapy."
    d. "The biggest risk I have during invasive health procedures is bleeding because of my anticoagulants."

## CASE STUDY

### INFECTIVE ENDOCARDITIS

#### Client Profile

Mr. B. is a 60-year-old man who is hospitalized with a suspected cerebrovascular accident.

#### Subjective Data

- Had a laparoscopic cholecystectomy a few weeks ago

#### Objective Data

- Neurological signs typical of a stroke
- Petechiae over chest
- Crescendo-decrescendo murmur present
- Rectal temperature 39.4°C (103°F)

## Critical Thinking Questions

1. What places Mr. B. at high risk for infective endocarditis?

2. What asymptomatic underlying cardiac conditions may Mr. B. have had that contributed to his infectious endocarditis?

3. Explain the cause of Mr. B.'s assessment findings.

4. What is the relevance of the endoscopic surgery he had a few weeks before this hospital admission?

5. What treatment would the nurse anticipate for Mr. B.?

6. Discuss how Mr. B.'s infective endocarditis could have been prevented.

7. Based on the assessment data presented, write one or more appropriate nursing diagnoses. Are there any collaborative problems?

# CHAPTER 37 NURSING MANAGEMENT: VASCULAR DISORDERS

1. When obtaining a health history from a 72-year-old man with peripheral arterial disease of the lower extremities, the nurse asks the client about a history of other atherosclerotic manifestations such as

   a. venous thrombosis.
   b. venous stasis ulcers.
   c. pulmonary embolism.
   d. carotid artery disease.

2. Match the following descriptions with the related types of aneurysms.

   _____ a. Pouch-like bulge of artery              1. Fusiform aneurysm

   _____ b. Disruption of all layers of an artery with    2. Saccular aneurysm
            bleeding
                                                    3. Pseudoaneurysm
   _____ c. Uniform, circumferential dilation of artery

3. A surgical repair is planned for a client who has a 5-cm abdominal aortic aneurysm. On physical assessment of the client, the nurse would expect to find

   a. hoarseness and dysphagia.
   b. severe back pain with flank ecchymosis.
   c. the presence of a bruit in the periumbilical area.
   d. weakness in the lower extremities progressing to paraplegia.

4. A thoracic aortic aneurysm is found when a client has a routine chest x-ray. The nurse anticipates that additional diagnostic testing to determine the size and structure of the aneurysm will include

   a. a CT scan.
   b. angiography.
   c. echocardiography.
   d. ultrasonography.

5. A client with a small abdominal aortic aneurysm is not a good surgical candidate. The nurse teaches the client that one of the best ways to prevent expansion of the lesion is to

   a. avoid strenuous physical exertion.
   b. control hypertension with prescribed therapy.
   c. comply with prescribed anticoagulant therapy.
   d. maintain a low-calcium diet to prevent calcification of the vessel.

6. During preoperative preparation of the client scheduled for an abdominal aortic aneurysm, the nurse establishes baseline data for the client knowing that

   a. post-operatively all physiological processes will be altered.
   b. the cause of the aneurysm is a systemic vascular disease.
   c. surgery will be cancelled if any physiological function is not normal.
   d. blood pressure and heart rate will be maintained below normal levels during the post-operative period.

258          Copyright © 2007, Elsevier Canada, Ltd. All rights reserved.

7. Complete the following statements.

   a. A(n) _____ aneurysm may be surgically treated by excising only the weakened area and suturing the artery closed.

   b. During conventional aortic aneurysm repair, a(n) _____ _____ is sutured to the aorta above and below the aneurysm, and the native aorta is replaced around the site.

   c. Repair of _____ aneurysms requires cross-clamping of the aorta proximal and distal to the aneurysm.

   d. A synthetic bifurcation graft is used in aneurysm repair when an abdominal aortic aneurysm extends into the _____ arteries.

   e. Repair of an aortic aneurysm by placing an aortic graft inside the aneurysm through the femoral artery is called the _____ _____ procedure.

   f. Major complications of aortic aneurysm repair are associated with involvement or obstruction of the _____ arteries.

8. During the client's acute post-operative period following repair of an aneurysm, the nurse should ensure that

   a. hypothermia is maintained to decrease oxygen need.
   b. the blood pressure and all peripheral pulses are evaluated at least every hour.
   c. IV fluids are administered at a rate to maintain an hourly urine output of 100 mL.
   d. the client's blood pressure is kept lower than baseline to prevent leaking at the suture line.

9. Following an ascending aortic aneurysm repair, the nurse monitors for and immediately reports

   a. shallow respirations and poor coughing.
   b. decreased drainage from the chest tubes.
   c. a change in level of consciousness and ability to speak.
   d. lower extremity pulses that are decreased from preoperative baseline.

10. Identify at least one observation made by the nurse that would indicate the presence of the following complications of aortic aneurysm repair.

    a. Graft thrombosis

    b. Myocardial ischemia

    c. Bowel infarction

    d. Graft infection

    e. Impaired renal perfusion

    f. Spinal cord ischemia

11. Following discharge teaching of a male client with an abdominal aortic aneurysm repair, the nurse determines that further instruction is needed when the client says,

    a. "I may have some permanent sexual dysfunction as a result of the surgery."
    b. "I may continue to have a poor appetite and irregular bowel patterns for a while."
    c. "I should take the pulses in my extremities and let the doctor know if they get too fast or too slow."
    d. "I must maintain a low-fat and low-cholesterol diet to help the new graft open."

12. During the nursing assessment of the client with a distal descending aortic dissection, the nurse would expect the client to manifest

    a. a cardiac murmur characteristic of aortic valve insufficiency.
    b. altered level of consciousness with dizziness and weak carotid pulses.
    c. severe hypertension and orthopnea and dyspnea of pulmonary edema.
    d. severe "ripping" back or abdominal pain with descending organ ischemia.

13. A client with a dissection of the arch of the aorta has a decreased level of consciousness and weak carotid pulses. The nurse anticipates that initial treatment of the client will include

    a. administration of packed RBCs to replace blood loss.
    b. immediate surgery to replace the torn area with a graft.
    c. administration of anticoagulants to prevent embolization.
    d. administration of antihypertensives to maintain a MAP of 70 to 80 mm Hg.

14. The nurse evaluates that treatment for the client with an uncomplicated aortic dissection is successful when

    a. pain is relieved.
    b. surgical repair is completed.
    c. renal output is maintained at 30 mL/hr.
    d. blood pressure is within normal range.

15. Complete the following statements.

    a. The classic ischemic pain of peripheral arterial disease is known as _____.

    b. Two serious complications of peripheral arterial disease that frequently lead to lower limb amputation are

       _____ and _____.

    c. A client with chronic arterial disease has a brachial systolic blood pressure of 132 mm Hg and an ankle

       systolic blood pressure of 102 mm Hg. The ankle-brachial index is _____ and indicates

       _____ (mild/moderate/severe) arterial disease.

    d. Surgery for peripheral arterial disease is indicated when the client has limb pain during _____.

16. Drug therapy for peripheral arterial disease to increase blood flow and prevent intermittent claudication includes the administration of

    a. ASA.
    b. cilostazol (Pletal).
    c. ticlopidine (Ticlid).
    d. clopidogrel (Plavix).

17. Match the following descriptions with the therapeutic procedures used for arterial occlusive disease.

_____ a. Removing obstructive plaques by opening the artery

_____ b. Helps prevent re-stenosis following angioplasty

_____ c. Often performed to reduce plaque size before angioplasty

_____ d. Surgical widening of the arterial lumen

_____ e. Best results in localized iliac and femoral artery lesions

_____ f. Autogenous vein or synthetic graft used to divert blood around occlusion

1. Percutaneous transluminal balloon angioplasty

2. Peripheral arterial bypass

3. Intravascular stent

4. Endarterectomy

5. Patch graft angioplasty

6. Atherectomy

18. A client with peripheral arterial disease has a nursing diagnosis of ineffective peripheral tissue perfusion. Appropriate teaching for the client includes instructions to

a. rest and sleep with the legs elevated.
b. soak the feet in warm water 30 minutes a day.
c. walk at least 30 minutes a day to the point of pain.
d. use nicotine replacement therapy as a substitute for smoking.

19. When teaching the client with peripheral disease about modifying risk factors associated with the condition, the nurse emphasizes that

a. amputation is the ultimate outcome if the client does not alter lifestyle behaviours.
b. risk-reducing behaviours initiated after angioplasty can stop the progression of the disease.
c. maintenance of normal body weight is the most important factor in controlling arterial disease.
d. modifications will reduce the risk of other atherosclerotic conditions such as coronary heart disease.

20. Indicate whether the following findings are characteristic of arterial disease (A) or venous disease (V).

_____ a. Paraesthesia

_____ b. Heavy ulcer drainage

_____ c. Edema around the ankles

_____ d. Gangrene over bony prominences on toes and feet

_____ e. Decreased peripheral pulses

_____ f. Brown pigmentation of the legs

_____ g. Thickened, brittle nails

_____ h. Ulceration around the medial malleolus

_____ i. Pallor on elevation of the legs

_____ j. Dull ache in calf or thigh

_____ k. Pruritus

21. A client with peripheral vascular disease has marked peripheral neuropathy. An appropriate nursing diagnosis for the client is

    a. risk for injury related to decreased sensation.
    b. impaired skin integrity related to decreased peripheral circulation.
    c. ineffective peripheral tissue perfusion related to decreased arterial blood flow.
    d. activity intolerance related to imbalance between oxygen supply and demand.

22. During care of the client following femoral bypass graft surgery, the nurse immediately notifies the physician if the client experiences

    a. fever and redness at the incision site.
    b. 2+ edema of the extremity and pain at the incision site.
    c. a loss of palpable pulses and numbness and tingling of the feet.
    d. decreasing ankle-brachial indices and serous drainage from the incision.

23. A client has chronic atrial fibrillation and develops an acute arterial occlusion at the iliac artery bifurcation. What are the six *P*s of acute arterial occlusion the nurse may find in the client?

    a. _____    c. _____    e. _____

    b. _____    d. _____    f. _____

24. Indicate whether the following manifestations and treatments are characteristic of thromboangiitis obliterans (Buerger's disease) (B) or arteriospastic disease (Raynaud's phenomenon) (R).

    _____ a. Involves small cutaneous arteries of the fingers and toes

    _____ b. Inflammation of midsized arteries and veins

    _____ c. Treated with calcium-channel blockers, especially nifedipine (Procardia)

    _____ d. Strongly associated with smoking

    _____ e. Predominant in young females

    _____ f. Episodes involve white, blue, and red colour changes of fingertips

    _____ g. Amputation of digits or legs below the knee may be necessary for ulceration and gangrene

    _____ h. Precipitated by exposure to cold, caffeine, and tobacco

    _____ i. Intermittent claudication of feet, arms, and hands may be present

    _____ j. Frequently associated with autoimmune disorders

25. Identify the factor(s) of Virchow's triad present in each of the following conditions associated with deep venous thrombosis (DVT).

    a. IV therapy

    b. Prolonged immobilization

    c. Estrogen therapy

    d. Abdominal surgery

    e. Smoking

    f. Pregnancy

26. Identify whether the following statements are true or false. If a statement is false, correct the bold word(s) to make the statement true.

    _____ a. The most common cause of superficial thrombophlebitis in the legs is **IV therapy**.

    _____ b. A tender, red, inflamed induration along the course of a subcutaneous vein is characteristic of a **deep venous thrombosis**.

    _____ c. A client with deep venous thrombosis is scheduled for surgical treatment. The nurse recognizes that surgery is most commonly performed for this condition to **insert a vena cava interruption device** to prevent pulmonary embolism.

    _____ d. The method of prevention of deep venous thrombosis in hospitalized clients that addresses all three aspects of Virchow's triad is the use of **elastic compression stockings**.

27. To help prevent embolization of the thrombus in a client with a DVT, the nurse teaches the client to

    a. dangle the feet over the edge of the bed q2–3h.
    b. ambulate for short periods three to four times a day.
    c. keep the affected leg elevated above the level of the heart.
    d. maintain bed rest until edema is relieved and anticoagulation is established.

28. Match the following anticoagulant drugs with their characteristics (answers may be used more than once).

    _____ a. Is only administered IV              1. Unfractionated heparin

    _____ b. No antidote for anticoagulant effect  2. Low-molecular-weight heparin

    _____ c. Vitamin K is antidote                 3. Hirudin derivatives

    _____ d. Is only administered SC               4. Coumarin derivatives

    _____ e. Routine coagulation tests not usually required

    _____ f. Protamine sulphate is antidote

    _____ g. May be administered IV or SC

    _____ h. Is only administered orally

    _____ i. INR used to monitor anticoagulant effect

29. The client with DVT is receiving therapy with heparin and asks the nurse if the drug will dissolve the clot in her leg. The best response of the nurse is

    a. "This drug will break up and dissolve the clot so that circulation in the vein can be restored."
    b. "The purpose of the heparin is to prevent growth of the clot or formation of new clots where the circulation is slowed."
    c. "Heparin won't dissolve the clot, but will inhibit the inflammation around the clot and delay the development of new clots."
    d. "The heparin will dilate the vein, preventing turbulence of blood flow around the clot that may cause it to break off and travel to the lungs."

30. A client with DVT is to be discharged on long-term warfarin (Coumadin) therapy and is taught about prevention and continuing treatment of DVT. The nurse determines that discharge teaching for the client has been effective when the client states,

    a. "I should expect that Coumadin will cause my stools to be somewhat black."
    b. "I should avoid all dark green and leafy vegetables while I am taking Coumadin."
    c. "Massaging my legs several times a day will help increase my venous circulation."
    d. "Swimming is a good activity to include in my exercise program to increase my circulation."

31. The nurse teaches the client with any venous disorder that the best way to prevent venous stasis and increase venous return is to

    a. walk.
    b. sit with the legs elevated.
    c. frequently rotate the ankles.
    d. continuously wear compression gradient stockings.

32. Number in sequence the processes that occur as venous stasis precipitates varicose veins leading to venous stasis ulcers.

    _____   a. Venous blood flow reverses

    _____   b. Edema forms

    _____   c. Venous pressure increases

    _____   d. Additional venous distension occurs

    _____   e. Blood supply to local tissues decreases

    _____   f. Venous valves become incompetent

    _____   g. Ulceration occurs

    _____   h. Capillary pressure increases

    _____   i. Veins dilate

33. The most important measure in the treatment of venous stasis ulcers is

    a. elevation of the limb.
    b. extrinsic compression.
    c. application of moist dressings.
    d. application of topical antibiotics.

34. A post-surgical client has an acute onset of dyspnea, tachycardia, and chest pain. While the physician is being notified, the nurse should

   a. elevate the head of the bed.
   b. administer oxygen at 6 L/min.
   c. elevate the lower extremities.
   d. start an IV line with $D_5W$ at a slow rate.

35. To determine the location of a pulmonary embolism, the nurse would expect the physician to order a(n)

   a. ECG.
   b. chest x-ray.
   c. perfusion lung scan.
   d. pulmonary angiogram.

# CASE STUDY

## ABDOMINAL AORTIC ANEURYSM (AAA)

### Client Profile

Mr. S. is a 73-year-old man who was brought to the local emergency department complaining of severe back pain.

### Subjective Data

- Has a known AAA, which has been followed with yearly abdominal ultrasounds
- Has smoked one pack per day for 52 years
- Has had occasional bouts of angina for the past three years

### Objective Data

- Has a pulsating abdominal mass
- BP 88/68 mm Hg
- Extremities are cool and clammy

## Critical Thinking Questions

1. What are Mr. S.'s risk factors for AAA?

2. Define the etiology of an AAA.

3. Which signs or symptoms make the nurse suspect that Mr. S. has a ruptured AAA rather than a non-ruptured AAA?

4. What is the first priority in this client's care?

5. What is the nurse's role in assisting the family in this critical situation?

6. What steps, if any, could have been taken to prevent the rupture of the AAA?

7. Based on the assessment data presented, write one or more appropriate nursing diagnoses. Are there any collaborative problems?

1. Identify the structures in the following illustrations.

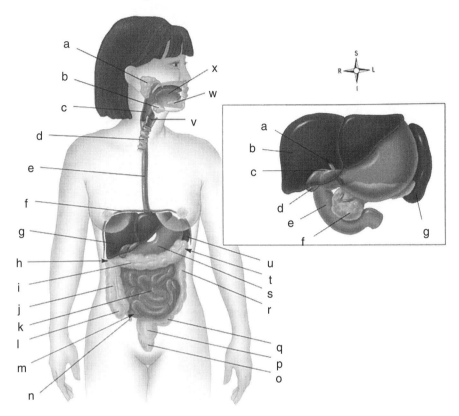

a. _____    i. _____    q. _____

b. _____    j. _____    r. _____

c. _____    k. _____    s. _____

d. _____    l. _____    t. _____

e. _____    m. _____    u. _____

f. _____    n. _____    v. _____

g. _____    o. _____    w. _____

h. _____    p. _____    x. _____

Inset:

a. _____    d. _____    g. _____

b. _____    e. _____

c. _____    f. _____

2. Identify the structures in the following illustration.

| | | |
|---|---|---|
| a. _____ | f. _____ | k. _____ |
| b. _____ | g. _____ | l. _____ |
| c. _____ | h. _____ | m. _____ |
| d. _____ | i. _____ | n. _____ |
| e. _____ | j. _____ | o. _____ |

3. A client receives atropine, an anticholinergic drug, in preparation for surgery. The nurse expects this drug to affect the gastrointestinal tract by

   a.   increasing gastric emptying.
   b.   relaxing pyloric and ileocecal sphincters.
   c.   decreasing secretions and peristaltic action.
   d.   depressing the nervous system of the GI tract.

4. A client with an inflamed gallbladder experiences pain after eating caused by contraction of the gallbladder. The mechanism responsible for this action is

   a.   production of bile by the liver.
   b.   production of secretin by the duodenum.
   c.   release of gastrin from the stomach antrum.
   d.   production of cholecystokinin by the duodenum.

5. A primary effect of removal of the stomach on nutritional status is

   a.   iron deficiency.
   b.   lactose intolerance.
   c.   protein malnutrition.
   d.   cobalamin (vitamin $B_{12}$) deficiency.

6. Identify whether the following statements are true or false. If a statement is false, correct the bold word(s) to make the statement true.

\_\_\_\_\_ a. The structure that prevents reflux of stomach contents into the esophagus is the **upper esophageal sphincter**.

\_\_\_\_\_ b. The nurse encourages the client with chronic constipation to attempt defecation after the first meal of the day because **gastrocolic and duodenocolic reflexes** increase colon peristalsis.

\_\_\_\_\_ c. A drug that blocks the release of secretions from the stomach **chief cells** will decrease gastric acidity.

\_\_\_\_\_ d. The secretion of hydrochloric acid and pepsinogen is stimulated by the **sight and smell** of food.

\_\_\_\_\_ e. Obstruction of the biliary tract is indicated by increased **unconjugated (indirect)** bilirubin levels in the blood.

\_\_\_\_\_ f. The major blood supply to the liver is the **portal vein**.

7. Match the following digestive substances with their descriptions.

\_\_\_\_\_ a. Gastrin               1. Converted to pepsin by acidity

\_\_\_\_\_ b. Intrinsic factor       2. Converts maltose to glucose

\_\_\_\_\_ c. Secretin              3. Increases gastric motility and secretion

\_\_\_\_\_ d. Bile                  4. Begins protein digestion

\_\_\_\_\_ e. Amylase              5. Responsible for absorption of cobalamin

\_\_\_\_\_ f. Enterokinase         6. Converts fats to fatty acids

\_\_\_\_\_ g. Pepsinogen           7. Stimulates pancreatic bicarbonate secretion

\_\_\_\_\_ h. Pepsin               8. Emulsifies fats

\_\_\_\_\_ i. Maltase              9. Converts trypsinogen to trypsin

\_\_\_\_\_ j. Lipase               10. Converts starch to disaccharides

8. The destruction of normal bowel bacteria by prolonged antibiotic therapy may cause

a. coagulation problems.
b. elevated serum ammonia levels.
c. impaired absorption of amino acids.
d. increased absorption of urobilinogen into the blood.

9. An obstruction at the sphincter of Oddi will affect the digestion of all nutrients because

a. bile is responsible for emulsification of all nutrients and vitamins.
b. intestinal digestive enzymes are released through the ampulla of Vater.
c. both bile and pancreatic enzymes enter the duodenum at the ampulla of Vater.
d. gastric contents can only pass to the duodenum when the sphincter of Oddi is open.

10. Identify the normal function of the liver that is impaired in the following findings in a client with liver disease.

   a. Hyperaldosteronism

   b. Hypoalbuminemia

   c. Increased serum ammonia

   d. Increased serum unconjugated bilirubin

   e. Purpura and petechiae

   f. Decreased serum cholesterol

   g. Male gynecomastia

11. A client experiences increased red blood cell destruction from a mechanical heart valve prosthesis. Describe what happens to the bilirubin that is released from the breakdown of hemoglobin from the red cells.



12. A clinical manifestation of age-related changes in the GI system the nurse would expect an older client to report is

   a. gastric hyperacidity.
   b. intolerance to fatty foods.
   c. yellowish tinge to the skin.
   d. reflux of gastric contents into the esophagus.

13. Identify one specific finding identified by the nurse during assessment of each of the client's functional health patterns that indicates a risk factor for gastrointestinal problems or the response of the client to a gastro-intestinal disorder.

   a. Health perception–health management

   b. Nutritional–metabolic

   c. Elimination

   d. Activity–exercise

   e. Sleep–rest

   f. Cognitive–perceptual

   g. Self-perception–self-concept

   h. Role–relationship

   i. Sexuality–reproductive

   j. Coping–stress tolerance

   k. Value–belief

14. A normal finding during physical assessment of the mouth is

    a. a red, slick appearance of the tongue.
    b. uvular deviation to the side on saying "Ahh."
    c. a thin, white coating of the dorsum of the tongue.
    d. scattered red, smooth areas on dorsum of tongue.

15. A normal finding on physical examination of the abdomen is

    a. auscultation of bruits.
    b. observation of visible palpations.
    c. percussion of liver dullness in the left midclavicular line.
    d. palpation of the spleen 1 to 2 cm below the left costal margin.

16. A client is admitted to the hospital with upper left quadrant pain. A possible source of the pain may be the

    a. liver.
    b. appendix.
    c. pancreas.
    d. gallbladder.

17. During auscultation of the abdomen

    a. the presence of borborygmi indicates hyperperistalsis.
    b. the bell of the stethoscope is used to auscultate high-pitched sounds.
    c. high-pitched, rushing, and tinkling bowel sounds are heard after eating.
    d. absence of bowel sounds for three minutes in each quadrant is reported as abnormal.

18. Complete the table below by indicating with check marks which of the following preparations are required for each of the diagnostic procedures listed.

    (1) NPO up to eight or more hours
    (2) Bowel emptying with laxatives, enemas, or both
    (3) Informed consent
    (4) Allergy to iodine ascertained

|  | (1) NPO | (2) Bowel | (3) Consent | (4) Allergy |
|---|---|---|---|---|
| UGI series |  |  |  |  |
| Barium enema |  |  |  |  |
| IV cholangiogram |  |  |  |  |
| Gallbladder ultrasonography |  |  |  |  |
| Hepatobiliary scintigraphy |  |  |  |  |
| Upper GI endoscopy |  |  |  |  |
| Colonoscopy |  |  |  |  |
| Endoscopic retrograde cholangiopancreatography |  |  |  |  |

19. The diagnostic test that is most specific for acute pancreatitis is
    a. serum amylase.
    b. abdominal ultrasonography.
    c. serum gamma-glutamyl transpeptidase (GGT).
    d. endoscopic retrograde cholangiopancreatography (ERCP).

20. A client's serum liver enzyme tests reveal an elevated aspartate aminotransferase (AST). The nurse recognizes that the elevated AST

    a. eliminates infection as a cause of liver damage.
    b. is diagnostic for liver inflammation and damage.
    c. may reflect tissue damage in organs other than the liver.
    d. may cause nervous system symptoms related to hepatic encephalopathy.

21. Match the nursing responsibilities indicated for the diagnostic procedures (answers may be used more than once).

    _____ a. Ensure no smoking morning of test

    _____ b. Monitor for LUQ pain and nausea/ vomiting

    _____ c. Observe for white stools

    _____ d. Monitor for rectal bleeding

    _____ e. Position to right side after test

    _____ f. Check for return of gag reflex

    _____ g. Monitor for internal bleeding

    _____ h. Check coagulation status before test

    _____ i. Insert nasogastric tube

    _____ j. Check temperature every 15 to 30 min for signs of perforation

    1. Barium swallow

    2. Gastric analysis

    3. Colonoscope

    4. Liver biopsy

    5. Gastroduodenoscopy

    6. Endoscopic retrograde cholangiopancreatography

# CHAPTER 39  NURSING MANAGEMENT: NUTRITIONAL PROBLEMS

1. A 30-year-old man's diet consists of 3000 calories with 120 g of protein, 160 g of fat, and 270 g of carbohydrate. He weighs 79 kg (174 lb) and is 178 cm (5 ft 11 in) tall.

   a. What percentage of total calories does each of the nutrients contribute to the man's diet?

      Protein

      Fat

      Carbohydrate

   b. According to *Canada's Food Guide to Healthy Eating*, how many calories would be recommended for him as an average adult?

   c. Using *Canada's Food Guide to Healthy Eating*, what changes could the nurse suggest to bring the man's diet more in line with nutrition recommendations?

2. Identify whether the following statements are true or false. If a statement is false, correct the bold word(s) to make the statement true.

   _____ a. Overnutrition resulting in obesity is a type of **malnutrition**.

   _____ b. The two nutrients most often lacking in the diet of a vegan are **vitamin B$_6$** and **folic acid**.

   _____ c. The major nutritional problem in Canada today is the high intake of **carbohydrate** in the diet.

   _____ d. **Marasmus** is a type of malnutrition that results from a deficiency of protein intake superimposed on a catabolic stress event.

3. The most common cause of secondary protein-calorie malnutrition in Canada is

   a. the unavailability of foods high in protein.
   b. a lack of knowledge about nutritional needs.
   c. a lack of money to purchase high-protein foods.
   d. an alteration in ingestion, digestion, absorption, or metabolism.

4. Describe the metabolism of nutrients used for energy during starvation within the given approximate time frames.

   a. First 18 hours

   b. 18 hours to five to nine days

   c. nine days to six weeks

   d. Over six weeks

5. Failure of the sodium-potassium pump during severe protein depletion may lead to

   a. ascites.
   b. anemia.
   c. hyperkalemia.
   d. hypoalbuminemia.

6. Identify whether the following statements are true or false. If a statement is false, correct the bold word(s) to make the statement true.

   _____ a. A client whose weight is 60 kg and who is 150 cm tall is classified as **Obese Class II** based on his BMI (Body Mass Index).

   _____ b. A client who is nutritionally fit on admission may develop nutritional problems during hospitalization because of dietary restrictions imposed by **diagnostic testing**.

   _____ c. Vitamin deficiencies in adults most commonly are clinically manifested by disorders of the **skin**.

   _____ d. Prolonged **antibiotic therapy** may contribute to vitamin deficiencies because of loss of bowel bacteria activity.

7. Use the following drugs or drug classifications to complete the sentences below.

erythropoietin                          phenothiazines
tricyclic antidepressants               phenytoin (Dilantin)
barbiturates                            warfarin (Coumadin)
monoamine oxidase inhibitors            calcium channel blockers
cholestyramine (Questran)

a. Drinking grapefruit juice will intensify the effects of _____.

b. Deficiency of all fat-soluble vitamins may occur with prolonged use of _____.

c. Green leafy vegetables, dairy products, and meat may decrease the effect of _____.

d. Riboflavin deficiency may occur with the use of _____ and

   _____.

e. Unless it is supplemented in the diet, folic acid deficiency may occur with the use of

   _____ and _____.

f. Aged cheese, fermented beverages, and smoked meats or poultry may cause a hypertensive crisis if taken

   with _____.

g. Folic acid and cobalamin deficiencies may decrease the effectiveness of _____.

8. During assessment of the client with protein-calorie malnutrition, the nurse would expect to find

   a. a flat or concave abdomen.
   b. increased sensitivity to cold.
   c. increased pulse and respiratory rate.
   d. increased reflexes and vibratory sense.

9. The nurse determines that the client with the highest risk for the nursing diagnosis of imbalanced nutrition: less than body requirements related to decreased ingestion is the client with

   a. tuberculosis infection.
   b. malabsorption syndrome.
   c. draining decubitus ulcers.
   d. severe anorexia secondary to radiation therapy.

10. The nurse monitors the laboratory results of the client with protein-calorie malnutrition during treatment. An indication of improvement in the client's condition is

   a. decreased lymphocytes.
   b. increased serum potassium.
   c. increased serum transferrin.
   d. decreased serum prealbumin.

11. When the nurse is concerned about the skeletal protein reserves of a client who has been hospitalized during cancer chemotherapy, the assessment of the client should include

    a. body mass index.
    b. height and weight.
    c. waist circumference.
    d. mid-upper arm circumference and triceps skin fold.

12. The nurse evaluates that client teaching about a high-calorie, high-protein diet has been effective when the client selects for breakfast from the hospital menu

    a. two poached eggs, hash brown potatoes, and whole milk.
    b. two slices of toast with butter and jelly, orange juice, and skim milk.
    c. three pancakes with butter and syrup, two slices of bacon, and apple juice.
    d. cream of wheat with two tablespoons skim milk powder, one-half grapefruit, and a high- protein milk-shake.

13. Upon admission to a long-term care facility, a 72-year-old woman's weight is 45.5 kg (100 lb) and she is 157.5 cm (5 ft 2 in) tall. Her BMI is calculated to be 18.22. The nurse hypothesizes that she

    a. is normal weight and at nutritional risk because of her age.
    b. is overweight and will need a reduction in either the quality or the quantity of her intake.
    c. is underweight and at increased risk of developing health problems.
    d. is underweight, but this is expected given her age.

14. When teaching the older adult about nutritional needs during aging, the nurse emphasizes that

    a. the need for all nutrients is decreased as one ages.
    b. fewer calories, but the same amount of protein, are required as one ages.
    c. fats, carbohydrates, and protein should be decreased, but vitamin and mineral intake should be increased.
    d. high-calorie oral supplements should be taken between meals to ensure that recommended nutrients are met.

15. When planning nutritional interventions for a healthy 83-year-old man, the nurse recognizes that the factor that is most likely to affect his nutritional status is

    a. living alone on a fixed income.
    b. changes in cardiovascular function.
    c. snacking between meals, resulting in obesity.
    d. an increase in gastrointestinal motility and absorption.

16. When considering tube feedings for a client with severe protein-calorie malnutrition, the nurse knows that an advantage of a gastrostomy tube over a nasogastric tube is that

    a. there is less irritation to the nasal and esophageal mucosa.
    b. the client experiences the sight and smells associated with eating.
    c. aspiration resulting from reflux of formulas into the esophagus is less common.
    d. routine checking for placement is not required because gastrostomy tubes do not become displaced.

17. Identify one nursing intervention that is indicated for each of the following desired outcomes of tube feeding.

    a. Prevention of aspiration

    b. Prevention of diarrhea

    c. Maintenance of tube patency

    d. Maintenance of tube placement

    e. Prevention of infection

18. Before administering a bolus of intermittent tube feeding to a client with a percutaneous endoscopic gastrostomy (PEG), the nurse aspirates 220 mL of gastric contents. The nurse should

    a. return the aspirate to the stomach and recheck the volume of aspirate in an hour.
    b. return the aspirate to the stomach and continue with the tube feeding as planned.
    c. discard the aspirate to prevent overdistending the stomach when the new feeding is given.
    d. notify the physician that the feedings have been scheduled too frequently to allow for stomach emptying.

19. Indicate whether the following characteristics of total parenteral nutrition (TPN) apply more to central parenteral nutrition (CPN) or peripheral parenteral nutrition (PPN).

    _____ a. Limited to 20% glucose

    _____ b. Tonicity of 1600 mOsm/L

    _____ c. Small fluid volumes

    _____ d. Supplements oral feedings

    _____ e. Long-term nutritional support

    _____ f. Phlebitis more common

    _____ g. May use peripherally inserted catheter (PIC)

20. An indication for TPN that is not appropriate for enteral tube feedings is

    a. head and neck cancer.
    b. hypermetabolic states.
    c. malabsorption syndrome.
    d. protein-calorie malnutrition.

21. What nursing interventions are indicated during TPN to prevent the following complications?

    a. Infection

    b. Hyperglycemia

    c. Air embolism

22. The nurse is caring for a client receiving 1000 mL of TPN solution over 24 hours. When it is time to change the solution, there is 150 mL remaining in the bottle. The most appropriate action by the nurse is to

    a. start the new solution and discard the unused solution.
    b. notify the physician for instructions regarding the infusion rate.
    c. open the IV line and infuse the remaining solution as quickly as possible.
    d. wait to change the solution until the remaining solution infuses at the prescribed rate.

23. The physician inserts a central catheter for administration of parenteral nutrition and orders the solution to be started when x-ray confirms proper placement of the catheter. Following the x-ray, radiology notifies the nurse that the catheter tip is in the superior vena cava. The most appropriate action by the nurse is to

    a. start the solution at the prescribed introductory rate.
    b. notify the physician that the catheter needs readjustment.
    c. continue to infuse the isotonic solution until further orders from the physician.
    d. gently push the catheter in 4 to 6 cm (2 to 3 in.) to reposition the tip in the right atrium.

24. The physician orders a 10% fat emulsion solution to be administered to a client who is currently receiving peripheral parenteral nutrition. The most appropriate action by the nurse is to

    a. administer the fat emulsion at the prescribed rate at a new, separate intravenous site.
    b. add the fat emulsion solution to the parenteral nutrition solution, since they are compatible.
    c. refrigerate the fat solution until the current bottle of parenteral nutrition has infused and then start the fat emulsion.
    d. connect the tubing of the fat emulsion below the filter on the parenteral nutrition tubing at the injection site closest to the client.

25. A client receiving a fat emulsion solution develops nausea, vomiting, and fever. The nurse recognizes that these symptoms may indicate

    a. a fat embolism.
    b. a fatty acid deficiency.
    c. a too-rapid infusion rate.
    d. an allergic reaction to the solution.

26. a. Use the nomogram in Figure 39-4 to determine the BMI for a client who is 165 cm (5 ft 5 in) tall and weighs

    91.8 kg (202 lb). _____

    b. What is the client's weight classification? _____

    c. This client has a waist circumference of 90 cm (35.4 in.). Does this indicate an increased or decreased risk of health problems?

27. Explain the rationale for the following interventions in the management of obesity.

    a. 800- to 1200-calorie diet

    b. Weight loss of 0.5–1 kg (approximately 1–2 lb) a week

    c. Keeping a diet diary

    d. Schedule several small meals a day

    e. Abstinence from alcohol

    f. Exercise program

    g. Behavioural-cognitive modification

28. Describe how the nurse would explain to the obese client about the following.

    a. The rapid weight loss of the first few days of dieting

    b. Why to weigh weekly rather than daily

    c. How gender influences weight loss

    d. Plateau periods

29. When medications are used in the treatment of obesity, it is important for the nurse to teach the client that

    a. over-the-counter diet aids are safer than other agents and can be useful in controlling appetite.
    b. diet and exercise are the most important in weight control, since drugs do not help change eating behaviours.
    c. all drugs used for weight control are capable of altering central nervous system function and should be used with caution.
    d. the primary effect of the medication is psychological, controlling the urge to eat in response to stress or feelings of rejection.

30. Match the following characteristics with the appropriate surgical procedures used for treatment of morbid obesity (answers may be used more than once).

    _____ a. Dumping syndrome common

    _____ b. Staple-created pouch with restricted outlet

    _____ c. A cosmetic procedure

    _____ d. Removes folds of adipose tissue

    _____ e. May require lifelong cobalamin supplementation

    _____ f. Staple-created gastric pouch with jejunal outlet

    _____ g. Distension of wall of pouch a complication

    1. Vertical banded gastroplasty

    2. Lipectomy

    3. Roux-en-Y gastric bypass

31. Identify whether the following statements are true or false. If a statement is false, correct the bold word(s) to make the statement true.

    _____ a. The **android** body fat distribution pattern is characterized by lower-body involvement and low waist circumference and skinfold thickness.

    _____ b. The highest risk for obesity associated with cardiovascular disease is seen in those individuals with **android** obesity.

    _____ c. **Primary** obesity results from the consumption of more food than required for normal physiological functions and growth.

32. The nurse plans care for the morbidly obese client recognizing that complications of obesity necessitate the cautious use of

    a. intravenous solutions.
    b. hypoglycemic agents.
    c. antihypertensive drugs.
    d. sedative and hypnotics.

33. During care of the morbidly obese client, it is important that the nurse

    a. avoid reference to the client's weight to avoid embarrassing the client.
    b. emphasize to the client how important it is to lose weight to maintain health.
    c. plan for necessary modifications in equipment and nursing techniques before initiating care.
    d. recognize that a full assessment of each body system may not be possible because of numerous layers of skinfolds.

34. A post-operative nursing intervention for the obese client who has undergone a vertical banded gastroplasty is

    a. irrigating and repositioning the nasogastric tube as needed.
    b. delaying ambulation until the client has enough strength to support self.
    c. keeping the client positioned on the side to facilitate respiratory function.
    d. using an extra-long or spinal needle to administer prescribed IM analgesics.

35. Dietary teaching for the client following a Roux-en-Y gastric bypass includes information regarding the need to

    a. gradually increase the amount of food ingested to preoperative levels.
    b. maintain a long-term liquid diet to prevent damage to the surgical site.
    c. avoid high-carbohydrate foods and limit fluids to prevent dumping syndrome.
    d. consume foods high in complex carbohydrate, protein, and fibre to add bulk to intestinal contents.

36. Identify the following characteristics of eating disorders as associated with anorexia nervosa (A), bulimia (B), or both (AB).

\_\_\_\_\_ a. Morbid fear of obesity

\_\_\_\_\_ b. Treated with psychotherapy

\_\_\_\_\_ c. Ignores feelings of hunger

\_\_\_\_\_ d. Binge eating with purging

\_\_\_\_\_ e. Feels fat even when emaciated

\_\_\_\_\_ f. Conceals abnormal eating habits

\_\_\_\_\_ g. Concerned about body image

\_\_\_\_\_ h. Self-induced starvation

37. An 18-year-old female client with anorexia nervosa is admitted to the hospital for treatment. On admission she weighs 37 kg (82 lb) and is 134.6 cm (5 ft 3 in) tall. Her lab results include the following: $K^+$ 2.8 mmol/L (2.8 mEq/L), Hg 89 g/L (8.9 g/dL), and BUN 22.8 mmol/L (64 mg/dL). In planning care for the client, the nurse gives the highest priority to the nursing diagnosis of

a. risk for injury related to dizziness and weakness secondary to anemia.
b. imbalanced nutrition: less than body requirements related to inadequate food intake.
c. risk for decreased cardiac output related to arrhythmias secondary to hypokalemia.
d. risk for impaired urinary elimination related to elevated BUN secondary to renal failure.

## CASE STUDY

### MALNUTRITION

### Client Profile

Mrs. M., a 62-year-old widow, has recently undergone radiation and chemotherapy following surgery for breast cancer. On a follow-up visit to the clinic, the nurse notes that Mrs. M. appears more thin and tired than usual.

### Subjective Data

- Says she has not had an appetite since the treatment for cancer was started
- Feels "weak" and "worn out"
- Thinks the treatment for cancer has not been effective
- Lives alone in an apartment in the inner city
- Immigrated from Russia 10 years ago
- Speaks, but does not read, English

### Objective Data

- Height 155 cm (62 in.); weight 41.8 kg (92 lb)
- BP 98/60, HR 60, RR 12
- Ulcerations of her buccal mucosal membranes and tongue
- Lab results:  Serum albumin 28 g/L (2.8 g/dL)
                Hg 100 g/L (10 g/dL); Hct 0.32 (32%)

**Critical Thinking Questions**

1. What additional assessment data should the nurse obtain from Mrs. M. related to her nutritional status?

2. What physical and psychosocial factors have contributed to Mrs. M.'s malnutrition?

3. What additional symptoms would the nurse expect to see based on Mrs. M.'s laboratory test results?

4. What complications of malnutrition are most likely to occur in Mrs. M. because of her history and clinical manifestations?

5. What instructions could the nurse give Mrs. M. regarding her diet that would be most therapeutic?

6. Based on the assessment data presented, write one or more appropriate nursing diagnoses. Are there any collaborative problems?

# CHAPTER 40 NURSING MANAGEMENT: UPPER GASTROINTESTINAL PROBLEMS

1. Identify whether the following statements are true or false. If a statement is false, correct the bold word(s) to make the statement true.

   _____ a. Immediately before the act of vomiting, activation of the **sympathetic nervous system** causes increased salivation, increased gastric mobility, and relaxation of the lower esophageal sphincter.

   _____ b. Stimulation of the vomiting centre by the chemoreceptor trigger zone (CTZ) is commonly caused by **stretch and distension of hollow organs**.

   _____ c. Vomiting may occur in response to psychological stress by stimulation of the vomiting centre from **the cerebral cortex**.

   _____ d. The acid–base imbalance most commonly associated with persistent vomiting is **metabolic acidosis** caused by loss of **bicarbonate**.

   _____ e. **Regurgitation** is not accompanied by nausea and is associated with increased intracranial pressure.

2. Laboratory findings that the nurse would expect in the client with persistent vomiting include

   a. ↓ pH, ↑ sodium, ↓ hematocrit.
   b. ↑ pH, ↓ chloride, ↓ hematocrit.
   c. ↑ pH, ↓ potassium, ↑ hematocrit.
   d. ↓ pH, ↓ potassium, ↑ hematocrit.

3. A client's vomitus is dark brown and has a coffee-ground appearance. The nurse recognizes that this emesis is characteristic of

   a. stomach bleeding.
   b. an intestinal obstruction.
   c. bile reflux into the stomach.
   d. active bleeding of the lower esophagus.

4. A client who has been vomiting for several days from an unknown cause is admitted to the hospital. The nurse anticipates collaborative care to include

   a. oral administration of broth and tea.
   b. administration of parenteral antiemetics.
   c. insertion of a nasogastric tube to suction.
   d. intravenous replacement of fluid and electrolytes.

5. A client treated for vomiting is to begin oral intake when the symptoms have subsided. To promote rehydration, the nurse plans to administer

   a. hot tea.
   b. Gatorade.
   c. cool water.
   d. warm broth.

6. Ondansetron (Zofran) is prescribed for a client with cancer-chemotherapy-induced vomiting. The nurse understands that this drug

   a. is a derivative of cannabis and has a potential for abuse.
   b. has a strong antihistamine effect that provides sedation and induces sleep.
   c. is used only when other therapies are ineffective because of side effects of anxiety and hallucinations.
   d. relieves vomiting centrally by action in the vomiting centre and peripherally by promoting gastric emptying.

7. Match the following characteristics of inflammations and infections of the mouth with their types (answers may be used more than once).

   _____ a. Viral infection related to upper respiratory infections and sun sensitivity

   _____ b. Staphylococcal infection that may occur with prolonged NPO status

   _____ c. Painful, bleeding gums with gingival necrosis and metallic-tasting saliva

   _____ d. Associated with prolonged high-dose antibiotic or corticosteroid therapy

   _____ e. Formation of abscesses with loosening of teeth

   _____ f. Infectious ulcers of mouth and lips with a defined erythematous base

   _____ g. White membranous lesions of mucosa of mouth and throat

   _____ h. Inflammation of mouth related to systemic disease and cancer chemotherapy

   _____ i. Shallow, painful vesicular ulcerations of lips and mouth

   _____ j. Results in decreased salivation and ear pain

   _____ k. Bacterial infection predisposed by fatigue, worry, and poor oral hygiene

   1. Gingivitis

   2. Vincent's infection

   3. Oral candidiasis

   4. Herpes simplex

   5. Aphthous stomatitis

   6. Parotitis

   7. Stomatitis

8. A client is scheduled for a biopsy of a painful tongue ulcer. Based on knowledge of risk factors for oral cancer, the nurse specifically asks the client about a history of

   a. excessive exposure to sunlight.
   b. recurrent herpes simplex infections.
   c. use of any type of tobacco products.
   d. difficulty swallowing and pain in the ear.

9. When caring for a client following a glossectomy with dissection of the floor of the mouth and a radical neck dissection for cancer of the tongue, the nurse's primary concern is maintaining

   a. relief of pain.
   b. a patent airway.
   c. a positive body image.
   d. tube feedings to provide nutrition.

10. A client with oral cancer has a history of heavy smoking, excessive alcohol intake, and personal neglect. During the client's early post-operative course, the nurse anticipates that the client may need

    a. oral nutritional supplements.
    b. drug therapy to prevent substance withdrawal symptoms.
    c. less pain medication because of cross-tolerance with CNS depressants.
    d. counselling about lifestyle changes to prevent recurrence of the tumour.

11. Identify four foods or beverages that decrease lower esophageal sphincter pressure that the nurse should teach the client with gastroesophageal reflux disease (GERD) to avoid.

    a.

    b.

    c.

    d.

12. Bethanechol (Duvoid) is added to the step-up drug regimen of a client with GERD. The nurse explains that the purpose of this drug is to

    a. act as a mechanical barrier to reflux.
    b. decrease the volume of gastric acid secretion.
    c. relieve heartburn by neutralizing hydrochloric acid.
    d. increase lower esophageal sphincter pressure and gastric emptying.

13. The nurse teaches the client with a hiatal hernia or GERD to control symptoms by

    a. drinking 300 to 350 mL (10 to 12 oz) of water with each meal.
    b. spacing six small meals a day between breakfast and bedtime.
    c. sleeping with the head of the bed elevated on 10- to 15-cm (4- to 6-inch) blocks.
    d. performing daily exercises of toe touching, sit-ups, and weight lifting.

14. A client is returned to the surgical unit following a laparoscopic fundoplication for repair of a hiatal hernia with an IV, NG tube to suction, and several small abdominal incisions. To prevent disruption of the surgical site, it is most important for the nurse to

    a. monitor for the return of peristalsis.
    b. position the client on the right side.
    c. maintain the patency of the NG tube.
    d. assess the abdominal wounds for drainage.

15. A client with esophageal cancer is scheduled for a partial esophagectomy. A nursing diagnosis that is likely to be of highest priority preoperatively is

    a. deficient fluid volume related to inadequate intake.
    b. impaired oral mucous membrane related to inadequate oral hygiene.
    c. imbalanced nutrition: less than body requirements related to dysphagia.
    d. ineffective therapeutic regimen maintenance related to lack of knowledge of disease process.

16. Following a client's esophagogastrostomy for cancer of the esophagus, it is important for the nurse to

    a. report any bloody drainage from the nasogastric tube.
    b. maintain the client in a semi-Fowler's or Fowler's position.
    c. monitor for abdominal distension that may disrupt the surgical site.
    d. expect to find decreased breath sounds bilaterally because of the surgical approach.

17. Match the following esophageal disorders with their descriptions.

    _____  a. Esophagitis

    _____  b. Esophageal diverticula

    _____  c. Esophageal strictures

    _____  d. Achalasia

    _____  e. Barrett's esophagus

    1. Absence of peristalsis of lower two thirds of esophagus with non-relaxing LES

    2. Inflammation of esophagus from irritants or gastric reflux

    3. Narrowing of esophagus from scarring

    4. Precancerous esophageal metaplasia associated with GERD

    5. Common site is above the upper esophageal sphincter

18. Complete the following sentences.

    a. The self-limiting type of gastritis most likely to occur in a university student who has an isolated drinking

       binge is _____ gastritis.

    b. _____ gastritis is associated with an increased risk for stomach cancer.

    c. A definite diagnosis of gastritis is made with the use of _____.

    d. The micro-organism that has a strong causative relation to both diffuse antral and multifocal gastritis is

       _____.

    e. A complication of chronic gastritis that results from the destruction and atrophy of acid-secreting cells is

       the loss of _____, leading to pernicious anemia.

    f. Drugs that contain _____ and _____ can reduce the bleeding and promote

       healing of erosive gastritis.

19. Nursing management of the client with chronic gastritis includes teaching the client to

    a. maintain a bland diet with six small meals a day.
    b. take antacids before meals to decrease stomach acidity.
    c. use NSAIDs other than ASA for any minor pain relief.
    d. eliminate alcohol and caffeine from the diet when symptoms occur.

20. Identify what type of bleeding is indicated by the following findings.

    a. Profuse bright-red hematemesis

    b. Coffee-ground emesis

    c. Melena

    d. Hematemesis with negative stool guaiac

21. During the nursing assessment of a client with upper GI bleeding, it is important to obtain a complete history of events leading to the bleeding episode. Match the following common causes of bleeding with the client situations that may be discovered during a nursing assessment.

    _____ a. Esophageal varices        1. Client with GERD

    _____ b. Stress ulcers             2. An older female client with arthritis

    _____ c. Esophagitis               3. Client with no history of GI symptoms

    _____ d. Mallory-Weiss syndrome    4. Client with cirrhosis of the liver

    _____ e. Hemorrhagic gastritis     5. Client with history of chronic atrophic gastritis

    _____ f. Drug-induced gastritis    6. Client with excessive alcohol intake

    _____ g. Cancer of the stomach     7. Client with severe retching and vomiting

    _____ h. Peptic ulcer              8. Client with severe burns

22. A client is admitted to the emergency department with profuse bright-red hematemesis. During the initial care of the client, the nurse's first priority is to

    a. perform a nursing assessment of the client's status.
    b. establish two intravenous sites with large-gauge catheters.
    c. obtain a thorough health history to assist in determining the cause of the bleeding.
    d. perform a gastric lavage with cool tap water in preparation for endoscopic examination and treatment.

23. A client with upper GI bleeding is treated with several drugs. The nurse recognizes that an agent that is used to decrease bleeding and decrease gastric acid secretions is

    a. ranitidine (Zantac).
    b. omeprazole (Losec).
    c. vasopressin (Pitressin).
    d. octreotide (Sandostatin).

24. In teaching clients at risk for upper GI bleeding to prevent bleeding episodes, the nurse stresses that

    a. all stools and vomitus must be tested for the presence of blood.
    b. the use of over-the-counter medications of any kind should be avoided.
    c. antacids should be taken with all prescribed medications to prevent gastric irritation.
    d. misoprostol should be used to protect the gastric mucosa in individuals with peptic ulcers.

25. The nurse evaluates that management of the client with upper GI bleeding is effective when assessment and laboratory findings reveal a

    a. decreasing BUN.
    b. normal hematocrit.
    c. urinary output of 20 mL/hr.
    d. urine specific gravity of 1.030.

26. When reviewing the medication history of a client with gastric bleeding, the nurse consults with the physician about changing the use of

    a. famotidine (Pepcid) to nizatidine (Axid).
    b. naproxen (Naprosyn) to valdecoxib (Bextra).
    c. aluminum hydroxide to sodium bicarbonate.
    d. diclofenac (Voltaren) to misoprostol.

27. Indicate whether the following characteristics are associated with gastric ulcers (G), duodenal ulcers (D), or both (B).

_____ a. Increased gastric secretion

_____ b. Superficial with smooth margins

_____ c. High recurrence rate

_____ d. Burning and cramping in mid-epigastric area

_____ e. Increased incidence with smoking, drug, and alcohol use

_____ f. Higher incidence in women in fifth and sixth decades

_____ g. Burning and gaseous pressure in high epigastrium

_____ h. Associated with psychological stress

_____ i. May cause hemorrhage, perforation, and obstruction

_____ j. Possible seasonal trend in occurrence

_____ k. Pain one to two hours after meals

_____ l. Increased incidence in persons from lower socio-economic class

_____ m. Associated with *H. pylori* infection

_____ n. Relief of pain with food

28. Match the following factors associated with the development of peptic ulcers with their probable pathophysiological mechanisms.

_____ a. *Helicobacter pylori*

_____ b. ASA and other NSAIDs

_____ c. Corticosteroids

_____ d. Vagal stimulation

_____ e. Severe physiological stress

_____ f. Nicotine

1. Decrease rate of mucous cell turnover

2. Ischemia of gastric mucosa

3. Generate ammonia in mucous layer

4. Decrease pancreatic bicarbonate secretion

5. Inhibit synthesis of mucus and prostaglandins

6. Hypersecretion of hydrochloric acid

29. Regardless of the precipitating factor, the injury to mucosal cells in peptic ulcers is caused by

a. acid back-diffusion into the mucosa.
b. ammonia formation in the mucosal wall.
c. breakdown of the gastric mucosal barrier.
d. the release of histamine from gastrointestinal cells.

30. The nurse expects a client with an ulcer of the posterior portion of the duodenum to experience

    a. pain that occurs after not eating all day.
    b. back pain that occurs two to four hours following meals.
    c. mid-epigastric pain that is unrelieved with antacids.
    d. high epigastric burning that is relieved with food intake.

31. Diagnostic testing is planned for a client with a suspected peptic ulcer. The nurse explains to the client that the most reliable test for determining the presence and location of an ulcer is a(n)

    a. endoscopy.
    b. gastric analysis.
    c. barium swallow.
    d. serological test for *H. pylori*.

32. The nurse teaches a client with newly diagnosed peptic ulcer disease to

    a. maintain a bland, soft, low-residue diet.
    b. use alcohol and caffeine in moderation and always with food.
    c. eat as normally as possible, eliminating foods that cause pain or discomfort.
    d. avoid milk and milk products because they stimulate gastric acid production.

33. Identify the rationale for treatment with nasogastric intubation for each of the following situations associated with peptic ulcer disease.

    a. Acute exacerbation

    b. Peritonitis

    c. Gastric outlet obstruction

34. A client who has peptic ulcer disease has the following medications ordered.

    Magnesium hydroxide/aluminum hydroxide (Mylanta) 15 mL PO 1 hr ac and 3 hr pc and hs
    Ranitidine (Zantac) 300 mg PO hs
    Sucralfate 1.0 g 1 hr ac and hs

    The client usually has meals at 7 AM, 12 noon, and 6 PM, and a bedtime snack at 10 PM.

    Plan an administration schedule that will be most therapeutic and acceptable to the client.

    **Times**

    a.  Mylanta

    b.  Ranitidine

    c.  Sucralfate

35. Match the following characteristics with the drugs used to treat or prevent peptic ulcer disease (answers may be used more than once).

   _____ a. Prevents conversion of pepsinogen to pepsin

   _____ b. Used in clients with verified *H. pylori*

   _____ c. Covers the ulcer, protecting it from hydroxide mixture erosion

   _____ d. Decreases gastric acid secretion by blocking ATPase enzyme

   _____ e. High incidence of side effects and contraindications

   _____ f. High dose and frequency stimulate release of gastrin

   _____ g. Reduce HCl acid secretion by blocking action of histamine

   _____ h. Antisecretory effects in clients using antiprostaglandin drugs

   _____ i. Has the greatest non-compliance

   _____ j. Decrease HCl acid secretion and gastric motility

   _____ k. Newer drugs in class more potent at reduced dosage

1. Famotidine (Pepcid)

2. Omeprazole (Losec)

3. Aluminum/magnesium hydroxide mixture

4. Sucralfate

5. Misoprostol

6. Amoxicillin/ clarithromycin/omeprazole

7. Anticholinergics

36. The nurse determines that teaching for the client with peptic ulcer disease has been effective when the client states

   a. "I should stop all my medications if I develop any side effects."
   b. "I should continue my treatment regimen as long as I have pain."
   c. "I have learned some relaxation strategies that decrease my stress."
   d. "I can buy whatever antacids are on sale because they all have the same effect."

37. A client with a history of peptic ulcer disease is hospitalized with symptoms of a perforation. During the initial assessment, the nurse would expect the client to report

   a. vomiting of bright-red blood.
   b. projectile vomiting of undigested food.
   c. sudden, severe upper abdominal pain and shoulder pain.
   d. hyperactive stomach sounds and upper abdominal swelling.

38. A client with a gastric outlet obstruction has been treated with nasogastric decompression. After the first 24 hours, the client develops nausea and increased upper abdominal bowel sounds. An appropriate action by the nurse is to

   a. check the patency of the NG tube.
   b. place the client in a recumbent position.
   c. assess the client's vital signs and circulatory status.
   d. encourage the client to breathe deeply and consciously relax.

39. When caring for a client with an acute exacerbation of a peptic ulcer, the nurse finds the client doubled up in bed with shallow, grunting respirations. The initial appropriate action by the nurse is to

    a. notify the physician.
    b. irrigate the client's NG tube.
    c. place the client in a high Fowler's position.
    d. assess the client's abdomen and vital signs.

40. Match the descriptions with the following surgical procedures used to treat peptic ulcer disease.

    _____  a. Often performed with a vagotomy to increase gastric emptying

    _____  b. Severing of a parasympathetic nerve to decrease gastric secretion

    _____  c. Removal of distal two thirds of stomach with anastomosis to jejunum

    _____  d. Removal of distal two thirds of stomach with anastomosis to duodenum

    1. Billroth I
    2. Billroth II
    3. Pyloroplasty
    4. Vagotomy

41. Following a Billroth II procedure, a client develops dumping syndrome. The nurse explains that the symptoms associated with this problem are caused by

    a. distension of the smaller stomach by too much food and fluid intake.
    b. hyperglycemia caused by uncontrolled gastric emptying into the small intestine.
    c. irritation of the stomach lining by reflux of bile salts because the pylorus has been removed.
    d. movement of fluid into the bowel because concentrated food and fluids move rapidly into the intestine.

42. The nurse determines that further dietary teaching is needed when a client with dumping syndrome says,

    a. "I should eat bread with every meal."
    b. "I should avoid drinking fluids with my meals."
    c. "I should eat smaller meals about six times a day."
    d. "I need to lie down for 30 to 60 minutes after my meals."

43. While caring for a client following a subtotal gastrectomy with a gastroduodenostomy anastomosis, the nurse determines that the nasogastric tube is obstructed. The nurse should

    a. replace the tube with a new one.
    b. irrigate the tube until return can be aspirated.
    c. reposition the tube and then attempt irrigation.
    d. notify the surgeon to reposition or replace the tube.

44. In promoting early detection of cancer of the stomach, the nurse focuses on identification of clients who are at risk because of

    a. achlorhydria.
    b. acute gastritis.
    c. heavy smoking.
    d. peptic ulcer disease.

45. During assessment of the client with gastric pain and discomfort, the nurse focuses on signs and symptoms that may differentiate cancer of the stomach from peptic ulcer disease. These findings include

    a. anorexia with weight loss.
    b. nausea, vomiting, and hematemesis.
    c. signs of anemia such as pallor, fatigue, and black tarry stools.
    d. pain that has previously been controlled with antacids becomes worse.

46. A client with cancer of the stomach at the lesser curvature undergoes a total gastrectomy with an esophago-jejunostomy. Post-operatively, the nurse teaches the client to expect

    a. rapid healing of the surgical wound.
    b. to be able to return to normal dietary habits.
    c. close follow-up for development of peptic ulcers in the jejunum.
    d. lifelong intramuscular or intranasal administration of cobalamin.

47. A large number of children at an elementary school have developed profuse diarrhea and bloody stools. The school nurse suspects food poisoning from the school cafeteria and requests analysis and culture of

    a. chicken.
    b. ground beef.
    c. commercially canned fish.
    d. salads with mayonnaise dressing.

## CASE STUDY

### GASTRIC CANCER

**Client Profile**

Mrs. E. is a 75-year-old retired garment worker who was diagnosed with gastric cancer two weeks ago. The home health nurse assigned to her case reads the following on her medical record.

**Subjective Data**

- Had a six-month history of epigastric discomfort, anorexia, nausea, vomiting, and an 11-kg (24-lb) weight loss
- Stated she has had "stomach problems" for a long time, and was diagnosed with gastritis 20 years ago
- Stated she was told that they could not take out the tumour because it was too far gone
- Stated, "I've always been a strong person, but now I'm just too tired to eat or do anything."

**Objective Data**

- Physical examination: palpable mass in left upper quadrant of the abdomen
- Diagnostic tests: Barium swallow, gastroscopy, and biopsy/cytology all confirmed the presence of a well-advanced tumour in the fundus of the stomach
- Laboratory tests: Decreased hemoglobin and hematocrit
              Serum albumin 24 g/L (2.4 g/dL)
- Appears emaciated, with areas of skin discoloration on her forearms

When the nurse visits Mrs. E., she has just returned from a radiation treatment and is holding a plastic emesis basin and tissues in her lap.

## Critical Thinking Questions

1. What pathophysiological changes occur in gastric cancer that lead to the symptoms experienced by Mrs. E.?

2. What subjective and objective data indicate the presence of malnutrition in Mrs. E.?

3. What other factors might be contributing to Mrs. E.'s malnutrition besides those described?

4. What other complications may develop as a result of Mrs. E's malnutrition?

5. What treatment plan should the nurse provide for Mrs. E. and her family?

6. Mrs. E. asks the nurse if anyone with her stage of gastric cancer has ever recovered. What is the nurse's best response to Mrs. E.?

7. Based on the assessment data presented, write one or more appropriate nursing diagnoses. Are there any collaborative problems?

1. Match the causes and findings with the appropriate classes of diarrhea (answers may be used more than once).

   _____ a. Irritable bowel syndrome        1. Decreased fluid absorption

   _____ b. Bowel resection or bypass       2. Increased fluid secretion

   _____ c. Stool positive for parasites    3. Motility disturbance

   _____ d. Radiation mucosal damage

   _____ e. Dumping syndrome

   _____ f. Antibiotic-induced *C. difficile*

   _____ g. Lactase deficiency

   _____ h. High stool fat and undigested protein

   _____ i. Foods and drugs containing sorbitol

2. The nurse identifies a need for additional teaching when a client with acute infectious diarrhea states,

   a. "I can use skin barrier creams or ointments around the anal area to protect my skin."
   b. "Gatorade is a good liquid to drink because it replaces the fluid and salts I have lost."
   c. "I must wash my hands after every bowel movement to prevent spreading the diarrhea to my family."
   d. "I may use over-the-counter loperamide (Imodium) or Parepectolin (paregoric, pectin, kaolin) as needed to control the diarrhea."

3. In instituting a bowel training program for a client with fecal incontinence, the nurse plans to

   a. teach the client to use a perianal pouch.
   b. place the client on a bedpan 30 minutes before breakfast.
   c. insert a rectal suppository at the same time every morning.
   d. assist the client to the bathroom at the time of the client's normal defecation.

4. Explain the significance of the following information obtained from the client with chronic constipation during the nursing assessment.

   a. Suppressing the urge to defecate while at work

   b. Thinks that there is a need for a daily bowel movement.

   c. History of hemorrhoids

   d. High dietary fibre with low fluid intake

5. The nurse teaches the client with chronic constipation that of the following foods, dietary fibre is highest in

   a. bananas.
   b. popcorn.
   c. dried beans.
   d. shredded wheat.

6. The preferred immediate treatment for an acute episode of constipation is

   a. soapsuds enemas.
   b. stimulant cathartics.
   c. stool-softening cathartics.
   d. tap water or hypertonic enemas.

7. A client is admitted to the emergency department with an acute abdomen. The nursing intervention that should be implemented first is

   a. measurement of vital signs to detect hypovolemic changes.
   b. administration of prescribed analgesics to promote client comfort and relieve anxiety.
   c. a thorough assessment of the onset, location, intensity, duration, and character of the pain.
   d. a physical assessment of the abdomen for distension, masses, abnormal pulsations, bowel sounds, and pigmentation changes.

8. For the following causes of acute abdomen, indicate whether surgery is indicated.

   _____ a. Foreign body perforation

   _____ b. Pancreatitis

   _____ c. Ruptured abdominal aneurysm

   _____ d. Ruptured ectopic pregnancy

   _____ e. Pelvic inflammatory disease

   _____ f. Acute ischemic bowel

9. A client returns to the surgical unit with a nasogastric tube to low intermittent suction, IV fluids, and a Jackson-Pratt drain at the surgical site following an exploratory laparotomy and repair of a bowel perforation. Four hours after admission, the client experiences nausea and vomiting. An appropriate nursing intervention for the client is to

   a. assess the abdomen for distension and bowel sounds.
   b. inspect the surgical site and drainage in the Jackson-Pratt.
   c. check the amount and character of gastric drainage, the patency of the NG tube, and the functions of the wall suction.
   d. administer prescribed dimenhydrinate (Gravol) to control the nausea and vomiting.

10. On the second post-operative day, a client who had an exploratory laparotomy complains of abdominal distension and gas pains. The client asks the nurse if this indicates damage to the bowel during surgery. The nurse's best response to the client is

   a. "Abdominal distension occurs as a normal response to inflammation and healing of the bowel."
   b. "Gas pains occur when a nasogastric tube is not used during surgery to remove air from the stomach."
   c. "This is a common complication of abdominal surgery but usually can be relieved by having a bowel movement."
   d. "This occurs because of bowel immobility caused by anaesthesia and manipulation of the intestine during surgery."

11. A post-operative client has a nursing diagnosis of pain related to immobility, medication, and decreased gut motility as evidenced by abdominal pain and distension and inability to pass flatus. An appropriate nursing intervention for the client is to

   a. have the client ambulate more frequently.
   b. assess the abdomen for bowel sounds.
   c. place the client in a high Fowler's position.
   d. withhold narcotics because they decrease bowel motility.

12. A 22-year-old client calls the outpatient clinic complaining of nausea and vomiting and right lower abdominal pain. The nurse advises the client to

   a. have the symptoms evaluated by a physician right away.
   b. use a heating pad to relax the muscles at the site of the pain.
   c. drink at least 2000 mL (two quarts) of juice to replace the fluid lost in vomiting.
   d. take a laxative to empty the bowel before examination at the clinic.

13. Identify whether the following statements are true or false. If a statement is false, correct the bold word(s) to make the statement true.

   _____ a. The nurse recognizes that surgery is indicated for the client with abdominal trauma when positive findings are obtained with **peritoneal lavage**.

   _____ b. The major complication of appendicitis is **colitis**.

   _____ c. The site of pain localization in appendicitis is known as **Rovsing's sign**.

   _____ d. Regardless of the cause of peritonitis the nurse would anticipate that treatment of the client would include **IV fluid replacement**.

   _____ e. The nurse advises the client with gastroenteritis to start increasing fluid intake as soon as **vomiting subsides**.

14. Match the following clinical manifestations with the pathophysiological changes that occur in cirrhosis (answers may be used more than once).

_____ a. Jaundice

_____ b. Testicular atrophy

_____ c. Anorexia and dyspepsia

_____ d. Spider angiomas

_____ e. Amenorrhea

_____ f. Peripheral neuropathy

_____ g. Dull, heavy, RUQ pain

_____ h. Male gynecomastia

_____ i. Petechiae and purpura

1. Decreased prothrombin production

2. Vascular congestion of spleen

3. Decreased estrogen metabolism

4. Stretching of liver capsule

5. Decreased bilirubin conjugation and excretion

6. Altered carbohydrate, protein, and fat metabolism

7. Decreased testosterone metabolism

8. Vitamin B deficiencies

15. Indicate whether the following characteristics of inflammatory bowel disease are most likely to be associated with ulcerative colitis (UC), Crohn's disease (CD), or both conditions (B).

_____ a. Presence of diarrhea

_____ b. Confined to large intestine

_____ c. Involves the entire thickness of the bowel wall

_____ d. Has periods of remission and exacerbation

_____ e. Can be cured with surgical colectomy

_____ f. Has segmented distribution

_____ g. Rectal bleeding

_____ h. Extraintestinal manifestations

_____ i. Risk of colon cancer

_____ j. Bowel perforation

_____ k. Formation of fistulas

_____ l. Unknown cause

_____ m. Abdominal pain

_____ n. Association with tumour necrosis factor-$\alpha$

16. Indicate what laboratory findings are expected in ulcerative colitis as a result of the following.

a. Bloody diarrhea

b. Cellular mucosal breakdown

c. Diarrhea and vomiting

d. Toxic megacolon

17. Extraintestinal symptoms that are seen in both ulcerative colitis and Crohn's disease are

a. uveitis and conjunctivitis.
b. pyoderma gangrenosum.
c. erythema nodosum and arthritis.
d. primary sclerosing cholangitis.

18. Match the following treatment modalities for inflammatory bowel disease with the appropriate rationale (answers may be used more than once).

\_\_\_\_\_  a. Corticosteroids

\_\_\_\_\_  b. Parenteral nutrition

\_\_\_\_\_  c. Cobalamin injections

\_\_\_\_\_  d. Antidiarrheal agents

\_\_\_\_\_  e. Sulphasalazine (Azulfidine)

\_\_\_\_\_  f. IV fluids

\_\_\_\_\_  g. 6-Mercaptopurine

\_\_\_\_\_  h. Nasogastric suction

\_\_\_\_\_  i. NPO

1. Promote bowel rest

2. Control inflammation

3. Correct malnutrition

4. Symptomatic relief of symptoms

5. Provide fluid and electrolyte management

19. A client with ulcerative colitis undergoes the first phase of a total colectomy with ileoanal anastomosis and formation of an ileal reservoir. On post-operative assessment of the client, the nurse would expect to find

a. a loop ileostomy.
b. a rectal tube set to low continuous suction.
c. an ileostomy stoma with a catheter in place to provide pouch irrigations.
d. a permanent ileostomy stoma in the right lower quadrant of the abdomen.

20. A client with ulcerative colitis has a total colectomy with formation of a terminal ileum stoma. An important nursing intervention for this client post-operatively is to

a. measure the ileostomy output to determine the status of the client's fluid balance.
b. change the ileostomy appliance every three to four hours to prevent leakage of drainage onto the skin.
c. emphasize that the ostomy is temporary and the ileum will be reconnected when the large bowel heals.
d. teach the client about the high-fibre, low-carbohydrate diet required to maintain normal ileostomy drainage.

21. A client with Crohn's disease is hospitalized with an acute exacerbation. The physician orders an elemental diet for the client. The nurse informs the client that an advantage of this diet is that it is

a. high in fat, promoting an emollient effect on the bowel.
b. absorbed in the proximal small bowel, promoting distal bowel rest.
c. milk based, correcting protein, calcium, and other nutritional deficits.
d. administered parenterally, resting the bowel and providing nutrients and electrolytes.

22. A client with inflammatory bowel disease has a nursing diagnosis of imbalanced nutrition: less than body requirements related to decreased nutritional intake and decreased intestinal absorption. Assessment data that support this nursing diagnosis are

    a. pallor and hair loss.
    b. frequent diarrheal stools.
    c. anorectal excoriation and pain.
    d. hypotension and urine output below 30 mL/hr.

23. Match the following intestinal obstructions with their descriptions.

    _____ a. Adhesions

    _____ b. Volvulus

    _____ c. Intussusception

    _____ d. Hernia

    _____ e. Vascular obstruction

    _____ f. Adynamic obstruction

    1. Atonic bowel

    2. Protrusion of bowel through fascial defect or abnormal opening

    3. Bands of scar tissue constrict the intestine

    4. Closed loop twisting of bowel on itself

    5. Bowel folding in on itself

    6. Emboli of arterial supply to the bowel

24. The fluid and electrolyte imbalances that occur with a low small bowel obstruction are a result of

    a. decreased secretion of intestinal fluids.
    b. loss of hydrochloric acid from persistent, copious vomiting.
    c. bleeding from a strangulated obstruction resulting in necrosis.
    d. movement of fluid and electrolytes from the bowel into the peritoneal cavity.

25. Identify whether the following statements are true or false. If a statement is false, correct the bold word(s) to make the statement true.

    _____ a. A rapid onset of projectile vomiting occurs with a **large bowel obstruction**.

    _____ b. Abdominal distension is the most apparent in an obstruction of the **large bowel**.

    _____ c. Fecal vomiting is most likely to occur in a **low small** bowel obstruction.

    _____ d. **Metabolic alkalosis** is most likely to occur with a low small bowel obstruction.

    _____ e. Sudden, severe constant abdominal pain is indicative of an **upper small** bowel obstruction.

    _____ f. Abdominal pain that is colicky and crampy, coming and going in waves, is characteristic of a **paralytic ileus**.

26. An important nursing intervention for the client with a small bowel obstruction who has a nasogastric tube is to

    a. offer ice chips to suck prn.
    b. provide mouth care every one to two hours.
    c. irrigate the tube with normal saline every eight hours.
    d. keep the client supine with the head of the bed elevated 30 degrees.

27. During a routine screening colonoscopy on a 56-year-old client, a rectosigmoidal polyp was identified and removed. The client asks the nurse if his risk for colon cancer is increased because of the polyp. The best response of the nurse is

    a. "It is very rare for polyps to become malignant, but you should continue to have routine colonoscopies."
    b. "Individuals with polyps have a 100% lifetime risk of developing colorectal cancer, and at an earlier age than those without polyps."
    c. "All polyps are abnormal and should be removed, but the risk for cancer depends on the type and whether malignant changes are present."
    d. "All polyps are premalignant and the source of most colon cancers. You will need to have a colonoscopy every six months to check for new polyps."

28. Early screening for detection of cancers of the right side of the colon in individuals over 50 years of age that should be done every year include

    a. serum CEA levels.
    b. flexible sigmoidoscopy.
    c. digital rectal examination.
    d. fecal testing for occult blood.

29. Describe how the structures of the colon are altered during an abdominal-perineal resection.

30. Upon examining a client eight hours after formation of a colostomy, the nurse would expect to find

    a. hypoactive, high-pitched bowel sounds.
    b. a pale pink to dark red, edematous stoma.
    c. a purplish stoma, shiny and moist with mucus.
    d. a small amount of liquid fecal drainage from the stoma.

31. A male client who has undergone an abdominal-perineal resection has a nursing diagnosis of risk for ineffective sexuality patterns. An appropriate nursing intervention for the client is to

    a. have the client's sexual partner reassure the client that he is still desirable.
    b. reassure the client that sexual function will return when healing is complete.
    c. remind the client that affection can be expressed in other ways besides sexual intercourse.
    d. explain that physical and emotional factors can affect sexual function but not necessarily the client's sexuality.

32. Describe the type of drainage expected from the stoma of each of the following.

    a.  Ileostomy

    b.  Descending colostomy

    c.  Transverse loop colostomy

33. The nurse plans teaching for the client with a colostomy, but the client refuses to look at the nurse or the stoma, stating "I just can't see myself with this thing." An appropriate nursing diagnosis for the client is

    a. self-care deficit related to refusal to care for colostomy.
    b. disturbed body image related to presence of colostomy stoma.
    c. ineffective coping related to feelings of helplessness and lack of coping skills.
    d. ineffective therapeutic regimen management related to lack of knowledge for care of colostomy.

34. In teaching a client about colostomy irrigation, the nurse tells the client to

    a. infuse 1500 to 2000 mL of warm tap water as irrigation fluid.
    b. allow 30 to 45 minutes for the solution and feces to be expelled.
    c. insert a firm plastic catheter 7.5 to 10 cm (3 to 4 in.) into the stoma opening.
    d. hang the irrigation bag on a hook about 90 cm (36 in.) above the stoma.

35. During an acute attack of diverticulitis, the client is

    a. monitored for signs of peritonitis.
    b. treated with daily medicated enemas.
    c. prepared for surgery to resect the involved colon.
    d. provided with a heating pad to apply to the left lower quadrant.

36. Match the types of hernias with their descriptions.

    _____    a. Reducible                    1. Obstructed intestinal flow and blood supply

    _____    b. Incarcerated                 2. Follows the spermatic cord or round ligament

    _____    c. Strangulated                 3. Weakness at the site of previous abdominal
                                                incision
    _____    d. Femoral
                                             4. Cannot be placed back into abdominal cavity
    _____    e. Inguinal
                                             5. Protrusion into femoral canal
    _____    f. Ventral
                                             6. Can be placed back into abdominal cavity

37. A nursing intervention that is indicated for a male client following an inguinal herniorrhaphy is

    a. applying heat to the inguinal area.
    b. elevating the scrotum with a scrotal support.
    c. applying a truss to support the operative site.
    d. encouraging the client to cough and breathe deeply.

38. The most common form of malabsorption syndrome is treated with

    a. administration of antibiotics.
    b. avoidance of milk and milk products.
    c. supplementation with pancreatic enzymes.
    d. avoidance of gluten found in wheat, barley, oats, and rye.

39. Short bowel syndrome is most likely to occur in the client with

    a. ulcerative colitis.
    b. irritable bowel syndrome.
    c. multiple, extensive resection of the small intestine.
    d. a colectomy performed for cancer of the bowel.

40. Match the following anorectal conditions with their descriptions.

    _____  a. Pilonidal sinus

    _____  b. Anorectal abscess

    _____  c. Anal fissure

    _____  d. Hemorrhoid

    _____  e. Anorectal fistula

    1. Engorged rectal vein around anal sphincter

    2. Ulcer in anal wall

    3. Tunnel leading from anus or rectum to perianal skin or buttocks

    4. Collection of perianal pus

    5. Sacrococcygeal hairy tract

41. Following anal surgery, the nurse advises the client to

    a. use daily laxatives to facilitate bowel emptying.
    b. apply ice packs to the perineum to prevent swelling.
    c. avoid having a bowel movement for several days until healing occurs.
    d. take warm sitz baths several times a day to promote comfort and cleaning.

# CASE STUDY

## CANCER OF THE RECTUM

### Client Profile

Mr. D., a 63-year-old married insurance salesman, has undergone an abdominal-perineal resection for cancer of the rectum. He is one day post-operative on the general surgical unit.

### Subjective Data

- Complains of pain in his abdominal and perineal incisions that is not well controlled even with his PCA machine
- Jokes about his stoma winking at him when the dressings are removed the first time and a temporary colostomy pouch is applied
- Refers to his stoma as "Jake"
- Tells his wife that "Jake" will be watching her
- Says he and his wife are worried about diet changes that may be required now that he has a colostomy

### Objective Data

- Stoma on left lower quadrant of abdomen, bright red, colostomy pouch has small amount of serosanguineous drainage
- Midline abdominal incision; no signs of infection; staples intact, incision edges well approximated
- Perineal incision sutured closed, two Jackson-Pratt drains to right and left lower abdomen with dressings, with large amount of serosanguineous drainage in bulbs
- All vital signs normal
- PCA orders of 1 mg morphine sulphate every 10 minutes, with 17 attempts in the past hour

### Critical Thinking Questions

1. What symptoms may have alerted Mr. D. to seek medical care for his cancer of the colon?

2. What care is indicated for Mr. D.'s perineal wound and abdominal drains?

3.  What are the primary goals of care for Mr. D.'s colostomy?

4.  What would be the nurse's evaluation of Mr. D.'s adjustment to his colostomy?

5.  What factors may be influencing the pain that Mr. D. is experiencing?

6.  What teaching will need to be accomplished with Mr. D. before his discharge?

7.  Based on the assessment data presented, write one or more appropriate nursing diagnoses.

# CHAPTER 42 NURSING MANAGEMENT: LIVER, BILIARY TRACT, AND PANCREAS PROBLEMS

1. Complete the following statements.

   a. The type of jaundice associated with gallstones is _____ jaundice, and the type of serum

      bilirubin that is elevated is most likely _____.

   b. Hemolytic jaundice is caused by _____, and the type of bilirubin elevated

      in the blood is _____.

   c. Jaundice resulting from failure of the liver to conjugate and excrete bilirubin is known as

      _____ jaundice and causes serum elevations of _____ bilirubin.

2. Match the following characteristics of viral hepatitis with their related types (answers may be used more than once).

   _____ a. IV drug use is mode of greatest transmission

   _____ b. Uncommon in Canada

   _____ c. Exists only with hepatitis B

   _____ d. Caused by a DNA virus

   _____ e. Most common cause of chronic hepatitis

   _____ f. Often causes asymptomatic anicteric hepatitis

   _____ g. Chronic carriers have increased risk for hepatocellular cancer

   _____ h. Has no chronic carrier state

   _____ i. No readily available diagnostic serology tests

   _____ j. Usual cause of hepatitis epidemics

   1. Hepatitis A (HAV)

   2. Hepatitis B (HBV)

   3. Hepatitis C (HCV)

   4. Hepatitis D (HDV)

   5. Hepatitis E (HEV)

3. Serological findings in viral hepatitis include both the presence of viral antigens and antibodies produced in response to the viruses. Identify the three antigens associated with active HBV and the corresponding antibodies for those antigens. (One of the antigens stimulates two antibodies.)

   | **Antigen** | **Antibodies** |
   | --- | --- |
   | a. (surface)_____ | _____ |
   | b. (e)_____ | _____ |
   | c. (core)_____ | _____ |
   | | _____ |

4. Complete the following sentences related to serological findings in viral hepatitis.

 a. In addition to HBV antigens and antibodies, the best indicator of active, ongoing HBV replication is the presence of _____ in the blood.

 b. The HBV antibody that is a marker of response to the HBV vaccine is _____.

 c. The HBV antibody that does not appear after immunization is _____.

 d. The HBV antigen that persists in chronic carrier states is _____.

 e. HAV antigens are not tested in the blood, but like HBV, they stimulate specific IgM and IgG antibodies. Acute HVA infection is indicated by _____ antibodies, whereas prior infection is indicated by _____ antibodies.

 f. Co-infection of HDV with HBV can be detected by testing for the _____ antibody.

 g. Several tests are used to determine the presence of HCV. The initial screening for acute or chronic HVC includes testing for the _____ antibody.

 h. A client with anti-HVC antibodies can have active, chronic, or prior HCV infection. The test that best indicates active disease and can also detect HVC in an immunosuppressed client is _____.

 i. A more sensitive antibody test for HCV includes the use of the _____.

5. The systemic effects of viral hepatitis are caused primarily by

 a. cholestasis.
 b. impaired portal circulation.
 c. toxins produced by the infected liver.
 d. activation of the complement system by antigen–antibody complexes.

6. During the pre-icteric phase of viral hepatitis, the nurse would expect the client to report

 a. pruritus and malaise.
 b. dark urine and easy fatigability.
 c. anorexia and right upper quadrant discomfort.
 d. constipation or diarrhea with light-coloured stools.

7. Fulminant hepatic failure as a complication of viral hepatitis is highest in those individuals with

 a. hepatitis A.
 b. hepatitis C.
 c. hepatitis B accompanied by hepatitis C.
 d. hepatitis B accompanied by hepatitis D.

8. Identify the prophylactic immunological agents that are used for the following.

   a. Pre-exposure protection to HBV

   b. Post-exposure protection to HBV

9. The family members of a client with hepatitis A ask if there is anything that will prevent them from developing the disease. The best response of the nurse is

   a. "No immunization is available for hepatitis A, nor are you likely to get the disease."
   b. "Only individuals who have had sexual contact with the client should receive immunization."
   c. "All family members should receive the hepatitis A vaccine to prevent or modify the infection."
   d. "Those who have had household or close contact with the client should receive immune globulin."

10. A client newly diagnosed with acute hepatitis B asks if there is drug therapy to treat the disease. The most appropriate response of the nurse is informing the client that

   a. there are no specific drug therapies that are effective for treating acute viral hepatitis.
   b. only chronic hepatitis C is treatable, primarily with antiviral agents and α-interferon.
   c. no drugs can be used for treatment of viral hepatitis because of the risk of additional liver damage.
   d. α-interferon combined with lamivudine (Heptovir) will decrease viral load and liver damage if taken for one year.

11. The nurse identifies a need for further teaching when the client with hepatitis B states,

   a. "I should avoid alcohol completely for as long as a year."
   b. "I must avoid all physical contact with my family until the jaundice is gone."
   c. "I should use a condom to prevent spread of the disease to my sexual partner."
   d. "I will need to rest several times a day, gradually increasing my activity as I tolerate it."

12. One of the most challenging nursing interventions to promote healing in the client with viral hepatitis is

   a. providing adequate nutritional intake.
   b. promoting strict bed rest during the icteric phase.
   c. providing pain relief without using liver-metabolized drugs.
   d. providing quiet diversional activities during periods of fatigue.

13. When caring for a client with autoimmune hepatitis, the nurse recognizes that unlike viral hepatitis, the client

   a. does not manifest hepatomegaly or jaundice.
   b. experiences less liver inflammation and damage.
   c. is treated with corticosteroids or other immunosuppressant agents.
   d. is usually an older adult who has used a wide variety of prescription and over-the-counter drugs.

14. Match the characteristics of cirrhosis with their related types (answers may be used more than once).

_____ a. Diffuse liver fibrosis

_____ b. Vascular congestion of liver

_____ c. Malnutrition related

_____ d. Associated with chemical toxicity

_____ e. Early fatty infiltration

_____ f. Viral induced

_____ g. Chronic biliary obstruction

1. Alcoholic

2. Post-necrotic

3. Biliary

4. Cardiac

15. Match the following clinical manifestations with the pathophysiological changes that occur in cirrhosis (answers may be used more than once).

_____ a. Jaundice

_____ b. Testicular atrophy

_____ c. Anorexia and dyspepsia

_____ d. Spider angiomas

_____ e. Amenorrhea

_____ f. Peripheral neuropathy

_____ g. Anemia, leukopenia, thrombocytopenia

_____ h. Dull, heavy, RUQ pain

_____ i. Male gynecomastia

_____ j. Petechiae and purpura

1. Decreased prothrombin production

2. Vascular congestion of spleen

3. Decreased estrogen metabolism

4. Stretching of liver capsule

5. Decreased bilirubin conjugation and excretion

6. Altered carbohydrate, protein, and fat metabolism

7. Decreased testosterone metabolism

8. Vitamin B deficiencies

16. Describe the pathophysiological changes of cirrhosis that cause the following.

a. Portal hypertension


b. Esophageal varices

17. Complete the following statements related to Figure 42-6 in the textbook.

   a. Portal hypertension and the resulting increased blood hydrostatic pressure cause leakage of plasma into the abdominal cavity from three major sources. These sources are _____,

   _____, and _____.

   b. Fluid also moves into the abdominal cavity, producing ascites because of decreased serum oncotic colloidal pressure. The decreased serum oncotic pressure is caused by _____.

   c. Fluid sequestering in the peritoneal cavity results in (increased/decreased) _____ vascular volume, (increased/decreased) _____ blood return to the heart, and (increased/decreased) _____ cardiac output.

   d. The change in cardiac output results in (increased/decreased) _____ kidney perfusion and secretion of _____ and _____, both of which increase fluid retention.

   e. The retained fluid has low oncotic colloidal pressure, and it escapes into the interstitial spaces, causing _____.

   f. Excessive fluid continues to be reabsorbed from the kidney because of the altered kidney perfusion and because _____ is not metabolized by the impaired liver.

   g. The changes in laboratory test results that relate to this process are _____ and _____.

18. Laboratory test results that the nurse would expect to find in a client with cirrhosis include

   a. serum albumin: 70 g/L (7.0 g/dL).
   b. bilirubin: total 54.7 $\mu$mol/L (3.2 mg/dL).
   c. serum cholesterol: 6.7 mmol/L (260 mg/dL).
   d. aspartate aminotransferase (AST): 0.1 $\mu$kat/L (6 U/L).

19. Identify the rationales for the following interventions in treating the cirrhotic client with ascites.

   a.  Bed rest

   b.  Salt-poor albumin

   c.  Diuretic therapy

   d.  Low-sodium diet

   e.  Paracentesis

   f.  Peritoneovenous shunts

20. The nurse recognizes early signs of hepatic encephalopathy in the client who

    a. manifests asterixis.
    b. becomes unconscious.
    c. has increasing oliguria.
    d. is irritable and lethargic.

21. Identify the rationales for the following interventions in treating the cirrhotic client with hepatic encephalopathy.

    a. Low-protein diet

    b. Lactulose

    c. Neomycin

    d. Eliminating blood from GI tract

22. A client with cirrhosis has a nursing diagnosis of disturbed body image. Common etiological factors for this diagnosis include

    a. jaundice and ascites.
    b. dyspnea and pruritus.
    c. alopecia and skin lesions.
    d. periorbital edema and decreased sensory perception.

23. A client with advanced cirrhosis has a nursing diagnosis of imbalanced nutrition: less than body requirements related to anorexia and inadequate food intake. An appropriate midday snack for the client would be

    a. peanut butter and salt-free crackers.
    b. popcorn with salt-free butter and herbal seasoning.
    c. canned chicken noodle soup with low-protein bread.
    d. a tomato sandwich with low-protein bread and salt-free butter.

24. A client with ascites is short of breath and has an increased respiratory rate. The nurse should

    a. notify the physician so a paracentesis can be performed.
    b. initiate oxygen therapy at 2 L/min to increase gas exchange.
    c. ask the client to cough and breathe deeply to clear respiratory secretions.
    d. place the client in Fowler's position to relieve pressure on the diaphragm.

25. During the treatment of the client with bleeding esophageal varices, it is most important that the nurse

    a. prepare the client for immediate portal shunting surgery.
    b. perform guaiac testing on all stools to detect occult blood.
    c. maintain the client's airway and prevent aspiration of blood.
    d. monitor for the cardiac stimulant effects of IV vasopressin and nitroglycerin.

26. A client with cirrhosis that is refractory to other treatments for esophageal varices undergoes a peritoneo-venous shunt. As a result of this procedure, the nurse would expect the client to experience

    a. an improved survival rate.
    b. decreased serum ammonia levels.
    c. improved metabolism of nutrients.
    d. improved hemodynamic function and renal perfusion.

27. In discussing long-term management with the client with alcoholic cirrhosis, the nurse advises the client that

    a. a daily exercise regimen is important to increase the blood flow through the liver.
    b. cirrhosis can be reversed if the client follows a regimen of proper rest and nutrition.
    c. abstinence from alcohol is the most important factor in improvement of the client's condition.
    d. the only over-the-counter analgesic that should be used for minor aches and pains is acetaminophen.

28. A client is hospitalized with metastatic cancer of the liver. The nurse plans care for the client based on the knowledge that

    a. chemotherapy is highly successful in the treatment of liver cancer.
    b. the client will undergo surgery to remove the involved portions of the liver.
    c. supportive care that is appropriate for all clients with severe liver damage is indicated.
    d. metastatic cancer of the liver is more responsive to treatment than primary carcinoma of the liver.

29. A client with cirrhosis asks the nurse about the possibility of a liver transplant. The best response of the nurse is

    a. "Liver transplants are only indicated in children with irreversible liver disease."
    b. "If you are interested in a transplant, you really should talk to your doctor about it."
    c. "Rejection is such a problem in liver transplants that it is seldom attempted in clients with cirrhosis."
    d. "Cirrhosis is an indication for transplantation in some cases. Have you talked to your doctor about this?"

30. Match the complications of acute pancreatitis with the pathophysiological mechanisms.

_____ a. Pseudocyst

_____ b. Pancreatic abscess

_____ c. Pleural effusion

_____ d. Tetany

_____ e. Hypovolemia

1. Combining of calcium with fatty acids during fat necrosis

2. Cavity continuous with pancreas filled with necrotic products and secretions

3. Pancreatic enzymes pass from peritoneal cavity through diaphragmatic lymph channels

4. Exudation of blood and plasma into retroperitoneal space

5. Extensive pancreatic necrosis with resultant fluid-filled cavity

31. When assessing a client with acute pancreatitis, the nurse would expect to find

 a. hyperactive bowel sounds.
 b. hypertension and tachycardia.
 c. severe mid-epigastric or LUQ pain.
 d. a temperature greater than 39°C (102°F).

32. Combined with clinical manifestations, the laboratory finding that is most commonly used to diagnose acute pancreatitis is

 a. increased serum lipase.
 b. increased serum amylase.
 c. increased urinary amylase.
 d. decreased renal amylase–creatine clearance ratio.

33. Management of acute peritonitis related to alcohol abuse includes

 a. surgery to remove the inflamed pancreas.
 b. replacement of pancreatic enzymes with meals.
 c. nasogastric suction to prevent gastric contents from entering the duodenum.
 d. endoscopic pancreatic sphincterotomy using retrograde cholangiopancreatography (ERCP).

34. The most effective means of suppressing pancreatic secretion during an episode of pancreatitis is the use of

 a. antibiotics.
 b. NPO status.
 c. antispasmodics.
 d. H$_2$R blockers or proton pump inhibitors.

35. A client with acute pancreatitis has a nursing diagnosis of pain related to distension of pancreas and peritoneal irritation. In addition to effective use of analgesics, the nurse should

 a. provide diversional activities to distract the client from the pain.
 b. provide small frequent meals to increase the client's tolerance to food.
 c. position the client on the side with the head of the bed elevated 45 degrees.
 d. have the client ambulate every three to four hours to increase circulation and decrease abdominal congestion.

36. The nurse determines that further discharge instruction is needed when the client with acute pancreatitis states,

    a. "I should observe for fat in my stools."
    b. "I must not use alcohol to prevent future attacks of pancreatitis."
    c. "I shouldn't eat salty foods or foods with high amounts of sodium."
    d. "I will need to continue to monitor my blood glucose levels until my pancreas is healed."

37. The client with chronic pancreatitis is more likely than the client with acute pancreatitis to

    a. need to abstain from alcohol.
    b. experience acute abdominal pain.
    c. have malabsorption and diabetes mellitus.
    d. require a high-carbohydrate, high-protein, low-fat diet.

38. A nursing intervention that is indicated in administration of pancreatic enzymes to the client with chronic pancreatitis is to

    a. have the client take the preparations with meals and snacks.
    b. dissolve the tablets in water before administration to activate the enzymes.
    c. monitor the client's blood glucose levels to evaluate the effectiveness of the enzymes.
    d. administer liquid enzymes through a straw to eliminate contact with the oral mucous membrane.

39. A risk factor associated with cancer of the pancreas is

    a. alcohol intake.
    b. cigarette smoking.
    c. exposure to asbestos.
    d. increased dietary intake of milk and milk products.

40. In a radical pancreaticoduodenectomy (Whipple procedure) for treatment of cancer of the pancreas, what anatomical structures are completely resected?

    a.

    b.

    What anatomical structures are partially resected?

    c.

    d.

    What anastomoses are made?

    e.

    f.

    g.

    h.

41. Identify whether the following statements are true or false. If a statement is false, correct the bold word(s) to make the statement true.

_____ a. **Cholelithiasis** is the most common disorder of the biliary system.

_____ b. Most gallstones are composed primarily of **calcium and bile salts**.

_____ c. If a gallstone blocks the cystic duct, the client will have brown stools and symptoms of **biliary colic**.

_____ d. Factors that cause stasis of bile flow lead to **cholecystitis**.

_____ e. Obstructive jaundice occurs when gallstones obstruct the **common bile duct**.

42. Of the following characteristics, identify those that are associated with cholelithiasis.

_____ a. Family history of gallbladder disease

_____ b. History of excessive alcohol intake

_____ c. Multiparous female

_____ d. Obesity

_____ e. High serum high-density lipoproteins

_____ f. Age over 40 years

_____ g. Use of estrogen or oral contraceptives

43. The client with an obstruction of the common bile duct has the following signs and symptoms. Identify the pathophysiological changes that cause these clinical manifestations.

a. Jaundice

b. Clay-coloured stools

c. Dark urine

d. Steatorrhea

e. Pain following fatty food intake

44. The client with suspected gallbladder disease is scheduled for an ultrasound of the gallbladder. The nurse explains to the client that this test

a. is non-invasive and is a very reliable method of detecting gallstones.
b. is used only when other tests cannot be used due to allergy to contrast media.
c. is an adjunct to liver function tests to determine if the gallbladder is inflamed.
d. will outline the gallbladder and the ductal system to enable visualization of stones.

45. Identify the rationale for the treatment of acute cholecystitis with the following interventions.

    a. NPO with nasogastric suction

    b. Pain management with meperidine (Demerol)

    c. Administration of antibiotics

    d. Administration of antispasmodics

46. Match the following descriptions with the treatments used for cholelithiasis.

    _____ a. External shock waves disintegrate
                stones

    _____ b. Stones removed through sphincter
                of Oddi

    _____ c. Cholesterol solvent injected directly
                into gallbladder

    _____ d. Administered orally to dissolve stones
                and reduce cholesterol saturation

    1. Endoscopic sphincterotomy

    2. Lithotripsy

    3. Methyl tertiary terbutal ether (MTBE)

    4. Chenodeoxycholic acid (CDCA)

47. The surgical treatment of choice for the client with symptomatic gallbladder disease is a

    a. cholecystotomy.
    b. choledocholithotomy.
    c. cholecystoduodenostomy.
    d. laparoscopic cholecystectomy.

48. Following a laparoscopic cholecystectomy, the nurse would expect the client to

    a. return to work in two to three weeks.
    b. be hospitalized for three to five days post-operatively.
    c. have four small abdominal incisions covered with small dressings.
    d. have a T-tube placed in the common bile duct to provide bile drainage.

49. A client with chronic cholecystitis asks the nurse if she will need to continue a low-fat diet after she has a cholecystectomy. The best response of the nurse is

    a. "A low-fat diet will prevent the development of further gallstones and should be continued."
    b. "Yes, because you will not have a gallbladder to store bile, you will not be able to digest fats adequately."
    c. "A low-fat diet is recommended for a few weeks after surgery until the intestine adjusts to receiving a continuous flow of bile."
    d. "Removal of the gallbladder will eliminate the source of your pain associated with fat intake so you may eat whatever you like."

50. Post-operatively, a client with an incisional cholecystectomy has a nursing diagnosis of ineffective breathing pattern related to splinted respirations secondary to a high abdominal incision. The nursing intervention that should be implemented first for this client is to

    a. assess lung sounds every two to four hours.
    b. provide analgesics to relieve incisional pain.
    c. assist the client to cough and breathe deeply every hour.
    d. position the client on the operative side to splint the incision.

51. To care for a T-tube in a client following a cholecystectomy, the nurse

    a. keeps the tube supported and free of kinks.
    b. attaches the tube to low continuous suction.
    c. clamps the tube when the client ambulates.
    d. irrigates the tube with 10 mL sterile saline every two to four hours.

52. During discharge instructions for a client following a laparoscopic cholecystectomy, the nursing advises the client to

    a. keep the incision areas clean and dry for at least a week.
    b. report the need to take pain medication for shoulder pain.
    c. report any bile-coloured or purulent drainage from the incisions.
    d. expect some post-operative nausea and vomiting for a few days.

## CASE STUDY

### ACUTE PANCREATITIS

### Client Profile

Mr. A. is a 55-year-old man admitted to the hospital with acute pancreatitis.

### Subjective Data

- Has severe abdominal pain in the LUQ, radiating to the back
- States he is nauseated and has been vomiting

### Objective Data

- Vital signs: Temp 38.3°C (101°F); HR 114; RR 26; BP 92/58
- Jaundice noted in sclera
- Laboratory values:     serum amylase 400 U/L
                         urinary amylase 3800 U/day
                         WBC count 20 x $10^9$/L (20 x $10^3$/μL)
                         blood glucose 10 mmol/L (180 mg/dL)
                         serum calcium 1.7 mmol/L (7 mg/dL)

### Collaborative Care

- NPO status
- NG tube to low, intermittent suction
- IV therapy with lactated Ringer's solution
- Meperidine (Demerol) IVPB
- Ranitidine (Zantac) IVPB

**Critical Thinking Questions**

1. Explain the pathophysiology of acute pancreatitis.

2. What are the most common causes of acute pancreatitis?

3. How do the results of Mr. A's laboratory values relate to the pathophysiology of acute pancreatitis?

4. What causes hypocalcemia in acute pancreatitis? How does the nurse assess for hypocalcemia?

5. Describe the characteristics of the pain that occurs in acute pancreatitis.

6. What complications can occur with acute pancreatitis?

7. Identify the purpose of each medication Mr. A. is taking.

8. Why is Mr. A. NPO? What is the purpose of the NG tube?

9. Based on the assessment data presented, write one or more appropriate nursing diagnoses. Are there any collaborative problems?

# CHAPTER *43* NURSING ASSESSMENT: URINARY SYSTEM

1. Using the following list of terms, identify the structures in the illustrations below (some of the terms will be used in both illustrations).

**List of Terms**

Adrenal gland
Aorta
Bladder
Cortex
Fibrous capsule
Kidney

Major calyx
Medulla
Minor caly
Papilla
Pyramid
Renal pelvis

Right renal artery
Right renal vein
Ureter
Urethra
Vena cava

a. _____    g. _____    m. _____

b. _____    h. _____    n. _____

c. _____    i. _____    o. _____

d. _____    j. _____    p. _____

e. _____    k. _____    q. _____

f. _____    l. _____    r. _____

2. Match the following functions with the appropriate site in the nephron (answers may be used more than once).

    \_\_\_\_\_ a. Active reabsorption of $Cl^-$ and passive reabsorption of $Na^+$

    \_\_\_\_\_ b. Formed from capillary network of afferent arterioles

    \_\_\_\_\_ c. Secretion of $H^+$ into filtrate

    \_\_\_\_\_ d. Reabsorption of water without ADH

    \_\_\_\_\_ e. Blood filtered into Bowman's capsule

    \_\_\_\_\_ f. Reabsorption of $Na^+$ in exchange for $K^+$

    \_\_\_\_\_ g. Reabsorption of most of electrolytes

    \_\_\_\_\_ h. Reabsorption of bicarbonate

    \_\_\_\_\_ i. Reabsorption of $Ca^{++}$ under parathyroid hormone influence

    \_\_\_\_\_ j. Reabsorption of glucose and amino acids

    \_\_\_\_\_ k. Reabsorption of water under ADH influence

1. Glomerulus

2. Proximal convoluted tubule

3. Descending loop of Henle

4. Ascending loop of Henle

5. Distal convoluted tubule

3. Identify whether the following statements are true or false. If a statement is false, correct the bold word(s) to make the statement true.

    \_\_\_\_\_ a. Glomerular filtration rate is primarily dependent on adequate **blood flow** and adequate **hydrostatic pressure**.

    \_\_\_\_\_ b. The primary function of the kidney is to **excrete nitrogenous waste products**.

    \_\_\_\_\_ c. **Water** is the primary substance reabsorbed in the collecting duct.

    \_\_\_\_\_ d. Atrial natriuretic factor (ANF) is secreted by the right atrium when atrial blood pressure is **low**, and it blocks the action of **aldosterone**.

    \_\_\_\_\_ e. Increased permeability in the **glomerulus** causes loss of proteins into the urine.

4. A client with an obstruction of the renal artery causing renal ischemia exhibits hypertension. One factor that may contribute to the hypertension is

    a. increased renin release.
    b. increased ADH secretion.
    c. decreased aldosterone secretion.
    d. increased synthesis and release of prostaglandins.

5. A clinical situation in which the increased release of erythropoietin would be expected is

    a. hypoxemia.
    b. hypotension.
    c. hyperkalemia.
    d. fluid overload.

6. Complete the following statements.

   a. The sites where urinary stones are most likely to obstruct the urinary system are at the

      _____ and the _____.

   b. The ureteral muscle fibre attachments into the bladder help prevent backflow of urine through the

      _____ junction.

   c. The volume of urine in the bladder that usually causes the urge to urinate is _____ mL.

   d. Total bladder capacity ranges from _____ mL to _____ mL.

   e. Absorption or leakage of urine wastes out of the urinary system is prevented by the cellular characteristics

      of the _____.

7. One factor that contributes to an increased incidence of urinary tract infections in women is

   a. the shorter length of the urethra.
   b. the larger capacity of the bladder.
   c. relaxation of pelvic floor muscles.
   d. the tight muscular support at the rhabdosphincter.

8. An age-related change in the kidney that leads to nocturia in an older adult is

   a. decreased renal mass.
   b. decreased detrusor muscle tone.
   c. decreased ability to conserve sodium.
   d. decreased ability to concentrate urine.

9. Identify one specific finding identified by the nurse during assessment of each of the client's functional health patterns that indicates a risk factor for urinary problems or a client response to a urinary disorder.

   a. Health perception–health management

   b. Nutritional–metabolic

   c. Elimination

   d. Activity–exercise

   e. Sleep–rest

   f. Cognitive–perceptual

   g. Self-perception–self-concept

   h. Role–relationship

   i. Sexuality–reproductive

   j. Coping–stress tolerance

   k. Value–belief

10. During physical assessment of the urinary system, the nurse

   a. auscultates the lower abdominal quadrants for fluid sounds.
   b. palpates an empty bladder at the level of the symphysis pubis.
   c. percusses the kidney with a firm blow at the posterior costovertebral angle.
   d. positions the client prone to palpate the kidneys with a posterior approach.

11. Match the following abnormal assessment findings with their descriptions.

   _____   a. Nocturia                  1. Blood in the urine

   _____   b. Dysuria                   2. Scanty urine output

   _____   c. Retention                 3. Can be caused by sneezing

   _____   d. Polyuria                  4. Urine containing gas

   _____   e. Enuresis                  5. Incontinence during sleep

   _____   f. Hematuria                 6. Painful urination

   _____   g. Oliguria                  7. No urine formation

   _____   h. Urgency                   8. Frequent urination at night

   _____   i. Anuria                    9. Inability to void

   _____   j. Hesitancy                 10. Large amount of urine output

   _____   k. Pneumaturia               11. Difficulty starting urine stream

   _____   l. Stress incontinence       12. Strong desire to urinate

12. A urinalysis of a urine specimen that is not processed within one hour may result in erroneous measurement of

   a. glucose.
   b. bacteria.
   c. specific gravity.
   d. white blood cells.

13. Urinalysis results that most likely indicate a urinary tract infection include

   a. colour yellow; protein 6 mg/dL; pH 6.8; $10^2$ bacteria.
   b. cloudy, yellow; WBC 50/hpf; pH 8.2; numerous casts.
   c. cloudy, brown; ammonia odour; specific gravity 1.030; RBC 3/hpf.
   d. clear; colourless; glucose trace; ketones trace; osmolality 500 mmol/kg (500 mOsm/kg).

14. A client who is being treated with diuretics for retained fluid would be expected to have a urine specific gravity of

   a. 1.002.
   b. 1.010.
   c. 1.025.
   d. 1.030.

15. Following a renal arteriogram, it is important that the nurse

    a. observe for gross bleeding in the urine.
    b. place the client in high Fowler's position.
    c. monitor the client for signs of allergy to the contrast medium.
    d. assess peripheral pulses in the involved leg every 30 to 60 minutes.

16. A client with an elevated BUN

    a. has decreased urea in the urine.
    b. may have non-renal tissue destruction.
    c. definitely has impaired renal function.
    d. will always have a rise in serum creatinine.

17. The test that is most specific for renal function is the

    a. renal scan.
    b. serum creatinine.
    c. blood urea nitrogen.
    d. creatinine clearance.

18. Identify the kidney function that is impaired in the following laboratory findings in a client with kidney disease.

    a. serum $Ca^{++}$: 1.8 mmol/L (7.2 mg/dL)

    b. Hg: 96 g/L (9.6 g/dL)

    c. serum creatinine: 150 $\mu$mol/L (1.70 mg/dL)

19. Following a renal biopsy, it is important that the nurse

    a. offer warm sitz baths to relieve discomfort.
    b. test urine for microscopic bleeding with a dipstick.
    c. expect the client to experience burning on urination.
    d. monitor the client for symptoms of a urinary infection.

20. Match the following nursing responsibilities with the appropriate diagnostic test (answers may be used more than once).

_____ a. Use dipstick and read results with colour chart

_____ b. Ensure informed consent obtained

_____ c. Explain that bladder will be filled with water to measure tone and stability

_____ d. Must start test with full bladder

_____ e. Keep client NPO 8 hr before test

_____ f. Insert catheter immediately after voiding

_____ g. Clean meatus before voiding

_____ h. First morning specimen is best

_____ i. Explain post-procedure pink urine normal

_____ j. Have client void, stop, void in container

_____ k. Discard first specimen at start; include voided specimen 24 hours later

_____ l. Use sterile container

_____ m. Assess for iodine sensitivity

1. Urinalysis

2. Creatinine clearance

3. Clean-catch urine specimen

4. Residual urine

5. Protein determination

6. Cystoscopy

7. Intravenous pyelogram

8. Cystometrogram

9. Urinary flow study

# CHAPTER 44 NURSING MANAGEMENT: RENAL AND UROLOGICAL PROBLEMS

1. Match the following characteristics with the appropriate classifications of urinary tract infection (UTI).

   _____ a. Occurs in otherwise normal urinary tract

   _____ b. Initially resistant to antibiotics

   _____ c. Bacterial colonization of bladder without symptoms

   _____ d. Exists in presence of obstruction or stones

   _____ e. Infection of kidney and/or kidney pelvis

   _____ f. Infection of bladder and/or urethra

   _____ g. Continuing infection because of development resistance

   _____ h. Reinfection following successful treatment of prior UTI

   1. Upper UTI

   2. Lower UTI

   3. Complicated UTI

   4. Uncomplicated UTI

   5. Recurrent UTI

   6. Unresolved bacteriuria

   7. Bacterial persistence

   8. Asymptomatic of resistant bacteriuria

2. The nurse identifies the client with the greatest risk for a urinary tract infection as a

   a. 37-year-old man with renal colic associated with kidney stones.
   b. 26-year-old pregnant woman who has a history of urinary tract infections.
   c. 69-year-old man who has urinary retention caused by benign prostatic hyperplasia.
   d. 72-year-old woman hospitalized with a stroke who has a Foley catheter because of urinary incontinence.

3. While caring for a 77-year-old woman who has a Foley catheter, the nurse monitors the client for development of a UTI. The clinical manifestations the client is most likely to experience include

   a. cloudy urine and fever.
   b. urethral burning and bloody urine.
   c. vague abdominal pain and disorientation.
   d. suprapubic pain and slight decline in body temperature.

4. A woman with no history of UTIs who is experiencing urgency, frequency, and dysuria comes to the clinic, where a dipstick and microscopic urinalysis indicate a bacteriuria. The nurse anticipates that the client will

   a. need to have a blood specimen drawn for a CBC and kidney function tests.
   b. not be treated with medication unless she develops fever, chills, and flank pain.
   c. be requested to obtain a clean-catch midstream urine specimen for culture and sensitivity.
   d. be treated empirically with trimethoprim-sulphamethasoxazole (TMP-SMX) for three days.

5. A female client with a UTI has a nursing diagnosis of risk for infection related to lack of knowledge regarding prevention of recurrence. The nurse includes in the teaching plan instructions to

   a. empty the bladder at least four times a day.
   b. urinate before and after sexual intercourse.
   c. drink 1000 mL of liquid every day.
   d. clean the urinary meatus with an anti-infective agent after voiding.

6. Acute pyelonephritis resulting from an ascending infection from the lower urinary tract occurs most often when

   a. the kidney is scarred and fibrotic.
   b. the organism is resistant to antibiotics.
   c. there is a pre-existing abnormality of the urinary tract.
   d. the client does not take all of the antibiotics for treatment of a UTI.

7. The client with acute pyelonephritis is more likely than the client with a lower UTI to have a nursing diagnosis of

   a. hyperthermia related to infection.
   b. acute pain related to dysuria and bladder spasms.
   c. impaired urinary elimination related to infection.
   d. risk for infection related to lack of knowledge regarding prevention of recurrence.

8. Identify whether the following statements are true or false. If a statement is false, correct the bold word(s) to make the statement true.

   _____ a. **Acute** pyelonephritis causes progressive destruction of nephrons resulting in chronic renal insufficiency.

   _____ b. In a client with acute pyelonephritis, an **IVP** may be performed **after** the infection is resolved to evaluate the urinary system for abnormalities.

   _____ c. Diagnosis of acute pyelonephritis always requires a **urine culture and sensitivity test.**

   _____ d. Following initial treatment of acute pyelonephritis, the client must have a follow-up **CBC**.

   _____ e. The most common cause of urethritis in men is **sexually transmitted infections**.

9. A client with suprapubic pain and symptoms of urinary frequency and urgency has two negative urine cultures. One assessment finding that would indicate interstitial cystitis is

   a. residual urine of greater than 200 mL.
   b. a large, atonic bladder on urodynamic testing.
   c. a voiding pattern that indicates psychogenic urinary retention.
   d. pain with bladder filling that is transiently relieved by urination.

10. When caring for the client with interstitial cystitis, the nurse teaches the client to

   a. avoid foods that make the urine more alkaline.
   b. use the dietary supplement calcium glycerophosphate (Prelief) to decrease bladder irritation.
   c. always keep a voiding diary to document pain, voiding frequencies, and patterns of nocturia.
   d. use high-potency vitamin therapy to decrease the autoimmune effects of the disorder.

11. Glomerulonephritis is characterized by glomerular damage caused by

   a. growth of micro-organisms in the glomeruli.
   b. release of bacterial substances toxic to the glomeruli.
   c. hemolysis of red blood cells circulating through the glomeruli.
   d. accumulation of immune complexes and complement in the glomeruli.

12. Indicate whether the following clinical manifestations of acute post-streptococcal glomerulonephritis (APSGN) are related to decreased glomerular filtration rate (GFR) or injury to the glomerular basement membrane (GBM).

_____ a. Periorbital edema

_____ b. Smoky urine

_____ c. Proteinuria

_____ d. Hypertension

_____ e. Increased BUN and creatinine

_____ f. Oliguria

13. Restriction of dietary protein may be indicated in management of acute post-streptococcal glomerulonephritis when the client has

a. hematuria.
b. proteinuria.
c. hypertension.
d. elevated BUN.

14. The nurse plans care for the client with acute post-streptococcal glomerulonephritis (APSGN) based on the knowledge that

a. most clients with APSGN recover completely or rapidly improve with conservative management.
b. chronic glomerulonephritis leading to renal failure is a common sequela to acute glomerulonephritis.
c. pulmonary hemorrhage may occur as a result of antibodies also attacking the alveolar basement membrane.
d. a large percentage of clients with APSGN develop rapidly progressive glomerulonephritis resulting in kidney failure.

15. The edema associated with nephrotic syndrome occurs as a result of

a. hypercoagulability.
b. hyperalbuminemia.
c. decreased plasma oncotic pressure.
d. decreased glomerular filtration rate.

16. An appropriate nursing diagnosis for the client with nephrotic syndrome is

a. risk for injury related to decreased clotting function.
b. risk for impaired skin integrity related to immobility.
c. risk for infection related to altered immune responses.
d. imbalanced nutrition: more than body requirements, related to high cholesterol intake.

17. Identify three HIV-associated renal syndromes.

a.

b.

c.

18. Number in sequence the following ascending pathological changes that occur in the urinary tract in the presence of a bladder outlet obstruction.

_____ a. Hydronephrosis

_____ b. Reflux of urine into ureter

_____ c. Bladder detrusor muscle hypertrophy

_____ d. Ureteral dilation

_____ e. Renal atrophy

_____ f. Trabeculation of muscle cells

_____ g. Hydroureter

_____ h. Diverticula formation

_____ i. Chronic pyelonephritis

19. Clients at risk for renal lithiasis can prevent the stones in many cases by

a. leading an active life.
b. limiting protein and acid foods in the diet.
c. drinking enough fluids to produce a urine output of 2 L/day.
d. taking prophylactic antibiotics to control urinary tract infections.

20. Match the following characteristics with their associated urinary tract calculi (answers may be used more than once).

_____ a. More common in women

_____ b. Genetic autosomal-recessive defect

_____ c. Often mixed with struvite and oxalate stones

_____ d. Frequently obstruct the ureter

_____ e. Always associated with UTI and urea-splitting bacteria

_____ f. Associated with gout

_____ g. Defective GI and kidney absorption

_____ h. Most common type of stone

_____ i. Often staghorn formation in kidney pelvis

_____ j. Most common in Jewish men

1. Calcium oxalate

2. Calcium phosphate

3. Struvite

4. Uric acid

5. Cystine

21. On assessment of the client with a renal calculi passing down the ureter, the nurse would expect the client to report

    a. dull, costovertebral flank pain.
    b. a history of chronic urinary tract infections.
    c. severe, colicky back pain radiating to the groin.
    d. a feeling of bladder fullness with urgency and frequency.

22. Prevention of calcium oxalate stones would include dietary restriction of

    a. milk and milk products.
    b. dried beans and dried fruits.
    c. liver, kidney, and sweetbreads.
    d. spinach, cabbage, and tomatoes.

23. Following lithotripsy for treatment of renal calculi, the client has a nursing diagnosis of risk for infection related to introduction of bacteria following manipulation of the urinary tract. An appropriate nursing intervention for the client is to

    a. monitor for hematuria.
    b. encourage high fluid intake.
    c. apply moist heat to the flank area.
    d. strain all urine through gauze or a special strainer.

24. Identify whether the following statements are true or false. If a statement is false, correct the bold word(s) to make the statement true.

    _____ a. Kidney injury should be suspected when a client suffering a sports injury has **gross hematuria**.

    _____ b. Benign and accelerated nephrosclerosis cause necrosis of the renal parenchyma and are treated with **anticoagulants**.

    _____ c. The most common manifestations of renal artery stenosis include **flank pain and hematuria**.

    _____ d. Renal vein thrombosis is most commonly treated with **surgical revascularization**.

    _____ e. Clients with urethral strictures may be taught to dilate the urethra by **self-catheterization** every few days.

25. In providing care for the client with adult-onset polycystic kidney disease, the nurse

    a. helps the client cope with the rapid progression of the disease.
    b. suggests genetic counselling resources for the children of the client.
    c. expects the client to have polyuria and poor concentration ability of the kidneys.
    d. implements appropriate measures for the client's deafness and blindness in addition to the renal problems.

26. Match the following metabolic and connective tissue diseases with the pathological renal changes that occur in the diseases.

_____ a. Diabetes mellitus

_____ b. Gout

_____ c. Amyloidosis

_____ d. Systemic lupus erythematosus

_____ e. Scleroderma

1. Connective tissue changes affecting the glomerulus

2. Diffuse and nodular glomerulosclerosis

3. Deposition of sodium urate crystals in interstitium and tubules

4. Vascular lesions with fibrosis

5. Deposition of hyaline substance in kidney

27. When obtaining a nursing history from a client with cancer of the urinary system, the nurse recognizes that a risk factor associated with cancer of both the kidney and the bladder is

a. smoking.
b. a family history of cancer.
c. chronic use of phenacetin.
d. chronic, recurrent nephrolithiasis.

28. The five-year survival rate for cancer of the kidney is usually low, primarily because

a. the only treatment modalities for the disease are palliative.
b. diagnostic tests are not available to detect tumours before they metastasize.
c. the classic symptoms of hematuria and palpable mass do not occur until the disease is advanced.
d. early metastasis to the brain impairs the client's ability to recognize the seriousness of symptoms.

29. A 60-year-old man with cancer of the bladder has laser photocoagulation for treatment of the tumour. Following the procedure, the nurse plans to

a. assess the client for symptoms of cystitis.
b. encourage the client to use warm sitz baths.
c. monitor the client for irritative bladder symptoms.
d. monitor urine output from the urinary catheter for hematuria.

30. Match the following characteristics with their associated types of urinary incontinence (answers may be used more than once).

    _____ a. Caused by overactivity of the
              detrusor muscle

    _____ b. Found following prostatectomy

    _____ c. Treated with Kegel exercises

    _____ d. Occurs with spinal cord lesions above S2

    _____ e. Involuntary urination with minimal
              warning

    _____ f. Common in post-menopausal women

    _____ g. Loss of urine caused by problems of mobility

    _____ h. Caused by outlet obstruction

    _____ i. Occurs without warning or stress equally during day and night

    _____ j. Bladder contracts reflexively, overriding central inhibition

    _____ k. Leakage of urine from overfull bladder

    _____ l. Involuntary urination with increased intra-abdominal pressure

    1. Stress incontinence

    2. Urge incontinence

    3. Overflow incontinence

    4. Reflex incontinence

    5. Functional incontinence

31. Indicate the type of incontinence the following drugs are used to treat and the rationale for their use.

    a. Estrogen replacement

    b. Anticholinergic drugs

    c. α-adrenergic blockers

    d. α-adrenergic agonists

32. To assist the client with stress incontinence, the nurse teaches the client to

    a. void every two hours to prevent leakage.
    b. use absorptive perineal pads to contain urine.
    c. perform pelvic floor muscle exercises four to five times a day.
    d. increase intra-abdominal pressure during voiding to fully empty the bladder.

33. Nursing care that applies to the management of all urinary catheters in hospitalized clients includes

    a. measuring urine output every one to two hours to ensure patency.
    b. turning the client frequently from side to side to promote drainage.
    c. using strict sterile technique during irrigation or opening of the collecting system.
    d. daily cleaning of the catheter insertion site with soap and water and application of an antimicrobial ointment.

34. A client has a right ureteral catheter placed following a lithotripsy for a stone in the ureter. In caring for the client after the procedure, the nurse

    a. milks or strips the catheter every two hours.
    b. measures ureteral urinary drainage every one to two hours.
    c. irrigates with catheter with 30 mL sterile saline q4h.
    d. encourages ambulation to promote urinary peristaltic action.

35. During assessment of the client who had a nephrectomy, the nurse would expect to find

    a. shallow, slow respirations.
    b. clear breath sounds in all lung fields.
    c. decreased breath sounds in the lower left lobe.
    d. decreased breath sounds in the right and left lower lobes.

36. Match the following urinary diversions with their descriptions.

    _____ a. Ileal conduit

    _____ b. Cutaneous ureterostomy

    _____ c. Kock pouch

    _____ d. Ureteroileosigmoidostomy

    1. Continent diversion created by formation of ileal pouch with stoma requiring catheterization

    2. Abdominal stoma formed from resected ileum into which ureters are implanted

    3. Stoma created from ureter(s) brought to abdominal wall

    4. Continent diversion in which ureters are attached to resected segment of ileum implanted into sigmoid colon

37. A client with bladder cancer undergoes cystectomy with formation of an ileal conduit. During the client's first post-operative day, the nurse plans to

    a. measure and fit the stoma for a permanent appliance.
    b. teach the client to self-catheterize the stoma every four to six hours.
    c. encourage high oral intake to flush mucus from the conduit.
    d. empty the drainage bag every two to three hours and measure the urinary output.

38. A teaching plan developed by the nurse for the client with a new ileal conduit or ureterostomy stoma includes instructions to

    a. clean the skin around the stoma with alcohol every day.
    b. use a wick to keep the skin dry during appliance changes.
    c. use sterile supplies and technique during care of the stoma.
    d. change the appliance every day and wash it with soap and warm water.

# CASE STUDY

## BLADDER CANCER

**Client Profile**

Mr. G. is a 55-year-old mechanic who had been healthy all of his life until he passed some blood in his urine and saw a urologist at his wife's insistence. A urine specimen for cytology revealed atypical cells, and a diagnosis of cancer of the bladder was made following a cystoscopy with biopsy of bladder tissue. Intravesical therapy with Bacille Calmette-Guérin (BCG) is planned.

**Subjective Data**

- Has smoked a pack of cigarettes a day since he was a teenager
- Says he dreads having the chemotherapy because he has heard cancer drugs cause such severe side effects

**Objective Data**

- Cystoscopy and biopsy results: moderately differentiated Jewett-Strong-Marshall stage A tumour on the left lateral bladder wall, with $T_2N_0M_0$ pathological stage; fulguration performed during cystoscopy
- Continues to have gross hematuria

## Critical Thinking Questions

1. What does staging of bladder tumours indicate?

2. What information and instructions would the nurse provide for Mr. G. about his intravesical therapy?

3. How can Mr. G. help prevent future bladder tumours from occurring?

4. How should the nurse explain the importance of follow-up cystoscopies?

5. What surgery may be indicated if the chemotherapy is not effective?

6. Based on the assessment data presented, write one or more appropriate nursing diagnoses. Are there any collaborative problems?

# CHAPTER 45 NURSING MANAGEMENT: ACUTE RENAL FAILURE AND CHRONIC KIDNEY DISEASE

1. Match the following conditions and characteristics with their associated etiologies of acute renal failure (answers may be used more than once).

   _____ a. Decreased cardiac output                1. Prerenal

   _____ b. Mechanical outflow obstruction          2. Intrarenal

   _____ c. Initial cause of most acute renal failure   3. Post-renal

   _____ d. Prostate cancer

   _____ e. Tubular obstruction by myoglobin

   _____ f. Hypovolemia

   _____ g. Renal stones

   _____ h. Nephrotoxic drugs

   _____ i. Bladder cancer

   _____ j. Renal vascular obstruction

   _____ k. Acute glomerulonephritis

   _____ l. Anaphylaxis

2. Complete the following statements related to acute tubular necrosis.

   a. Acute tubular necrosis is a type of acute renal failure that results primarily from _____ and

      _____.

   b. Renal ischemia leads to acute tubular necrosis by disrupting the _____ and causing patchy

      destruction of the _____.

   c. Nephrotoxic agents cause necrosis of the _____ that sloughs off and blocks the

      _____.

   d. Acute tubular necrosis from nephrotoxic injury is more likely to be reversible because the

      _____ is usually not initially destroyed.

3. Diagram the processes that occur when hypovolemia and decreased renal blood flow lead to decreased glomerular filtration rate (GFR) and tubular dysfunction with ultimate oliguria by filling in the blanks with the following terms.

Angiotensin-aldosterone system                    Renal artery vasoconstriction
Decreased glomerular capillary pressure           Renin
Decreased renal blood flow

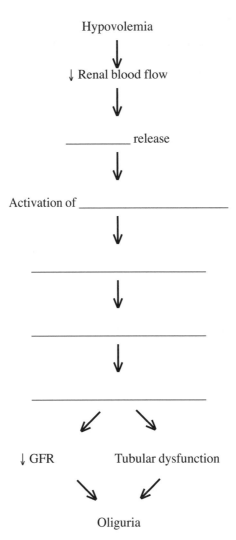

4. Diagram the processes that occur during kidney ischemia that continue to further decrease glomerular filtration rate and injure kidney cells by filling in the blanks with the following terms.

Tubular dysfunction/damage          Decreased tubular blood flow
Decreased glomerular filtration rate     Increased tissue pressure

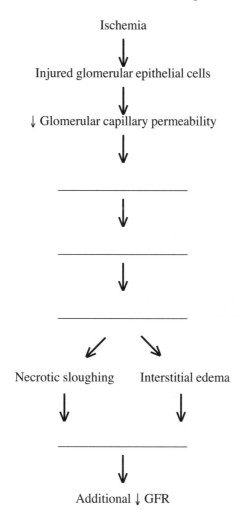

Ischemia

↓

Injured glomerular epithelial cells

↓

↓ Glomerular capillary permeability

↓

_____

↓

_____

↓

_____

↙        ↘

Necrotic sloughing     Interstitial edema

↓              ↓

_____

↓

Additional ↓ GFR

5. The nurse determines that a client with oliguria has prerenal oliguria when

   a. urine testing reveals a low specific gravity.
   b. the causative factor is malignant hypertension.
   c. urine testing reveals a high sodium concentration.
   d. reversal of the oliguria occurs with fluid replacement.

6. Tubular damage is indicated in the client with acute renal failure by a urinalysis finding of

   a. hematuria.
   b. specific gravity fixed at 1.010.
   c. urine sodium of 12 mmol/L (12 mEq/L).
   d. osmolality of 1000 mmol/kg (1000 mOsm/kg).

7. Metabolic acidosis occurs in the oliguric phase of acute renal failure as a result of impaired

    a. ammonia synthesis.
    b. excretion of sodium.
    c. excretion of bicarbonate.
    d. conservation of potassium.

8. Although both BUN and serum creatinine levels are increased in renal failure, a BUN of 30.3 mmol/L (85 mg/dL) and a serum creatinine of 336 $\mu$mol/L (3.8 mg/dL) would most likely occur in a client with acute renal failure caused by

    a. massive trauma.
    b. bladder obstruction.
    c. congestive heart failure.
    d. acute glomerulonephritis.

9. The nurse determines that a client with acute renal failure is in the recovery phase when the client experiences

    a. a return to normal weight.
    b. a urine output of 3700 mL/day.
    c. decreasing BUN and creatinine levels.
    d. decreasing sodium and potassium levels.

10. While caring for the client in the oliguric phase of acute renal failure, the nurse monitors the client for associated collaborative problems, notifying the physician when

    a. urine output is 300 mL/24 hr.
    b. edema occurs in the feet, legs, and sacral area.
    c. the cardiac monitor reveals a depressed T wave and a sagging ST segment.
    d. the client experiences increasing muscle weakness and abdominal cramping.

11. Identify whether the following statements are true or false. If a statement is false, correct the bold word(s) to make the statement true.

    _____ a. The most common cause of death in acute renal failure is **irreversible metabolic acidosis**.

    _____ b. Serum **potassium** and **urea** are increased during catabolism of body protein.

    _____ c. During the oliguric phase of acute renal failure, daily fluid intake is limited to **1000** mL plus the prior day's measurable fluid loss.

    _____ d. Dietary sodium and potassium during the oliguric phase of acute renal failure are managed according to the client's **urinary output**.

    _____ e. One of the most important nursing measures in managing fluid balance in the client in acute renal failure is **accurate daily weights**.

12. A 68-year-old man with a history of congestive heart failure secondary to hypertension has acute renal failure resulting from the effects of nephrotoxic diuretics. Currently his serum potassium is 6.2 mmol/L (6.2 mEq/L) with cardiac changes, his BUN is 38.6 mmol/L (108 mg/dL), his creatinine is 362 $\mu$mol/L (4.1 mg/dL), and his serum $HCO_3^-$ is 14 mEq/L (14 mmol/L). He is somnolent and disoriented. What three criteria for treatment with dialysis does he meet?

    a.

    b.

    c.

13. A client with acute renal failure has a serum potassium level of 6.8 mmol/L (6.8 mEq/L) and the following arterial blood gas results: pH 7.28, $PaCO_2$ 30 mm Hg, $PaO_2$ 86 mm Hg, $HCO_3^-$ 18 mmol/L (18 mEq/L). The nurse recognizes that treatment of the acid–base problem would cause a decrease in the

    a. pH.
    b. potassium level.
    c. bicarbonate level.
    d. carbon dioxide level.

14. In replying to a client's questions about the seriousness of her chronic kidney disease, the nurse knows that the stage of chronic kidney disease is based on

    a. the total daily urine output.
    b. the glomerular filtration rate.
    c. serum creatinine and urea levels.
    d. the degree of altered mental status.

15. A client with a creatinine clearance test of 30 mL/minute would have a glomerular filtration rate of _____ and stage _____ chronic kidney disease.

    a. 3 mL/min/17.3 $m^2$; 5
    b. 10 mL/min/17.3 $m^2$; 4
    c. 30 mL/min/17.3 $m^2$; 3
    d. 60 mL/min/17.3 $m^2$; 2

16. List two clinical manifestations and their pathophysiological causes that can be noted by the nurse when performing physical assessment of the following systems on the client with chronic renal disease.

| | **Findings** | **Cause** |
|---|---|---|
| a. Skin | | |
| b. Cardiovascular | | |
| c. Respiratory | | |
| d. GI | | |
| e. Neurological | | |

17. List the alterations that occur in at least 10 serum laboratory values in chronic renal disease.

a.                                        f.

b.                                        g.

c.                                        h.

d.                                        i.

e.                                        j.

18. The nurse identifies a nursing diagnosis of risk for injury: fracture related to alterations in calcium and phosphorus metabolism for a client with chronic renal disease. The pathological process directly related to the risk for fractures is

a. loss of aluminum through the impaired kidneys.
b. deposition of calcium phosphate in the soft tissues of the body.
c. impaired vitamin D activation resulting in decreased GI absorption of calcium.
d. increased release of parathyroid hormone in response to decreased calcium levels.

19. A client with chronic renal insufficiency weighs 70 kg and has the following laboratory results: creatinine clearance 18 mL/min; potassium 6.2 mmol/L (6.2 mEq/L); BUN 26.8 mmol/L (75 mg/dL); serum creatinine 557 µmol/L (6.3 mg/dL). An appropriate dietary modification for the client is

a. a protein restriction of 70 g/day.
b. a potassium restriction of 2–3 g/day.
c. a sodium restriction of 1000 mg/day.
d. unlimited intake of breads and cereals.

20. In implementing care for the client on peritoneal dialysis, the nurse recognizes that dietary needs include an increased amount of

a. fats.
b. protein.
c. calories.
d. carbohydrates.

21. The most appropriate snack for the nurse to offer the client with chronic renal disease is

a. raisins.
b. ice cream.
c. dill pickles.
d. hard candy.

22. Match the following drugs with their use in chronic kidney disease (answers may be used more than once).

   _____ a. Erythropoietin

   _____ b. IV glucose and insulin

   _____ c. Nifedipine (Procardia)

   _____ d. Sevelamer (Remagel)

   _____ e. Sodium polystyrene sulfonate (Kayexalate)

   _____ f. Furosemide (Lasix)

   _____ g. Calcium acetate (PhosLo)

   _____ h. 10% calcium gluconate IV

   1. Treatment of hyperkalemia

   2. Treatment of hyperphosphatemia

   3. Treatment of anemia

   4. Treatment of hypertension

23. Identify whether the following statements are true or false. If a statement is false, correct the bold word(s) to make the statement true.

   _____ a. A nutrient that is commonly supplemented for the client on dialysis because it is dialyzable is **iron**.

   _____ b. The syndrome that includes all the signs and symptoms seen in the various body systems in chronic kidney disease is **azotemia**.

   _____ c. The use of calcium-based phosphate binders in the client with chronic kidney disease is contraindicated when serum **phosphate** levels are increased.

   _____ d. The use of **morphine** is contraindicated in the client with chronic kidney disease because accumulation of its metabolites may cause seizures.

24. During the nursing assessment of the client with renal insufficiency, the nurse asks the client specifically about a history of

   a. angina.
   b. asthma.
   c. hypertension.
   d. rheumatoid arthritis.

25. When teaching a client with chronic kidney disease about prevention of complications, the nurse instructs the client to

   a. monitor for proteinuria daily with a urine dipstick.
   b. weigh daily and report a gain of greater than 2 kg (4 lb).
   c. take calcium-based phosphate binders on an empty stomach.
   d. perform self-catheterization every four hours to accurately measure I&O.

26. The client with end-stage renal disease tells the nurse that she hates the thought of being tied to the machine, but is also glad to start dialysis because she will be able to eat and drink what she wants. Based on this information, the nurse identifies the nursing diagnosis of

   a. self-esteem disturbance related to dependence on dialysis.
   b. anxiety related to perceived threat to health status and role functioning.
   c. ineffective management of therapeutic regimen related to lack of knowledge of treatment plan.
   d. risk for imbalanced nutrition: more than body requirements, related to increased dietary intake.

27. Indicate whether the following characteristics are associated with peritoneal dialysis (PD) or hemodialysis (HD).

    _____ a. Requires vascular access

    _____ b. Increased hyperlipidemia

    _____ c. Lowers serum triglycerides

    _____ d. Portable system

    _____ e. Less cardiovascular stress

    _____ f. More protein loss

    _____ g. Intensifies anemia

    _____ h. Rapid fluid and creatinine loss

    _____ i. Requires fewer dietary restrictions

28. The dialysate for peritoneal dialysis contains

    a. electrolytes in an equal concentration to the blood.
    b. calcium in a lower concentration than in the blood.
    c. sodium in a higher concentration than in the blood.
    d. glucose in a higher concentration than in the blood.

29. Complete the following statements.

    a. An exchange in peritoneal dialysis includes the phases of _____, _____,

    and _____.

    b. The amount of peritoneal dialysate used for one exchange is usually _____ litre(s).

    c. The client using _____ peritoneal dialysis usually dialyzes during sleep and leaves the fluid

    in the abdomen during the day.

30. To prevent the most common serious complication of peritoneal dialysis, it is important for the nurse to

    a. infuse the dialysate slowly.
    b. use strict aseptic technique in the dialysis procedures.
    c. have the client empty the bowel before the inflow phase.
    d. reposition the client frequently and promote deep breathing.

31. The composition of the periotoneal dialysate solution requires careful monitoring of the client who also has

    a. diabetes.
    b. liver disease.
    c. congestive heart failure.
    d. chronic obstructive pulmonary disease.

32. Match the characteristics with the type of vascular access sites (answers may be used more than once).

    _____ a. Two to four weeks required for healing          1. External AV shunt

    _____ b. Least likely to thrombose                       2. AV fistula

    _____ c. Usually used for temporary access               3. AV graft
            for continuous renal replacement theory

    _____ d. May lead to distal ischemia

    _____ e. Most prone to infection

    _____ f. Four to six weeks required for healing

33. A client on hemodialysis develops a thrombus of a subcutaneous AV graft requiring its removal. While waiting for a replacement graft or fistula, the client is most likely to have

    a. an external access shunt.
    b. a percutaneous femoral vein cannula.
    c. a percutaneous subclavian vein cannula.
    d. a Silastic catheter tunnelled subcutaneously to the jugular vein.

34. A client with end-stage renal failure is scheduled for hemodialysis following healing of an AV fistula. The nurse explains that during dialysis

    a. he will be able to visit, read, sleep, or watch TV while reclining in a chair.
    b. he will be placed on a cardiac monitor to detect any adverse effects that might occur.
    c. the dialyzer will remove and hold part of his blood for 20 to 30 minutes to remove the waste products.
    d. a large catheter with two lumens will be inserted into the fistula to send blood to and return it from the dialyzer.

35. The nurse evaluates the patency of an AV graft by

    a. palpating for pulses distal to the graft site.
    b. auscultating for the presence of a bruit at the site.
    c. evaluating the colour and temperature of the extremity.
    d. assessing for the presence of numbness and tingling distal to the site.

36. A client returns from her initial hemodialysis treatment with nausea, confusion, twitching, and jerking. The pathophysiological mechanism of dialysis responsible for these signs and symptoms is a

    a. loss of blood into the dialyzer caused by heparin use.
    b. rapid removal of vascular volume causing hypovolemia.
    c. high osmotic gradient in the brain causing cerebral edema.
    d. neuromuscular hypersensitivity resulting from fluid and sodium loss.

37. A client in acute renal failure is a candidate for continuous renal replacement therapy (CRRT). The most common indication for use of CRRT is

    a. azotemia.
    b. pericarditis.
    c. hyperkalemia.
    d. fluid overload.

38. A client rapidly progressing toward end-stage renal disease asks about the possibility of a kidney transplant. In responding to the client, the nurse knows that contraindications to kidney transplantation include

    a. hepatitis C infection.
    b. coronary artery disease.
    c. refractory hypertension.
    d. extensive vascular disease.

39. A client in end-stage renal disease is being evaluated for a kidney transplant from a live related donor. Results of histocompatibility testing that would indicate the best match of the client and the donor include

    a. ABO compatibility and no HLA match.
    b. ABO compatibility and six-HLA match.
    c. ABO compatibility and negative antibody cross-match.
    d. HLA-identical match and positive antibody cross-match.

40. During the immediate post-operative care of the recipient of a kidney transplant, the nurse expects to

    a. regulate fluid intake hourly based on urine output.
    b. find urine-tinged drainage on the abdominal dressing.
    c. medicate the client frequently for incisional flank pain.
    d. remove the Foley catheter to evaluate the ureteral implant.

41. Signs and symptoms of chronic rejection of the kidney are caused by

    a. recurrence of the original kidney disease.
    b. gradual occlusion of the renal blood vessels.
    c. T-cytotoxic cell attack on the foreign kidney.
    d. destruction of kidney tissue by sensitized antibodies.

42. Signs and symptoms of acute rejection that the nurse should teach the client to observe for include

    a. tachycardia and headache.
    b. fever and painful transplant site.
    c. severe hypotension and weight loss.
    d. recurrent urinary tract infections and oral yeast infections.

# CASE STUDY

## KIDNEY TRANSPLANT

### Client Profile

Ms. B. had end-stage renal disease secondary to hypertension. She underwent hemodialysis for two years and then received a cadaveric renal transplant one year ago. She had one episode of acute rejection three months after transplant. Her baseline creatinine has been 106 to 115 mmol/L (1.2 to 1.3 mg/dL). She came to the clinic complaining of decreased urinary output, fever, and tenderness at the transplant site. She is admitted to the hospital for a kidney biopsy.

### Subjective Data

- Tells the nurse if she loses this kidney, she does not think she can stand to go back on dialysis

### Objective Data

- Laboratory findings:  serum creatinine 265 μmol/L (3 mg/dL)
  BUN 25 mmol/L (70 mg/dL)
  glucose 404 mg/dl (22.4 mmol/L)
  $K^+$ 5.1 mmol/L (5.1 mEq/L)
  $HCO_3^-$ 18 mmol/L (18 mEq/L)
- Blood pressure 150/90 mm Hg

### Collaborative Care

- Muromonab-CD3 (Orthoclone OKT3) therapy initiated for 10 days
- Mycophenolate mofetil (Cellcept)
- Methylprednisolone (Solu-Medrol)
- Furosemide (Lasix)
- Nifedipine (Procardia)
- Sodium bicarbonate
- Tacrolimus (Prograf)
- Insulin

### Critical Thinking Questions

1. Explain the physiology of acute rejection.

2. Identify the abnormal diagnostic study results and why each would occur. What significance do the abnormal results have for nursing care?

3. Explain the rationale for Ms. B.'s collaborative care. How does each immunosuppressive medication work? (See Chapter 13.)

4. What clinical manifestations may develop as a result of immunosuppressive therapy? What nursing care is indicated?

5. Explain the long-term problems of a client with a kidney transplant.

6. Based on the assessment data presented, write one or more appropriate nursing diagnoses. Are there any collaborative problems?

1. Identify the glands in the following illustration.

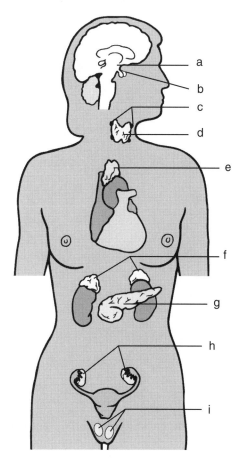

a. _____    f. _____

b. _____    g. _____

c. _____    h. _____

d. _____    i. _____

e. _____

2. Match the following hormones with their secretory glands (answers may be used more than once).

\_\_\_\_\_   a.  Thyroxin ($T_4$)

\_\_\_\_\_   b.  Cortisol

\_\_\_\_\_   c.  Glucagon

\_\_\_\_\_   d.  Prolactin

\_\_\_\_\_   e.  Progesterone

\_\_\_\_\_   f.  Growth hormone

\_\_\_\_\_   g.  Tri-iodothyronine ($T_3$)

\_\_\_\_\_   h.  Melanocyte-stimulating hormone

\_\_\_\_\_   i.  Insulin

\_\_\_\_\_   j.  TSH

\_\_\_\_\_   k.  Calcitonin

\_\_\_\_\_   l.  Gonadotropic hormones

\_\_\_\_\_   m.  Somatostatin

\_\_\_\_\_   n.  Epinephrine/norepinephrine

\_\_\_\_\_   o.  ACTH

\_\_\_\_\_   p.  ADH

1. Anterior pituitary

2. Posterior pituitary

3. Thyroid

4. Parathyroid

5. Beta cells of islets of Langerhans

6. Alpha cells of islet of Langerhans

7. Delta cells of islet of Langerhans

8. Adrenal cortex

9. Adrenal medulla

10. Ovaries

3. Identify whether the following statements are true or false. If a statement is false, correct the bold word(s) to make the statement true.

\_\_\_\_\_   a.  Overproduction of the **adrenal cortex** may cause masculinization in women.

\_\_\_\_\_   b.  Two hormones that have all cells as target tissue include **growth hormone** and **TSH**.

\_\_\_\_\_   c.  Epinephrine and norepinephrine are considered **hormones** when they are secreted by the adrenal medulla and are considered **neurotransmitters** when they are secreted by nerve cells.

\_\_\_\_\_   d.  In a person who normally works a night shift from 11:00 PM to 7:00 AM and sleeps from 8:00 AM to 3:00 PM, a serum analysis of cortisol taken at 7:30 AM would reveal a **false high** cortisol level.

\_\_\_\_\_   e.  An example of a complex negative feedback system is the regulation of **insulin**.

\_\_\_\_\_   f.  Hormones that act on the anterior pituitary gland to stimulate tropic hormone secretion are known as **releasing hormones**.

\_\_\_\_\_   g.  Endocrine glands that have negative feedback systems to the hypothalamus include the **pancreas** and the **parathyroid gland**.

\_\_\_\_\_   h.  **Androgens** secreted by the adrenal cortex are responsible for sex drive in women.

\_\_\_\_\_   i.  The mechanism for the action of **protein hormones** is binding to receptors inside the cell.

4. Match each hormone with the primary factor that stimulates its secretion and the primary factor that inhibits its secretion (factors may be used more than once).

| **Stimulate** | **Inhibit** | **Hormone** | **Primary Factor** |
|---|---|---|---|
| ＿＿ | ＿＿ | a. TSH or thyrotropin | 1. Increased stress |
| ＿＿ | ＿＿ | b. Corticotropin-releasing hormone | 2. Increased serum thyroxin |
| ＿＿ | ＿＿ | c. ADH | 3. Decreased serum $T_3$ |
| ＿＿ | ＿＿ | d. FSH | 4. Increased serum cortisol |
| ＿＿ | ＿＿ | e. Calcitonin | 5. Increased serum estrogen |
| ＿＿ | ＿＿ | f. Aldosterone | 6. Decreased serum estrogen |
| ＿＿ | ＿＿ | g. Glucagon | 7. Increased serum glucose |
| ＿＿ | ＿＿ | h. Parathyroid hormone | 8. Decreased serum glucose |
| ＿＿ | ＿＿ | i. Insulin | 9. Increased serum calcium |
| | | | 10. Decreased serum calcium |
| | | | 11. Decreased arterial BP |
| | | | 12. Increased arterial BP |
| | | | 13. Increased plasma osmolality |
| | | | 14. Decreased plasma osmolality |

5. The normal response to increased serum osmolality is release of

    a. aldosterone from the adrenal cortex, which stimulates sodium excretion by the kidney.
    b. ADH from the posterior pituitary gland, which stimulates the kidney to reabsorb water.
    c. mineralocorticoids from the adrenal gland, which stimulate the kidney to excrete potassium.
    d. calcitonin from the thyroid gland, which increases bone resorption and decreases serum calcium levels.

6. The hormone that increases calcium resorption from the bones and kidney and increases absorption for the intestine is

    a. TSH.
    b. calcitonin.
    d. aldosterone.
    d. parathyroid hormone.

7. Hormones of one gland influence the function of hormones of another gland. This is demonstrated by the fact that

    a. increased insulin levels inhibit the secretion of glucagon.
    b. increased testosterone levels inhibit the release of estrogen.
    c. increased cortisol levels stimulate the secretion of insulin.
    d. increased atrial natriuretic hormone levels inhibit the secretion of aldosterone.

8. Following the ingestion of a high-protein, carbohydrate-free meal

   a. both insulin and glucagon are inhibited because blood glucose levels are unchanged.
   b. insulin is released to facilitate breakdown of amino acids into glucose and glucagon is inhibited.
   c. insulin is inhibited by low glucose levels and glucagon is released to promote gluconeogenesis.
   d. glucagon is released to promote gluconeogenesis and insulin is released to facilitate movement of amino acids into muscle cells.

9. In a client with an elevated serum cortisol, the nurse would expect other laboratory findings to reveal

   a. hyponatremia.
   b. hyperkalemia.
   c. hypoglycemia.
   d. decreased serum triglycerides.

10. Two effects of hypokalemia on the endocrine system are

    a. decreased insulin and aldosterone release.
    b. decreased glucagon and increased cortisol release.
    c. decreased release of atrial natriuretic factor and increased ADH release.
    d. decreased release of parathyroid hormone and increased calcitonin release.

11. Manifestations of endocrine problems in the older adult that are commonly attributed to the aging process are

    a. tremors and paraesthesias.
    b. fatigue and mental impairment.
    c. fluid retention and hypertension.
    d. hyperpigmentation and oily skin.

12. Common non-specific manifestations that may alert the nurse to endocrine dysfunction include

    a. goitre and alopecia.
    b. exophthalmos and tremors.
    c. weight loss, fatigue, and depression.
    d. polyuria, polydipsia, and polyphagia.

13. Identify one specific finding identified by the nurse during assessment of each of the client's functional health patterns that indicates a risk factor for endocrine problems or a client response to an actual endocrine problem.

   a. Health perception–health management

   b. Nutritional–metabolic

   c. Elimination

   d. Activity–exercise

   e. Sleep–rest

   f. Cognitive–perceptual

   g. Self-perception–self-concept

   h. Role–relationship

   i. Sexuality–reproductive

   j. Coping–stress tolerance

   k. Value–belief

14. A potential adverse effect of palpation of the thyroid gland is

   a. carotid artery obstruction.
   b. damage to the cricoid cartilage.
   c. release of excessive thyroid hormone into circulation.
   d. hoarseness from pressure on the recurrent laryngeal nerve.

15. Complete the following sentences related to abnormal assessment findings of the endocrine system.

   a. Tetanic muscle spasms are associated with hypofunction of the _____ gland.

   b. Hyperpigmentation is associated with hypofunction of the _____ gland.

   c. Exophthalmos is associated with excessive secretion of the _____ gland.

   d. Moon face is associated with _____ secretion of the adrenal gland.

   e. A goitre is associated with either hyper- or hypofunction of the _____ gland.

   f. An increase in hand and foot size is associated with excessive secretion of _____ hormone.

   g. Striae are associated with excessive secretion of the _____ gland.

   h. Heat intolerance is associated with _____ secretion of the thyroid gland.

16. A client has a low serum T$_3$ level, and the physician orders a TSH level. If the TSH level is elevated, this indicates that

    a. the cause of the low T$_3$ is most likely primary hypothyroidism.
    b. the negative feedback system is failing to stimulate the anterior pituitary gland.
    c. the client has an underactive thyroid gland that is not receiving TSH stimulation.
    d. there is most likely a tumour of the anterior pituitary gland that is causing increased production of TSH.

17. To ensure accurate results of a fasting blood glucose analysis, the nurse has the client fast for at least

    a. two hours.
    b. four hours.
    c. eight hours.
    d. 12 hours.

18. Match the following diagnostic studies with the descriptions.

    _____ a. five-hour glucose tolerance test

    _____ b. Growth hormone stimulation test

    _____ c. Serum phosphate

    _____ d. 17-ketosteroids

    _____ e. ACTH stimulation test

    _____ f. Glycosylated hemoglobin

    _____ g. Water deprivation test

    _____ h. ACTH (dexamethasone)

    1. Normal response is drop in blood glucose to <2.2 mmol/L (40 mg/dL)

    2. Normal response is decreased cortisol

    3. Normal response is increased plasma cortisol

    4. Evaluates hypoglycemia

    5. Decreases indicate hyperparathyroidism

    6. Differentiates causes of polyuria

    7. Evaluates glucose control over time

    8. Evaluates steroid hormone function suppression test

# CHAPTER 47  NURSING MANAGEMENT: DIABETES MELLITUS

1. Although the primary function of insulin is to promote glucose transport from the blood into the cell, insulin also

    a. enhances breakdown of adipose tissue for energy.
    b. stimulates hepatic glycogenolysis and gluconeogenesis.
    c. prevents the transport of triglycerides into adipose tissue.
    d. accelerates the transport of amino acids into cells and their synthesis into protein.

2. Complete the following statements:

    a. Tissues that require insulin for glucose transport are _____ and _____ tissues.

    b. During the development of type 1 diabetes, the β-cell response to the hyperglycemia can be identified in

       the blood and urine by the presence of _____.

    c. Two hormones released during physical and emotional stress that are counterregulatory to insulin are

       _____ and _____.

    d. The type of diabetes that is strongly related to human leukocyte antigen types is _____.

3. Indicate whether the following mechanisms of diabetes are characteristic of the pathophysiology of type 1 (1) or type 2 (2) diabetes.

    _____ a. Insulin resistance

    _____ b. β-cell secretory exhaustion

    _____ c. Inherited defect in insulin receptors

    _____ d. Production of islet cell antibodies

    _____ e. Genetic susceptibility for antibody production

    _____ f. Inappropriate glucose production by the liver

    _____ g. β-cell destruction

    _____ h. Impaired glucose tolerance occurs gradually

    _____ i. Compensatory increased insulin production

4. Describe the process that occurs to cause the following classic diabetes symptoms.

    a. Polyuria

    b. Polydipsia

    c. Polyphagia

5. The nurse identifies that the risk for developing diabetes is highest in

   a. a 62-year-old obese white man.
   b. an obese, 50-year-old Asian woman.
   c. a child whose father has type 1 diabetes.
   d. a 34-year-old woman whose parents both have type 2 diabetes.

6. When caring for a client with metabolic syndrome (insulin resistance syndrome), the nurse plans teaching to decrease the client's risk for

   a. hypertension.
   b. hypoglycemia.
   c. cardiovascular disease.
   d. hyperglycemic non-ketotic syndrome.

7. A 52-year-old client admitted to the hospital with vomiting and diarrhea has a fasting blood sugar (FBS) of 28.4 mmol/L (512 mg/dL) and an arterial pH of 7.38. He is diagnosed with diabetes mellitus and treated with insulin and IV fluids. The nurse recognizes that it is most likely that this client

   a. will require insulin treatment only during stress.
   b. is demonstrating the abrupt onset of type 1 diabetes.
   c. will require long-term insulin therapy to control the diabetes.
   d. has enough endogenous insulin to prevent diabetic ketoacidosis with the hyperglycemia.

8. During routine health screening, a client is found to have a fasting plasma glucose (FPG) of 7.33 mmol/L (132 mg/dL). At a following visit, a diagnosis of diabetes would be made based on

   a. glucosuria of 3+.
   b. an FPG of 7 mmol/L (126 mg/dL).
   c. a random plasma glucose of 11.7 mmol/L (210 mg/dL) without symptoms.
   d. a two-hour oral glucose tolerance test (OGTT) of 10.5 mmol/L (190 mg/dL).

9. The nurse determines that a client with a two-hour OGTT of 28 mmol/L (144 mg/dL) has

   a. diabetes.
   b. impaired fasting glucose.
   c. impaired glucose tolerance.
   d. elevated glycosolated hemoglobin.

10. When teaching the client with diabetes about insulin administration, the nurse instructs the client to

   a. pull back on the plunger after inserting the needle to check for blood.
   b. clean the skin at the injection site with an alcohol swab before each injection.
   c. consistently use the same size of the appropriate strength insulin syringe to avoid dosing errors.
   d. rotate injection sites from arms to thighs to abdomen with each injection to prevent lipodystrophies.

11. A client with type 1 diabetes uses 20 U of 30/70 (regular/NPH) in the morning and at 6:00 P.M. When teaching the client about this regimen, the nurse stresses that

   a. hypoglycemia is most likely to occur before the noon meal.
   b. flexibility in food intake is possible since there is 24-hour insulin availability.
   c. a set meal pattern with a bedtime snack is necessary to prevent hypoglycemia.
   d. premeal glucose checks are required to determine needed changes in daily dosing.

12. Lispro insulin (Humalog) with NPH insulin is ordered for a client with newly diagnosed type 1 diabetes. The nurse knows that when Humalog insulin is used, it should be administered

    a. only once a day.
    b. one hour before meals.
    c. 30 to 45 minutes before meals.
    d. at mealtime or within 15 minutes of meals.

13. A client with diabetes is learning to mix regular insulin and NPH insulin in the same syringe. The nurse determines that additional teaching is needed when the client

    a. withdraws the NPH dose into the syringe first.
    b. injects air equal to the NPH dose into the NPH vial first.
    c. removes any air bubbles after withdrawing the first insulin.
    d. adds air equal to the insulin dose into the regular vial and withdraws the dose.

14. The home care nurse should intervene to correct a client whose insulin administration includes

    a. warming a prefilled refrigerated syringe in the hands before administration.
    b. storing syringes prefilled with NPH and regular insulin needle-upward in the refrigerator.
    c. placing the insulin bottle currently in use in a small container on the bathroom countertop.
    d. mixing an evening dose of Humalog insulin with insulin glargine in the same syringe for administration.

15. The major advantage of using an insulin pump or intensive insulin therapy is that

    a. tight glycemic control can be maintained.
    b. errors in insulin dosing are less likely to occur.
    c. complications of insulin therapy are prevented.
    d. frequent blood glucose monitoring is unnecessary.

16. A client taking insulin has a glucose level of 12 mmol/L (216 mg/dL) on awakening in the morning. The nurse advises the client to

    a. increase the evening insulin dose to prevent the dawn phenomenon.
    b. use a single-dose insulin regimen with an intermediate-acting insulin.
    c. monitor the glucose level at bedtime, between 2 and 4 A.M., and on arising.
    d. decrease the evening insulin dosage to prevent night hypoglycemia and the Somogyi effect.

17. Match the following oral antihyperglycemic agents with their descriptions (answers may be used more than once).

_____ a. Decreases endogenous glucose production

_____ b. Should be taken within 30 minutes of each meal

_____ c. Decreases glycogenolysis

_____ d. Fewer adverse effects with second-generation agents

_____ e. Rapid and short-acting release of insulin from pancreas

_____ f. Delays glucose absorption from the GI tract

_____ g. Stimulates production and release of insulin

_____ h. Increases glucose uptake, especially in muscles

_____ i. Primary effect is decreased glucose production by liver

_____ j. Not effective against fasting hyperglycemia

_____ k. Taken with first bite of each meal

1. Insulin secretagogue: Sulphonylurea

2. Insulin secretagogue: Non-sulphonylurea

3. Biguanide

4. α-glucosidase inhibitor

5. Thiazolidinedione

18. One of the disadvantages of the use of oral antihyperglycemic agents in comparison with the use of insulin is that

a. hypoglycemic episodes are more common and prolonged than with the use of insulin.
b. more frequent blood glucose monitoring is necessary to evaluate the effect of oral antihyperglycemic agents.
c. clients may assume that their diabetes is not serious and that dietary modifications and meal planning are not important.
d. the use of other medications may cause interactions, potentiating the glucose-lowering effect of oral anti-hyperglycemic agents.

19. In nutritional management of all types of diabetes, it is important for the client to

a. eat three meals per day at regular times.
b. restrict calories to promote moderate weight loss.
c. eliminate sucrose and other simple sugars from the diet.
d. limit saturated fat intake to 30% of dietary calorie intake.

20. Goals of nutritional therapy for the client with type 2 diabetes includes maintenance of

a. ideal body weight.
b. normal serum glucose and lipid levels.
c. a special diabetic diet using dietetic foods.
d. five small meals per day with a bedtime snack.

21. To prevent hyperglycemia or hypoglycemia with exercise, the nurse teaches the client using glucose-lowering agents that exercise should be undertaken

a. only after a 10- to 15-g carbohydrate snack is eaten.
b. about one hour after eating when blood glucose levels are rising.
c. when glucose monitoring reveals that the blood glucose is in the normal range.
d. when blood glucose levels are high, because exercise always has a hypoglycemic effect.

22. The nurse assesses the client with diabetes' technique of self-monitoring of blood glucose (SMBG) three months after initial instruction. An error in the performance of SMBG noted by the nurse that requires intervention is

    a. doing the SMBG before and after exercising.
    b. puncturing the finger on the side of the finger pad.
    c. cleaning the puncture site with alcohol before the puncture.
    d. holding the hand down for a few minutes before the puncture.

23. Ideally, the goal of client diabetes education is to

    a. make all clients responsible for the management of their disease.
    b. involve the client's family and significant others in the care of the client.
    c. enable the client to become the most active participant in the management of the diabetes.
    d. to provide the client with as much information as soon as possible to prevent complications of diabetes.

24. A nurse working in an ambulatory clinic plans a screening program for diabetes. Recommendations for screening would include

    a. OGTT for all ethnic populations every year.
    b. FPG for all individuals at age 40 and then every three years.
    c. testing all people before the age of 21 for islet cell antibodies.
    d. testing for type 2 diabetes only in overweight or obese individuals.

25. A client with diabetes calls the clinic because she is experiencing nausea and flu-like symptoms. The nurse advises the client to

    a. administer the usual insulin dosage.
    b. hold fluid intake until the nausea subsides.
    c. come to the clinic immediately for evaluation and treatment.
    d. monitor the blood glucose q1-2h and call if the glucose rises over 8 mmol/L (144 mg/dL).

26. Ketoacidosis occurs as a complication of diabetes when

    a. illnesses causing nausea and vomiting lead to bicarbonate loss with body fluids.
    b. the glucose level becomes so high that osmotic diuresis promotes fluid and electrolyte loss.
    c. an insulin deficit causes the body to metabolize large amounts of fatty acids rather than glucose for energy.
    d. the client skips meals after taking insulin leading to rapid metabolism of glucose and breakdown of fats for energy.

27. Number in sequence from 1 to 8 the processes of potassium imbalance in diabetic ketoacidosis (DKA).

    _____ a. Treatment with insulin increases glucose metabolism and decreases fat metabolism

    _____ b. Decreased $H^+$ ions in the blood

    _____ c. $K^+$ from the cells moves into blood in exchange for $H^+$ ions

    _____ d. Movement of $K^+$ back into cells

    _____ e. $K^+$ excreted in urine with osmotic diuresis

    _____ f. Increased serum $K^+$ concentration

    _____ g. Total body $K^+$ deficit

    _____ h. Increased $H^+$ ions present in form of acidic ketones and acetone

28. List five signs and symptoms that are present in DKA that are not seen in hyperglycemic hyperosmolar non-ketotic syndrome (HHNS).

    a.                                    d.

    b.                                    e.

    c.

29. The treatment for diabetic ketoacidosis (DKA) and hyperglycemic hyperosmolar non-ketotic syndrome (HHNS) differ primarily in that

    a. DKA requires administration of bicarbonate to correct acidosis.
    b. potassium replacement is not necessary in management of HHNS.
    c. HHNS requires greater fluid replacement to correct the dehydration.
    d. administration of glucose is withheld in HHNS until the blood glucose reaches a normal level.

30. The nurse is alerted to the possibility of hypovolemic shock occurring in the client with HHNS by the presence of

    a. an increase in CVP.
    b. deep, rapid respirations.
    c. a change from polyuria to oliguria.
    d. depressed ST segment and T waves on cardiac monitoring.

31. Indicate whether the following characteristics are associated with hypoglycemia (1), hyperglycemia (2), or both (3).

    _____   a. Slurred speech and irritability

    _____   b. Headache

    _____   c. Nausea and vomiting

    _____   d. Too much exercise without food

    _____   e. Increased food intake

    _____   f. Cold, clammy skin

    _____   g. Precipitated by stress

    _____   h. Changes in vision

32. A client with diabetes is found unconscious at home and a family member calls the clinic. After determining that no glucometer is available, the nurse advises the family member to

    a. administer 10 U regular insulin SC.
    b. administer glucagon 1 mg IM or SC.
    c. try to arouse the client to drink some orange juice.
    d. call for an ambulance to transport the client to a medical facility.

33. Two days following a self-managed hypoglycemic episode at home, the client tells the nurse that his blood glucose levels since the episode have been between 4 and 5 mmol/L (72 and 90 mg/dL). The best response of the nurse is

    a. "That is a good range for your glucose levels."
    b. "You should call your physician because you need to have your insulin increased."
    c. "That level is too low in view of your recent hypoglycemia, and you should increase your food intake."
    d. "You should only take half your insulin dosage for the next few days to get your glucose level back to normal."

34. In diabetes, atherosclerotic disease affecting the cerebrovascular, cardiovascular, and peripheral vascular systems

    a. can be prevented by tight glucose control.
    b. occurs with a higher frequency and earlier onset than in the non-diabetic population.
    c. is caused by the hyperinsulinemia related to insulin resistance common in type 2 diabetes.
    d. cannot be modified by reduction of risk factors such as smoking, obesity, and high fat intake.

35. Match the following characteristics as they relate to complications of diabetes (answers may be used more than once).

    _____ a. Male impotence (erectile dysfunction)        1. Microangiopathy

    _____ b. Diffuse and nodular glomerulosclerosis        2. Macroangiopathy

    _____ c. Related to altered lipid metabolism of        3. Autonomic neuropathy
             diabetes
                                                             4. Sensory neuropathy
    _____ d. Micro-aneurysms and destruction of retinal
             capillaries

    _____ e. Atrophy of small muscles of the hands

    _____ f. Capillary and arteriole basement membrane
             thickening specific to diabetes

    _____ g. Pain and paraesthesia of legs

    _____ h. Ulceration and amputation of lower extremities

    _____ i. Shin spots—dermopathy

    _____ j. Delayed gastric emptying

    _____ k. Ischemic heart disease

36. Following the teaching of foot care to a client with diabetes, the nurse determines that additional instruction is needed when the client says,

    a. "I should wash my feet daily with soap and warm water."
    b. "I should always wear shoes to protect my feet from injury."
    c. "If my feet are cold, I should wear socks instead of using a heating pad."
    d. "I'll know if I have sores or lesions on my feet because they will be painful."

37. A 72-year-old woman is diagnosed with diabetes. The nurse recognizes that management of diabetes in the older adult

    a. may not require as tight glucose control as in younger individuals with diabetes.

    b. is usually not treated unless the client becomes severely hyperglycemic.

    c. does not include treatment with insulin because of limited dexterity and vision.

    d. usually requires that a younger family member be responsible for care of the client.

## CASE STUDY

### HYPOGLYCEMIA

**Client Profile**

Ms. W. was brought to the first aid tent provided for participants in a charity marathon. She is a 24-year-old woman with type I diabetes, well maintained on a regimen of self-monitoring of blood glucose, insulin, and nutrition.

**Subjective Data**

- States she feels cold, has a headache, and her fingers feel numb
- Took her usual insulin dose this morning but was unable to eat her entire breakfast due to lack of time
- Completed the entire marathon in a personal-best time

**Objective Data**

- Has slurred speech and unsteady gait
- Pulse 120 beats/min
- Appears confused
- Capillary blood glucose level 2.7 mmol/L (48 mg/dL)

### Critical Thinking Questions

1. Describe what Ms. W. could have done to prevent this hypoglycemic event.

2. What is the etiology of the signs and symptoms displayed by Ms. W.?

3. How would you expect to treat her hypoglycemia?

4. What teaching is appropriate for this client once her condition has been stabilized?

5. What adjustments in her diabetic regimen could Ms. W. make to allow her to continue with her exercise habits?

6. Based on the assessment data presented, write one or more appropriate nursing diagnoses. Are there any collaborative problems?

1. A client suspected of having acromegaly has an elevated plasma growth hormone level. In acromegaly, the nurse would also expect the client's diagnostic results to include

   a. hyperinsulinemia.
   b. a plasma glucose of less than 3.9 mmol/L (70 mg/dL).
   c. decreased growth hormone levels with an oral glucose challenge test.
   d. a serum somatomedin C (insulin-like growth factor-1) of more than 300 μg/L (300 ng/mL).

2. During assessment of the client with acromegaly, the nurse would expect the client to report

   a. infertility.
   b. dry, irritated skin.
   c. undesirable changes in appearance.
   d. an increase in height of 5 to 7.5 cm (2 to 3 in.) a year.

3. A client with acromegaly is treated with a transsphenoidal hypophysectomy. Post-operatively, the nurse

   a. ensures that any clear nasal drainage is tested for glucose.
   b. maintains the client flat in bed to prevent cerebrospinal fluid leakage.
   c. assists the client with toothbrushing q4h to keep the surgical area clean.
   d. encourages deep breathing and coughing to prevent respiratory complications.

4. Identify whether the following statements are true or false. If a statement is false, correct the bold word(s) to make the statement true.

   _____ a. Drugs used in the primary treatment of acromegaly are effective because they **block the action** of growth hormone.

   _____ b. A client with diabetes mellitus who undergoes a hypophysectomy will require a **larger** dose of insulin than preoperatively.

   _____ c. Pituitary tumours causing either hyperpituitarism or hypopituitarism may cause **visual changes and disturbances**.

   _____ d. **Hyposecretion** of FSH is associated with the onset of menopause.

   _____ e. Early hypofunction of the pituitary gland usually results in non-specific symptoms primarily because there are no obvious manifestations of **growth hormone** deficiencies in adults.

5. Identify five hormones that are replaced when panhypopituitarism results from radiation therapy or total hypophysectomy as treatment for pituitary tumours.

   a.

   b.

   c.

   d.

   e.

6. In the following diagram of the pathophysiology of antidiuretic hormone (ADH) problems, indicate in the appropriate blanks whether the processes are increased (↑) or decreased (↓) in syndrome of inappropriate ADH (SIADH) and diabetes insipidus (DI).

7. During care of the client with syndrome of inappropriate ADH (SIADH), the nurse should

   a. monitor neurological status q2h or more often if needed.
   b. keep the head of the bed elevated to prevent ADH release.
   c. teach the client receiving treatment with diuretics to restrict sodium intake.
   d. notify the physician if the client's blood pressure decreases more than 20 mm Hg from baseline.

8. A client with SIADH is treated with water restriction and administration of IV fluids. The nurse evaluates that treatment has been effective when the client experiences

   a. increased urine output, decreased serum sodium, and increased urine specific gravity.
   b. increased urine output, increased serum sodium, and decreased urine specific gravity.
   c. decreased urine output, increased serum sodium, and decreased urine specific gravity.
   d. decreased urine output, decreased serum sodium, and increased urine specific gravity.

9. In a client with central diabetes insipidus, administration of aqueous vasopressin during a water deprivation test will result in a

   a. decrease in body weight.
   b. increase in urinary output.
   c. decrease in blood pressure.
   d. increase in urine osmolality.

10. A client with diabetes insipidus is treated with nasal desmopressin. The nurse recognizes that the drug is not having an adequate therapeutic effect when the client experiences

    a.  headache and weight gain.
    b.  nasal irritation and nausea.
    c.  a urine specific gravity of 1.002.
    d.  an oral intake greater than urinary output.

11. When caring for a client with nephrogenic diabetes insipidus, the nurse would expect treatment to include

    a.  fluid restriction.
    b.  thiazide diuretics.
    c.  a high-sodium diet.
    d.  chlorpropamide (Diabinese).

12. Identify whether the following statements are true or false. If a statement is false, correct the bold word(s) to make the statement true.

    \_\_\_\_\_   a.  The two most common forms of hyperthyroidism are **Graves' disease** and **toxic adenoma**.

    \_\_\_\_\_   b.  Exophthalmos may occur in **any form of hyperthyroidism**.

    \_\_\_\_\_   c.  Clinical manifestations of hyperthyroidism occur as a result of **increased metabolic rate** and **an increased number of β-adrenergic receptors**.

    \_\_\_\_\_   d.  Diagnostic testing in the client with Graves' disease will reveal an **increased TSH level** and a radioactive iodine uptake of **0.05 (5%)**.

    \_\_\_\_\_   e.  Goitrogens are substances that **promote** thyroid function and are **encouraged** for clients with hypothyroidism.

13. A client with Graves' disease asks the nurse what caused the disorder. The best response of the nurse is

    a.  "The cause of Graves' disease is not known, although it is thought to be genetic."
    b.  "It is usually associated with goitre formation from an iodine deficiency over a long period of time."
    c.  "Antibodies develop against thyroid tissue and destroy it, causing a deficiency of thyroid hormones."
    d.  "In genetically susceptible persons antibodies form that attack thyroid tissue and stimulate overproduction of thyroid hormones."

14. A client is admitted to the hospital in thyrotoxic crisis. On physical assessment of the client, the nurse would expect to find

    a.  hoarseness and laryngeal stridor.
    b.  bulging eyeballs and arrhythmias.
    c.  elevated temperature and signs of heart failure.
    d.  lethargy progressing suddenly to impairment of consciousness.

15. Match the following characteristics and rationales for the uses of the drugs used in treatment of hyperthyroidism (answers may be used more than once).

_____ a. Should be taken with a straw to avoid staining the teeth

_____ b. Is not used in women of childbearing age

_____ c. Decreases release of thyroid hormones

_____ d. Often used with iodine to produce euthyroid before surgery

_____ e. May cause agranulocytosis

_____ f. Used to decrease size and vascularity of thyroid gland preoperatively

_____ g. Used to control sympathetic symptoms

_____ h. Blocks peripheral conversion of $T_4$ to $T_3$

_____ i. Decreases thyroid secretion by damaging thyroid gland

_____ j. Indications of toxicity are excessive salivation and skin reactions

_____ k. Often causes hypothyroidism over time

1. Propylthiouracil (PTU)

2. Potassium iodide (SSKI)

3. Propranolol (Inderal)

4. Radioactive iodine

16. Identify one nursing diagnosis that is appropriate for the client with the following manifestations of hyperthyroidism.

   a. Exophthalmos

   b. Weight loss and hunger

   c. Hair loss and vitiligo

   d. Exhaustion and dyspnea

17. Preoperative instructions for the client scheduled for a subtotal thyroidectomy includes teaching the client

   a. how to support the head with the hands when moving.
   b. that coughing should be avoided to prevent pressure on the incision.
   c. that the head and neck will need to remain immobile until the incision heals.
   d. that any tingling around the lips or in the fingers after surgery is expected and temporary.

18. Identify the rationale for having the following items immediately available in the client's room following a thyroidectomy.

   a. Tracheostomy tray

   b. Calcium salts for IV administration

   c. Oxygen equipment

19. When providing discharge instructions to a client following a subtotal thyroidectomy, the nurse advises the client to

   a. never miss a daily dose of thyroid replacement therapy.
   b. avoid regular exercise until thyroid function is normalized.
   c. avoid eating foods such as soybeans, turnips, and rutabagas.
   d. use warm salt water gargles several times a day to relieve throat pain.

20. Match the following characteristics with their related disorders.

   _____ a. Viral-induced hyperthyroidism

   _____ b. Autoimmune fibrous and lymphocytic replacement of thyroid gland

   _____ c. Enlarged thyroid gland

   _____ d. Lymphocytic infiltration of thyroid gland that may occur postpartum

   _____ e. Bacterial or fungal infection of thyroid gland

   _____ f. Malignant or benign deformity of the thyroid gland

   1. Goitre

   2. Thyroid nodules

   3. Hashimoto's thyroiditis

   4. Subacute granulomatous thyroiditis

   5. Silent thyroiditis

   6. Acute thyroiditis

21. Causes of primary hypothyroidism in adults include

   a. malignant or benign thyroid nodules.
   b. surgical removal or failure of the pituitary gland.
   c. surgical removal or radiation of the thyroid gland.
   d. autoimmune-induced atrophy of the thyroid gland.

22. The nurse has identified the following nursing diagnoses for a client who is hypothyroid. For each nursing diagnosis, identify an appropriate etiology for the diagnosis and at least two common signs or symptoms of hypothyroidism that support the diagnosis.

    a.  Disturbed sleep pattern related to _____ as manifested by

        _____ and _____.

    b.  Imbalanced nutrition: more than body requirements related to _____ as

        manifested by _____ and _____.

    c.  Disturbed thought processes related to _____ as manifested by

        _____ and _____.

    d.  Activity intolerance  related to _____ as manifested by

        _____ and _____.

23. Physical changes of hypothyroidism that must be monitored when replacement therapy is started include

    a.  achlorhydria and constipation.
    b.  slowed mental processes and lethargy.
    c.  anemia and increased capillary fragility.
    d.  decreased cardiac contractility and coronary atherosclerosis.

24. A client with hypothyroidism is treated with levothyroxine (Synthroid). When teaching the client about the therapy, the nurse

    a.  explains that caloric intake must be reduced when drug therapy is started.
    b.  provides written instruction for all information related to the medication therapy.
    c.  assures the client that a return to normal function will occur with replacement therapy.
    d.  informs the client that medications must be taken until hormone balance is re-established.

25. Indicate whether the following clinical manifestations are characteristic of hyperparathyroidism (1) or hypoparathyroidism (2).

    _____  a. Decreased bone density

    _____  b. Muscle spasms and stiffness

    _____  c. Psychomotor retardation

    _____  d. Calcium nephrolithiasis

    _____  e. Anorexia and abdominal pain

    _____  f. Decreased contractility of myocardium

    _____  g. Laryngeal spasm

    _____  h. Skeletal pain

    _____  i. Abdominal cramping

    _____  j. Cardiac irritability

26. An appropriate nursing intervention for the client with hyperparathyroidism is to

    a. pad side rails as a seizure precaution.
    b. increase fluid intake to 3000 to 4000 mL/day.
    c. maintain bed rest to prevent pathological fractures.
    d. monitor the client for Trousseau's phenomenon and Chvostek's sign.

27. When the client with parathyroid disease experiences symptoms of hypocalcemia, a measure that can be used to temporarily raise serum calcium levels is to

    a. administer IV normal saline.
    b. have the client rebreathe in a paper bag.
    c. administer furosemide (Lasix) as ordered.
    d. administer oral phosphorus supplements.

28. A client with hypoparathyroidism as a result of surgical treatment of hyperparathyroidism is preparing for discharge. The nurse teaches the client that

    a. milk and milk products should be increased in the diet.
    b. parenteral replacement of PTH will be required for life.
    c. calcium supplements with vitamin D can effectively maintain calcium balance.
    d. bran and whole grain foods should be used to prevent GI effects of replacement therapy.

29. A client is admitted to the hospital with a diagnosis of Cushing's syndrome. On physical assessment of the client, the nurse would expect to find

    a. hypertension, peripheral edema, and petechiae.
    b. weight loss, buffalo hump, and moon face with acne.
    c. abdominal and buttock striae, truncal obesity, and hypotension.
    d. anorexia, signs of dehydration, and hyperpigmentation of the skin.

30. To prevent complications in the client with Cushing's syndrome, the nurse monitors the client for

    a. hypotension.
    b. hypoglycemia.
    c. cardiac arrhythmias.
    d. decreased cardiac output.

31. A client is scheduled for a bilateral adrenalectomy. During the post-operative period, the nurse would expect administration of corticosteroids to be

    a. reduced to promote wound healing.
    b. withheld until symptoms of hypocortisolism appear.
    c. increased to promote an adequate response to the stress of surgery.
    d. reduced because excessive hormones are released during surgical manipulation of the glands.

32. A client with Addison's disease comes to the emergency department with complaints of nausea, vomiting, diarrhea, and fever. The nurse would expect collaborative care to include

    a. parenteral injections of ACTH.
    b. IV administration of vasopressors.
    c. IV administration of hydrocortisone.
    d. IV administration of $D_5W$ with 20 mEq KCl.

33. The nurse determines that the client in acute adrenal insufficiency is responding favourably to treatment when

    a. the client appears alert and oriented.
    b. the client's urinary output has increased.
    c. pulmonary edema is reduced as evidenced by clear lung sounds.
    d. laboratory tests reveal serum elevations of potassium and glucose and a decrease in sodium.

34. During discharge teaching for the client with Addison's disease, the nurse identifies a need for additional instruction when the client says,

    a. "I should always call the doctor if I develop vomiting or diarrhea."
    b. "If my weight goes down, my dosage of steroid is probably too high."
    c. "I should double or triple my steroid dose if I undergo rigorous physical exercise."
    d. "I need to carry an emergency kit with injectable hydrocortisone in case I can't take my medication by mouth."

35. A client who is on corticosteroid therapy for treatment of an autoimmune disorder has the following additional drugs ordered. How is the need for these drugs related to the effects of glucocorticosteroids?

    a. Furosemide (Lasix)

    b. Ranitidine (Zantac)

    c. Alendronate (Fosamax)

    d. Insulin

    e. Potassium

    f. Isoniazid (INH)

36. A client with mild iatrogenic Cushing's syndrome is on an alternate-day regimen of corticosteroid therapy. The nurse explains to the client that this regimen

    a. maintains normal adrenal hormone balance.
    b. prevents ACTH release from the pituitary gland.
    c. minimizes hypothalamic-pituitary-adrenal suppression.
    d. increases the therapeutic effect of the drug.

37. When caring for a client with primary hyperaldosteronism, the nurse would question a physician's order for the use of

    a. furosemide (Lasix).
    b. amiloride (Midamor).
    c. spironolactone (Aldactone).
    d. aminoglutethimide (Cytadren).

38. The most important nursing intervention during the medical and surgical treatment of the client with a pheochromocytoma is

    a. administering IV fluids.
    b. monitoring blood pressure.
    c. monitoring I&O and daily weights.
    d. administering β-adrenergic blocking agents.

# CASE STUDY

## CUSHING'S SYNDROME

### Client Profile

Mr. H. is a 26-year-old elementary school teacher. He seeks the advice of his physician because of changes in his appearance over the past year.

### Subjective Data

- Complains of weight gain, particularly through his midsection, easy bruising, and edema of his feet, lower legs, and hands
- Has been having increasing insomnia

### Objective Data

- Physical examination: BP 150/110; 2+ edema of lower extremities; purplish striae on abdomen; thin extremities with thin, friable skin; severe acne of the face and neck
- Blood analysis: glucose 9.3 mmol/L (167 mg/dL), WBC $13.6 \times 10^9$/L ($13.6 \times 10^3$/μL, lymphocytes 0.12 (12%), RBC $6.6 \times 10^{12}$/L ($6.6 \times 10^6$ μL), $K^+$ 3.2 mmol/L (3.2 mEq/L)

### Critical Thinking Questions

1. Discuss the probable causes of the alterations in Mr. H.'s blood values.

2. Explain the pathophysiology of Cushing's syndrome.

3. What diagnostic testing would identify the cause of Mr. H.'s Cushing's syndrome?

4. What is the usual treatment of Cushing's syndrome?

5. What is meant by a "medical adrenalectomy"?

6. What are the major nursing responsibilities in the care of this client?

7. Based on the assessment data presented, write one or more appropriate nursing diagnoses. Are there any collaborative problems?

1. Identify the structures in the following illustrations by filling in the blanks on the next page with the correct answers from the list of terms below (some terms will be used in both illustrations).

**List of Terms**

Anterior cul-de-sac
Anus
Body (corpus) of uterus
Cowper's gland
Cervix
Clitoris
Corpus cavernosum
Corpus spongiosum
Ductus deferens
Ejaculatory duct

Epididymis
Fallopian tube
Fornix of vagina
Fundus of uterus
Glans
Labia majora
Labia minora
Penis
Posterior cul-de-sac
Prostate gland

Rectum
Round ligament
Scrotum
Seminal vesicle
Symphysis pubis
Testis
Ureter
Urethra
Urinary bladder
Vagina

a. _____

b. _____

c. _____

d. _____

e. _____

f. _____

g. _____

h. _____

i. _____

j. _____

k. _____

l. _____

m. _____

n. _____

o. _____

p. _____

q. _____

r. _____

s. _____

t. _____

u. _____

v. _____

w. _____

x. _____

y. _____

z. _____

aa. _____

bb. _____

cc. _____

dd. _____

ee. _____

ff. _____

gg. _____

hh. _____

2. Using the list of terms below, identify the structures in the following illustrations.

### List of Terms

| | |
|---|---|
| Alveoli | Nipple |
| Anus | Pectoralis major muscle |
| Areola | Perineum |
| Clitoris | Prepuce |
| Labia majora | Urethra |
| Labia minora | Vagina |
| Mons pubis | Vestibule |

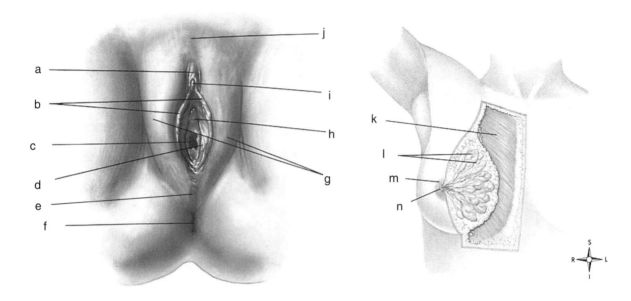

a. _____    h. _____

b. _____    i. _____

c. _____    j. _____

d. _____    k. _____

e. _____    l. _____

f. _____    m. _____

g. _____    n. _____

3. Number in sequence from 1 to 8 the passage of sperm through, and the formation of semen in, the structures of the male reproductive system.

_____ a. Ductus deferens

_____ b. Urethra

_____ c. Epididymis

_____ d. Prostate gland

_____ e. Seminiferous tubules

_____ f. Cowper's glands

_____ g. Seminal vesicles

_____ h. Ejaculatory duct

4. Match the following descriptions with the structures of the female breast.

_____ a. Pigmented centre of breast

_____ b. Erectile tissue containing pores

_____ c. Carry milk from alveoli to lactiferous sinuses

_____ d. Major composition of non-lactating breast

_____ e. Store milk during lactation

_____ f. Sebaceous-like gland on areola

_____ g. Secrete milk during lactation

_____ h. Anchor glandular tissue, skin, and muscles

1. Alveoli

2. Montgomery's tubercles

3. Lactiferous sinuses

4. Areola

5. Ligaments of Cooper

6. Ducts

7. Adipose tissue

8. Nipple

5. Identify whether the following statements are true or false. If a statement is false, correct the bold word(s) to make the statement true.

_____ a. The normal process of destruction of oocytes throughout the female life span is known as **atresia**.

_____ b. Fertilization of an ovum by a sperm occurs in the **uterus**.

_____ c. A Pap smear should include cells from the **ectocervix**.

_____ d. Mobility of sperm into the uterus is promoted by **thin, watery cervical mucus** at the time of ovulation.

_____ e. A middle-aged woman is considered to be in menopause when she has not had a menstrual period for **two years**.

6. Match the descriptions with the reproductive hormones (answers may be used more than once).

_____ a. Called ICSH in males           1. FSH

_____ b. Stimulated by elevated estrogen levels    2. LH

_____ c. Produced by testes            3. Prolactin

_____ d. Elevated at onset of menopause    4. Estrogen

_____ e. Produced by corpus luteum    5. Progesterone

_____ f. Stimulates testosterone production    6. Testosterone

_____ g. Required for female sex characteristics    7. ICSH

_____ h. Needed for growth of mammary glands    8. GnRH

_____ i. Needed for male sex characteristics

_____ j. Decreased by increased testosterone levels

_____ k. Responsible for ovarian follicle maturation

_____ l. Responsible for spermatogenesis

_____ m. Maintains implanted egg

_____ n. Completes follicle maturation

7. Match the events of the menstrual cycle with their associated phases (answers may be used more than once).

_____ a. Corpus luteum secretes estrogen    1. Follicular phase

_____ b. Estrogen secreted by follicles    2. Luteal phase

_____ c. FSH secretion suppressed    3. Menstrual phase

_____ d. GnRH secreted

_____ e. Ischemia of the endometrium

_____ f. LH released

_____ g. Release of mature ovum

_____ h. FSH released

8. A 52-year-old woman tells the nurse that she thinks she has started menopause and asks what changes she can expect. The nurse explains that

    a. she is at increased risk for dyspareunia because of changes in the vaginal epithelium.
    b. after menopause she will only stop menstruating; there are no other significant changes that she should worry about.
    c. post-menopausal women are likely to have difficulty with sexual pleasure because of drastic changes in the female sexual response.
    d. she should use hormone replacement therapy to prevent the many uncomfortable and pathological effects of ovarian failure.

9. A 72-year-old male client asks the nurse whether it is normal for him to become impotent at his age. The best response of the nurse includes the information that

    a. most decreased sexual function in older adults is due to psychological stress.
    b. physiological changes of aging may require increased stimulation for an erection to occur.
    c. although the penis decreases in size in older males, there should be no change in sexual function.
    d. benign changes in the prostate gland that occur with aging can cause a decreased ability to attain an erection.

10. When obtaining information related to reproductive function from a female client, the nurse knows that sensitive issues may best be discussed by first asking about

    a. sexual practices.
    b. obstetric history.
    c. menstrual history.
    d. use of recreational drugs.

11. List one problem associated with each of the following that may be identified during assessment of the reproductive system.

    a. Rubella

    b. Mumps

    c. Diabetes mellitus

    d. Antihypertensive agents

12. Identify one specific finding identified by the nurse during assessment of each of the client's functional health patterns that indicates a risk factor for reproductive problems or a client response to an actual reproductive problem.

   a. Health perception–health management

   b. Nutritional–metabolic

   c. Elimination

   d. Activity–exercise

   e. Sleep–rest

   f. Cognitive–perceptual

   g. Self-perception–self-concept

   h. Role–relationship

   i. Sexuality–reproductive

   j. Coping–stress tolerance

   k. Value–belief

13. A 58-year-old man has difficulty starting a urinary stream, and benign prostatic hyperplasia (BPH) is suspected. Assessment of the client for the presence of BPH involves

   a. palpation of the scrotum and testes for a mass.
   b. palpating the base of the penis for enlargement.
   c. palpating the inguinal ring while the client bears down.
   d. a digital rectal examination to palpate the prostate gland.

14. When assessing an aging adult male, the nurse notes as normal the finding of

   a. decreased penis size.
   b. decreased pubic hair.
   c. a decrease in scrotal colour.
   d. unilateral breast enlargement.

15. During examination of the breast, the nurse establishes the presence of nipple and skin retraction by

   a. compressing the nipple.
   b. lying the client supine with her hand above and behind her head.
   c. systematically palpating the breast tissue in a circular or spoke pattern.
   d. asking the client to lift her hands above her head and then press her hands on her hips while seated.

16. During examination of the female reproductive system, the nurse notes as abnormal the finding of

   a. clear vaginal discharge.
   b. perineal episiotomy scars.
   c. non-palpable Skene's ducts.
   d. diamond pubic hair distribution.

17. A 36-year-old woman calls the clinic to schedule a pelvic examination and Pap smear. The nurse informs the client that

   a. she should douche the day before the test.
   b. the examination should be scheduled in the middle of her menstrual cycle.
   c. she should not have sexual intercourse for 48 hours before the examination.
   d. the examination must be performed during the secretory phase of the menstrual cycle, after ovulation.

18. Match the following laboratory tests with their purposes.

   _____  a. Urine HCG                          1. Identifies secondary gonadal failure

   _____  b. Serum estradiol                     2. Used for rapid diagnosis of gonorrhea

   _____  c. Serum FSH                           3. Specific antibody test for syphilis

   _____  d. VDRL                                4. Measures ovarian function

   _____  e. Fluorescent treponemal antibody     5. Detects pregnancy
          absorption (FTAAbs)
                                                 6. Used to detect prostate cancer
   _____  f. Urine FSH assay
                                                 7. Non-specific antibody test for syphilis
   _____  g. Gram's stain                           screening

   _____  h. Alpha-fetoprotein (AFP)             8. Tumour marker for testicular cancer

   _____  i. PSA                                 9. Used to validate menopause

19. Following a dilation and curettage (D&C), it is important for the nurse to assess the client for the complication of

   a. infection.
   b. hemorrhage.
   c. urinary retention.
   d. perforation of the bladder.

20. Diagnostic tests of the reproductive system that are operative procedures requiring surgical anaesthesia include

   a. culdoscopy and conization.
   b. colposcopy and breast biopsy.
   c. laparoscopy and endometrial biopsy.
   d. dilation with curettage and contrast mammography.

21. The fertility test that requires the couple to have sexual intercourse at the time of ovulation and come for testing two to eight hours after intercourse is the

   a. Huhner test.
   b. semen analysis.
   c. endometrial biopsy.
   d. hysterosalpingogram.

# CHAPTER 50 NURSING MANAGEMENT: BREAST DISORDERS

1. The nurse encourages all women to perform breast self-examination (BSE) primarily because

   a. most breast lesions are discovered by women themselves.
   b. breast lesions can be felt before they are evident on a mammogram.
   c. BSE has been shown to reduce mortality in breast cancer in women under age 50.
   d. early detection and treatment of breast cancer is the most significant factor in survival rates.

2. Identify the guidelines for breast surveillance practices established by the Canadian Cancer Society (CCS).

   a.

   b.

   c.

   d.

3. When planning teaching of BSE, the nurse knows that a woman is more likely to perform regular breast self-examination when

   a. the perceived risk for breast cancer is high.
   b. she knows what to do if a lesion is detected.
   c. active practice by the woman increases her confidence in her skill.
   d. she is aware of the statistics related to breast cancer survival and mortality.

4. The diagnostic test that is most accurate and advantageous in terms of time and expense in diagnosing malignant breast disorders is

   a. mammography.
   b. open surgical biopsy.
   c. fine-needle aspiration.
   d. stereotactic core biopsy.

5. While examining a client's breasts, the nurse notes multiple, bilateral mobile lumps. To assess the client further, the most appropriate question of the nurse is

   a. "Do you have a high caffeine intake?"
   b. "When did you last have a mammogram?"
   c. "Is there a history of breast cancer in your mother or sisters?"
   d. "Do the size and tenderness of the lumps change with your menstrual cycle?"

6. While teaching the client with fibrocystic changes in the breast, the nurse explains to the client that this condition is significant because fibrocystic changes

   a. commonly become malignant over time.
   b. make it more difficult to examine the breasts.
   c. will eventually cause atrophy of breast tissue.
   d. can be controlled with hormone replacement therapy.

7. Match the following descriptions with their related benign breast disorders (answers may be used more than once).

_____ a. Almost always self-limiting and disappears

_____ b. Peaks at age 40

_____ c. Most common between ages 21 and 25

_____ d. Occurs most often during lactation

_____ e. Associated with increased conversion of androgens to estrogen

_____ f. Associated with breast trauma

_____ g. Multicoloured, sticky nipple discharge

_____ h. Caused by increased estrogen production in those 13 to 17 years old

_____ i. Common cause is *S. aureus*

_____ j. Involves ducts in subareolar area

_____ k. Usually resolves in 6 to 12 months

_____ l. Wart-like growth in mammary ducts near nipple

_____ m. Well-delineated, very mobile tumours

1. Fibroadenoma

2. Mastitis

3. Intraductal papilloma

4. Ductal ectasia

5. Fat necrosis

6. Prepubescent gynecomastia

7. Senescent gynecomastia

8. The risk for breast cancer is highest in women who

a. are obese.
b. are over the age of 60.
c. have fibrocystic breast changes.
d. have an inherited aberration of the BRCA1 or 2 gene.

9. The nurse would be most concerned when examination of a client's breasts revealed

a. a large, tender, movable mass in the upper inner quadrant.
b. an immobile, hard, non-tender lesion in the upper outer quadrant.
c. a 2- to 3-cm, firm, defined, mobile mass in the lower outer quadrant.
d. a painful, immobile mass with reddened skin in the upper outer quadrant.

10. The best prognosis is indicated in the client with breast cancer when diagnostic studies reveal

a. negative axillary lymph nodes.
b. aneuploid DNA tumour content.
c. cells with high S-phase fractions.
d. an estrogen and progesterone receptor–negative tumour.

11. Recurrence or metastasis of breast cancer occurs

    a. most often at sites distant from the breast.
    b. only through the lymphatic chains draining the breast.
    c. most commonly to the bowel and reproductive organs.
    d. in clients who have small tumours with negative axillary lymph nodes.

12. The physician of a client with a positive biopsy of a 2-cm breast tumour has recommended a lumpectomy with radiation therapy or a modified radical mastectomy as treatment. The client says she does not know how to choose and asks the female nurse what she would do if she had to make the choice. The best response of the nurse is

    a. "It doesn't matter what I would do. It is a decision you have to make for yourself."
    b. "There are advantages and disadvantages of both procedures. What do you know about these procedures?"
    c. "I would choose the modified radical mastectomy because it would ensure the entire tumour was removed."
    d. "The lumpectomy maintains a nearly normal breast but the survival rate is not as good as it is with a mastectomy."

13. A client undergoing either a mastectomy or a lumpectomy for treatment of breast cancer can usually also expect to undergo

    a. chemotherapy.
    b. radiation therapy.
    c. hormonal therapy.
    d. axillary node dissection.

14. Identify the type of radiation therapy (primary, adjunctive to surgery, high-dose brachytherapy, or palliative) related to the following situations.

    a. Used to treat possible local residual cancer cells post-mastectomy

    b. Used to reduce tumour size and stabilize metastatic lesions for pain relief

    c. Alternative to traditional radiation therapy for early stage breast cancer

    d. Follows local excision of tumour

    e. Used to reduce the size of a tumour before other therapy

    f. May be completed in five days

15. Systemic chemotherapy is indicated in treatment of clients with breast cancer

    a. only for estrogen receptor–negative tumours.
    b. only when there is evidence of node involvement.
    c. only for post-menopausal clients with nodal involvement.
    d. in premenopausal women even when no nodal involvement is present.

16. A client with a positive breast biopsy tells the nurse that she has read about tamoxifen (Nolvadex) in magazines and asks about its use. The best response of the nurse includes the information that

    a. tamoxifen is used only to prevent the development of new primary tumours.
    b. tamoxifen is the primary treatment for breast cancer if axillary lymph nodes are positive for cancer.
    c. tamoxifen is the treatment of choice after surgery if the tumour has receptors for estrogen on its cells.
    d. because tamoxifen has been shown to increase the risk for uterine cancer, it is used only when other treatment has not been successful.

17. During the immediate post-operative period following a mastectomy, the nurse initially institutes exercises for the affected arm by

    a. performing full passive ROM exercises to the affected arm.
    b. having the client brush or comb her hair with the affected arm.
    c. asking the client to flex and extend the fingers and wrist of the operative side.
    d. having the client crawl her fingers up the wall, raising her arm above her head.

18. Following a modified radical mastectomy, a client develops lymphedema of the affected arm. The nurse teaches the client to

    a. avoid skin softening agents on the arm.
    b. protect the arm from any type of trauma.
    c. abduct and adduct the arm at the shoulder hourly.
    d. keep the arm positioned so that it is in straight and dependent alignment.

19. A client undergoing surgery and radiation for treatment of breast cancer has a nursing diagnosis of disturbed body image related to absence of the breast. An appropriate nursing intervention for the client is to

    a. provide the client with information about surgical breast reconstruction.
    b. restrict visitors and phone calls until the client feels better about herself.
    c. arrange for a Reach to Recovery visitor or similar resource available in the community.
    d. encourage the client to obtain a permanent breast prosthesis as soon as she is discharged from the hospital.

20. A 56-year-old client is undergoing a mammoplasty for breast reconstruction following a mastectomy one year ago. During the preoperative preparation of the client, it is important that the nurse

    a. determine why the client is choosing reconstruction surgery rather than the use of an external prosthesis.
    b. ensure that the client has realistic expectations about the outcome and possible complications of the surgery.
    c. inform the client that implants used for breast reconstruction have been shown to cause immune-related diseases.
    d. let the client know that although the shape will be different from the other breast, the nipple can be reconstructed from other erectile tissue.

21. A client undergoing a modified radical mastectomy for cancer of the breast is going to use tissue expansion and an implant for breast reconstruction. The nurse knows that

    a. weekly injections of water or saline into the expander will be required.
    b. the expander cannot be placed until healing from the mastectomy is complete.
    c. this method of breast reconstruction uses the client's own tissue to replace breast tissue.
    d. the nipple from the affected breast will be saved to be grafted onto the reconstructed breast.

## CASE STUDY

### METASTATIC BREAST CANCER

#### Client Profile

Mrs. T., a 57-year-old married lawyer, was found to have a 4 × 6 cm firm, fixed mass in the upper, outer quadrant of the right breast during a routine physical examination, and a stereotactic core biopsy indicated a malignant tumour. Although the surgeon recommended a mastectomy because of the size of the tumour, Mrs. T. chose to have a lumpectomy. Now, three weeks post-operative, she is scheduled for chemotherapy.

#### Subjective Data

- Never had routine mammography
- Never practised breast self-examination
- States she deserves to have breast cancer for being so careless about her health
- Chose to have a lumpectomy to remove the tumour in spite of the large size because she believes her breasts are critical in her relationship with her husband

#### Objective Data

- Physical examination
  Right breast: healed lumpectomy breast incision and right axillary incision
  Limited ROM of right arm
  Port of central venous catheter in place on left upper chest

- Diagnostic studies
  Pathology: estrogen receptor–positive infiltrating ductal carcinoma; eight of twelve lymph nodes positive for malignant cells
  Staging: stage IIIB carcinoma of the right breast

- Clinical course
  Lumpectomy performed to remove tumour three weeks ago
  Chemotherapy with CAF protocol planned—cyclophosphamide (Cytoxan), doxorubicin (Adriamycin), and 5-fluorouracil (5-FU)

**Critical Thinking Questions**

1. Why is chemotherapy indicated for Mrs. T.?

2. Compare the three chemotherapeutic agents planned for Mrs. T. with respect to classification type, cell specificity, and common side effects.

3. What can the nurse do to help Mrs. T. reduce or manage the common physical effects of the chemotherapy?

4. What does the finding that Mrs. T.'s tumour is estrogen receptor-positive mean? What additional treatment modalities might this suggest?

5.  How could the nurse help Mrs. T. cope with her feelings of guilt and maintain a positive relationship with her husband?

6.  What are some possible reasons that Mrs. T. did not perform BSE or have mammography performed?

7.  What teaching by the nurse is indicated for Mrs. T. regarding follow-up care related to recurrence of the breast cancer?

8.  Based on the assessment data presented, write one or more appropriate nursing diagnoses. Are there any collaborative problems?

# CHAPTER *51* NURSING MANAGEMENT: SEXUALLY TRANSMITTED INFECTIONS

1. The current incidence of sexually transmitted infections (STIs) is related in part to

    a. increased virulence of organisms causing STIs.
    b. an increase in the recognition of homosexuality.
    c. the use of oral agents and intrauterine devices as contraceptives.
    d. development of resistance of micro-organisms to common antibiotics.

2. Match the following micro-organisms with the disease they cause.

    _____ a. *Treponema pallidum*          1. Gonorrhea

    _____ b. *Chlamydia trachomatis*       2. Genital herpes

    _____ c. *Neisseria gonorrhoeae*       3. Syphilis

    _____ d. Human papillomavirus          4. Non-gonococcal urethritis

    _____ e. Herpes simplex virus          5. Genital warts

3. A female client with a purulent vaginal discharge is seen at an outpatient clinic. The nurse would expect a diagnosis of gonorrhea to

    a. be treated with benzathine penicillin G.
    b. indicate the presence of pelvic inflammatory disease.
    c. be confirmed with a Gram's stain smear of the exudate.
    d. be treated with ceftriaxone (Rocephin) and doxycycline (Vibramycin).

4. A 22-year-old woman with multiple sexual partners seeks care after several weeks of experiencing painful and frequent urination and vaginal discharge. Although the results of a culture of cervical secretions are not yet available, the nurse explains to the client that she will be treated as if she has gonorrhea and chlamydia in order to prevent

    a. obstruction of the fallopian tubes.
    b. endocarditis and aortic aneurysms.
    c. disseminated gonococcal infection.
    d. polyarthritis and generalized adenopathy.

5. Indicate whether the following clinical manifestations of syphilis are characteristic of primary (P), secondary (S), latent (L), or tertiary (T) syphilis.

_____    a. Condyloma lata

_____    b. Aortic valve insufficiency

_____    c. Destructive skin, bone, and soft tissue lesions

_____    d. Chancre

_____    e. Mental deterioration

_____    f. Generalized adenopathy

_____    g. Absence of symptoms with a positive fluorescent treponemal antibody (FTAAbs) test

_____    h. Tabes dorsalis

_____    i. Generalized cutaneous rash

_____    j. Saccular aneurysms

6. A premarital blood test for syphilis reveals that a woman has a positive VDRL test. The nurse advises the client that

a. a single dose of penicillin will cure the syphilis.
b. she should question her fiancé about prior sexual contacts.
c. additional testing to detect specific anti-treponomal antibodies is necessary.
d. a lumbar puncture to evaluate cerebrospinal fluid is necessary to rule out active syphilis.

7. The nurse encourages serological testing for HIV in the client with syphilis primarily because

a. syphilis is more difficult to treat in clients with HIV infection.
b. the presence of HIV infection increases the risk of contracting syphilis.
c. CNS involvement is more common in clients with HIV infection and syphilis.
d. the incidence of syphilis is highest in those with high rates of sexual promiscuity and drug abuse.

8. In establishing screening programs for populations at high risk for chlamydial infections, the nurse recognizes that in women, *C. trachomatis* infection most often results in

a. cervicitis.
b. no symptoms.
c. acute urethritis.
d. liver inflammation.

9. A male client returns to the clinic with a recurrent urethral discharge after being treated for a chlamydial infection two weeks ago. Which statement of the client indicates the most likely cause of the recurrence of his infection?

a. "I took the vibramycin twice a day for a week."
b. "I haven't told my girlfriend about my infection yet."
c. "I had a couple of beers while I was taking the medication."
d. "I've only had sexual intercourse once since my medication was finished."

10. A diagnosis of chlamydial infection is made in a male client with a purulent urethral discharge when

    a. cultures for chlamydial organisms are positive.
    b. direct fluorescent antibody (DFA) tests are positive.
    c. Gram's stain smears and cultures are negative for gonorrhea.
    d. signs and symptoms of epididymitis or proctitis are also present.

11. Identify whether the following statements are true or false. If a statement is false, correct the bold word(s) to make the statement true.

    _____ a. Herpes simplex virus type 2 (HSV-2) is capable of causing **only genital lesions**.

    _____ b. The primary symptoms of genital herpes include painful **vesicular lesions that rupture and ulcerate.**

    _____ c. Treatment with acyclovir can **cure** genital herpes.

    _____ d. To prevent transmission of genital herpes, **condoms should be used** when lesions are present.

    _____ e. Recurrent symptomatic genital herpes may be precipitated by **sexual activity** and **stress**.

12. During the physical assessment of a female client with human papillomavirus infection, the nurse would expect to find

    a. purulent vaginal discharge.
    b. a painless, indurated lesion on the vulva.
    c. painful perineal vesicles and ulcerations.
    d. multiple, coalescing grey warts in the perineal area.

13. It is most important for the nurse to teach the female client with genital warts to

    a. have an annual Pap test.
    b. apply topical acyclovir faithfully as directed.
    c. have her sexual partner treated for the condition.
    d. use a contraceptive to prevent pregnancy, which may exacerbate the disease.

14. Based on the incidence of sexually transmitted infections (STIs) in Canada, the nurse informs individuals who have unprotected sexual activity with multiple partners that they are at highest risk for contracting

    a. syphilis.
    b. gonorrhea.
    c. chlamydia.
    d. genital warts.

15. Indicate what treatment or precautions should be taken during pregnancy or delivery when the client has active

    a. syphilis.
    b. gonorrhea.
    c. genital herpes.
    d. chlamydia.
    e. genital warts.

16. The nurse counsels the sexually active individual that the best prevention of STIs includes

    a. using condoms with a spermicidal jelly.
    b. voiding immediately following intercourse.
    c. substituting oral-anal intercourse for vaginal intercourse.
    d. thorough hand washing after contact with genitals.

17. The client who is most likely to have a nursing diagnosis of risk for non-compliance is the client with

    a. syphilis.
    b. gonorrhea.
    c. genital herpes.
    d. HPV infection.

## CASE STUDY

### GONORRHEA

**Client Profile**

Jack, a 20-year-old university student, had intercourse with a prostitute while on vacation. He returned home three days later and had intercourse with his fiancée, Ann. The next day he began to experience symptoms of a sexually transmitted infection.

**Subjective Data**

- Experiences pain and burning on urination
- Has a yellowish-white discharge from his penis
- Expresses concern over the possibility of having gonorrhea and what this diagnosis would mean in his relationship with his fiancée

**Objective Data**

- Positive Gram's stain for *N. gonorrhoeae*

### Critical Thinking Questions

1. Jack asks the nurse's advice on how to tell his fiancée about the diagnosis. What should the nurse's advice be?

2. What symptoms will Ann have if she has been infected?

3.  What physical examinations and laboratory procedures are required to establish a diagnosis of gonorrhea in Jack and Ann?

4.  What measures can be used to assist the couple in coping with the psychological implications of the infection?

5.  What treatment will be prescribed for Jack and Ann?

6.  What are the possible complications of untreated gonorrhea in men and in women?

7.  Based on the assessment data presented, write one or more appropriate nursing diagnoses. Are there any collaborative problems?

# CHAPTER 52 NURSING MANAGEMENT: FEMALE REPRODUCTIVE PROBLEMS

1. A couple seeks assistance from an infertility specialist for evaluation of their infertility. The nurse informs the couple that during the initial visit they can expect

   a. physical examinations and review of menstrual history.
   b. assessment of tubal patency with a hysterosalpingogram.
   c. pelvic ultrasonography for the woman and semen analysis for the man.
   d. post-coital testing to evaluate sperm numbers and motility in cervical and vaginal secretions.

2. An infertile couple is instructed in at-home ovulation testing using basal body temperature. The nurse explains that this testing

   a. can identify the need for intrauterine insemination as a result of anovulation.
   b. requires that the temperature be taken by the same route every morning on awakening before any activity.
   c. is an easy, non-stressful way to determine when ovulation occurs and when to have intercourse if pregnancy is desired.
   d. indicates when ovulation occurs by revealing a sharp rise in temperature followed by a drop in basal body temperature.

3. In working with couples with infertility, it is important for the nurse to

   a. inform the couple that most infertility can be successfully treated.
   b. warn the couple that treatment may exceed their financial resources.
   c. explain that most infertility results from causative factors in the woman.
   d. encourage the couple to participate in a support group for infertile couples.

4. A client with a 10-week pregnancy is admitted to the emergency department with vaginal bleeding and abdominal cramping. The nurse recognizes that

   a. the client will be scheduled for an immediate D&C.
   b. the client will recover quickly when the bleeding stops.
   c. the client is most likely experiencing a spontaneous abortion.
   d. treatment of the client with bed rest is usually successful in preventing further bleeding.

5. Premenstrual syndrome (PMS) is most likely to be diagnosed in a woman

   a. who has symptoms only when oral contraceptives are used.
   b. whose symptoms can be controlled with the use of progesterone.
   c. whose symptoms can be correlated with altered serum levels of estrogen and progesterone.
   d. who has the same symptom pattern following ovulation for two to three consecutive menstrual cycles.

6. When teaching a client with PMS about management of the disorder, the nurse focuses on the need to

   a. supplement the diet with vitamins C and E.
   b. use estrogen supplements during the luteal phase.
   c. limit dietary intake of caffeine, salt, and refined sugar.
   d. limit exercise and physical activity when symptoms are present.

7. The rationale for the regular use of non-steroidal anti-inflammatory drugs (NSAIDs) during the first several days of the menstrual period for women who have primary dysmenorrhea is that these drugs

    a. suppress ovulation and the production of prostaglandins that occur with ovulation.
    b. cause uterine relaxation and small vessel constriction, preventing cramping and abdominal congestion.
    c. inhibit the production of prostaglandins believed to be responsible for menstrual pain and associated symptoms.
    d. block the release of luteinizing hormone, preventing the increase in progesterone associated with maturation of the corpus luteum.

8. Match the following characteristics with their related menstrual irregularities (answers may be used more than once).

    _____ a. Common cause is use of hormonal contraceptives

    _____ b. May be caused by strenuous exercise or severe dieting

    _____ c. Bleeding or spotting between menstrual periods

    _____ d. May be associated with endometrial cancer

    _____ e. Increased duration or amount of menstrual bleeding

    _____ f. Excessive bleeding at irregular intervals

    _____ g. Absence of menses

    1. Amenorrhea
    2. Menorrhagia
    3. Metrorrhagia
    4. Menometrorrhagia

9. A young woman who runs vigorously as a form of exercise has not had a menstrual period in more than six months. The nurse advises her that

    a. normal periods will return when she stops running.
    b. uterine balloon therapy may be necessary to promote uterine sloughing of the overgrown endometrium.
    c. progesterone or birth control pills should be used to prevent persistent overgrowth of the endometrium.
    d. unopposed progesterone production causes an overgrowth of the endometrium that increases her risk for endometrial cancer.

10. A client with abdominal pain and irregular vaginal bleeding is admitted to the hospital with a suspected ectopic pregnancy. The most appropriate nursing intervention for the client is to

    a. provide analgesics for pain relief.
    b. monitor her vital signs and pain frequently.
    c. explain the need for frequent blood samples for $\beta$-HCG monitoring.
    d. offer support for the client's emotional response to the loss of the pregnancy.

11. Identify whether the following statements are true or false. If a statement is false, correct the bold word(s) to make the statement true.

_____ a. During the **perimenopausal** period a woman experiences cessation of menses.

_____ b. Menopause occurs in response to decreasing levels of **FSH**.

_____ c. Physical responses directly related to decreased estrogen during menopause include **hot flashes** and **atrophic vaginitis**.

_____ d. If estrogen replacement is used by a post-menopausal woman with a uterus, it is important that progesterone be taken to decrease the risk for **endometrial cancer**.

_____ e. Research contributing to evidence-based practice indicates that hormone replacement with estrogen and progesterone increases the risk for **cardiovascular disease**.

12. Identify four beneficial effects and four potential risks related to HRT that should be discussed with a woman during perimenopause.

**Benefits**

a. _____

b. _____

c. _____

d. _____

**Risks**

e. _____

f. _____

g. _____

h. _____

13. To prevent osteoporosis and cardiovascular disease, the nurse teaches the post-menopausal client to

a. supplement her diet with vitamin E.
b. maintain a high-protein, low-fat diet.
c. maintain a calcium intake of 800 mg daily.
d. engage in regular aerobic, weight-bearing exercise.

14. A woman with manifestations of menopause does not want to use hormone replacement and asks the nurse about the use of alternative and complementary therapies. The nurse suggests that the phytoestrogen that appears to be the most effective and least toxic is

a. valerian.
b. dong quai.
c. soy products.
d. black cohosh.

15. On admission of a victim of sexual assault to the emergency department, the first priority of the nurse is to

a. contact a rape victim support person for the client.
b. assess the client for urgent medical problems.
c. question the client about the details of the assault.
d. inform the client what procedures and treatments will be performed.

16. To prepare a sexually assaulted woman for physical examination, the nurse first

    a. ensures that a signed informed consent is obtained from the client.
    b. provides a private place for the client to talk about what happened to her.
    c. administers prophylaxis for sexually transmitted infections and tetanus.
    d. instructs the client not to wash, eat, drink, or urinate before the examination.

17. Match the following characteristics with the related infections (answers may be used more than once).

    _____ a. Pruritic, frothy greenish or grey discharge

    _____ b. May be treated with OTC antifungal
            agents

    _____ c. Thick, white, cottage-cheese–like discharge

    _____ d. Treated with regimens for chlamydia

    _____ e. Fishy-smelling watery discharge

    _____ f. Intense itching and dysuria

    _____ g. Hemorrhagic cervix and vagina

    _____ h. Severe recurrent infections associated with
            HIV infection

    _____ i. Mucopurulent discharge and post-coital spotting

    1. Vulvovaginal candidiasis

    2. Trichomoniasis

    3. Bacterial vaginosis

    4. Cervicitis

18. A client is diagnosed and treated for a *Gardnerella vaginalis* infection at a clinic. For her treatment to be effective, the nurse tells the client that

    a. her sexual partner must also be examined and treated.
    b. her sexual partner must use a condom during intercourse.
    c. she should wear minipads to prevent reinfection as long as she has vaginal drainage.
    d. the vaginal cream must be used at bedtime when she lies down to prevent its loss from the vagina.

19. A young woman is admitted to the hospital with acute pelvic inflammatory disease (PID). During the nursing history, the nurse notes as a significant risk factor the client's

    a. lack of any method of birth control.
    b. sexual activity with multiple partners.
    c. use of a vaginal sponge for contraception.
    d. recent antibiotic-induced monilial vaginitis.

20. In implementing care for the client with acute PID, the nurse

    a. performs vaginal irrigations every four hours.
    b. promotes bed rest in a semi-Fowler's position.
    c. instructs the client to use tampons to control vaginal drainage.
    d. has the client ambulate frequently to promote drainage of exudate.

21. A 20-year-old client with PID is crying and tells the nurse that she is afraid she will not be able to have children as a result of the infection. The nurse's best response to the client is

    a. "I would not worry about that right now. Our immediate concern is to cure the infection you have."
    b. "The possibility of infertility following PID is high. Would you like to talk about what it means to you?"
    c. "Sterility following PID is possible, but not common, and it is too soon to know what the effects will be."
    d. "The infection can cause more serious complications such as abscesses and shock that you should be more concerned about."

22. Identify whether the following statements are true or false. If a statement is false, correct the bold word(s) to make the statement true.

    _____ a. The presence of ectopic uterine tissue that bleeds and causes pelvic and abdominal adhesions and cysts is known as **uterine leiomyoma**.

    _____ b. Two gynecological conditions that subside with the onset of menopause are **endometriosis** and **cervical polyps**.

    _____ c. Polycystic ovary syndrome results when eggs are not released monthly from the ovaries as a result of increased production of **LH** and decreased production of **FSH**.

    _____ d. Treatments of endometriosis and leiomyomas depend on the severity of the symptoms and **the woman's desire to maintain fertility**.

    _____ e. Danazol (Danacrine) and Lupron (gonadotropin-releasing hormone analogue) are used to treat endometriosis and leiomyomas to create a **pseudopregnancy**.

    _____ f. The most common symptom of cervical polyps is **menorrhagia**.

    _____ g. An **ovarian cyst** may cause severe pain if twisting of the pedicle occurs.

23. A client with a stage 0 cervical cancer identified from a Pap smear asks the nurse what this finding means. The nurse's response includes the information that

    a. malignant cells have extended beyond the cervix but not to the pelvic wall.
    b. abnormal cells are present but are confined to the epithelial layer of the cervix.
    c. atypical cells characteristic of inflammation, but not necessarily malignancy, are present.
    d. this is a common finding on the Pap test and she will be examined frequently to see if the abnormal cells spread beyond the cervix.

24. Fertility and normal reproductive function can be maintained when a cancer of the cervix is treated with

    a. external radiation therapy.
    b. internal radiation implants.
    c. conization or laser surgery.
    d. cryotherapy or subtotal hysterectomy.

25. A post-menopausal woman of 10 years calls the clinic because of vaginal bleeding. The nurse schedules a visit for the client and informs her to expect to have

    a. an abdominal x-ray.
    b. an endometrial biopsy.
    c. a laser treatment to the cervix.
    d. only a routine pelvic examination and Pap test.

26. A client has been diagnosed with cancer of the ovary. In planning care for the client, the nurse recognizes that treatment indicated for the client depends on

    a. results of a direct-needle biopsy of the ovary.
    b. results of a laparoscopy with multiple biopsies.
    c. whether the client desires to maintain fertility.
    d. the findings of metastasis by ultrasonography or CT scan.

27. Indicate whether the following factors are associated with an increased risk for cervical cancer (C), endometrial cancer (E), ovarian cancer (O), or vaginal cancer (V).

    _____  a. Obesity

    _____  b. BRCA gene mutations

    _____  c. Smoking

    _____  d. Early sexual activity

    _____  e. Intrauterine exposure to estrogen (DES)

    _____  f. Unopposed estrogen-only replacement therapy

    _____  g. Human papillomavirus infection

    _____  h. Early menarche and late menopause

    _____  i. Low socio-economic status

    _____  j. Family history

28. During assessment of the client with vulvar cancer, the nurse would expect to find

    a. soreness and itching of the vulva.
    b. labial lesions with purulent exudate.
    c. severe excoriation of the labia and perineum.
    d. painless, firm nodules embedded in the labia.

29. A 44-year-old woman undergoing a total abdominal hysterectomy asks if she will need to take estrogen until she reaches the age of menopause. The best response of the nurse is

    a. "You are close enough to normal menopause that you probably won't need additional estrogen."
    b. "Yes, it will help prevent the more intense symptoms caused by surgically induced menopause."
    c. "Since your ovaries won't be removed, they will continue to secrete estrogen until your normal menopause."
    d. "There are so many risks associated with estrogen replacement therapy that it is best to begin menopause now."

30. While caring for a client on her second post-operative day following an abdominal panhysterectomy, the nurse would be most concerned if the client

    a. complains of abdominal distension and gas pains.
    b. complains of pain in her calf when her leg is extended.
    c. says she feels depressed and has periodic crying spells.
    d. has not voided for four hours following removal of the in-dwelling catheter.

31. A nursing diagnosis of disturbed body image is likely to be most appropriate for the client undergoing a

    a. vaginectomy
    b. hemivulvectomy.
    c. pelvic exenteration.
    d. radical hysterectomy.

32. During treatment with an intrauterine radioactive implant, the client

    a. may ambulate in the room as desired.
    b. should have all care provided by the same nurse.
    c. can have unlimited duration of visits and number of visitors.
    d. is restricted to bed rest with turning from side to side.

33. When teaching a client with problems of pelvic support to perform Kegel exercises, the nurse tells the client to

    a. contract her muscles as if trying to stop the flow of urine.
    b. tighten the lower abdominal muscles over the bladder area.
    c. squeeze all the perineal muscles as if trying to close the vagina.
    d. lie on the floor and do leg lifts to strengthen the abdominal muscles.

34. Match the following uterine structure abnormalities with their descriptions.

    _____ a. Uterine prolapse               1. Opening between vagina and bladder

    _____ b. Cystocele                      2. Protrusion of rectum through vaginal wall

    _____ c. Rectocele                      3. Protrusion of bladder through vaginal wall

    _____ d. Vesicovaginal fistula          4. Opening between rectum and vagina

    _____ e. Rectovaginal fistula           5. Displacement of uterus through vagina

35. An appropriate outcome for a client who undergoes an anterior colporrhaphy is that the client will

    a. maintain normal bowel patterns.
    b. adjust to temporary ileal conduit.
    c. urinate within eight hours post-operatively.
    d. experience healing of excoriated vaginal and vulvar tissues.

# CASE STUDY

## ACUTE PELVIC INFLAMMATORY DISEASE

### Client Profile

Ms. R., a 23-year-old unmarried woman, has a recent history of gonorrhea. For the past two weeks she has had a heavy purulent vaginal discharge and general malaise. Concerned that her symptoms appear to be worsening, Ms. R. makes an appointment at the gynecological clinic.

### Subjective Data

- Experiences an increase in lower abdominal pain during vaginal examination
- Expresses concern over worsening of her condition and the effect this will have on future child-bearing ability

### Objective Data

- Vital signs: T 38.3°C (101°F), HR 90, RR 18, BP 110/58
- Physical examination: heavy, purulent vaginal discharge
- Diagnostic studies: vaginal discharge positive for *N. gonorrhoeae*
- Admitted to the hospital for monitoring, IV fluids, and antibiotic therapy

### Critical Thinking Questions

1. What route does the gonococcus take in the development of PID?

2. What are the clinical manifestations of acute PID?

3. How would Ms. R.'s infection be managed if it were decided to treat her as an outpatient? What instructions should she receive?

4. How does chronic PID compare with acute PID?

5. What measures should the nurse take to prevent extension of the infection?

6. How should the nurse respond to Ms. R.'s concern over the effect of this infection on her future child-bearing ability?

7. Based on the assessment data presented, write one or more appropriate nursing diagnoses. Are there any collaborative problems?

# CHAPTER *53* NURSING MANAGEMENT: MALE REPRODUCTIVE PROBLEMS

1. A client asks the nurse what the difference between benign prostatic hyperplasia (BPH) and cancer of the prostate is. The best response of the nurse includes the information that BPH is

   a. a benign tumour that does not spread beyond the prostate gland.
   b. a precursor to prostate cancer but does not yet show any malignant changes.
   c. an enlargement of the gland caused by an increase in the size of existing cells.
   d. a benign enlargement of the gland due to an increase in the number of normal cells.

2. When taking a nursing history from a client with BPH, the nurse would expect the client to report

   a. nocturia, dysuria, and bladder spasms.
   b. urinary frequency, hematuria, and perineal pain.
   c. urinary hesitancy, post-void dribbling, and weak urinary stream.
   d. urinary urgency with a forceful urinary stream and cloudy urine.

3. The extent of urinary obstruction caused by BPH can be determined by

   a. a cystometrogram.
   b. transrectal ultrasonography.
   c. urodynamic flow studies.
   d. post-voiding catheterization.

4. The effect of finasteride (Proscar) in the treatment of BPH is

   a. reduction in the size of the prostate gland.
   b. relaxation of the smooth muscle of the urethra.
   c. increased bladder tone that promotes bladder emptying.
   d. relaxation of the bladder detrusor musculature, promoting urine flow.

5. On admission to the ambulatory surgical centre, a client with BPH informs the nurse that he is going to have a steel tube placed in his urethra to hold it open. The nurse recognizes that the client will need

   a. monitoring for post-operative urinary retention.
   b. teaching about the effects of general anaesthesia.
   c. to be informed of the possibility of short-term incontinence.
   d. instruction about home management of an in-dwelling catheter.

6. Match the following therapies used for BPH with their characteristics (answers may be used more than once).

    _____ a. Involves an external incision

    _____ b. Results in delayed sloughing of tissue

    _____ c. Most common surgical procedure to treat BPH

    \_\_\_\_ d. Use of low-wave radiofrequency to precisely destroy prostate tissue

    _____ e. Resectoscopic excision and cauterization of prostate tissue

    _____ f. Incisions made into prostate around bladder neck

    _____ g. Most effective long-term treatment of BPH

    _____ h. Use of microwave heat to destroy prostate tissue

    _____ i. Can be used on clients taking anticoagulants

    _____ j. Indicated for very large prostate gland

    _____ k. Temporary solution to obstructive problems

    _____ l. Inappropriate for men with rectal problems

1. Transurethral resection prostatectomy (TURP)

2. Transurethral incision of the prostate (TUIP)

3. Simple open prostatectomy

4. Transurethral microwave thermotherapy (TUMT)

5. Laser prostatectomy

6. Transurethral needle ablation (TUNA)

7. A health promotion intervention for detecting BPH in men over 50 is an annual

    a. urinalysis.
    b. PSA level.
    c. cystoscopy.
    d. digital rectal examination.

8. Before undergoing prostate surgery, the client should be informed that

    a. some degree of urinary incontinence will occur with all prostatectomies.
    b. all prostatectomies except TUIP result in some degree of retrograde ejaculation.
    c. erectile dysfunction will result if a vasectomy is performed with the prostatectomy.
    d. he will be discharged with an in-dwelling catheter to maintain urinary output until healing is complete.

9. Following a TURP, a client has a continuous bladder irrigation. Four hours after surgery, the catheter drainage contains thick, bright red clots and tissue. The nurse should

    a. release the traction on the catheter.
    b. manually irrigate the catheter until the drainage is clear.
    c. clamp the drainage tube and notify the client's physician.
    d. increase the rate of the irrigation and take the client's vital signs.

10. A client with continuous bladder irrigation following a prostatectomy tells the nurse he has bladder spasms and leaking of urine around the catheter. The nurse should first

    a. slow the rate of the irrigation.
    b. assess the catheter and drainage tube for clots.
    c. encourage the client to try to urinate around the catheter.
    d. administer a belladonna and opium suppository as prescribed.

11. The nurse provides discharge teaching to a client following a TURP and determines that the client understands the instructions when he says,

    a. "I should use daily enemas to avoid straining until healing is complete."
    b. "At least I don't have to worry about developing cancer of the prostate now."
    c. "I should avoid heavy lifting, climbing, and driving until my follow-up visit."
    d. "Every day I should drink 10 to 12 glasses of liquids such as coffee, tea, or soft drinks."

12. Identify three findings in the following areas that are present in the client with prostatic cancer that differ from findings in BPH.

    a. Prostatic palpation

    b. Blood tests

    c. Extraurinary symptoms

13. A client with prostate cancer is scheduled for a radical prostatectomy with a perineal approach. The nurse assesses the client's knowledge about the complications resulting from this surgery, primarily because of the high post-operative incidence of

    a. urinary retention.
    b. incisional infection.
    c. erectile dysfunction.
    d. loss of libido and gynecomastia.

14. Identify whether the following statements are true or false. If a statement is false, correct the bold word(s) to make the statement true.

    _____  a. A **radical prostatectomy** is a treatment option for all clients with prostatic cancer except those with stage D tumours.

    _____  b. The preferred hormonal therapy for treatment of prostate cancer includes **estrogen** and **androgen-receptor blockers**.

    _____  c. Early detection of cancer of the prostate is increased with annual rectal examinations and **serum prostatic acid phosphatase (PAP) measurements**.

    _____  d. Because of the variety of treatment options available for cancer of the prostate, it is common for a client to have a nursing diagnosis of **decisional conflict**.

    _____  e. An annual prostate examination is recommended starting at **age 50** for men because early prostate cancer screening may reduce the mortality rate by as much as 35%.

    _____  f. **Chronic bacterial prostatitis** manifests with symptoms of urinary tract infection with a swollen, very tender prostate gland.

    _____  g. Drainage of the prostate through intercourse, masturbation, and prostatic massage is indicated for management of **chronic prostatitis**.

15. Match the following terms with their descriptions.

    _____ a. Testicular torsion          1. Painful, prolonged erection

    _____ b. Hydrocele                    2. Ventral urinary meatus

    _____ c. Phimosis                     3. Complication of mumps

    _____ d. Epispadias                   4. Twisted spermatic cord

    _____ e. Cryptorchidism               5. Removal of penile foreskin

    _____ f. Varicocele                   6. Inflammation of the prepuce

    _____ g. Epididymitis                 7. Sperm-filled cyst of epididymis

    _____ h. Priapism                     8. Scrotal lymphedema

    _____ i. Orchitis                     9. Inflammation of the epididymis

    _____ j. Hypospadias                 10. Dorsal urinary meatus

    _____ k. Spermatocele                11. Testicular vein dilation

    _____ l. Circumcision                12. Undescended testicle

16. Serum tumour markers that may be elevated on diagnosis of cancer of the testicle and used to monitor the response to therapy include

    a. tumour necrosis factor (TNF) and C-reactive protein (CRP).
    b. alpha-fetoprotein (AFP) and human chorionic gonadotropin (HCG).
    c. prostate-specific antigen (PSA) and prostate acid phosphatase (PAP).
    d. carcinoembryonic antigens (CEA) and antinuclear antibodies (ANA).

17. When teaching a client testicular self-examination, the nurse instructs the client to report a finding of

    a. an irregular-feeling epididymis.
    b. one testis that is larger than the other.
    c. the spermatic cord within the testicle.
    d. a firm, non-tender nodule on the testis.

18. The nurse teaches the client having a vasectomy that following the procedure

    a. the amount of ejaculate will be noticeably decreased.
    b. he may have difficulty maintaining an erection for several months.
    c. contraception must be used for six to eight weeks.
    d. the testes will gradually decrease production of sperm and testosterone.

19. A client seeking medical intervention for erectile dysfunction should be thoroughly evaluated primarily because

    a. treatment of erectile dysfunction is based on the cause of the problem.
    b. psychological counselling can reverse the problem in 80–90% of the cases.
    c. new invasive and experimental techniques currently used have unknown risks.
    d. most treatments for erectile dysfunction are contraindicated in clients with systemic diseases.

20. A functional erection requires desire, adequate blood supply, nerve innervation, and hormone balance. Identify two conditions or factors that may alter each of these requirements.

    a. Desire

    b. Blood supply

    c. Innervation

    d. Hormones

21. Match the following treatment modalities for erectile dysfunction with their characteristics (answers may be used more than once).

    _____ a. Blood drawn into corporeal bodies and held with a ring

    _____ b. Indicated for hypogonadism

    _____ c. Relaxes smooth muscle in penis

    _____ d. Direct application of drugs that increase blood flow in penis

    _____ e. Devices implanted into corporeal bodies to firm the penis

    _____ f. Should be avoided in those using nitrates

    _____ g. Contraindicated in prostate cancer

    _____ h. May cause priapism

    1. Parenteral testosterone

    2. Intracavernosal self-injection of vasoactive drugs

    3. Vacuum constriction device (VCD)

    4. Penile implants

    5. Sildenafil (Viagra)

## CASE STUDY

### TESTICULAR CANCER

**Client Profile**

Following a shower last evening, 19-year-old Jerry was performing his routine testicular self-examination when he discovered a firm lump on his left testis. After a medical examination, he was admitted to the hospital for a left orchiectomy and lymph node resection.

**Subjective Data**

- Has a history of an undescended left testis, which was surgically corrected at age four
- Expresses concern about surgery and how it will affect him
- Asks about his prognosis and chances for recovery after the surgery
- Denies back pain

**Objective Data**

- Very firm, non-tender nodule on left testis
- Local lymph node enlargement
- No gynecomastia noted
- Biopsy revealed seminoma germ cell tumour

**Critical Thinking Questions**

1. Explain the development and risk factors for cancer of the testes.

2. How does cancer of the testis differ from a spermatocele on examination?

3. What is Jerry's prognosis if the malignancy is in early stages?

4. What blood tests for tumour markers should be done preoperatively and are indicated for long-term follow-up care, and why?

5. How can the nurse help Jerry deal with the psychological components of his illness?

6. What effect will this surgery have on Jerry's sexual functioning?

7. Based on the assessment data presented, write one or more appropriate nursing diagnoses. Are there any collaborative problems?

1.  Using the list of terms below, identify the structures in the following illustration.

**List of Terms**

Axon
Axon hillock
Collateral axon
Dendrites
Gemmule
Golgi apparatus
Mitochrondrion
Myelin sheath
Neuron cell body
Nissl bodies
Node of Ranvier
Nucleolus
Nucleus
Schwann cell
Synaptic knobs
Telodendria

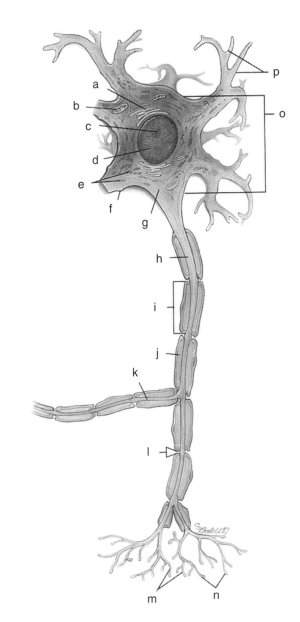

a. _____   g. _____   m. _____

b. _____   h. _____   n. _____

c. _____   i. _____   o. _____

d. _____   j. _____   p. _____

e. _____   k. _____

f. _____   l. _____

2.  Using the following list of terms, identify the structures in the illustration below.

### List of Terms

Anterior corticospinal tract
Anterior horn
Anterior spinocerebellar tract
Anterior spinothalamic tract
Central canal
Fasciculus cuneatus

Fasciculus gracilis
Lateral corticospinal tract
Lateral spinothalamic tract
Posterior horn
Posterior spinocerebellar tract
Posterolateral tract of Lissauer

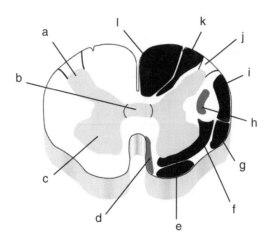

a. _____

b. _____

c. _____

d. _____

e. _____

f. _____

g. _____

h. _____

i. _____

j. _____

k. _____

l. _____

3. Crossword Puzzle

**Across**

3. Synaptic _____; spaces where neurotransmitters cross from neuron to neuron
6. Junction between two neurons
9. Produces myelin sheath of nerve fibres in CNS
11. Component of white matter
12. Part of the cell body of a neuron
14. Action _____; event that causes depolarization
15. Innermost meningeal mater
16. Site where cranial nerve V arises
17. Assessed in part with orientation and memory
18. Basic unit of the nervous system

**Down**

1. Gaps in peripheral nerve axons
2. Help form blood–brain barrier
3. Protective fluid of CNS
4. Lower extremity (abb.)
5. Produces myelin sheath of peripheral nerves
7. Carries impulses from nerve cell body
8. May occur with damage to peripheral axons
10. Carries impulses to nerve cell body
13. Area of brain concerned with emotions and aggression
14. Common symptom of disease
15. By mouth
16. Orally

4. Identify whether the following statements are true or false. If a statement is false, correct the bold word(s) to make the statement true.

    \_\_\_\_\_    a. Neuroglial cells that line the ventricles and assist in production of cerebral spinal fluid (CSF) are called **microglia**.

    \_\_\_\_\_    b. During depolarization of a nerve cell, **sodium** moves into the cell, creating a **positive** intracellular environment relative to the outside.

    \_\_\_\_\_    c. Breakdown of ATP for the sodium-potassium pump is required to move sodium **into the cell** and potassium **out of the cell** during repolarization.

    \_\_\_\_\_    d. When an action potential reaches the end of an axon and releases an **excitatory** neurotransmitter, the permeability of $K^+$ and $Cl^-$ at the receptor site is increased.

    \_\_\_\_\_    e. The transmission of an action potential at a synapse depends on the **number** of presynaptic cells releasing neurotransmitters and the **frequency** of the release of neurotransmitters.

5. A client has a lesion involving the fasciculus gracilis/cuneatus of the spinal cord. The nurse would expect the client to experience loss of

    a. pain and temperature sensations.
    b. touch, deep pressure, vibration, and position sense.
    c. unconscious information about body position and muscle tension.
    d. voluntary muscle control from the cerebral cortex to the peripheral nerves.

6. Lower motor neurons differ from upper motor neurons primarily in that lesions of the lower motor neurons

    a. cause hyporeflexia and flaccidity.
    b. affect motor control of the lower body.
    c. arise in structures above the spinal cord.
    d. interfere with reflex arcs in the spinal cord.

7.  Match the following functions with the associated area of the brain.

    _____    a.  Major relay centre for sensory and motor input to
                  cerebrum

    _____    b.  Responsible for arousal

    _____    c.  Controls initiation, execution, and completion of
                  voluntary and automatic movements

    _____    d.  Controls judgement, insight, and reasoning

    _____    e.  Regulates respiratory, vasomotor, and cardiac functions

    _____    f.  Sound and visual interpretation

    _____    g.  Maintains trunk stability and equilibrium

    _____    h.  Registers visual images

    _____    i.  Integrates somatic and special sensory inputs

    _____    j.  Related to emotion and sexual response

    _____    k.  Regulates endocrine and autonomic functions

    _____    l.  Responsible for verbal expression

    1.  Anterior frontal lobe

    2.  Temporal lobe

    3.  Parietal lobe

    4.  Occipital lobe

    5.  Limbic system

    6.  Broca's area

    7.  Basal ganglia

    8.  Thalamus

    9.  Hypothalamus

    10. Reticular activating system

    11. Medulla

    12. Cerebellum

8.  Spinal nerves of the peripheral nervous system differ from cranial nerves in that

    a.  only spinal nerves occur in pairs.
    b.  cranial nerves affect only the sensory and motor function of the head and neck.
    c.  the cell bodies of all cranial nerves are located in the brain while cell bodies of spinal nerves are located in
        the spinal cord.
    d.  all spinal nerves contain both afferent sensory and efferent motor fibres, while cranial nerves contain one
        or the other or both.

9. Indicate whether the following descriptions are characteristic of the sympathetic nervous system (S) or the parasympathetic nervous system (P).

_____ a. Preganglionic cells bodies are located in spinal segments T1-L2

_____ b. Norepinephrine released by most post-ganglionic fibres

_____ c. Responsible for conservation and restoration of energy stores

_____ d. Cause pupillary constriction and accommodation for near vision

_____ e. Necessary for ejaculation in men

_____ f. Acetylcholine released at both preganglionic and post-ganglionic nerve endings

_____ g. Increase heart rate and dilate coronary arteries

_____ h. Relax sphincters of the GI and GU tract

_____ i. Necessary for penile erection

_____ j. Preganglionic cells bodies located in brainstem and sacral spinal segment

_____ k. Responsible for some effects of cranial nerves III and X

10. A client has an atherosclerotic plaque in the middle cerebral artery. The nurse recognizes that

a. assessment will reveal distended jugular veins.
b. cerebral circulation may be maintained through the circle of Willis.
c. the client may develop a loss of temporal and parietal lobe function.
d. increased pressure in the middle cerebral artery will back up into the vertebral arteries.

11. Match the supportive and protective structures of the nervous system with their characteristics.

_____ a. Skull

_____ b. Vertebral column

_____ c. Cerebrospinal fluid (CSF)

_____ d. Blood–brain barrier

_____ e. Ventricles

_____ f. Falx cerebri

_____ g. Arachnoid layer

_____ h. Pia mater

_____ i. Tentorium cerebelli

1. Produce and circulate CSF

2. Forms a space with pia mater through which blood vessels and nerves pass

3. Separates cerebrum from the posterior fossa

4. Provides for flexibility while protecting spinal cord

5. Inner layer of meninges

6. Protects brain from external trauma

7. Protects against harmful blood-borne agents

8. Prevents expansion of brain tissue into adjacent hemisphere

9. Cushions the brain and spinal cord and provides nutrients

12. During neurological assessment of the older adult, the nurse would expect to find

    a. absent deep tendon reflexes.
    b. below-average intelligence score.
    c. decreased sensation of touch and temperature.
    d. decreased frequency of spontaneous awakening.

13. Identify three factors that should be considered when taking the history of a client with a neurological problem.

    a.

    b.

    c.

14. During the nursing history of a client with a neurological problem, the nurse notes as significant the client's report of

    a. kidney stones.
    b. a recent cholecystectomy.
    c. the use of ASA for control of headache.
    d. a fainting episode associated with a severe menopausal hot flash.

15. Identify one specific finding identified by the nurse during assessment of each of the client's functional health patterns that indicates a risk factor for neurological problems or a client response to an actual neurological problem.

    a. Health perception–health management

    b. Nutritional–metabolic

    c. Elimination

    d. Activity–exercise

    e. Sleep–rest

    f. Cognitive–perceptual

    g. Self-perception–self-concept

    h. Role–relationship

    i. Sexuality–reproductive

    j. Coping–stress tolerance

    k. Value–belief

16. During a neurological assessment, the nurse obtains most of the data related to mental status

    a. during the nursing history.
    b. by asking the client specific problem-solving questions.
    c. noting behaviours while the client is unaware of the nurse's presence.
    d. by asking the client to complete a written standardized mental examination.

17. Match the following cranial nerves with their methods of evaluation (evaluation methods may be used more than once, and some nerves may be tested with more than one method).

_____ a. Olfactory (I)

_____ b. Optic (II)

_____ c. Oculomotor (III)

_____ d. Trochlear (IV)

_____ e. Trigeminal (V)

_____ f. Abducens (VI)

_____ g. Facial (VII)

_____ h. Cochlear branch of acoustic (VIII)

_____ i. Glossopharyngeal (IX)

_____ j. Vagus (X)

_____ k. Spinal accessory (XI)

_____ l. Hypoglossal (XII)

1. Resistive shoulder shrug

2. Smile, frown, and close eyes

3. Light touch to face

4. Confrontation

5. Tongue protrusion

6. Corneal reflex test

7. Identify odours

8. Pupillary response

9. Oblique eye movement

10. Salt and sugar discrimination

11. Gag reflex

12. Lateral eye movement

13. Ticking watch

18. During an assessment of the motor system, the nurse finds that the client has a staggering gait and an abnormal arm swing. The nurse uses this information to

a. protect the client from injury due to falls.
b. assist the client to cope with the disability.
c. plan a rehabilitation program for the client.
d. help establish a diagnosis of cerebellar dysfunction.

19. Match the assessment methods that may elicit the following abnormal findings.

_____ a. Cotton wisp

_____ b. Plantar stimulation

_____ c. Sharp end of pin

_____ d. Heel-to-shin test

_____ e. Hold arms forward at shoulder with palms up

_____ f. Passive ROM to limbs

_____ g. Applying dual stimulus a few millimetres apart on tips of fingers

_____ h. Simultaneously stimulating opposite sides of the body

_____ i. Have client stand with feet close together and close eyes

_____ j. Tuning fork to bony prominences

1. Hypertonia

2. Loss of position sense

3. Lack of vibratory sense

4. Absence of two-point discrimination

5. Analgesia

6. Absence of light touch

7. Sensory extinction

8. Extension of the toes

9. Lack of coordination

10. Pronator drift

20. The normal response to striking the triceps tendon with a reflex hammer is

a. forearm pronation.
b. extension of the arm.
c. flexion of the arm at the elbow.
d. flexion and supination of the elbow.

21. Normal deep tendon reflexes are graded

a. 1/5.
b. 2/5.
c. 3/5.
d. 4/5.

22. To prepare a client for a lumbar puncture, the nurse

a. sedates the client with medication before the test.
b. withholds beverages containing caffeine for eight hours.
c. has the client sit on the side of the bed, leaning on a padded overbed table.
d. positions the client in a lateral recumbent position with the hips, knees, and neck flexed.

23. Following a lumbar puncture, the nurse assesses the client for

a. headache.
b. lower limb paralysis.
c. allergic reactions to the dye.
d. hemorrhage from the puncture site.

24. Nursing care of the client following a myelogram includes

    a. restricting fluids until the client is ambulatory.
    b. keeping the client positioned flat in bed for at least several hours.
    c. positioning the client with the head of the bed elevated 30 degrees.
    d. providing mild analgesics for pain associated with the insertion of needles.

25. The neurological diagnostic test that has the highest risk of complications and requires frequent monitoring of neurological and vital signs following the procedure is

    a. myelography.
    b. cerebral angiography.
    c. electroencephalography.
    d. transcranial Doppler sonography.

26. In noting the results of an analysis of cerebrospinal fluid, the nurse identifies as an abnormal finding

    a. a pH of 7.35.
    b. WBCs of 0.006/L (6/$\mu$L).
    c. clear, colourless appearance.
    d. glucose of 1.7 mmol/L (30 mg/dL).

1. Identify two ways the following three volume components of intracranial pressure (ICP) can be changed to adapt to small increases in intracranial pressure.

    a. Cerebrospinal fluid (CSF)

    b. Brain tissue

    c. Blood tissue

2. Complete the following statements related to intracranial pressure.

    a. Normal intracranial pressure ranges from _____ to _____ mm Hg.

    b. Autoregulation to maintain constant blood flow to the brain becomes ineffective when the mean arterial

       pressure (MAP) is below _____ mm Hg and the brain becomes _____. Autoregulation also

       becomes ineffective when MAP is greater than _____ mm Hg because the vessels are maximally

       _____.

    c. The cerebral perfusion pressure (CPP) is the blood pressure needed to ensure blood flow to the brain.

       Normal CPP is _____ mm Hg. Calculate the cerebral perfusion pressure (CPP) of a client

       whose blood pressure is 106/52 and ICP is 14 mm Hg: _____ mm Hg.

    d. A client with an ICP of 34 mm Hg and a systemic blood pressure of 108/64 has a CPP of

       _____ mm Hg.

    e. Cerebral ischemia and neuronal death occurs when CPP is less than _____ mm Hg. Cellular ischemia

       and death result when CPP is less than _____ mm Hg.

3. The relationship of intracranial pressure to volume is affected by the brain's elastance and compliance in that

    a. as volume in the brain increases, there is decreased elastance.
    b. a decrease in compliance occurs as volume and pressure increase.
    c. with high elastance, an increase in volume does not increase intracranial pressure.
    d. with high compliance, a small increase in volume results in high changes in pressure.

4. Indicate whether the following factors increase (I) or decrease (D) cerebral blood flow.

    _____ a. $PaCO_2$ of 30 mm Hg.

    _____ b. $PaO_2$ of 45 mm Hg.

    _____ c. decreased MAP

    _____ d. increased ICP

    _____ e. arterial blood pH of 7.3

5. Match the common causes of cerebral edema with their related types (answers may be used more than once).

    _____ a. SIADH                                  1. Vasogenic

    _____ b. Increased permeability of blood–        2. Cytotoxic
                brain barrier
                                                       3. Interstitial
    _____ c. Cerebral hypoxia

    _____ d. Ingested toxins

    _____ e. Hydrocephalus

6. In the following events that occur in the progression of increased intracranial pressure (ICP), indicate whether the event is directly **caused by** (CB) increased ICP or is a **cause of** (CO) increased ICP (see Fig. 55-3).

    _____ a. Tissue edema from initial insult

    _____ b. Edema of necrotic tissue

    _____ c. Compression of blood vessels

    _____ d. Vasodilation

    _____ e. Brainstem compression and herniation

7. The earliest signs of increased ICP the nurse should assess for include

    a. Cushing's triad.
    b. unexpected vomiting.
    c. decreasing level of consciousness.
    d. dilated pupil with sluggish response to light.

8. The nurse recognizes the presence of Cushing's triad in the client with

    a. increased pulse, irregular respiration, increased blood pressure.
    b. increased pulse, decreased respiration, increased pulse pressure.
    c. decreased pulse, irregular respiration, increased pulse pressure.
    d. decreased pulse, increased respiration, decreased systolic blood pressure.

9. Increased intracranial pressure in the left cerebral cortex caused by intracranial bleeding causes displacement of brain tissue to the right hemisphere beneath the falx cerebri. The nurse knows that this is referred to as

   a. uncal herniation.
   b. tentorial herniation.
   c. cingulate herniation.
   d. temporal lobe herniation.

10. A client has ICP monitoring with an intraventricular catheter. A priority nursing intervention for the client is

   a. aseptic technique to prevent infection.
   b. constant monitoring of ICP waveforms.
   c. removal of CSF to maintain normal ICP.
   d. sampling CSF to determine abnormalities.

11. Identify whether the following statements are true or false. If a statement is false, correct the bold word(s) to make the statement true.

   _____ a. During intracranial pressure monitoring, the client may be at risk for development of increased ICP when the height of the **P2 wave** is higher than the **P1 wave**.

   _____ b. P waves of ICP are normal and reflect changes in intracranial pressure with the **respiratory** cycle.

   _____ c. **A waves** in ICP waveforms indicate a sharp rise in ICP.

   _____ d. A complication of removal of CSF during intracranial pressure monitoring to control ICP is **ventricular collapse**.

12. Match the following treatments used to manage increased ICP with their effects.

   _____ a. Oxygen administration          1. Decreased CSF production with decreased ICP

   _____ b. Mild hyperventilation          2. Decreased cerebral metabolism with decreased ICP

   _____ c. Osmotic diuretics              3. Prevention of hypoxia

   _____ d. Loop diuretics                 4. Decreased volume of brain water

   _____ e. Dexamethasone (Decadron)       5. Cerbral arterial vasoconstriction

   _____ f. Barbiturates                   6. Decreased lesion edema

13. Metabolic and nutritional needs of the client with increased intracranial pressure are best met with

   a. enteral feedings that are low in sodium.
   b. the simple glucose available in $D_5W$ IV solutions.
   c. a fluid restriction that promotes a moderate dehydration.
   d. balanced, essential nutrition in a form that the client can tolerate.

14. The three criteria for the definition of coma are that the client is unable to

    a.

    b.

    c.

15. A client with an intracranial problem does not open his eyes to any stimulus, has no verbal response except muttering when stimulated, and flexes his arm in response to painful stimuli. The nurse records the client's Glasgow Coma Scale score as

    a. 6.
    b. 7.
    c. 8.
    d. 11.

16. When assessing the body functions of a client with increased intracranial pressure, the nurse should initially assess

    a. corneal reflex testing.
    b. extremity strength testing.
    c. pupillary reaction to light.
    d. circulatory and respiratory status.

17. Cranial nerve III originating in the midbrain is assessed by the nurse for an early indication of pressure on the brainstem by

    a. assessing for nystagmus.
    b. testing the corneal reflex.
    c. testing pupillary reaction to light.
    d. testing for oculocephalic (doll's eyes) reflex.

18. A client has a nursing diagnosis of altered cerebral tissue perfusion related to cerebral edema. An appropriate nursing intervention for the client is

    a. avoiding positioning the client with neck and hip flexion.
    b. maintaining hyperventilation to a $PaCO_2$ of 15 to 20 mm Hg.
    c. clustering nursing activities to provide periods of uninterrupted rest.
    d. routine suctioning to prevent accumulation of respiratory secretions.

19. A client with increased intracranial pressure is positioned in a lateral position with the head of the bed elevated 30 degrees. The nurse evaluates a need for lowering the head of the bed when the client experiences

    a. ptosis of the eyelid.
    b. unexpected vomiting.
    c. a decrease in motor functions.
    d. decreasing level of consciousness.

20. An unconscious client with increased intracranial pressure is on ventilatory support. The nurse notifies the physician when ABG results reveal a

    a. pH of 7.43.
    b. $SaO_2$ of 94%.
    c. $PaO_2$ of 50 mm Hg.
    d. $PaCO_2$ of 30 mm Hg.

21. While caring for a client with increased intracranial pressure, the nurse monitors intake and output and urine specific gravity. A finding that indicates the presence of a posterior pituitary disturbance that may cause an increase in ICP is

    a. increased urinary output and increased urine specific gravity.
    b. decreased urinary output and increased urine specific gravity.
    c. increased urinary output and decreased urine specific gravity.
    d. decreased urinary output and decreased urine specific gravity.

22. While the nurse performs ROM on an unconscious client with increased intracranial pressure, the client experiences severe decerebrate posturing reflexes. The nurse should

    a. use restraints to protect the client from injury.
    b. administer CNS depressants to lightly sedate the client.
    c. perform the exercises less frequently because posturing can increase ICP.
    d. continue the exercises because they are necessary to maintain musculoskeletal function.

23. Match the following types of head injury with their descriptions.

    _____ a. Linear skull fracture

    _____ b. Depressed skull fracture

    _____ c. Compound skull fracture

    _____ d. Comminuted skull fracture

    _____ e. Basilar skull fracture

    _____ f. Posterior fossa fracture

    _____ g. Frontal lobe skull fracture

    _____ h. Orbital skull fracture

    _____ i. Parietal skull fracture

    _____ j. Temporal skull fracture

    _____ k. Cerebral concussion

    _____ l. Cerebral contusion

    1. Depressed skull fracture and scalp lacerations with communication to intracranial cavity

    2. Temporary, minor injury with transient reduction in neural activity and LOC

    3. Possible pneumocranium, CSF rhinorrhea

    4. Fractured skull without alteration in fragments

    5. Bruising of brain, often associated with coup-contrecoup injury

    6. May involve dural tear with CSF otorrhea, vertigo, and Battles' sign

    7. Multiple linear fracture with fragmentation of bone

    8. Causes periorbital ecchymosis

    9. Inward indentation of skull with possible pressure on brain

    10. Cortical blindness or visual field defects

    11. Boggy temporal muscle because of extravasation of blood

    12. May cause deafness, loss of taste, CSF otorrhea

24. A client with a head injury has bloody drainage from the ear. To determine if CSF is present in the drainage, the nurse

    a. examines the tympanic membrane for a tear.
    b. tests the fluid with a glucose-identifying strip or stick.
    c. tests the fluid for a halo sign on a white 4 × 4 dressing.
    d. collects 5 mL of fluid in a test tube and sends it to the laboratory for analysis.

25. The nurse suspects the presence of an arterial epidural hematoma in the client who experiences

    a. failure to regain consciousness following a head injury.
    b. a rapid deterioration of neurological function within 24 to 48 hours following a head injury.
    c. non-specific, non-localizing progression of alteration in LOC occurring over weeks or months.
    d. unconsciousness at the time of a head injury with a brief period of consciousness followed by a decrease in LOC.

26. Skull x-rays and a CT scan provide evidence of a depressed parietal fracture with a subdural hematoma in a client admitted to the emergency department following an automobile accident. In planning care for the client, the nurse anticipates that

    a. the client will receive life-support measures until the condition stabilizes.
    b. immediate burr holes will be made to rapidly decompress the intracranial cavity.
    c. the client will be treated conservatively with close monitoring for changes in neurological status.
    d. the client will be taken to surgery for a craniotomy for evacuation of blood and decompression of the cranium.

27. When a client is admitted to the emergency department following a head injury, the nurse's first priority in management of the client is

    a. maintaining cervical spine precautions.
    b. determining the presence of increased ICP.
    c. monitoring for changes in neurological status.
    d. establishing IV access with a large-bore catheter.

28. A 54-year-old man is recovering from a skull fracture with a subacute subdural hematoma. He has return of motor control and orientation but appears apathetic and has reduced awareness of his environment. When planning discharge of the client, the nurse explains to the client and the family that

    a. continuous improvement in the client's condition should occur until he has returned to pre-trauma status.
    b. the client's complete recovery may take years, and the family should plan for his long-term dependent care.
    c. the client is likely to have long-term emotional and mental changes that may require continued professional help.
    d. role changes in family members will be necessary because the client will be dependent on his family for care and support.

29. Identify whether the following statements are true or false. If a statement is false, correct the bold word(s) to make the statement true.

_____ a. Without treatment, **only malignant** brain tumours will cause death, as a result of increased growth leading to increased ICP and compression of vital brain centres.

_____ b. Symptoms of visual disturbances and seizures may indicate a tumour of the **temporal** lobe.

_____ c. The most common malignant brain tumour is **an astrocytoma**.

_____ d. Tumours that are considered inoperable are those located in the **upper brainstem** or **deep in the dominant hemisphere**.

_____ e. Radiation therapy for brain tumours may cause serious **increases in ICP**.

30. Assisting the family to understand what is happening to the client is an especially important role of the nurse when the client has a tumour of the

    a. ventricles.
    b. frontal lobe.
    c. parietal lobe.
    d. occipital lobe.

31. Match the following types of cranial surgery with their descriptions.

_____ a. Burr holes            1. Excision of cranial bone without replacement

_____ b. Craniotomy           2. Three-dimensional targeting of cranial tissue

_____ c. Craniectomy          3. Placement of tubes to redirect CSF from one area to another

_____ d. Cranioplasty         4. Opening into cranium with a drill to remove blood and fluid

_____ e. Sterotactic surgery  5. Replacement of part of the cranium with an artificial plate

_____ f. Shunt procedures     6. Opening into cranium with removal of bone flap to open dura

32. For the client undergoing a craniotomy, the nurse provides information about the use of wigs and hairpieces or other methods to disguise hair loss

    a. during preoperative teaching.
    b. if the client asks about their use.
    c. in the immediate post-operative period.
    d. when the client expresses negative feelings about his or her appearance.

33. It is most important that the nurse position the client who has had a craniectomy with an anterior fossae incision

    a. on the unoperated side.
    b. flat, with the head slightly hyperextended.
    c. with the head of the bed elevated 15 degrees.
    d. on either side, with the head elevated 30 degrees.

34. Successful achievement of client outcomes for the client with cranial surgery would best be indicated by

    a. ability to return home in six days.
    b. ability to meet all self-care needs.
    c. acceptance of residual neurological deficits.
    d. absence of signs and symptoms of increased intracranial pressure.

35. Indicate whether the following descriptions are characteristic of meningitis (M) or encephalitis (E).

    _____    a. Most frequently caused by bacteria

    _____    b. Is an inflammation of the brain

    _____    c. May be transmitted by insect vectors

    _____    d. CSF production is increased

    _____    e. Almost always has a viral cause

    _____    f. Involves an inflammation of pia mater and arachnoid layer

    _____    g. Has a rapid onset of symptoms

    _____    h. Cerebral edema is a major problem

    _____    i. Exudate may impair normal CSF flow and absorption

36. A client is admitted to the hospital with possible bacterial meningitis. During the initial assessment, the nurse questions the client about a recent history of

    a. mosquito or tick bites.
    b. chicken pox or measles.
    c. cold sores or fever blisters.
    d. an upper respiratory infection.

37. Classic symptoms of bacterial meningitis include

    a. papilledema and psychomotor seizures.
    b. high fever, nuchal rigidity, and severe headache.
    c. behavioural changes with memory loss and lethargy.
    d. positive Kernig's and Brudzinski's signs and hemiparesis.

38. Management of the client with bacterial meningitis includes

    a. administering antibiotics immediately following collection of specimens for culture.
    b. waiting for results of a CSF culture to identify an organism before initiating treatment.
    c. providing symptomatic and supportive treatment because drug therapy is not effective in treatment.
    d. performing skull x-rays and CT scans to determine the extent of the disease before treatment is started.

39. Vigorous control of fever in the client with meningitis is required to prevent complications. Identify four undesirable effects of fever in the client with meningitis.

    a.

    b.

    c.

    d.

40. On physical examination of a client with headache and fever, the nurse would suspect a brain abscess when the client has

    a. seizures.
    b. nuchal rigidity.
    c. focal symptoms.
    d. signs of increased ICP.

## CASE STUDY

### NEUROLOGICAL COMPLICATIONS

**Client Profile**

Steven K., a 16-year-old unrestrained driver, suffered a compound fracture of the skull and facial fractures in a motor vehicle accident. On admission to the hospital, he was immediately taken to surgery for evacuation of a right subdural hematoma in the temporal region and repair of facial fractures. On the fourth post-operative day, the nurse obtains the following findings during assessment of Steven.

**Subjective Data**

- Increasingly difficult to rouse

**Objective Data**

- Glasgow Coma Scale decreased from 10 to 5
- Signs of nuchal rigidity
- Temperature 39°C (102.2°F), BP 110/60, HR 114
- ICP ranges between 20 and 30 mm Hg despite CSF drainage and mannitol

### Critical Thinking Questions

1. What is the probable cause of Steven's change in neurological status?

2. What were the contributing factors that put Steven at risk for complications after a head injury and surgery?

3. Discuss the pathophysiological basis for the symptoms exhibited by Steven.

4. On the basis of the nursing assessment, what are the priority interventions?

5. Discuss the possible areas for organisms to gain access to the meninges in the case of Steven.

6. Based on the assessment data presented, write one or more appropriate nursing diagnoses. Are there any collaborative problems?

# CHAPTER 56  NURSING MANAGEMENT: STROKE

1. In promoting health maintenance for prevention of strokes, the nurse understands that the highest risk for the most common type of stroke is present in

   a. men who are physically inactive.
   b. women who smoke.
   c. individuals with hypertension and diabetes.
   d. those who are obese with high dietary fat intake.

2. A thrombus that develops in a cerebral artery does not always cause a loss of neurological function because

   a. the body can dissolve atherosclerotic plaques as they form.
   b. some tissues of the brain do not require constant blood supply to prevent damage.
   c. circulation through the circle of Willis may provide blood supply to the affected area of the brain.
   d. neurological deficits occur only when major arteries are occluded by thrombus formation around an atherosclerotic plaque.

3. A client comes to the emergency department immediately after experiencing numbness of the face and an inability to speak, but while the client awaits examination, the symptoms disappear and the client requests discharge. The nurse stresses that it is important for the client to be evaluated, primarily because

   a. the client has probably experienced an asymptomatic lacunar stroke.
   b. the symptoms are likely to return and progress to worsening neurological deficit in the next 24 hours.
   c. neurological deficits that are transient occur most often as a result of small hemorrhages that clot.
   d. the client has probably experienced a transient ischemic attack (TIA), which is a sign of progressive cerebral vascular disease.

4. Match the characteristics with their related type of stroke (answers may be used more than once).

   _____ a. Onset unrelated to activity

   _____ b. Rupture of atherosclerotic vessels

   _____ c. Carries the poorest prognosis

   _____ d. Type most often signalled by TIAs

   _____ e. Most common cause of sudden death

   _____ f. Creates mass that compresses brain

   _____ g. Symptoms of meningeal irritation

   _____ h. Commonly occur during or after sleep

   _____ i. Quick onset and resolution

   _____ j. Caused by rupture of intracranial aneurysm

   _____ k. Strong association with hypertension

   _____ l. Associated with sudden, severe headache

   _____ m. Associated with endocardial disorders

   1. Thrombotic

   2. Embolic

   3. Intracerebral hemorrhage

   4. Subarachnoid hemorrhage

432

5. A client with right-sided paraesthesias and hemiparesis is hospitalized and diagnosed with a thrombotic stroke. Over the next 72 hours the nurse plans care with the knowledge that the client

   a. is ready for aggressive rehabilitation.
   b. will show gradual improvement of the initial neurological deficits.
   c. may show signs of deteriorating neurological function as cerebral edema increases.
   d. should not be turned or exercised to prevent extension of the thrombus and increased neurological deficits.

6. The neurological functions that are affected by a stroke are primarily related to

   a. the amount of tissue area involved.
   b. the rapidity of the onset of symptoms.
   c. the brain area perfused by the affected artery.
   d. the presence or absence of collateral circulation.

7. Indicate whether the following manifestations of a stroke are more likely to occur with right brain damage (R) or left brain damage (L).

   _____    a. Aphasia

   _____    b. Left homonymous hemianopsia

   _____    c. Agnosia

   _____    d. Quick and impulsive behaviour

   _____    e. Inability to remember words

   _____    f. Neglect of the left side of the body

8. Identify whether the following statements are true or false. If a statement is false, correct the bold word(s) to make the statement true.

   _____    a. **Receptive** aphasia is characterized by a lack of comprehension of both verbal and written language.

   _____    b. **Dysarthria** results from a disturbance in Broca's area and is an impairment in speaking and writing.

   _____    c. A lesion that affects both Wernicke's area and Broca's area is most likely to cause **global** aphasia.

   _____    d. A **non-fluent dysphagia** is characterized by the presence of speech that contains little meaningful communication.

   _____    e. The long-term effect of paralysis of an extremity resulting from a stroke is **flaccidity**.

9. A client is admitted to the hospital with a left hemiplegia. To determine the size, location, and whether a stroke is ischemic or hemorrhagic the nurse anticipates that the physician will request a

   a. CT scan.
   b. lumbar puncture.
   c. cerebral arteriogram.
   d. positron emission tomography (PET).

10. A carotid endarterectomy is being considered as treatment for a client who has had several TIAs. The nurse explains to the client that this surgery

   a. is used to restore blood circulation to the brain following an obstruction of a cerebral artery.
   b. involves intracranial surgery to join a superficial extracranial artery to an intracranial artery.
   c. involves removing an atherosclerotic plaque in the carotid artery to prevent an impending stroke.
   d. is used to open a stenosis in a carotid artery with a balloon and stent to restore cerebral circulation.

11. The incidence of ischemic stroke in clients with TIAs and other risk factors is reduced with the administration of

   a. furosemide (Lasix).
   b. lovastatin (Mevacor).
   c. daily low-dose ASA.
   d. nimodipine (Nimotop).

12. An essential intervention in the emergency management of the client with a stroke is

   a. intravenous fluid replacement.
   b. administration of osmotic diuretics to reduce cerebral edema.
   c. initiation of hypothermia to decrease the oxygen needs of the brain.
   d. maintenance of respiratory function with a patent airway and oxygen administration.

13. A diagnosis of a ruptured cerebral aneurysm has been made in a client with manifestations of a stroke. The nurse anticipates that treatment options that would be evaluated for the client include

   a. hyperventilation therapy.
   b. surgical clipping of the aneurysm.
   c. administration of hyperosmotic agents.
   d. administration of thrombolytic therapy.

14. During the acute phase of a stroke, the nurse assesses the client's vital signs and neurological status q4h. A cardiovascular sign that the nurse would see as the body attempts to increase cerebral blood flow is

   a. hypertension.
   b. fluid overload.
   c. cardiac arrythmias.
   d. $S_3$ and $S_4$ heart sounds.

15. Identify four nursing diagnoses in which impaired neuromotor function can be an etiological factor.

   a.

   b.

   c.

   d.

16. A nursing intervention that is indicated for the client with hemiplegia is

   a. the use of a footboard to prevent plantar flexion.
   b. immobilization of the affected arm against the chest with a sling.
   c. positioning the client in bed with each joint lower than the joint proximal to it.
   d. having the client perform passive ROM of the affected limb with the unaffected limb.

17. A newly admitted client who has suffered a right brain stroke has a nursing diagnosis of disturbed visual sensory perception related to homonymous hemianopsia. Early in the care of the client, the nurse should

    a. place objects on the right side within the client's field of vision.
    b. approach the client from the left side to encourage the client to turn the head.
    c. place objects on the client's left side to assess the client's ability to compensate.
    d. patch the affected eye to encourage the client to turn the head to scan the environment.

18. Four days following a stroke, a client is to start oral fluids and feedings. Before feeding the client, the nurse should first

    a. check the client's gag reflex.
    b. order a soft diet for the client.
    c. raise the head of the bed to a sitting position.
    d. evaluate the client's ability to swallow small sips of ice water.

19. An appropriate food for a client with a stroke who has mild dysphagia is

    a. fruit juices.
    b. pureed meat.
    c. scrambled eggs.
    d. fortified milkshakes.

20. A client who has suffered a stroke is experiencing urinary incontinence. Nursing management of the client includes

    a. limiting fluid intake to 1000 mL/day.
    b. taking the client to the bathroom q4h.
    c. determining the pattern and cause of the incontinence.
    d. using incontinence briefs to reduce the effects of incontinence.

21. To promote communication during rehabilitation of the client with aphasia, an appropriate nursing intervention is to

    a. use gestures, pictures, and music to stimulate client responses.
    b. talk about activities of daily living that are familiar to the client.
    c. structure statements so that the client does not have to respond verbally.
    d. use flash cards with simple words and pictures to promote language recall.

22. A client with a right hemisphere stroke has a nursing diagnosis of unilateral neglect related to sensory–perceptual deficits. During the client's rehabilitation, it is important for the nurse to

    a. avoid positioning the client on the affected side.
    b. place all objects for care on the client's unaffected side.
    c. teach the client to consciously care for the affected side.
    d. protect the affected side from injury with pillows and supports.

23. A client with a stroke has a right-sided hemiplegia. The nurse prepares family members to help control behaviour changes seen with this type of stroke by teaching them to

    a. ignore undesirable behaviours manifested by the client.
    b. provide directions to the client verbally in small steps.
    c. distract the client from inappropriate emotional responses.
    d. supervise all activities before allowing the client to pursue them independently.

24. The nurse can assist the client and the family in coping with the long-term effects of a stroke by

   a. informing family members that the client will need assistance with almost all ADLs.
   b. explaining that the client's pre-stroke behaviour will return as improvement progresses.
   c. encouraging the client and family members to seek assistance from family therapy or stroke support groups.
   d. helping the client and family understand the significance of residual stroke damage to promote problem solving and planning.

## CASE STUDY

### STROKE

#### Client Profile

Mrs. C., a 38-year-old married woman, was admitted unconscious to the hospital after her family could not rouse her in the morning. She was accompanied by her husband and three daughters, ages 10, 13, and 15.

#### Subjective Data

- Has no history of hypertension or other health problems
- Had complained of a headache the day before she developed unconsciousness

#### Objective Data

- Diagnostic tests reveal a subarachnoid hemorrhage
- Vital signs: BP 150/82; RR 16; HR 56, T 38.3°C (101°F)
- Glasgow Coma Scale score: 5

#### Critical Thinking Questions

1. What diagnostic tests would be indicated to determine the cause of Mrs. C.'s unconsciousness?

2. What signs of increased intracranial pressure are present in Mrs. C.?

3. What should the family be told to expect in terms of Mrs. C.'s condition?

4. What nursing interventions have the highest priority for Mrs. C. at this stage of her illness?

5. What treatment modalities indicated for thrombotic strokes are contraindicated for Mrs. C.?

6. What therapeutic options are available for the client with a hemorrhagic stroke resulting from a ruptured aneurysm?

7. Based on the assessment data presented, write one or more appropriate nursing diagnoses. Are there any collaborative problems?

# CHAPTER 57  NURSING MANAGEMENT: CHRONIC NEUROLOGICAL PROBLEMS

1. Match the following characteristics with their related type of headache (answers may be used more than once).

   _____ a. Activation of trigeminal nerve causes facial vasomotor symptoms and pain

   _____ b. Chronic, dull, persisting intermittently over months or years

   _____ c. Strong family history

   _____ d. Bilateral pressure or tightness sensation

   _____ e. Commonly recur several times a day for several weeks

   _____ f. May occur with or between migraine headaches

   _____ g. Severe, steady, penetrating head pain

   _____ h. Causes agitation, restlessness

   _____ i. May be accompanied by systemic edema, nausea, and vomiting

   _____ j. Abrupt onset lasting 30 to 90 minutes

   _____ k. Unilateral or bilateral throbbing pain

   _____ l. Prodrome phase followed by headache phase

   1. Tension-type

   2. Migraine

   3. Cluster

2. The most important method of diagnosing functional headaches is

   a. electromyography (EMG).
   b. CT scan.
   c. cerebral blood flow studies.
   d. a thorough history of the headache.

3. Drug therapy for acute migraine and cluster headaches that appears to alter the pathophysiological process includes

   a. serotonin antagonists such as methysergide (Sansert).
   b. tricyclic antidepressants such as amitriptyline (Elavil).
   c. β-adrenergic blockers such as propranolol (Inderal).
   d. vasoconstrictors such as sumatriptan (Imitrex).

4. A nursing intervention that is appropriate for the client with a nursing diagnosis of anxiety related to lack of knowledge of etiology and treatment of headache is to

   a. help the client examine lifestyle patterns and precipitating factors.
   b. administer medications as ordered to relieve pain and promote relaxation.
   c. provide a quiet, dimly lit environment to reduce stimuli that increase muscle tension and anxiety.
   d. support the client's use of counselling or psychotherapy to enhance conflict resolution and stress reduction.

438

5. During the nursing assessment of a client with a headache, the nurse recognizes that the headache may be organic when the headache is associated with

   a. projectile vomiting.
   b. visual disturbances.
   c. weakness and paralysis.
   d. paraesthesias and confusion.

6. Generalized seizures differ from partial seizures in that

   a. partial seizures are confined to one side of the brain and remain focal in nature.
   b. generalized seizures result in loss of consciousness, while partial seizures do not.
   c. generalized seizures result in temporary residual deficits during the post-ictal phase.
   d. generalized seizures have no warning or aura because the entire brain is affected at the onset.

7. Match the following characteristics with their related types of seizures (answers may be used more than once).

   _____ a. Also known as petit mal seizure                    1. Generalized tonic-clonic

   _____ b. Sudden, excessive jerk of body that                2. Typical absence
            may hurl the person to the ground
                                                                 3. Atypical absence
   _____ c. Often involve behavioural, emotional,
            and cognitive functions with altered                4. Myoclonic
            consciousness
                                                                 5. Atonic
   _____ d. Often accompanied by incontinence,
            tongue or cheek biting                              6. Simple partial

   _____ e. Brief staring spell accompanied by                 7. Complex partial
            peculiar behaviour during seizure
            or post-ictal confusion

   _____ f. Focal motor, sensory, or autonomic
            symptoms without loss of consciousness

   _____ g. Also known as grand mal seizure

   _____ h. Falling spell from loss of muscle tone
            accompanied by brief unconsciousness

   _____ i. Staring spell lasting a few seconds

   _____ j. Psychomotor seizures with repetitive behaviours and lip smacking

   _____ k. Alterations in memory, sexual sensations, and distortions of visual or auditory sensations

   _____ l. Loss of consciousness, stiffening of the body with subsequent jerking of extremities

   _____ m. Known as temporal lobe seizures

   _____ n. Very brief and may occur in clusters

8. Identify whether the following statements are true or false. If a statement is false, correct the bold word(s) to make the statement true.

_____ a. **Status epilepticus** is the effect that occurs when frequent seizures produce permanent changes in neuron excitability, increasing the likelihood of more seizures.

_____ b. Status epilepticus is most serious in **tonic-clonic seizures** because it can cause ventilatory insufficiency and hypoxemia.

_____ c. Permanent brain damage may occur from status epilepticus of **any type of** seizures.

_____ d. The most useful tool for diagnosing epilepsy is **the EEG**.

_____ e. Immediate medical care should be sought for **all** seizures.

_____ f. A tonic-clonic seizure with loss of consciousness that is preceded by an aura is a **partial** seizure that generalizes.

9. A client admitted to the hospital following a generalized tonic-clonic seizure asks the nurse what caused the seizure. The best response of the nurse is

a. "So many factors can cause epilepsy that it is impossible to say what caused your seizure."
b. "Epilepsy is an inherited disorder. Does anyone else in your family have a seizure disorder?"
c. "In seizures, some type of trigger causes sudden, abnormal bursts of electrical brain activity."
d. "Scar tissue in the brain alters the chemical balance, creating uncontrolled electrical discharges."

10. A client with a seizure disorder is being evaluated for surgical treatment of the seizures. The nurse recognizes that one of the requirements for surgical treatment is

a. identification of scar tissue that can be removed.
b. an adequate trial of drug therapy that had unsatisfactory results.
c. development of toxic syndromes from long-term use of antiseizure drugs.
d. the presence of symptoms of cerebral degeneration from repeated seizures.

11. The nurse teaches the client taking antiseizure drugs that the method most commonly used to measure compliance and to monitor for toxicity is

a. monthly EEGs.
b. a daily seizure log.
c. urine testing for drug levels.
d. blood testing for drug levels.

12. When teaching a client with a seizure disorder about the medication regimen, it is most important for the nurse to stress that

a. the client should increase the dosage of the medication if stress is increased.
b. if gingival hypertrophy occurs the drug should be stopped and the physician notified.
c. stopping the medication abruptly may increase the intensity and frequency of seizures.
d. most over-the-counter and prescription drugs are safe to take with anticonvulsant drugs.

13. The nurse finds a client in bed having a generalized tonic-clonic seizure. During the seizure activity, the nurse should

a. turn the client to the side.
b. suction the client and administer oxygen.
c. insert an oral airway into the client's mouth.
d. restrain the client's extremities to prevent soft tissue and bone injury.

14. Following a generalized tonic-clonic seizure, the client is tired and sleepy. The nurse should

    a. suction the client before allowing him to rest.
    b. allow the client to sleep as long as he feels sleepy.
    c. stimulate the client to increase his level of consciousness.
    d. check the client's level of consciousness every 15 minutes for an hour.

15. During the diagnosis and long-term management of a seizure disorder, the nurse recognizes that one of the major needs of the client is assistance to

    a. manage the complicated drug regimen of seizure control.
    b. cope with the effects of negative social attitudes toward epilepsy.
    c. adjust to the very restricted lifestyle required by a diagnosis of epilepsy.
    d. learn to minimize the effect of the condition in order to obtain employment.

16. Match the chronic neurological disorders with their pathophysiological descriptions.

    _____ a. Multiple sclerosis
    _____ b. Parkinson's disease
    _____ c. Myasthenia gravis
    _____ d. Huntington's disease
    _____ e. Amyotropic lateral sclerosis

    1. Degeneration of motor neurons in brainstem and spinal cord
    2. Deficiency of acetylcholine and GABA in basal ganglia and extrapyramidal system
    3. Immune-mediated inflammatory destruction of myelin and replacement with glial scar tissue
    4. Autoimmune antibody destruction of cholinergic receptors at the neuromuscular junction
    5. Degeneration of dopamine-producing neurons in substantia nigra of midbrain and basal ganglia

17. A 38-year-old woman has newly diagnosed multiple sclerosis (MS) and asks the nurse what is going to happen to her. The best response of the nurse is

    a. "You need to plan for a continuous loss of movement, sensory functions, and mental capabilities."
    b. "Most people with MS have periods of attacks and remissions, with progressively more nerve damage over time."
    c. "You will most likely have a steady course of chronic progressive nerve damage that will change your personality."
    d. "It is common for people with MS to have an acute attack of weakness and then not have any other symptoms for years."

18. During assessment of a client admitted to the hospital with an acute exacerbation of MS, the nurse would expect to find

    a. tremors, dysphasia, and ptosis.
    b. bowel and bladder incontinence and loss of memory.
    c. motor impairment, visual disturbances, and paraesthesias.
    d. excessive involuntary movements, hearing loss, and ataxia.

19. The nurse explains to a client newly diagnosed with MS that the diagnosis is made primarily by

    a. MRI findings.
    b. T cell analysis of the blood.
    c. analysis of cerebrospinal fluid.
    d. history and clinical manifestations.

20. Mitoxantrone (Novantrone) is being considered as treatment for a client with progressive-relapsing MS. The nurse explains that a disadvantage of this drug compared with other drugs used for multiple sclerosis is that it

    a. must be given subcutaneously every day.
    b. has a lifetime dose limit due to cardiac toxicity.
    c. is an anticholinergic agent that causes urinary incontinence.
    d. is an immunosuppressant agent that increases the risk for infection.

21. A client with MS has a nursing diagnosis of self-care deficit related to muscle spasticity and neuromuscular deficits. In providing care for the client, it is most important for the nurse to

    a. teach the family members how to adequately care for the client's needs.
    b. encourage the client to maintain social interactions to prevent social isolation.
    c. promote the use of assistive devices so the client can participate in self-care activities.
    d. perform all activities of daily living for the client in order to conserve the client's energy.

22. A client with newly diagnosed MS has been hospitalized for evaluation and initial treatment of the disease. Following discharge teaching, the nurse evaluates that additional instruction is needed when the client says,

    a. "It is important for me to avoid exposure to those with upper respiratory infections."
    b. "When I begin to feel better, I should stop taking the prednisone to prevent side effects."
    c. "I plan to use vitamin supplements and a high-protein diet to help manage my condition."
    d. "I must plan with my family how we are going to manage my care if I become more incapacitated."

23. List the classic triad of signs associated with Parkinson's disease and identify one consequence in client function for each of the signs.

    a.

    b.

    c.

24. A client with a tremor is evaluated for Parkinson's disease. The nurse explains to the client that Parkinson's disease can be confirmed by

    a. CT and MRI scans.
    b. relief of symptoms with administration of dopaminergic agents.
    c. the presence of tremors that increase during voluntary movement.
    d. a cerebral angiogram that reveals the presence of cerebral atherosclerosis.

25. An observation of the client made by the nurse that is most indicative of Parkinson's disease is

    a. large and embellished handwriting.
    b. weakness in one leg resulting in a limping walk.
    c. difficulty arising from a chair and beginning to walk.
    d. the onset of muscle spasms occurring with voluntary movement.

26. A client with Parkinson's disease is started on levodopa. The nurse explains that this drug

    a. stimulates dopamine receptors in the basal ganglia.
    b. promotes the release of dopamine from brain neurons.
    c. is a precursor of dopamine that is converted into dopamine in the brain.
    d. prevents the excessive breakdown of dopamine in the peripheral tissues.

27. An appropriate nursing intervention to promote speech and swallowing in a client with Parkinson's disease is

    a. massaging the facial and neck muscles.
    b. keeping the client upright.
    c. encouraging deep breaths before speaking or attempting to swallow.
    d. suctioning the client to remove pooled secretions and prevent aspiration.

28. To reduce the risk for falls in the client with Parkinson's disease, the nurse teaches the client to

    a. use an elevated toilet seat.
    b. use a walker or cane for support.
    c. consciously lift the toes when stepping.
    d. rock side to side to initiate leg movements.

29. A client with myasthenia gravis is admitted to the hospital with respiratory insufficiency and severe weakness. A diagnosis of cholinergic crisis is made when

    a. the client's respiration is impaired because of muscle weakness.
    b. administration of edrophonium (Tensilon) increases muscle weakness.
    c. the edrophonium (Tensilon) test results in improved muscle contractility.
    d. electromyography reveals decreased response to repeated stimulation of muscles.

30. During care of a client in myasthenic crisis, the nurse's first priority for the client is maintenance of

    a. mobility.
    b. nutrition.
    c. respiratory function.
    d. verbal communication.

31. A client at the clinic for a routine health examination mentions that she is exhausted because her legs bother her so much at night that she cannot sleep. The nurse questions the client further about her leg symptoms with the knowledge that if she has "restless legs syndrome"

    a. the condition can be readily diagnosed with electromyography.
    b. other more serious nervous system dysfunctions may be present.
    c. dopaminergic agents are often effective in managing the symptoms.
    d. the symptoms can be controlled by vigorous exercise of the legs during the day.

32. When providing care for a client with amyotrophic lateral sclerosis (ALS), the nurse recognizes that one of the most distressing problems experienced by the client is

    a. painful spasticity of the face and extremities.
    b. retention of cognitive function with total degeneration of motor function.
    c. uncontrollable, writhing, twisting movements of the face, limbs, and body.
    d. the knowledge that there is a 50% chance the disease has been passed to any offspring.

33. In providing care for clients with chronic, progressive neurological disease, the major goal of treatment that the nurse works toward is to

    a. meet the client's personal care needs.
    b. return the client to normal neurological function.
    c. maximize neurological functioning as long as possible.
    d. prevent the development of additional chronic diseases.

## CASE STUDY

### MULTIPLE SCLEROSIS

**Client Profile**

Ms. S., a 32-year-old white woman, born and raised in Ottawa, is diagnosed with multiple sclerosis after an episode of numbness and tingling on the left side of her body that started several months ago. Two years ago she had an episode of optic neuritis in the right eye.

**Subjective Data**

- Difficulty seeing out of the right eye
- Numbness and tingling on the left side that worsens in hot weather
- Tires easily
- Used all sick days at work; concerned about losing her job and her ability to care for her three-year-old son

**Objective Data**

- Crying softly during the interview
- Appears tense and anxious
- Prolonged visual evoked response in right eye
- MRI scan of head shows several plaques in white matter

### Critical Thinking Questions

1. What is the pathophysiology of multiple sclerosis?

2. What precipitating factors for multiple sclerosis are present in Ms. S.'s life?

3. Why did it take so long for a definitive diagnosis to be made for Ms. S.?

4. What teaching plan should be developed for Ms. S.?

5. What treatment would be appropriate for Ms. S.?

6. Based on the assessment data presented, write one or more appropriate nursing diagnoses for Ms. S. Are there any collaborative problems?

1. The nurse assesses a post-operative client who has Parkinson's disease for early signs of delirium based on the knowledge that

    a. anticholinergic medications used to treat Parkinson's disease can precipitate delirium in older adults.
    b. older clients are more likely to develop delirium and most clients with Parkinson's disease are older adults.
    c. decreased levels of dopamine in the CNS found in Parkinson's disease have also been shown to be related to the onset of delirium.
    d. the decreased production of acetylcholine in clients with Parkinson's disease may also be responsible for development of delirium.

2. A client with metastatic cancer develops delirium. The nurse recognizes that a factor of the client's disease that may be related to development of delirium is

    a. decreased production of WBC.
    b. decreased antibody production.
    c. decreased production of platelets.
    d. increased production of cytokines.

3. A 72-year-old woman is hospitalized in the intensive care unit (ICU) with pneumonia secondary to COPD. She has a fever, productive cough, and adventitious breath sounds throughout her lungs. In the past 24 hours her fluid intake was 1000 mL and her urine output was 700 mL. She was diagnosed with early stage Alzheimer's disease six months ago but has been able to maintain her ADLs with supervision. Identify at least six risk factors for the development of delirium in this client.

    a.

    b.

    c.

    d.

    e.

    f.

4. A 68-year-old man is admitted to the emergency department with multiple blunt traumas following a one-vehicle car accident. He is restless; disoriented to person, place, and time; and agitated. He resists attempts at examination and calls out the name "Janice." The nurse suspects delirium rather than dementia in this client based on

    a. the fact that he would not have been allowed to drive if he had dementia.
    b. his hyperactive behaviour, which differentiates his condition from the hypoactive behaviour of dementia.
    c. the report of emergency personnel that he was non-communicative when they arrived at the accident scene.
    d. the report of his family that although he has heart disease and is "very hard of hearing," this behaviour is unlike him.

5. The management of a client with delirium includes

   a.  the use of restraints to protect the client from injury.
   b.  the use of short-acting benzodiazepines to sedate the client.
   c.  identification and treatment of underlying causes when possible.
   d.  administration of high doses of an antipsychotic drug such as haloperidol (Haldol).

6. Identify the following manifestations of cognitive impairment as primarily characteristic of delirium (DL) or dementia (DM).

   _____  a.  Delusions and hallucinations common

   _____  b.  Impaired judgements

   _____  c.  Sleep–wake cycle reversed

   _____  d.  Distorted thinking and perception

   _____  e.  Inability to perform purposeful acts

   _____  f.  Lucid intervals

   _____  g.  Insidious onset with prolonged course and duration

   _____  h.  Struggles to perform well with mental status testing

   _____  i.  Fluctuating impaired orientation

   _____  j.  Generally normal alertness

7. Identify whether the following statements are true or false. If a statement is false, correct the bold word(s) to make the statement true.

   _____  a.  The two major causes of dementia are **neurodegenerative conditions** and **multi-infarction**.

   _____  b.  **Neurodegenerative** dementia can be diagnosed by brain lesions identified with neuroimaging techniques.

   _____  c.  Dementia caused by hepatic or renal **encephalopathy** is potentially reversible.

   _____  d.  Dementia resulting from **vascular** causes can be prevented.

   _____  e.  A genetic mutation that has been found in some clients with Alzheimer's disease causes over-production of **tau proteins**.

8. A client with dementia has manifestations of depression. The nurse knows that treatment of the client with antidepressants will most likely

   a.  improve cognitive function.
   b.  not alter the course of either condition.
   c.  cause interactions with the drugs used to treat the dementia.
   d.  be contraindicated because of the CNS depressant effect of antidepressants.

9. The wife of a client who is manifesting deterioration in memory asks the nurse whether her husband has Alzheimer's disease. The nurse explains that a diagnosis of Alzheimer's disease is made when

   a. a CT scan of the brain indicates brain atrophy.
   b. a urine test indicates elevated levels of isoprostanes.
   c. all other possible causes of dementia have been eliminated.
   d. blood analysis reveals increased amounts of amyloid-beta protein.

10. The nurse uses the Mini-Mental State Examination to evaluate a client with cognitive impairment, primarily because this test

    a. is a good tool to evaluate mood and thought processes.
    b. indicates cognitive impairment if the score is more than 30 points.
    c. can help document the degree of cognitive impairment in delirium and dementia.
    d. is useful for initial evaluation of mental status, but additional tools are needed to evaluate cognition changes over time.

11. Collaborative care of clients with Alzheimer's disease focuses on

    a. replacement of deficient acetylcholine in the brain.
    b. drug therapy to enhance cognition and control undesirable behaviours.
    c. the use of memory-enhancing techniques to delay disease progression.
    d. prevention of other chronic diseases that hasten the progression of Alzheimer's disease.

12. Match each of the following medications used in the management of Alzheimer's disease with its classification and use.

| | | **Medication** | **Classification** |
|---|---|---|---|
| ____ | ____ | a. amitriptyline (Elavil) | 1. Cholinesterase inhibitors |
| ____ | ____ | b. haloperidol (Haldol) | 2. Selective serotonin reuptake inhibitors |
| ____ | ____ | c. donepezil (Aricept) | 3. Tricyclic antidepressants |
| ____ | ____ | d. lorazepam (Ativan) | 4. Conventional antipsychotics |
| ____ | ____ | e. risperidone (Risperdal) | 5. Atypical antipsychotics |
| ____ | ____ | f. oxazepam (Serax) | 6. Benzodiazepines |
| ____ | ____ | g. doxepin (Sinequan) | 7. Non-benzodiazepine sedative-hypnotics |
| ____ | ____ | h. fluoxetine (Prozac) | **Use** |
| ____ | ____ | i. olanzapine (Zyprexa) | 8. Improved cognition |
| ____ | ____ | j. rivastigmine (Exelon) | 9. Behaviour management |
| ____ | ____ | k. sertraline (Zoloft) | 10. Treatment of depression |
| | | | 11. Treatment of sleep disturbances |

13. A client with moderate Alzheimer's disease has a nursing diagnosis of disturbed thought processes related to effects of dementia. An appropriate nursing intervention for the client is

    a. posting clocks and calendars in the client's environment.
    b. monitoring the client's activity to maintain a safe client environment.
    c. establishing and consistently following a daily schedule with the client.
    d. stimulating thought processes by asking the client questions about recent activities.

14. The caregiver for a client with Alzheimer's disease expresses an inability to make decisions, concentrate, or sleep. The nurse determines that the caregiver

    a. is also developing signs of Alzheimer's disease.
    b. is manifesting symptoms of caregiver role strain.
    c. needs a period of respite from the care of the client.
    d. should ask other family members to participate in the client's care.

15. The wife of a man with moderate Alzheimer's disease has a nursing diagnosis of social isolation related to diminishing social relationships and behavioural problems of the client with Alzheimer's disease. A nursing intervention that would be appropriate to provide respite care and allow the wife to have satisfactory contact with significant others is to

    a. help the wife arrange for adult day care for the client.
    b. encourage permanent placement of the client in an Alzheimer's unit of a long-term care facility.
    c. refer the wife to a home health agency to arrange daily home nursing visits to assist with the client's care.
    d. arrange for hospitalization of the client for three or four days so that the wife can visit out-of-town friends and relatives.

## CASE STUDY

### ALZHEIMER'S DISEASE

### Client Profile

Mr. D. is a 79-year-old man whose wife noticed that he had become increasingly forgetful over the past three years. Recently he was diagnosed with Alzheimer's disease.

### Subjective Data

- Wanders out of the house at night
- States that he "sees things that aren't there"
- Is able to dress, bathe, and feed himself
- Has trouble figuring out how to use his electric razor
- His wife is distressed about his cognitive decline
- His wife says she is depressed and cannot watch him at night and get rest herself

### Objective Data

- CT scan: moderate cerebral atrophy

## Critical Thinking Questions

1. What pathophysiological changes are associated with Alzheimer's disease?

2. How is a diagnosis of Alzheimer's disease made?

3. What progression of symptoms should Mr. D.'s wife be told to expect over the course of the disease?

4. What suggestions can the nurse make to relieve some of the stress on the wife?

5.  What community resources might be available to Mr. D. and his wife?

6.  Based on the assessment data presented, write one or more appropriate nursing diagnoses for Mr. D. Are there any collaborative problems?

7.  Based on the assessment data presented, write one or more appropriate nursing diagnoses for Mr. D.'s wife. Are there any collaborative problems?

1. Identify whether the following statements are true or false. If a statement is false, correct the bold word(s) to make the statement true.

   _____ a. Trigeminal neuralgia affects the **sensory branches of the trigeminal nerve**, while Bell's palsy affects the **motor branches of the facial nerve**.

   _____ b. Herpes simplex virus infection is strongly associated as a precipitating factor in the development of **trigeminal neuralgia**.

   _____ c. **Antiseizure drugs** are the drugs of choice for treatment of Bell's palsy.

   _____ d. Gentle upward massage of the face may be indicated to maintain circulation in the client with **trigeminal neuralgia**.

   _____ e. A special need of clients with both trigeminal neuralgia and Bell's palsy is **oral hygiene**.

   _____ f. Severe withdrawal behaviours and suicidal tendencies may be seen in clients with **trigeminal neuralgia**.

2. In planning care for the client with trigeminal neuralgia, the nurse sets the highest priority on the client outcome of

   a. relief of pain.
   b. protection of the cornea.
   c. maintenance of nutrition.
   d. maintenance of positive body image.

3. Surgical intervention is being considered for a client with trigeminal neuralgia. The nurse recognizes that the procedure that has the least residual effects with a positive outcome is

   a. glycerol rhizotomy.
   b. suboccipital craniotomy.
   c. microvascular decompression.
   d. percutaneous radiofrequency rhizotomy.

4. In providing care for a client with an acute attack of trigeminal neuralgia, the nurse should

   a. carry out all hygiene and oral care for the client.
   b. use conversation to distract the client from pain.
   c. maintain a quiet, comfortable, draft-free environment.
   d. have the client examine the mouth after each meal for residual food.

5. A client is admitted to the hospital with Guillain-Barré syndrome. She had a weakness in her feet and ankles that has progressed to weakness with numbness and tingling in both legs. During the acute phase of her illness, the nurse recognizes that

   a. the most important aspect of care is to monitor the client's vital capacity and ABGs.
   b. early treatment with corticosteroids can suppress the immune response and prevent ascending nerve damage.
   c. although voluntary motor neurons are damaged by the inflammatory response, the autonomic nervous system is unaffected by the disease.
   d. the most serious complication of this condition is ascending demyelination of the peripheral nerves of the lower brainstem and cranial nerves.

6. A client with Guillain-Barré syndrome asks if he is going to die as the paralysis spreads toward his chest. In responding to the client, the nurse knows that

   a. clients who require ventilatory support almost always die.
   b. death occurs when nerve damage affects the brain and meninges.
   c. most clients with Guillain-Barré syndrome make a complete recovery.
   d. if death can be prevented, residual paralysis and sensory impairment are usually permanent.

7. Match the following characteristics with their related condition (answers may be used more than once).

   _____  a. Results in progressive locomotor ataxia.

   _____  b. Inhibits transmission of acetylcholine
             at myoneural junction

   _____  c. Transmitted through traumatic wound contamination

   _____  d. Initially manifests with GI symptoms with
             subsequent GI absorption of neurotoxin

   _____  e. Primary prevention is immunization

   _____  f. May involve a meningoencephalitic infection

   _____  g. Blocks inhibitory transmitters in spinal cord and brain

   _____  h. Prevented by boiling food for 10 minutes

   _____  i. Severe, conscious, continuous tonic convulsions with apnea

   _____  j. Degenerative changes in spinal cord and brainstem

   _____  k. Motor and sensory loss

   1. Botulism

   2. Tetanus

   3. Neurosyphilis

8. In planning community education for prevention of spinal cord injuries, the nurse targets

   a. elderly men.
   b. teenage females.
   c. elementary school-aged children.
   d. adolescent and young adult men.

9. A client has a complete spinal cord transection at the C7 level. During the acute period, the nurse would expect the client to have

   a. paraplegia with a flaccid paralysis.
   b. tetraplegia with total sensory loss.
   c. total hemiplegia with sensory and motor loss.
   d. flaccid tetraplegia with loss of pressure sensation.

10. Match the syndromes of incomplete spinal cord lesions with their descriptions.

_____ a. Central cord syndrome

_____ b. Anterior cord syndrome

_____ c. Brown-Sequard syndrome

_____ d. Posterior cord syndrome

_____ e. Caudio equina syndrome/ conus medullaris syndrome

1. Spinal cord damage resulting in ipsilateral motor paralysis and contralateral loss of pain and sensation below level of lesion

2. Damage to the most distal cord and nerve roots, resulting in flaccid paralysis of the lower limbs and areflexic bowel and bladder

3. Rare cord damage resulting in loss of proprioception below level of lesion with retention of motor control and temperature and pain sensation

4. Often caused by flexion injury with acute compression of cord resulting in complete motor paralysis and loss of pain and temperature sensation below the level of injury

5. Cord damage common in cervical region resulting in greater weakness in upper extremities than lower

11. An initial incomplete spinal cord injury often results in complete cord damage because of

a. edematous compression of the cord above the level of the injury.
b. continued trauma to the cord resulting from damage to stabilizing ligaments.
c. infarction and necrosis of the cord caused by edema, hemorrhage, and metabolites.
d. mechanical transection of the cord by sharp vertebral bone fragments after the initial injury.

12. A client with a spinal cord injury has spinal shock. The nurse plans care for the client based on the knowledge that

a. rehabilitation measures cannot be initiated until spinal shock has resolved.
b. the client will need continuous monitoring for hypotension, tachycardia, and hypoxemia.
c. resolution of spinal shock is manifested by spasticity, hyperreflexia, and reflex emptying of the bladder.
d. the client will have complete loss of motor and sensory functions below the level of the injury, but autonomic functions are not affected.

13. Two days following a spinal cord injury, a client asks continuously about the extent of impairment that will result from the injury. The best response of the nurse is

a. "You will have more normal function when spinal shock resolves and the reflex arc returns."
b. "The extent of your injury cannot be determined until the secondary injury to the cord is resolved."
c. "When your condition is more stable, an MRI will be done that can reveal the extent of the cord damage."
d. "Because long-term rehabilitation can affect the return of function it will be years before we can tell what the complete effect will be."

14. Indicate the lowest level of acute spinal cord injury at which the following effects occur.

a. GI hypomotility with paralytic ileus and gastric distension

b. Loss of all respiratory muscle function

c. Respiratory diaphragmatic breathing

d. Hypofunction and distension of bladder and bowel

15. A client is hospitalized following a spinal cord injury at the level of C8. A priority of nursing care for the client is monitoring for

    a. return of reflexes.
    b. bradycardia with hypoxemia.
    c. effects of sensory deprivation.
    d. fluctuations in body temperature.

16. Match the following activities with the highest level of spinal cord injury at which the activity can be expected (not all answers will be used).

    _____ a. Ambulate with crutches and leg braces                1. C1–C3

    _____ b. Push wheelchair on flat surfaces                      2. C4

    _____ c. Maintain bowel and bladder continence                3. C5

    _____ d. Have normal respiratory function                     4. C6

    _____ e. Drive electric wheelchair with chin control          5. C7–C8

    _____ f. Be independent in self-care and wheelchair use       6. T1–T6

                                                                  7. T6–T12

                                                                  8. L1–L2

                                                                  9. L3–L4

17. One indication for surgical therapy of the client with a spinal cord injury is when

    a. there is incomplete cord lesion involvement.
    b. the ligaments that support the spine are torn.
    c. a high cervical injury causes loss of respiratory function.
    d. evidence of continued compression of the cord is apparent.

18. A client is admitted to the emergency department with a possible cervical spinal cord injury following an automobile accident. During the admission of the client, the nurse places the highest priority on

    a. maintaining a patent airway.
    b. assessing the client for head and other injuries.
    c. maintaining immobilization of the cervical spine.
    d. assessing the client's motor and sensory function.

19. Immobilization and traction of the client with a cervical spinal cord injury most frequently requires the use of

    a. kinetic beds.
    b. hard cervical collars.
    c. skeletal traction with skull tongs.
    d. sternal-occipital-mandibular immobilizer (SOMI) brace.

20. The current standard of care for spinal cord injury within the first eight hours of injury is treatment with

    a. dopamine (Intropin).
    b. high-volume IV fluids.
    c. dexamethasone (Decadron).
    d. methylprednisolone (Medrol).

21. During the assessment of a client with a spinal cord injury, the nurse determines that the client has a poor cough with diaphragmatic breathing. Based on this finding, the nurse

    a. uses tracheal suctioning to remove secretions.
    b. assesses lung sounds and respiratory parameters q1–2h.
    c. places the client prone to promote drainage of respiratory secretions.
    d. explains to the client that mechanical ventilation will be necessary to maintain respiratory function.

22. Following a T2 spinal cord injury, the client develops paralytic ileus. While this condition is present, the nurse anticipates that the client will need

    a. IV fluids.
    b. tube feedings.
    c. nasogastric suctioning.
    d. total parenteral nutrition.

23. Urinary function during the acute phase of spinal cord injury is maintained with

    a. an in-dwelling catheter.
    b. intermittent catheterization.
    c. insertion of a suprapubic catheter.
    d. use of incontinent pads to protect the skin.

24. A week following a spinal cord injury at T2, a client experiences movement in his leg and tells the nurse he is recovering some function. The nurse's best response to the client is

    a. "It is really still too soon to know if you will have a return of function."
    b. "That could be a really positive finding. Can you show me the movement?"
    c. "That's wonderful. We will start exercising your legs more frequently now."
    d. "I'm sorry, but the movement is only a reflex and does not indicate normal function."

25. A client with a spinal cord lesion at C8 tells the nurse that he has a headache and feels flushed and warm. The first action of the nurse is to

    a. check the client's temperature.
    b. take the client's blood pressure.
    c. elevate the head of the client's bed.
    d. assess the client for a distended bladder or rectum.

26. Two weeks following a spinal cord injury, the client has a neurogenic bladder. The nurse recognizes that a neurogenic bladder

    a. has no reflex detrusor contractions.
    b. has sensory function but no motor function.
    c. has hyperactive reflect detrusor contractions.
    d. requires diagnostic evaluation to determine the best management interventions.

27. The preferred method of long-term management of a neurogenic bladder in a paraplegic client is

    a. surgical urinary diversion.
    b. in-dwelling catheterization.
    c. suprapubic catheterization.
    d. intermittent self-catheterization.

28. In counselling clients with spinal cord lesions regarding sexual function, the nurse advises a male client with a complete lower motor neuron lesion that he

    a. is most likely to have reflexogenic erections, and may experience orgasm if ejaculation occurs.
    b. may have uncontrolled reflex erections, but that orgasm and ejaculation are usually not possible.
    c. has a lesion with the greatest possibility of successful psychogenic erection with ejaculation and orgasms.
    d. will probably be unable to have either psychogenic or reflexogenic erections, with no ejaculation or orgasm.

29. During the client's process of grieving for the losses resulting from spinal cord injury, the nurse

    a. helps the client understand that working through the grief will be a lifelong process.
    b. should assist the client to move through all stages of the mourning process to acceptance.
    c. lets the client know that anger directed at the staff or the family is not a positive coping mechanism.
    d. facilitates the grieving process so that it is completed by the time the client is discharged from rehabilitation.

30. A client with a metastatic tumour of the spinal cord is scheduled for removal of the tumour by a laminectomy. In planning post-operative care for the client, the nurse recognizes that

    a. most cord tumours cause autodestruction of the cord as in traumatic injuries.
    b. metastatic tumours are commonly extradural lesions that can be removed completely.
    c. radiation therapy is routinely administered following surgery for all malignant spinal cord tumours.
    d. because complete removal of intramedullary tumours is not possible, the surgery is considered palliative.

## CASE STUDY

### SPINAL CORD INJURY

### Client Profile

Susan M. is a 16-year-old high-school student who sustained a C7 spinal cord injury when she dove into a lake while swimming with her friends. Susan was admitted directly to the ICU.

### Subjective Data

• Has patchy sensation in her upper extremities

### Objective Data

• Very weak bicep and tricep strength bilaterally
• Moderate strength in both of her lower extremities
• Bowel and bladder control present
• X-rays show no fracture dislocation of the spine
• Placed on bed rest with a hard cervical collar
• Methylprednisolone administered per protocol

**Critical Thinking Questions**

1. What spinal cord syndrome is Susan experiencing?

2. What is the physiological reason that Susan can move her lower extremities better than her upper extremities?

3. Why does Susan have a spinal cord injury without having sustained any spinal fracture?

4. What is the rationale for the use of the methylprednisolone?

5. What psychological problems are anticipated?

6. What can be done to begin long-term plans for Susan?

7. Based on the assessment data presented, write one or more appropriate nursing diagnoses. Are there any collaborative problems?

1. Using the list of terms below, identify the structures in the following illustration.

**List of Terms**

Articular cartilage          Epiphyseal growth plate
Bone marrow               Epiphysis
Cancellous bone         Medullary cavity
Cortical bone             Metaphysis
Diaphysis                 Periosteum

a. _____      f. _____

b. _____      g. _____

c. _____      h. _____

d. _____      i. _____

e. _____      j. _____

2. Using the terms below, identify the structures in the following illustration.

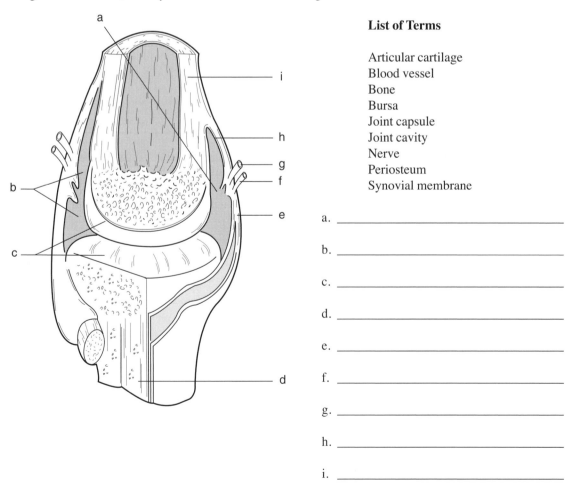

**List of Terms**

Blood vessels
Canaliculi
Haversian canal
Haversian system (osteon)
Periosteum

a. _____

b. _____

c. _____

d. _____

e. _____

3. Using the terms below, identify the structures in the following illustration.

**List of Terms**

Articular cartilage
Blood vessel
Bone
Bursa
Joint capsule
Joint cavity
Nerve
Periosteum
Synovial membrane

a. _____

b. _____

c. _____

d. _____

e. _____

f. _____

g. _____

h. _____

i. _____

4.  Word Search: Find the words that are described by the clues given below. The words may be located horizontally, vertically, or diagonally, and may be reversed.

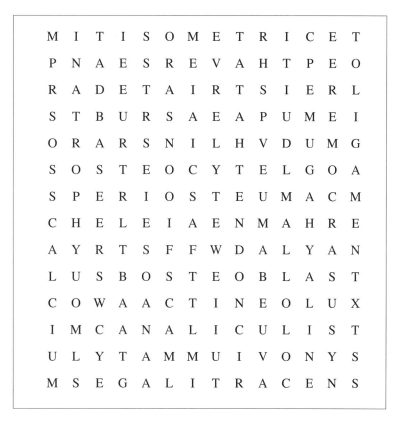

```
M  I  T  I  S  O  M  E  T  R  I  C  E  T
P  N  A  E  S  R  E  V  A  H  T  P  E  O
R  A  D  E  T  A  I  R  T  S  I  E  R  L
S  T  B  U  R  S  A  E  A  P  U  M  E  I
O  R  A  R  S  N  I  L  H  V  D  U  M  G
S  O  S  T  E  O  C  Y  T  E  L  G  O  A
S  P  E  R  I  O  S  T  E  U  M  A  C  M
C  H  E  L  E  I  A  E  N  M  A  H  R  E
A  Y  R  T  S  F  F  W  D  A  L  Y  A  N
L  U  S  B  O  S  T  E  O  B  L  A  S  T
C  O  W  A  A  C  T  I  N  E  O  L  U  X
I  M  C  A  N  A  L  I  C  U  L  I  S  T
U  L  Y  T  A  M  M  U  I  V  O  N  Y  S
M  S  E  G  A  L  I  T  R  A  C  E  N  S
```

a.   System of structural unit of compact bone
b.   Contractile unit of myofibrils
c.   Cancellous bone at end of long bones
d.   Mature bone cell
e.   Attaches muscles to bone
f.   Connective tissue covering bone
g.   Lining of joint capsule
h.   Muscle contraction that produces hypertrophy
i.   Mineral responsible for muscle contraction
j.   Canals extending from lacunae to connect osteocytes
k.   Bone cell responsible for resorption of bone
l.   Decrease in size of muscle
m.   Thin myofibril filaments
n.   Small sacs of connective tissue lined with synovium and synovial fluid
o.   Bone cell responsible for formation of bone
p.   Lack of blood supply makes this tissue slow healing
q.   Connects bone to bone at joint
r.   Connective tissue surrounding muscle
s.   Most common type of cartilage tissue
t.   Characteristic of skeletal muscle

5.  In performing ROM with a client, the nurse puts each joint through its full movement. Match the type of movements that can be performed on the following joints (answers may be used more than once, and joints may have more than one movement).

_____ a. Knee                          1. Flexion/extension

_____ b. Hip                           2. Abduction/adduction

_____ c. Thumb                         3. Circumduction

_____ d. Radioulnar joint              4. Rotation

_____ e. Shoulder

_____ f. Elbow

_____ g. Wrist

6.  While having his height measured during a routine health examination, a 79-year-old man asks the nurse why he is "shrinking." The nurse explains that decreased height occurs with aging because

    a. decreased muscle mass results in a stooped posture.
    b. loss of cartilage in the knees and hip joints causes a loss of height.
    c. long bones become less dense and shorten as bone tissue compacts.
    d. vertebrae become more compressed with thinning of intervertebral disks.

7.  A 78-year-old woman has a physiological change related to aging in her joints. An appropriate nursing diagnosis related to common changes of aging in the skeletal system is

    a. fatigue.
    b. risk for injury.
    c. impaired physical mobility.
    d. risk for impaired skin integrity.

8.  When obtaining information about the client's use of medications, the nurse recognizes that both bone and muscle function may be impaired when the client reports taking

    a. corticosteroids.
    b. oral hypoglycemic agents.
    c. potassium-depleting diuretics.
    d. non-steroidal anti-inflammatory drugs (NSAIDs).

9. Identify one specific finding made by the nurse during assessment of each of the client's functional health patterns that indicates a risk factor for musculoskeletal problems or a client response to an actual musculoskeletal problem.

   a. Health perception–health management

   b. Nutritional–metabolic

   c. Elimination

   d. Activity–exercise

   e. Sleep–rest

   f. Cognitive–perceptual

   g. Self-perception–self-concept

   h. Role–relationship

   i. Sexuality–reproductive

   j. Coping–stress tolerance

10. During muscle-strength testing, the client has active movement against gravity and some resistance to pressure. The nurse scores this finding as

   a. 2.
   b. 3.
   c. 4.
   d. 5.

11. On observation of the client, the nurse notes the presence of a gait disturbance. To further evaluate the client, the nurse should

   a. palpate the hips for crepitation.
   b. measure the length of the limbs.
   c. evaluate the degree of leg movement.
   d. compare the muscle mass of one leg with that of the other.

12. A client with severe joint immobility is receiving physiotherapy and exercise therapy. To evaluate the effect of the treatment the nurse may assess joint range of motion with a(n)

   a. myometer.
   b. ergometer.
   c. goniometer.
   d. arthrometer.

13. Match the following assessment abnormalities with their descriptions.

| | | | |
|---|---|---|---|
| _____ | a. Lordosis | 1. | Partial joint dislocation |
| _____ | b. Varus | 2. | Shortening of muscle or ligament |
| _____ | c. Ankylosis | 3. | Convex curve of the spine |
| _____ | d. Subluxation | 4. | Grating sensation between bones |
| _____ | e. Ganglion | 5. | Angulation of bone away from midline |
| _____ | f. Scoliosis | 6. | Fluid-filled cyst |
| _____ | g. Valgus | 7. | Angulation of bone toward the midline |
| _____ | h. Crepitation | 8. | Lateral curvature of the spine |
| _____ | i. Contracture | 9. | Fixed joint |
| _____ | j. Kyphosis | 10. | Concave curve of the spine |

14. Complete the following statements.

a. The most common diagnostic test used to assess musculoskeletal disorders is _____.

b. Insertion of a needle into a joint for aspiration and analysis of synovial fluid is known as a(n)

_____.

c. A test that is specific for visualization of intervertebral disc abnormalities is a(n) _____.

d. A fast, precise measurement of the bone mass of the spine, forearm, and total body calcium to evaluate

osteoporosis can be obtained with the use of _____.

e. The study in which needles are inserted into muscles to measure electrical activity of muscles is a(n)

_____.

f. The enzyme that is most predominant in skeletal muscle is _____ _____.

15. Identify three serological tests that may be positive or elevated in rheumatoid arthritis.

a.

b.

c.

1. A 72-year-old man tells the nurse that he cannot perform most of the physical activities he could do five years ago because of overall joint aches and pains. To prevent further deconditioning and the risk for developing musculoskeletal problems, the nurse can advise the client to

   a. avoid the use of canes and walkers because they increase dependence on ambulation aids.
   b. limit weight-bearing exercise to prevent stress on fragile bones and possible hip fractures.
   c. increase his activity by more frequently climbing stairs.
   d. use ASA or ibuprofen as prescribed by the physician to decrease inflammation and pain so that exercise can be maintained.

2. The nurse teaches individuals that one of the best ways to prevent musculoskeletal injuries during physical exercise is to

   a. increase muscle strength with daily isometric exercises.
   b. avoid exercising on concrete or hard pavement surfaces.
   c. perform stretching and warm-up exercises before exercise.
   d. wrap susceptible joints with elastic bandages or adhesive tape before exercise.

3. Match the following types of musculoskeletal soft-tissue injuries with their definitions.

   _____ a. Sprain

   _____ b. Strain

   _____ c. Dislocation

   _____ d. Subluxation

   _____ e. Repetitive strain injury

   _____ f. Bursitis

   _____ g. Carpal tunnel syndrome

   _____ h. Meniscus injury

   _____ i. Impingement syndrome

   _____ j. Rotator cuff injury

   1. Inflammation of synovial membrane sac at friction sites

   2. Incomplete separation of articular surfaces of joint due to ligament injury

   3. Compression of median nerve in wrist

   4. Entrapment of soft-tissue structures under coracoacromial arch of shoulder

   5. Tear within muscles or ligaments of shoulder

   6. Complete separation of articular surface of joint due to ligament injury

   7. Cartilage compression and tearing associated with rotational stress

   8. Tearing of a ligament

   9. Tendon and muscle strain with inflammation and decreased circulation

   10. Stretching of muscle and fascia sheath

4. Application of RICE (rest, ice, cold compression, and elevation) is indicated for initial management of

   a. muscle spasms.
   b. sprains and strains.
   c. repetitive strain injury.
   d. dislocations and subluxations.

5. During the recovery phase of acute musculoskeletal soft-tissue injuries, management of the affected limb includes

    a. gradual, gentle exercise.
    b. immobilization and rest.
    c. alternating use of cold and heat.
    d. administration of anti-inflammatory drugs.

6. Match the following types of fractures with their descriptions.

    _____ a. Avulsion                1. Bone fragments driven into each other

    _____ b. Comminuted              2. One side splintered and other side bent

    _____ c. Open                    3. Line of fracture twists along shaft of bone

    _____ d. Oblique                 4. Results from pulling effect of tendons or ligaments

    _____ e. Impacted                5. Fracture with communication with external environment

    _____ f. Pathological            6. Slanted fracture line

    _____ g. Greenstick              7. Fracture fragment overrides other bone fragment

    _____ h. Displaced               8. Fracture with more than two fragments

    _____ i. Transverse              9. Spontaneous fracture at site of bone disease

    _____ j. Spiral                  10. Line of fracture at right angle to longitudinal axis

7. Match the characteristics of the fracture healing process with their stages (answers may be used more than once).

    _____ a. Invasion of osteoblasts and deposition        1. Hematoma
              of calcium
                                                           2. Granulation
    _____ b. Closure of space between bone fragments
                                                           3. Callus formation
    _____ c. Semi-solid blood clot at ends of fragments
                                                           4. Ossification
    _____ d. Absorption of excess cells
                                                           5. Consolidation
    _____ e. Phagocytosis of necrotic byproducts
                                                           6. Remodelling
    _____ f. Deposition and absorption of bone in
              response to stress

    _____ g. Organization of hematoma into fibrous network

    _____ h. First stage to prevent movement at fracture site

    _____ i. Return to pre-injury strength and shape

    _____ j. Formation of osteoid

    _____ k. Stage at which radiographic union first apparent

8. A client is brought to the emergency department following a fall while rock climbing that injured his left lower leg. The nurse identifies the presence of a fracture based on the cardinal sign of

   a. muscle spasms.
   b. obvious deformity.
   c. edema and swelling.
   d. pain and tenderness.

9. A client with a fractured femur experiences the complication of malunion. The nurse recognizes that with this complication

   a. the fracture heals in an unsatisfactory position.
   b. the fracture fails to heal properly despite treatment.
   c. fracture healing progresses more slowly than expected.
   d. loss of bone substances occurs as a result of immobilization.

10. Identify whether the following statements are true or false. If a statement is false, correct the bold word(s) to make the statement true.

   _____    a. Realignment of bone fragments into anatomical position is known as **fixation**.

   _____    b. **Traction** may be used to both reduce a fracture and immobilize a fracture.

   _____    c. The disadvantage of open reduction and internal fixation of a fracture is that the client has an increased risk for **complications related to immobility**.

   _____    d. Pressure causing circulatory, nerve, and skin impairment is most likely to occur with the use of **skeletal** traction.

   _____    e. Countertraction with Russell's traction may be achieved by elevating **the head of the bed**.

   _____    f. A cast or splint is a type of **external fixation**.

11. In planning care for the client in traction, the nurse knows that elevation of the buttocks and back off the bed for linen changes, bedpan use, and skin care is possible for the client with

   a. pelvic traction.
   b. Buck's traction.
   c. Russell's traction.
   d. balanced suspension traction.

12. When assessing the traction of a client with a fracture femur, the nurse recognizes that a correction should be made if

   a. the weights are touching the floor.
   b. the ropes are in the centre of the pulley.
   c. the client exercises the unaffected limb.
   d. the client is lying flat in the centre of the bed.

13. A client with a fractured femur has a hip spica cast applied. While the cast is drying, the nurse should

   a. elevate the legs above the level of the heart for 24 hours.
   b. turn the client to both sides and prone to supine every two hours.
   c. cover the cast with a light blanket to avoid chilling from evaporation.
   d. assess the client frequently for abdominal pain, nausea, and vomiting.

14. A client is admitted with an open fracture of the tibia following a bicycle accident. During assessment of the client, the nurse questions the client specifically about

   a. any previous injuries to the leg.
   b. the status of tetanus immunization.
   c. the use of antibiotics in the last month.
   d. whether the injury was exposed to dirt or gravel.

15. A client has fallen in the bathroom of the hospital room and complains of pain in the right upper arm and elbow. Before splinting the injury, the nurse knows that emergency management of a possible fracture should include

   a. elevation of the arm.
   b. application of ice to the site.
   c. notification of the physician.
   d. neurovascular checks below the site of the injury.

16. To assess for neurological status in a client with a fractured humerus, the nurse asks the client to

   a. evert, invert, dorsiflex, and plantar flex the foot.
   b. abduct, adduct, and oppose the fingers, and pronate and supinate the hand.
   c. assess the location, quality, and intensity of pain below the site of the injury.
   d. assess the colour, temperature, capillary refill, peripheral pulses, and presence of edema in the extremity.

17. A client is discharged from the outpatient clinic following application of a synthetic fibreglass long arm cast for a fractured ulna. Before discharge, the nurse instructs the client to

   a. never get the cast wet.
   b. move the shoulder and fingers frequently.
   c. place tape petals around the edges of the cast when it is dry.
   d. use a sling to support the arm at waist level for the first 48 hours.

18. A client with a long leg cast is allowed to ambulate with crutches with no weight bearing on the affected leg. The nurse teaches the client to use a

   a. swing-to gait.
   b. two-point gait.
   c. four-point gait.
   d. swing-through gait.

19. A client with a fractured tibia accompanied by extensive soft-tissue damage initially has a splint applied and held in place with an elastic bandage. An early sign that would alert the nurse that the client is developing compartment syndrome is

   a. paralysis of the toes.
   b. absence of peripheral pulses.
   c. progressive pain unrelieved by usual analgesics.
   d. the skin over the injury site is blanched when the bandage is removed.

20. Identify the problems that are indicated by each of the six Ps characteristic of an impending compartment syndrome.

    a.

    b.

    c.

    d.

    e.

    f.

21. Surgical treatment that is indicated for compartment syndrome is

    a. fasciotomy.
    b. amputation.
    c. internal fixation.
    d. release of tendons.

22. A fat embolism is most likely to occur

    a. 24 to 48 hours following a fractured tibia.
    b. 36 to 72 hours following a skull fracture.
    c. four to five days following a fractured femur.
    d. five to six days following a pelvic fracture.

23. The nurse suspects a fat embolism rather than a pulmonary embolism from a venous thrombosis in the client with a fracture who develops

    a. tachycardia and dyspnea.
    b. a sudden onset of chest pain.
    c. ECG changes and decreased $PaO_2$.
    d. petechiae around the neck and upper chest.

24. Match the following characteristics with the related type of fracture (answers may be used more than once).

_____ a. Possible radial nerve and brachial artery damage

_____ b. Moving the client may cause serious injury from bone fragments

_____ c. Often occurs when breaking a fall with an outstretched hand

_____ d. Airway patency is a major concern

_____ e. Balanced suspension traction and hip spica cast are treatment options

_____ f. Hanging arm cast may be used to reduce the fracture

_____ g. Most often a compression fracture

_____ h. High incidence of fat embolism and compartment syndrome

_____ i. Drastic change in appearance requires supportive care

_____ j. Fractured distal radius and possible styloid process of ulna

_____ k. Most serious complication is displacement of fracture

_____ l. May be accompanied by intra-abdominal lacerations and ruptures

_____ m. Vulnerable site because of lack of anterior muscle covering

_____ n. Internal fixation with intermedullary rod or compression plates preferred

_____ o. Halo apparatus may be used for immobilization

1. Colles' fracture

2. Fractured humerus

3. Fractured pelvis

4. Femoral shaft fracture

5. Fractured tibia

6. Stable vertebral fracture

7. Facial fractures

25. Identify whether the following statements are true or false. If a statement is false, correct the bold word(s) to make the statement true.

_____ a. **Extracapsular** hip fractures often occur in individuals with osteoporosis and minor injury.

_____ b. An **intertrochanteric** fracture of the hip occurs between the greater and lesser trochanter.

_____ c. Avascular necrosis is a serious complication of displaced **subtrochanteric** fractures.

_____ d. The preferred treatment of extracapsular fractures is **pinning or nailing** while intracapsular fractures are usually repaired with **hip prostheses**.

_____ e. **Intracapsular** hip fractures are also known as fractures of the neck of the femur.

26. An older woman is admitted to the emergency department after falling at home. The nurse suspects a fractured hip when assessment of the client reveals

    a. inability to move the toes and ankle.
    b. edema of the thigh extending to the knee.
    c. internal rotation of the leg with groin pain.
    d. shortening and external rotation of the leg.

27. A client with an extracapsular hip fracture is admitted to the orthopedic unit and placed in Russell's traction. The nurse explains to the client that the purpose of the traction is to

    a. pull bone fragments back into alignment.
    b. immobilize the leg until healing is complete.
    c. reduce pain and muscle spasms before surgery.
    d. prevent damage to the blood vessels at the fracture site.

28. A client with a fractured right hip has an open reduction and internal fixation of the fracture. Post-operatively, the nurse plans to

    a. get the client up to the chair the first post-operative day.
    b. position the client only on the back and the side specified by the surgeon.
    c. keep leg abductor splints on the client except when bathing.
    d. have the client ambulate with partial weight bearing by discharge.

29. Discharge instructions for the client who received a hip prosthesis include

    a. restrict walking for two to three months.
    b. take a bath rather than a shower to prevent falling.
    c. keep the leg internally rotated while sitting and standing.
    d. have a family member put on the client's shoes and socks.

30. When preparing a client for discharge following fixation of a mandibular fracture, the nurse determines that teaching has been successful when the client says,

    a. "I can keep my mouth moist by sucking on hard candy."
    b. "I should cut the wires with scissors if I begin to vomit."
    c. "I may use a bulk-forming laxative if my liquid diet causes constipation."
    d. "I should use a moist swab to clean my mouth every time I eat something."

31. A left above-the-knee amputation (AKA) is scheduled for a diabetic client with ischemic gangrene of three toes. The client asks why they cannot just amputate her toes. The best response of the nurse is

    a. "A prosthesis is easier to fit with this type of amputation."
    b. "The amputation must be high enough to have good circulation for healing."
    c. "There is infection in your lower leg that you cannot see that must be removed."
    d. "An amputation at this level will help prevent further circulatory problems in your leg."

32. A client who suffered a traumatic below-the-elbow amputation in a boating accident is withdrawn, does not look at the arm, and asks to be left alone. An appropriate nursing diagnosis of the client includes

    a. impaired adjustment.
    b. disturbed body image.
    c. impaired social interaction.
    d. ineffective individual coping.

33. A client complains of pain in the foot of a leg that was recently amputated. The nurse recognizes that the pain

    a. is caused by swelling at the incision.
    b. should be treated with ordered analgesics.
    c. will become worse with the use of a prosthesis.
    d. can be managed with diversion since it is psychological.

34. An immediate prosthetic fitting during surgery is used for a client with a traumatic below-the-knee amputation (BKA). During the immediate post-operative period, it is most important for the nurse to

    a. assess the site for hemorrhage.
    b. monitor the client's vital signs.
    c. elevate the residual limb on pillows.
    d. have the client flex and extend the knee every hour.

35. The nurse positions a client with an above-the-knee amputation with a delayed prosthetic fitting prone several times a day to

    a. prevent flexion contractures.
    b. assess the posterior skin flap.
    c. reduce edema in the residual limb.
    d. relieve pressure on the incision site.

36. A client who had a below-the-knee amputation is to be fitted with a temporary prosthesis. It is most important for the nurse to teach the client to

    a. inspect the residual limb daily for irritation.
    b. apply an elastic shrinker before applying the prosthesis.
    c. perform ROM exercises to the affected leg four times a day.
    d. apply alcohol to the residual limb every morning and evening to toughen the skin.

37. Match the following joint surgeries with their uses.

    _____ a. Synovectomy

    _____ b. Osteotomy

    _____ c. Debridement

    _____ d. Arthroplasty

    _____ e. Arthrodesis

    1. Reconstruction or replacement of a joint to relieve pain and correct deformity

    2. Surgical fusion of a joint to relieve pain

    3. Used in rheumatoid arthritis to remove the tissue involved in joint destruction

    4. Correction of bone deformity by removal of a wedge or slice of bone

    5. Arthroscopic removal of degenerative tissue in joints

38. A 65-year-old client has undergone a right total hip arthroplasty with a cemented prosthesis for treatment of severe osteoarthritis of the hip. Client activity that the nurse anticipates on the client's first or second postoperative day includes

    a. transfer from bed to chair bid only.
    b. turning from back to side specified by the surgeon q2h only.
    c. crutch walking with non-weight bearing on the operative leg.
    d. ambulation and weight bearing on the right leg with a walker.

39. When positioning the client with a total hip arthroplasty, it is important that the nurse maintains the affected extremity in

    a. adduction and flexion.
    b. extension and abduction.
    c. abduction and internal rotation.
    d. adduction and external rotation.

40. Following a knee arthroplasty, a client has a continuous passive motion machine for the affected joint. The nurse explains to the client that this device is used to

    a. relieve edema and pain at the incision site.
    b. promote early joint mobility and increase knee flexion.
    c. prevent venous stasis and the formation of a deep venous thrombosis.
    d. improve arterial circulation to the affected extremity to promote healing.

41. A client with severe ulnar deviation of the hands undergoes an arthroplasty with reconstruction and replacement of finger joints. Post-operatively, it is most important for the nurse to

    a. position the fingers lower than the elbow.
    b. perform neurovascular assessments of the fingers q2–4h.
    c. encourage the client to gently flex, extend, abduct, and adduct the fingers q4h.
    d. remind the client that function of the hands is more important than their cosmetic appearance.

## CASE STUDY

### FRACTURE

### Client Profile

Mr. A., a 30-year-old telephone lineman, was seen in the emergency department after falling from a pole. His right lower extremity was splinted with a cardboard splint and a large bulky dressing.

### Subjective Data

- Complains of severe pain in the right leg
- Expresses concern about notifying his wife about the accident and his whereabouts
- Asks how long he will be off work

### Objective Data

- Avulsion of soft tissue on the anterolateral aspect of the tibia
- Obvious deformity, marked swelling, and ecchymosis in region of injury

## Critical Thinking Questions

1. Was the immobilization of the fracture at the scene of the accident appropriate?

2. What is the appropriate nursing neurovascular assessment of the injured extremity?

3. What are the probable therapeutic and nursing interventions to prevent infection?

4. What specific nursing actions should the nurse implement to alleviate Mr. A.'s pain?

5. How would the nurse answer Mr. A.'s question about time off from work based on the stages of fracture healing?

6. How should the nurse notify Mrs. A. about her husband's accident?

7. Based on the assessment data presented, write one or more appropriate nursing diagnoses. Are there any collaborative problems?

# CHAPTER 62 NURSING MANAGEMENT: MUSCULOSKELETAL PROBLEMS

1. A client with chronic osteomyelitis has been hospitalized for surgical removal of the infection. The nurse explains to the client that surgical treatment is necessary because

   a. the process of involucrum blocks the vascular supply to the bone.
   b. removal of the infection prevents the need for bone and skin grafting.
   c. formation of avascular scar tissue has led to a protected area of bacterial growth.
   d. antibiotics are not effective against micro-organisms that cause chronic osteomyelitis.

2. A nursing intervention that is carried out to prevent the development of complications in the client with osteomyelitis is

   a. providing ROM q4h to the involved extremity.
   b. handling the involved extremity gently during movement.
   c. using careful and appropriate disposal of soiled dressings.
   d. measuring the circumference of the affected extremity daily.

3. A client who experienced an open fracture of the humerus two weeks ago is having increased pain at the fracture site. To determine the causative agent if the client has developed an acute osteomyelitis at the site, the nurse would expect testing to include

   a. x-rays.
   b. a CT scan.
   c. a bone biopsy.
   d. WBC and erythrocyte sedimentation rate (ESR).

4. Following two weeks of IV antibiotic therapy, a client with acute osteomyelitis of the tibia is prepared for discharge from the hospital. The nurse determines that additional instruction is needed when the client says,

   a. "I will need to continue antibiotic therapy for four to eight weeks."
   b. "I should notify the physician if the pain in my leg becomes worse."
   c. "I shouldn't bear weight on my affected leg until healing is complete."
   d. "I can use a heating pad on my lower leg for comfort and to promote healing."

5. During a follow-up visit to a client with acute osteomyelitis treated with IV antibiotics, the home care nurse is told by the client's wife that she can hardly get the client to eat because his mouth is so sore. In checking the client's mouth, the nurse would expect to find

   a. a dry, cracked tongue with a central furrow.
   b. white, curd-like membranous lesions of the mucosa.
   c. ulcers of the mouth and lips surrounded by a reddened base.
   d. single or clustered vesicles on the tongue and buccal mucosa.

6. Match the following characteristics with their related types of bone cancer (answers may be used more than once).

\_\_\_\_\_ a. Involves medullary cavity of long bones

\_\_\_\_\_ b. Involves bones with active marrow

\_\_\_\_\_ c. Arises in cancellous ends of long bones

\_\_\_\_\_ d. Often brought to attention by injury

\_\_\_\_\_ e. Replacement of bone marrow by malignant plasma cells

\_\_\_\_\_ f. Extremely malignant and metastasizes early

\_\_\_\_\_ g. Locally destructive lesion without metastasis

1. Multiple myeloma

2. Osteosarcoma

3. Osteoclastoma

4. Ewing's sarcoma

7. A 24-year-old client with a 12-year history of Becker's muscular dystrophy is hospitalized with congestive heart failure. A nursing intervention that would be appropriate for this client and any client with muscular dystrophy is

a. to feed and bathe the client to avoid exhausting the muscles.
b. frequent repositioning to avoid skin and respiratory complications.
c. to provide hand weights for the client to exercise the upper extremities.
d. using orthopedic braces to promote ambulation to prevent muscle wasting.

8. Identify whether the following statements are true or false. If a statement is false, correct the bold word(s) to make the statement true.

\_\_\_\_\_ a. **Chemotherapy** may be used in the management of all primary bone tumours.

\_\_\_\_\_ b. The most common cause of low back pain is **herniation of an intervertebral disc**.

\_\_\_\_\_ c. Use of **NSAIDs** for chronic low back pain is important in being able to maintain exercise and activity throughout the day.

\_\_\_\_\_ d. The low back pain associated with a **lumbosacral instability** is usually accompanied by buttock and leg pain along the sciatic nerve.

\_\_\_\_\_ e. **Degenerative disk disease** is a major factor in the development of herniated intervertebral discs.

9. The nurse teaches the client with an acute episode of low back pain to

a. perform daily exercise as a lifelong routine.
b. sit in a chair with the hips lower than the knees.
c. avoid occupations in which the use of the body is required.
d. sleep on the abdomen or on the back with the legs extended.

10. To help prevent the client with chronic low back pain from assuming sick-role behaviours, the nurse

a. teaches the client alternative methods of pain control.
b. encourages activity and ambulation within the client's limitations.
c. discusses the nature of chronic pain and the need for lifestyle adjustments.
d. monitors for decreased muscle strength that indicates the development of complications.

11. A client with a herniated intravertebral disc and acute back pain is treated conservatively with rest and drug therapy. An important nursing intervention during this time is to

    a. monitor neurological signs q4h.
    b. encourage foot and leg exercises q2–4h.
    c. assess the client's use of body mechanics to identify teaching needs.
    d. maintain the client in a semi-recumbent position with the head slightly elevated and the knees flexed.

12. A laminectomy and spinal fusion is performed on a client with a herniated lumbar intervertebral disc. During the post-operative period, the nurse notifies the physician when the client experiences

    a. paralytic ileus.
    b. urinary incontinence.
    c. greater pain at the graft site than at the lumbar incision site.
    d. leg and arm movement and sensation unchanged from preoperative status.

13. Before repositioning the client to the side after a lumbar laminectomy, the nurse

    a. raises the head of the bed 30 degrees.
    b. has the client flex the knees and hips.
    c. places a pillow between the client's legs.
    d. has the client grasp the side rail on the opposite side of the bed.

14. Match the following foot problems with their characteristics (answers may be used more than once).

    _____ a. Breakdown of metatarsal arch

    _____ b. Papilloma growth on sole of foot

    _____ c. Local thickening of skin caused by pressure on bony prominences

    _____ d. Deformity of second toe with callus on dorsum of proximal interphalangeal joint

    _____ e. Tumour on nerve tissue between third and fourth metatarsal heads

    _____ f. Lateral angulation of large toe toward second toe

    _____ g. Metatarsal joint support used in conservative treatment

    _____ h. May be trimmed with razor or scalpel after softening

    _____ i. Surgical treatment is removal of bursal sac and bony enlargement

    _____ j. Thickening of skin on weight-bearing part of foot

    1. Hallux valgus (bunion)
    2. Hammer toe
    3. Morton's neuroma
    4. Pes planus
    5. Corn
    6. Callus
    7. Plantar wart

15. In promoting healthy feet, the nurse recognizes the factor that is associated with most foot problems is

    a. poor foot hygiene.
    b. congenital deformities.
    c. improperly fitting shoes.
    d. peripheral vascular disease.

16. Match the following metabolic bone diseases with their characteristics (answers may be used more than once).

    _____ a. Loss of total bone mass and substance     1. Osteomalacia

    _____ b. Results from vitamin D deficiency     2. Paget's disease

    _____ c. Replacement of normal marrow with     3. Osteoporosis
              vascular connective tissue

    _____ d. Generalized bone decalcification with bone deformity

    _____ e. Most common in bones of spine, hips, and wrists

    _____ f. Abnormal remodelling and resorption of bone

    _____ g. Bowed legs and cranial enlargement

17. The nurse determines that the woman with the highest risk for osteoporosis is a

    a. 60-year-old aerobic instructor.
    b. 65-year-old on estrogen therapy.
    c. 45-year-old obese black woman.
    d. 55-year-old cigarette smoker of Asian descent.

18. Identify three methods of preventing osteoporosis in post-menopausal women.

    a.

    b.

    c.

# CASE STUDY

## HERNIATED INTRAVERTEBRAL DISK

### Client Profile

Howard Brown is a 38-year-old truck driver who slipped on a wet floor at work and landed on his buttocks.

### Subjective Data

- Experienced immediate, severe lower back pain, with pain radiating into his right buttock
- Had worsening of pain in three days, with pain radiating down his entire leg into his foot
- Experienced tingling of his toes
- Rested at home for two weeks without relief
- Smokes one pack of cigarettes a day

### Objective Data

- Is 161 cm (5 ft 3 in) tall; weighs 115 kg (253 lb)
- Diagnostic studies: MRI revealed a large herniated disc at L 4-5 level.

### Collaborative Care

- Underwent microdiscectomy at L 4–5
- Expected discharge two days after surgery

### Critical Thinking Questions

1. What risk factors for low back pain does Mr. Brown have?

2. What preoperative teaching is indicated for Mr. Brown?

3. What post-operative activity restrictions will Mr. Brown need to follow?

4. What post-operative nursing assessments should be made?

5. What discharge teaching should be implemented with Mr. Brown?

6. Based on the assessment data presented, write one or more nursing diagnoses. Are there any collaborative problems?

# CHAPTER 63 NURSING MANAGEMENT: ARTHRITIS AND CONNECTIVE TISSUE DISEASES

1. A 60-year-old woman has pain on motion in her fingers and asks the nurse whether this is just a result of aging. The best response of the nurse includes the information that

   a. joint pain with functional limitation is a normal change that affects all people to some extent.
   b. joint pain that develops with age is usually related to previous trauma or infection of the joints.
   c. this is a symptom of a systemic arthritis that eventually affects all joints as the disease progresses.
   d. changes in the cartilage and bones of joints may cause symptoms of pain and loss of function in some people as they age.

2. Number in sequence from 1 to 6 the pathophysiological processes that occur in osteoarthritis (OA).

   _____ a. Erosion of articular surfaces

   _____ b. Joint space narrows

   _____ c. Incongruity in joint surfaces leads to reduction in motion

   _____ d. Joint cartilage becomes yellow and rough

   _____ e. Osteophytes formed at joint margins

   _____ f. Cartilage becomes softer and less elastic

3. Identify whether the following statements are true or false. If a statement is false, correct the bold word(s) to make the statement true.

   _____ a. **Bouchard's nodes** are reddened, tender protuberances found at the distal interphalangeal joints in some clients with osteoarthritis.

   _____ b. The pain of latent osteoarthritis is most commonly caused by **swelling and stretching of soft tissue around the joint**.

   _____ c. Joint stiffness in OA can be caused by **crepitation**.

   _____ d. First-line drug therapy used in the management of osteoarthritis is **ASA**.

   _____ e. Pain and immobility of osteoarthritis may be aggravated by **falling barometric pressure**.

4. To preserve function and the ability to perform activities of daily living, the nurse teaches the client with osteoarthritis to

   a. avoid exercise that involves the affected joints.
   b. plan and organize less stressful ways to perform tasks.
   c. maintain normal activities during an acute episode to prevent loss of function.
   d. use mild analgesics to control symptoms when performing tasks that cause pain.

5. A client with osteoarthritis uses NSAIDs to decrease pain and inflammation. The nurse teaches the client that common side effects of these drugs include

   a. allergic reactions, fever, and oral lesions.
   b. fluid retention, hypertension, and bruising.
   c. skin rashes, gastric irritation, and headache.
   d. prolonged bleeding time, blood dyscrasias, and hepatic damage.

6. A client with osteoarthritis asks the nurse whether he could try glucosamine and chondroitin for control of his symptoms. The best response of the nurse includes the information that

   a. although these substances may not help, there is no evidence that they can cause any untoward effects.
   b. glucosamine should not be used by clients with diabetes because it can decrease blood glucose levels.
   c. these supplements are a fad that has not been shown to reduce pain or increase joint mobility in clients with OA.
   d. only dosages of these supplements available by prescription are high enough to provide any benefit in treatment of OA.

7. A client taking ibuprofen (Motrin) for treatment of OA has good pain relief but is experiencing increased dyspepsia and nausea with the drug's use. The nurse knows that an appropriate alternative with fewer GI effects than ibuprofen would be
   a. diclofenac sodium and misoprostol (Arthrotec).
   b. naproxen (Naprosyn).
   c. prednisone.
   d. indomethacin (Indocin).

8. The basic pathophysiological process of rheumatoid arthritis is

   a. destruction of joint cartilage and bones by an autoimmune process.
   b. initiated by a viral infection that destroys the synovial membranes of joints.
   c. the presence of HLA-DR4 antigen that causes inflammatory responses throughout the body.
   d. an immune response that activates complement and produces inflammation of joints and other organ systems.

9. Indicate whether the following descriptions are most characteristic of osteoarthritis (O), rheumatoid arthritis (R), or both (B).

   _____ a. Most commonly occurs in women

   _____ b. Affects knees, hips, and spine

   _____ c. Asymmetric involvement of joints

   _____ d. Joint pain, stiffness, and limitation of motion

   _____ e. Inflammatory synovial fluid

   _____ f. Joint stiffness in morning and after periods of inactivity

   _____ g. Firm, subcutaneous, non-tender nodules

   _____ h. Normal erythrocyte sedimentation rate (ESR)

   _____ i. Anemia and weight loss

   _____ j. Associated with normal life expectancy

   _____ k. Associated with autoantibodies to abnormal IgG

10. Number in sequence the pathophysiological processes of rheumatoid arthritis.

    _____ a. Invasion of joint capsule by granulation inflammatory tissue

    _____ b. Calcification of fibrous tissue

    _____ c. Joint inflammation

    _____ d. Formation of pannus at juncture of synovium and cartilage

    _____ e. Joint capsule occluded by tough fibrous connective tissue

    _____ f. Bony ankylosis of joint with total immobilization

    _____ g. Swelling of synovial membrane

11. During the physical assessment of the client with moderate rheumatoid arthritis, the nurse would expect to find

    a. hepatomegaly.
    b. Heberden's nodes.
    c. spindle-shaped fingers.
    d. crepitus on joint movement.

12. Laboratory findings that the nurse would expect to be present in the client with rheumatoid arthritis include

    a. polycythemia.
    b. increased IgG.
    c. increased ESR.
    d. decreased WBC.

13. A 70-year-old client is being evaluated for symptoms of rheumatoid arthritis. The nurse recognizes that a major problem in the management of rheumatoid arthritis in the older adult is that

    a. rheumatoid arthritis is usually more severe in older adults.
    b. older clients are not as likely to comply with treatment regimens.
    c. drug interactions and toxicity are more likely to occur with multidrug therapy.
    d. laboratory and other diagnostic tests are not effective in identifying rheumatoid arthritis in older adults.

14. After teaching a client with rheumatoid arthritis about the prescribed therapeutic regimen, the nurse determines that further instruction is needed when the client says,

    a. "It is important for me to perform my prescribed exercises every day."
    b. "I should perform most of my daily chores in the morning when my energy level is highest."
    c. "An ice pack to a joint for ten minutes may help relieve pain and inflammation when I have an acute flare."
    d. "I can use assistive devices such as padded utensils, electric can openers, and elevated toilet seats to protect my joints."

15. A client recovering from an acute exacerbation of rheumatoid arthritis tells the nurse she is too tired to bathe. The nurse should

    a. give the client a bed bath to conserve her energy.
    b. allow the client a rest period before showering with the nurse's help.
    c. tell the client that she can skip bathing if she will walk in the hall later.
    d. inform the client that it is important for her to maintain self-care activities.

16. Characteristics of spondyloarthritides associated with the HLA-B27 antigen include

    a. absence of extra-articular disease.
    b. symmetric polyarticular arthritis.
    c. presence of rheumatoid factor and autoantibodies.
    d. high involvement of sacroiliac joints and the spine.

17. An important nursing intervention for the client with ankylosing spondylitis is to teach the client to

    a. wear roomy shoes with good orthotic support.
    b. sleep on the side with the knees and hips flexed.
    c. keep the spine slightly flexed while sitting, standing, or walking.
    d. perform chest-cage stretching and deep chest breathing exercises.

18. Match the following characteristic with their related rheumatic disorders (answers may be used more than once).

    _____ a. High association with stress and
             irritable bowel syndrome

    _____ b. Characteristic symptom of erythema
             migrans

    _____ c. Methotrexate is a treatment of choice

    _____ d. Fever and extra-articular symptoms
             present in full attack

    _____ e. Infection of a joint often caused by
             hematogenous route

    _____ f. Inflammation and dysfunction of
             salivary and lacrimal glands

    _____ g. Diagnosed by finding of hypersensitive
             tender points

    _____ h. An inflammatory polyarthritis associated
             with psoriasis

    _____ i. Increased risk in persons with decreased
             host resistance and prior joint disease

    _____ j. Lymphatic infiltration of bone marrow and
             visceral organs may occur

    _____ k. Systemic infection with migratory
             polyarthritis that may involve cardiac and
             neurological function

    _____ l. Self-limiting reactive arthritis following
             enteric or venereal infections

    1. Psoriatic arthritis

    2. Reiter's syndrome

    3. Septic arthritis

    4. Lyme disease

    5. Sjögren's syndrome

    6. Fibromyalgia

19. A client is seen at the outclient clinic for a sudden onset of inflammation and severe pain in the great toe. A diagnosis of gout is made on the basis of

    a. a family history of gout.
    b. elevated urine uric acid levels.
    c. elevated serum uric acid levels.
    d. the presence of sodium urate crystals in synovial fluid.

20. During treatment of the client with an acute attack of gout, the nurse would expect to administer

    a. ASA.
    b. colchicine.
    c. allopurinol (Zyloprim).
    d. probenecid (Benuryl).

21. A client with gout is treated with drug therapy to prevent future attacks. The nurse teaches the client that it is most important to

    a. avoid all foods high in purine, such as organ meats.
    b. have periodic determination of serum uric acid levels.
    c. perform active ROM of all joints that have been affected by gout.
    d. increase the dosage of medication with the onset of an acute attack.

22. The pathophysiology of systemic lupus erythematosus (SLE) is characterized by

    a. destruction of constituents of the cell nucleus by autoantibodies.
    b. overproduction of collagen, which disrupts the functioning of internal organs.
    c. formation of abnormal IgG that attaches to cellular antigens, activating complement.
    d. increased activity of T-suppressor cells with B cell hypoactivity, resulting in an immunodeficiency.

23. Identify the most common clinical manifestations of SLE that may occur in each of the following organ systems.

    a. Skin

    b. Musculoskeletal

    c. Cardiac

    d. Pulmonary

    e. Renal

    f. Central nervous

    g. Hematological

24. A client with newly diagnosed SLE asks the nurse how the disease will affect her life. The best response of the nurse is

    a. "You can plan to have a near-normal life as SLE rarely causes death."
    b. "It is difficult to tell since the disease is so variable in its severity and progression."
    c. "Lifespan is shortened somewhat in people with SLE, but the disease can be controlled with long-term use of corticosteroids."
    d. "Most people with SLE have alternating periods of remissions and exacerbations with rapid progression to permanent organ damage."

25. During an acute exacerbation, a client with SLE is treated with corticosteroids. The nurse would expect the steroids to begin to be tapered when serum laboratory results indicate

    a. increased RBC.
    b. decreased ESR.
    c. decreased anti-DNA.
    d. increased complement.

26. Teaching that the nurse plans for the client with SLE includes

    a. ways to avoid exposure to sunlight.
    b. increasing dietary protein and carbohydrate intake.
    c. the necessity of genetic counselling before planning a family.
    d. the use of non-pharmacological pain interventions instead of analgesics.

27. During an acute exacerbation of SLE, the client has a nursing diagnosis of impaired skin integrity. An appropriate nursing intervention for the client is to

    a. clean the skin with mild soap and water and keep it dry.
    b. apply moisturizing lotion to the skin several times a day.
    c. use a mild astringent on the face to stimulate circulation.
    d. teach the client to use cosmetics to minimize the skin changes.

28. During assessment of the client with systemic sclerosis, the nurse would expect to find

    a. cool, cyanotic fingers with thinning skin over the joints.
    b. swan-neck deformity or ulnar drift deformity of the hands.
    c. low back pain, stiffness, and limitation of spine movement.
    d. expressionless facial features with pursed lips and a small mouth.

29. When caring for the client with CREST syndrome associated with systemic sclerosis, the nurse teaches the client to

    a. avoid exposure to the sun or other UV light.
    b. maintain a fluid intake of at least 3000 mL/day.
    c. monitor and keep a log of daily blood pressure.
    d. protect the hands and feet from cold exposure and injury.

30. During the acute phase of dermatomyositis, an appropriate client outcome is

    a. performs active ROM qid.
    b. relates improvement in pain.
    c. does not experience aspiration.
    d. maintains absolute rest of affected joints.

31. A 56-year-old man develops symptoms of dermatomyositis. The client asks the nurse why his physician has ordered so many screening diagnostic examinations. The best response of the nurse includes the information that

    a. the disease is often precipitated by a hidden, latent infection.
    b. dermatomyositis in older men is often associated with a malignancy.
    c. extensive diagnostic testing is required to determine the effects of the disease on internal organs.
    d. symptoms of dermatomyositis are so rare in older persons that diagnosis requires extensive testing.

32. During assessment of the client diagnosed with fibromyalgia syndrome (FMS), the nurse would expect the client to report

    a. generalized muscle twitching and spasms.
    b. non-restorative sleep with resulting fatigue.
    c. profound and progressive muscle weakness that limits ADLs.
    d. widespread musculoskeletal pain that is accompanied by inflammation and fever.

33. One criterion for a diagnosis of FMS is

    a. fiber atrophy found on muscle biopsy.
    b. elimination of all other causes of musculoskeletal pain.
    c. the presence of the manifestations of chronic fatigue syndrome.
    d. the elicitation of pain upon palpation of at least 11 of 18 identified tender points.

34. One important nursing intervention for the client with FMS is to teach the client to

    a. rest the muscles as much as possible to avoid triggering pain.
    b. plan night-time sleep and naps to obtain 12–14 hours of sleep a day.
    c. use stress-management techniques such as biofeedback, guided imagery, or tai chi.
    d. try the use of food supplements such as glucosamine and chondroitin for relief of pain.

35. A client with debilitating fatigue has been diagnosed with chronic fatigue syndrome. List the four major criteria that must be present for this diagnosis to be made.

    a.

    b.

    c.

    d.

# CASE STUDY

### RHEUMATOID ARTHRITIS

**Client Profile**

Mrs. M. is a 36-year-old obese white woman who has rheumatoid arthritis. When her symptoms began to interfere with her daily activities, she sought medical help.

**Subjective Data**

- Has painful, stiff hands and feet
- Feels tired all of the time
- Reports an intermittent low-grade fever
- Takes naproxen (Naprosyn) 500 mg twice daily
- Wears a copper bracelet on the advice of a neighbour

**Objective Data**

- Hands show mild ulnar drift and puffiness
- Temperature 37.8°C (100°F)
- Admitted to the hospital for examination and comprehensive treatment plan
- Methotrexate therapy is to be initiated

## Critical Thinking Questions

1. How might the nurse explain the pathophysiology of rheumatoid arthritis to Mrs. M.?

2. What manifestations does Mrs. M. have that suggest the diagnosis of rheumatoid arthritis?

3. What results may be expected from methotrexate therapy? What are the nursing responsibilities related to methotrexate therapy?

4. What suggestions may be offered to Mrs. M. concerning home management and joint protection?

5. How can the nurse help Mrs. M. recognize ineffective, unproved methods of treatment?

6. What other sources of information regarding arthritis might the nurse suggest to Mrs. M.?

7. Based on the assessment data presented, write one or more appropriate nursing diagnoses. Are there any collaborative problems?

# CHAPTER 64 NURSING MANAGEMENT: CRITICAL CARE

1. A primary difference in the skills of a certified critical care nurse compared with nurses certified in medical-surgical nursing is an ability to

   a. diagnose and treat life-threatening diseases.
   b. detect and manage early complications of health problems.
   c. provide intensive psychological support to the client and family.
   d. use advanced technology to assess and maintain physiological function.

2. Identify which of the common three reasons clients are admitted to the ICU apply in the following situations.

   a. Client with diabetic ketoacidosis

   b. Client with non-displaced skull fracture who is alert and oriented

   c. Post-operative client with mitral valve replacement

   d. Comatose client who had an anaphylactic reaction with cardiopulmonary arrest at home with re-establishment of cardiac function

3. A nursing intervention that is indicated for the client in the ICU who has a nursing diagnosis of anxiety related to ICU environment and sensory overload is

   a. eliminating unnecessary alarms and overhead paging.
   b. providing flexible visiting schedules for family members.
   c. administering sedatives or psychotropic drugs to promote rest.
   d. allowing the client to do as much self-care in daily activities as possible.

4. The critical care nurse includes family members of the client in the ICU as part of the healthcare team primarily because

   a. the costs of critical care will affect the entire family.
   b. family members are responsible for making healthcare decisions for the client.
   c. the extent of the family members' involvement affects the client's clinical course.
   d. family members that are ignored are more likely to question the client's quality of care.

5. Review the concepts of cardiac output (CO), preload, and afterload by indicating whether the following conditions cause an increase or a decrease in the parameters under normal conditions.

   a. If heart rate (HR) is decreased, CO is _____.

   b. If stroke volume (SV) is increased, CO is _____.

   c. A decrease in preload will _____ SV.

   d. An increase in fluid administration will _____ preload.

   e. A decrease in afterload causes _____ CO.

   f. Increased systemic vascular resistance (SVR) _____ afterload.

6. During hemodynamic monitoring, the nurse finds that the client has a decreased CO with unchanged pulmonary artery occlusive pressure (PAOP), HR, and SVR. The nurse identifies that the client has a decrease in

    a. SV.
    b. preload.
    c. afterload.
    d. contractility.

7. Before taking hemodynamic measurements, the monitoring equipment must be referenced by

    a. confirming that when pressure in the system is zero, the equipment reads zero.
    b. positioning the stopcock nearest the transducer level with the phlebostatic axis.
    c. placing the transducer on the left side of the chest at the fourth intercostal space.
    d. placing the client in a left lateral position with the transducer level with the top surface of the mattress.

8. Identify whether the following statements are true or false. If a statement is false, correct the bold word(s) to make the statement true.

    \_\_\_\_\_ a. When a client has an arterial catheter placed for arterial blood gas (ABG) sampling, the low pressure alarm must be activated to detect **disconnection** of the line.

    \_\_\_\_\_ b. A pulmonary artery flow-directed catheter has a balloon at the distal tip that floats into the **left side of the heart**.

    \_\_\_\_\_ c. The pressure obtained when the balloon of the pulmonary artery catheter is inflated reflects the preload of the **right ventricle**.

    \_\_\_\_\_ d. In the absence of mitral value impairment, the left ventricular end-diastolic pressure is reflected by the **wedge**.

    \_\_\_\_\_ e. A decrease in $SVO_2$ (mixed venous blood) when arterial oxygenation, hemoglobin, and tissue perfusion are unchanged indicates **increased oxygen consumption**.

9. In preparing the client for insertion of a pulmonary artery catheter, the nurse

    a. obtains informed consent from the client.
    b. places the client in a high Fowler's position.
    c. ensures that the client has continuous ECG monitoring.
    d. performs an Allen test to confirm adequate ulnar artery perfusion.

10. Describe the techniques the nurse uses to obtain the following data from the pulmonary artery catheter.

    a. PAOP

    b. Thermodilution CO

11. A client in the ICU with hemodynamic monitoring has the following values:

BP 90/68 mm Hg
HR 124
PAOP 22 mm Hg
CO 3.2 L/min
RAP (CVP) 14 mm Hg
Pulmonary artery pressure 38/20 mm Hg

a. Calculate the additional values that can be determined from these findings.

MAP                    PAP

SV                     SVR

b. What interpretation can the nurse make about the client's circulatory status and cardiac function from these values?

12. A client has $SVO_2$ of 52%, CO of 4.8 L/min, $SpO_2$ of 95%, and unchanged hemoglobin level. The nurse should assess the client for

a. arrhythmias.
b. pain or movement.
c. pulmonary edema.
d. signs of septic shock.

13. The nurse observes a pulmonary artery wedge pressure waveform on the monitor when the balloon of the client's pulmonary artery catheter is deflated. The nurse recognizes that

a. the client is at risk for embolism because of occlusion of the catheter with a thrombus.
b. the client is developing pulmonary edema that has increased the pulmonary artery pressure.
c. the client is at risk for an air embolus because the injected air cannot be withdrawn into the syringe.
d. the catheter must be immediately repositioned to prevent pulmonary infarction or pulmonary artery rupture.

14. The use of the intra-aortic balloon pump (IABP) would be indicated for the client with

a. an insufficient aortic valve.
b. a dissecting aortic aneurysm.
c. accelerating or crescendo angina.
d. generalized peripheral vascular disease.

15. Identify whether the following statements are true or false. If a statement is false, correct the bold word(s) to make the statement true.

_____ a. The rapid deflation of the intra-aortic balloon causes a decreased **preload**.

_____ b. During intra-aortic counterpulsation, the balloon is inflated during **diastole**.

_____ c. A primary effect of the intra-aortic balloon pump is increased **systolic** pressure.

16. To prevent arterial trauma during the use of the IABP, the nurse should

    a. reposition the client q2h.
    b. check the site for bleeding every hour.
    c. prevent hip flexion of the cannulated leg.
    d. cover the insertion site with an occlusive dressing.

17. A client who is hemodynamically stable is weaned from the IABP. The nurse should

    a. decrease the augmentation pressure to zero.
    b. stop the machine when hemodynamic parameters are satisfactory.
    c. stop the infusion flow through the catheter when weaning is initiated.
    d. continue the pumping every third or fourth beat until the balloon is removed.

18. Ventricular assist devices are designed to

    a. provide permanent, total circulatory support when the left ventricle fails.
    b. temporarily partially or totally support circulation until a donor heart can be obtained.
    c. support circulation only when clients cannot be weaned from cardiopulmonary bypass.
    d. reverse the effects of circulatory failure in clients with acute myocardial infarction in cardiogenic shock.

19. A comatose client with a possible cervical spine injury is intubated with a nasal endotracheal tube. The nurse recognizes that in comparison with an oral endotracheal tube, a nasal tube

    a. requires the placement of a bite block.
    b. is more likely to cause laryngeal trauma.
    c. requires greater respiratory effort in breathing.
    d. provides for easier suctioning and secretion removal.

20. In preparing an alert client in the ICU for oral endotracheal intubation, the nurse

    a. tells the client that the tongue should be extruded while the tube is inserted.
    b. explains that gagging and feelings of suffocation may be experienced during insertion of the tube.
    c. positions the client supine with the head hanging over the edge of the bed to align the mouth and trachea.
    d. informs the client that while it will not be possible to talk during insertion of the tube, speech will be possible after it is correctly placed.

21. A client has an oral endotracheal tube inserted to relieve an upper airway obstruction and to facilitate secretion removal. The first responsibility of the nurse immediately following placement of the tube is to

    a. suction the tube to remove secretions.
    b. mark the tube where it exits the mouth.
    c. secure the tube to the face with adhesive tape.
    d. assess for bilateral breath sounds and symmetric chest movement.

22. The nurse uses the minimal occluding volume (MOV) to inflate the cuff on an endotracheal tube to minimize the incidence of

    a. infection.
    b. hypoxemia.
    c. tracheal necrosis.
    d. accidental extubation.

23. Complete the following statements related to the client with an endotracheal tube.

    a.  After inflating an endotracheal tube cuff, the nurse monitors the cuff pressure every _____ hours with

        a manometer to verify that the cuff pressure is _____ mm Hg.

    b.  Equipment that should be at the bedside for all clients undergoing endotracheal intubation includes

        _____ equipment and a _____.

    c.  A catheter used to suction an endotracheal tube should be no larger than _____ the diameter of

        the ET tube.

    d.  When suctioning an endotracheal tube, the nurse uses a suction pressure of _____ to _____ mm Hg.

    e.  During endotracheal tube suctioning, each suction pass should be no longer than _____ seconds.

    f.  To prevent hypoxemia during endotracheal suctioning, the nurse always _____ the client

        before and after suctioning.

24. The nurse suctions the client's endotracheal tube when the client

    a.  has peripheral crackles in all lobes.
    b.  has not been suctioned for two hours.
    c.  has coarse rhonchi over central airways.
    d.  needs stimulation to cough and breathe deeply.

25. While suctioning the endotracheal tube of a spontaneously breathing client, the nurse notes that the client develops bradycardia with premature ventricular contractions. The nurse should

    a.  stop the suctioning and assess the client for spontaneous respirations.
    b.  attempt to resuction the client with reduced suction pressure and pass time.
    c.  stop suctioning and ventilate the client with a bag-valve-mask (BVM) with 100% oxygen until the heart rate returns to baseline.
    d.  stop the suctioning and ventilate the client with slow, small-volume breaths using the BVM device.

26. Identify two precautions the nurse should take during mouth care of the client with an oral endotracheal tube to prevent and detect tube dislodgement.

    a.

    b.

27. A client with an oral endotracheal tube has a nursing diagnosis of risk for aspiration related to presence of artificial airway. An appropriate nursing intervention for this client is to

    a.  monitor the client for an inability to speak.
    b.  inflate the cuff during tube feedings and mouth care.
    c.  keep the ventilator tubing cleared of condensed water.
    d.  use a small-bore, blunt ring-tipped catheter to suction the oropharynx.

28. When extubation of the client is being performed, it is most important to

    a. observe the client for respiratory distress after tube removal.
    b. have the client cough to remove secretions before extubation.
    c. perform tracheal suctioning immediately following removal of the tube.
    d. obtain a blood specimen for ABGs immediately after the tube is removed.

29. Mechanical ventilation is indicated when a client in respiratory distress has a

    a. $PaCO_2$ of 50 mm Hg.
    b. tidal volume of 8 mL/kg.
    c. resting minute ventilation of 5L/min.
    d. maximal inspiratory pressure of –15 cm $H_2O$.

30. Indicate whether the following are characteristic of negative pressure ventilators (N), positive pressure ventilators (P), or both (B).

    _____ a. Reduce intrathoracic pressure causing air to be pulled into lungs

    _____ b. Require an artificial airway

    _____ c. Expiration is passive as machine cycles off

    _____ d. Most similar to physiological ventilation

    _____ e. Applied to outside of the body

    _____ f. Can provide control and assist-control ventilatory modes

    _____ g. Most frequently used with acutely ill clients

    _____ h. Frequently used in the home for neuromuscular or nervous system disorders

31. Match the following types of positive pressure ventilators with their descriptions (answers may be used more than once).

    _____ a. Indicated for clients at risk for barotrauma          1. Volume ventilator

    _____ b. Preset volume of gas delivered with                   2. Pressure ventilator
              pressure-limiting valve

    _____ c. Inspiration terminated when preset airway
              pressure achieved

    _____ d. Volume of gas delivery limited if
              obstructions or asynchronous breathing present

    _____ e. Consistent volume and oxygen
              concentrations delivered despite lung resistance

32. Identify the ventilatory settings and modes described below.

    a. Positive pressure applied through the entire respiratory cycle _____ _____

    b. Client self-regulates the rate and depth of spontaneous respirations but may also receive preset volume

       and frequency breaths by ventilator_____ _____

    c. Ventilator delivers gas independent of client's ventilatory efforts _____ _____

    d. Positive pressure applied only during inspiration that supplies a rapid flow of gas _____

       _____

    e. Preset tidal volume delivered at set frequency but can be delivered more frequently if client attempts to

       inhale _____ _____

    f. Positive pressure applied to airway during exhalation _____ _____

    g. Delivery of small tidal volumes at a rapid respiratory rate _____ _____

    h. Prolonged inspiration and shortened expiration set to promote alveolar expansion and prevent

       collapse _____ _____

33. A client in acute respiratory failure is receiving assist-control mechanical ventilation with PEEP of 10 cm
    $H_2O$. A sign that alerts the nurse to undesirable effects of increased airway and thoracic pressure is

    a. decreased $PaO_2$.
    b. increased crackles.
    c. decreased blood pressure.
    d. decreased spontaneous respirations.

34. The nurse recognizes that a factor that is commonly responsible for sodium and fluid retention in the client on
    mechanical ventilation is

    a. increased ADH release.
    b. increased release of atrial natriuretic factor.
    c. increased insensible water loss via the airway.
    d. decreased renal perfusion with release of renin.

35. A client with chronic COPD who is on mechanical assist-control ventilation has $PaCO_2$ of 40 mm Hg, $PaO_2$
    of 70 mm Hg, and pH of 7.45. The nurse determines that

    a. the client is responding optimally to the ventilator settings.
    b. the ventilator setting for rate or volume should be decreased.
    c. PEEP is indicated to increase the $PaO_2$ and improve gas exchange.
    d. an inverse-ratio ventilation manoeuvre should be set on the ventilator.

36. A client receiving mechanical ventilation is very anxious and agitated, and neuromuscular blocking agents are used to promote ventilation. The nurse recognizes that

   a. the client will be too sedated to be aware of the details of care.
   b. visitors should be encouraged to provide stimulation and diversion.
   c. the client should always be addressed and explanations of care given.
   d. communication will not be possible with the use of neuromuscular blocking agents.

37. Identify five problems associated with inadequate nutrition in the client receiving prolonged mechanical ventilation.

   a.

   b.

   c.

   d.

   e.

38. The nurse determines that alveolar hypoventilation is occurring in a client on a ventilator when

   a. the client develops cardiac arrhythmias.
   b. auscultation reveals an air leak around the ET cuff.
   c. ABG results show a $PaCO_2$ of 32 mm Hg and a pH of 7.47.
   d. the client tries to breathe faster than the ventilator setting.

39. When weaning a client from a ventilator, the nurse plans

   a. to decrease the delivered $FIO_2$ concentration.
   b. intermittent trials of spontaneous ventilation followed by ventilatory support to provide rest.
   c. substitution of ventilator support with a manual resuscitation bag if the client becomes hypoxemic.
   d. to implement weaning procedures round-the-clock until the client does not experience ventilatory fatigue.

40. A client is to be discharged to home with mechanical ventilation. Before discharge, it is most important for the nurse to

   a. teach the family members to care for the client with a home ventilator.
   b. stress the advantages for the client in being cared for in the home environment.
   c. help the family plan for the time and financial resources required for home care.
   d. have the family arrange for round-the-clock home health nurses for the first several weeks.

# CASE STUDY

## CRITICALLY ILL CLIENT

### Client Profile

Mr. V., age 42, has a history of HIV infection with the development of manifestations of AIDS two years ago. He has been hospitalized and treated twice for *Pneumocystis carinii* pneumonia and is now admitted to the ICU with suspected cryptococcal meningitis. Intracranial pressure (ICP) monitoring is instituted, and an arterial line and flow-directed pulmonary artery catheter are inserted. Endotracheal intubation with assist-control mechanical ventilation at 12 breaths per minute, 15 cm $H_2O$ PEEP, and $FIO_2$ of 50% is established. (Note: This client is very critically ill and requires review of intracranial pressure, septic shock, multiple organ dysfunction syndrome, and respiratory failure.)

### Subjective Data

- Friend relates that Mr. V. had two generalized tonic-clonic seizures in the two hours before admission.

### Objective Data

- Glasgow Coma Scale score: 6
- ICP: 22 mm Hg
- Vital signs: T 39°C (102.2°F), HR 80, RR 26/min, BP 100/46 mm Hg
- Arterial blood gases: $PaO_2$ 65 mm Hg, $PaCO_2$ 32 mm Hg, $HCO_3$ 16 mmol/L (16 mEq/L), pH 7.26
- Other lab: glucose 12.6 mmol/L (228 mg/dL), lactate 3 mmol/L (3 mEq/L), WBC 18.5 x $10^9$/L (18.5 x $10^3$/μL)
- Hemodynamic monitoring values: CO 6 L/min, PAP 8 mm Hg, PAOP 15 mm Hg, SVR 530 dyne/sec/cm$^{-5}$, $SvO_2$ 90%, $SaO_2$ 92%
- Skin warm and dry
- Foley catheter inserted with 30 mL urine return

### Critical Thinking Questions

1. What are the best indicators to use in Mr. V.'s case to monitor his hemodynamic status?

2. What effect might the use of PEEP have on Mr. V.'s intracranial pressure?

3. What is Mr. V.'s MAP? What MAP would be necessary to promote tissue and cerebral perfusion and yet not increase ICP?

4. What drugs and fluids would be indicated for Mr. V.'s treatment?

5. How may Mr. V.'s condition be complicated by gastrointestinal ischemia?

6. Explain the processes that account for the abnormal assessment findings in Mr. V.

7. Based on the assessment data presented, write one or more appropriate nursing diagnoses. Are there any collaborative problems?

# CHAPTER 65 NURSING MANAGEMENT: SHOCK AND MULTIPLE ORGAN DYSFUNCTION SYNDROME

1. The key factor in describing any type of shock is

   a. hypoxemia.
   b. hypotension.
   c. vascular collapse.
   d. inadequate tissue perfusion.

2. Match each type of shock with its major classification.

   _____ a. Anaphylactic shock          1. Low blood flow

   _____ b. Cardiogenic shock           2. Maldistribution of blood

   _____ c. Hypovolemic shock

   _____ d. Neurogenic shock

   _____ e. Septic shock

3. Match the following precipitating factors with their related types of shock (answers may be used more than once).

   _____ a  Acute myocardial infarction     1. Neurogenic

   _____ b. Insect bites                    2. Cardiogenic

   _____ c. Burns                           3. Anaphylactic

   _____ d. Severe pain                     4. Septic

   _____ e. Ventricular arrhythmias         5. Hypovolemic

   _____ f. Spinal cord injury

   _____ g. Hemorrhage

   _____ h. Urinary tract infection

   _____ i. Vaccines

   _____ j. Ruptured spleen

   _____ k. Epidural block

   _____ l. Severe vomiting and diarrhea

   _____ m. Peritonitis

   _____ n. Pulmonary embolism

4. Identify whether the following statements are true or false. If a statement is false, correct the bold word(s) to make the statement true.

_____    a. **Cardiogenic shock** is characterized by increased systemic vascular resistance (SVR), decreased cardiac output (CO), and decreased pulmonary artery pressure (PAP).

_____    b. In septic shock, bacterial endotoxins cause vascular changes that result in **decreased systemic vascular resistance** with **increased cardiac output**.

_____    c. Bradycardia with hypotension is characteristic of **neurogenic shock**.

_____    d. In anaphylactic shock, death may occur as a result of **respiratory** failure.

_____    e. Hypovolemic shock from **relative hypovolemia** may occur with diabetes insipidus.

_____    f. Hemodynamic monitoring in the client with cardiogenic shock will reveal an **increased** PAWP and a **decreased** cardiac index.

5. Complete the following pathophysiological mechanisms that occur in the compensated stage of hypovolemic shock, filling the blanks with the following words or phrases. (See Figure 65-6.)

| | |
|---|---|
| Aldosterone secretion | Increased serum osmolality |
| Alpha-adrenergic stimulation | Increased venous return to heart |
| Beta-adrenergic stimulation | Release of ADH |
| Decreased capillary hydrostatic pressure | Renal water reabsorption |
| Increased blood pressure | Renin release |
| Increased heart strength and rate | |

a. Decreased blood pressure → _____ → Fluid movement into intravascular space.

b. Decreased blood pressure → Activation of sympathetic nervous system → _____

   → Decreased blood flow to lungs, skin, and GI tract.

c. Decreased blood pressure → Activation of sympathetic nervous system → _____ →

   Coronary vasodilation and _____.

d. Decreased kidney perfusion → _____ → Increased angiotensin I.

e. Increased angiotensin II → _____ → Increased renal sodium reabsorption.

f. Increased angiotensin II → Venous and arterial vasoconstriction → _____ and

   _____.

g. Increased renal sodium reabsorption → _____ → _____

h. Increased ADH → _____ → Increased blood volume.

6. From the data presented in question 5, identify six clinical manifestations that may be evident in a client in the compensated stage of shock.

   a.

   b.

   c.

   d.

   e.

   f.

7. When caring for a client with shock, the nurse knows that alterations in coagulation are more likely to manifest earlier and more severely in the client with

   a. septic shock.
   b. neurogenic shock.
   c. hypovolemic shock.
   d. anaphylactic shock.

8. Progressive tissue hypoxia leading to anaerobic metabolism and metabolic acidosis is characteristic of the progressive stage of shock. Identify what changes occur in the following tissues to cause this increasing tissue hypoxia.

   a. Renal

   b. Lung

   c. Capillaries

   d. Cardiac

9. The major pathophysiological characteristic of the irreversible or refractory stage of shock is

   a. cardiac failure.
   b. renal insufficiency.
   c. ischemia of the intestinal mucosa.
   d. failure of compensatory mechanisms.

10. An intervention that is appropriate in the emergency management of any type of shock is

    a. vasopressor therapy.
    b. high-volume fluid resuscitation.
    c. administration of high-flow oxygen (100%).
    d. endotracheal intubation and mechanical ventilation.

11. An abnormal finding that is common in early, compensated shock is

    a. metabolic acidosis.
    b. increased serum sodium.
    c. decreased blood glucose.
    d. increased serum potassium.

12. In late, irreversible shock in a client with massive thermal burns the nurse would expect the client's laboratory results to reveal

    a. respiratory alkalosis.
    b. increased liver enzymes.
    c. decreased urine specific gravity.
    d. decreased hemoglobin and hematocrit.

13. A client with hypovolemic shock is receiving lactated Ringer's for fluid replacement therapy. During this therapy, it is most important for the nurse to monitor the client's

    a. serum pH.
    b. serum sodium.
    c. serum potassium.
    d. hemoglobin and hematocrit.

14. A client in shock weighs 90 kg (198 lb). Adequate fluid volume replacement in this client would be indicated

    by minimum urine output of _____ mL/hr.

15. Large amounts of crystalloid fluids are administered to a client in septic shock to maintain adequate blood volume. As a result of this therapy, the nurse would expect the client to experience

    a. decreased CO.
    b. systemic edema.
    c. decreased PAWP.
    d. decreased urinary output.

16. When caring for a client in cardiogenic shock, the nurse recognizes that the metabolic demands of turning and moving the client exceed the oxygen supply when hemodynamic monitoring reveals a change in

    a. $SvO_2$ from 62% to 54%.
    b. SV from 52 to 68 mL/beat.
    c. CO from 4.2 L/min to 4.8 L/min.
    d. SVR from 1300 to 1120 dyne sec/cm$^{-5}$.

17. During administration of intravenous norepinephrine (Levophed), the nurse should assess the client for

    a. hypotension.
    b. marked diuresis.
    c. metabolic alkalosis.
    d. decreased tissue perfusion.

18. When administering any vasoactive drug during the treatment of shock, the nurse knows that the goal of the therapy is to

    a. increase urine output to 50 mL/hr.
    b. maintain a MAP of at least 60 mm Hg.
    c. dilate vessels to improve tissue perfusion.
    d. constrict vessels to maintain blood pressure.

19. Identify two medical therapies that are specific to each of the following types of shock.

    a. Cardiogenic

    b. Hypovolemic

    c. Septic

    d. Anaphylactic

20. Identify four drugs and their actions that are used in treatment of cardiogenic shock and that are not generally used for other types of shock.

    | **Drug** | **Actions** |
    | --- | --- |
    | a. | |
    | b. | |
    | c. | |
    | d. | |

21. The most important nursing responsibility in the prevention of shock is

    a. frequently monitoring all clients' vital signs.
    b. using aseptic technique for all invasive procedures.
    c. being aware of the potential for shock in all clients at risk.
    d. teaching clients health promotion activities to prevent shock.

22. Five indicators of tissue perfusion that should be monitored in critically ill clients are

    _____, _____, _____, _____, and

    _____.

23 . Match each assessment area with the frequency with which the nurse should monitor its status when caring for an unstable client in the acute phases of shock (some answers may not be used).

    _____ a. Renal function                    1. Continuously

    _____ b. HR, BP, CVP, and PAP              2. q15min

    _____ c. Neurological function             3. q1h

    _____ d. GI function                       4. q2h

    _____ e. Respiratory rate and rhythm       5. q4h

    _____ f. Oxygen saturation                 6. q8h

    _____ g. Breath sounds

    _____ h. Electrocardiogram

    _____ i. Response to medication and fluid administration

    _____ j. Normal body temperature

24. A client in the progressive stage of shock has rapid, deep respirations. The nurse determines that the client's hyperventilation is compensating for a metabolic acidosis when the client's arterial blood gas results include

    a. pH 7.42, $PaO_2$ 80 mm Hg.
    b. pH 7.48, $PaO_2$ 69 mm Hg.
    c. pH 7.38, $PaCO_2$ 30 mm Hg.
    d. pH 7.32, $PaCO_2$ 48 mm Hg.

25. A client in shock has a nursing diagnosis of fear related to severity of condition and perceived threat of death as manifested by verbalization of anxiety about condition and fear of death. An appropriate nursing intervention for the client is to

    a. administer anti-anxiety agents.
    b. call a member of the clergy to visit the client.
    c. allow family members to visit as much as possible.
    d. inform the client of the current plan of care and its rationale.

26. Identify whether the following statements are true or false. If a statement is false, correct the bold word(s) to make the statement true.

    _____ a. Systemic inflammatory response syndrome (SIRS) is always present in a client with **sepsis**.

    _____ b. Multiple organ dysfunction syndrome (MODS) **may occur independently** from SIRS.

    _____ c. All clients with septic shock develop **MODS**.

    _____ d. A client with direct multiple organ damage from massive trauma experiences **primary** MODS.

    _____ e. A common initial mediator that causes endothelial damage leading to SIRS and MODS is **endotoxin**.

    _____ f. Generally, the first organ system affected by mediator-induced injury in SIRS and MODS is the **central nervous system**.

27. Match the following clinical findings with their related primary pathophysiological processes of SIRS and MODS (answers may be used more than once).

    _____ a. Decreased preload

    _____ b. Metabolic acidosis

    _____ c. Warm skin

    _____ d. Prolonged prothrombin time

    _____ e. Cerebral edema and increased intracranial pressure

    _____ f. Translocation of GI bacteria

    _____ g. Decreased serum protein and albumin

    _____ h. Stress ulcers

    _____ i. Cardiac arrhythmias

    _____ j. Decreased serum potassium

    _____ k. Decreased serum calcium, phosphate, and magnesium

    1. Increased capillary permeability

    2. Impaired liver function

    3. Gastrointestinal ischemia

    4. Vasodilation

    5. Release of aldosterone

    6. Impaired kidney function

28. The nurse recognizes that SIRS is present in the client who manifests

    a. a $PaCO_2$ of 48 mm Hg and a WBC of 13 x $10^9$/L (13 x $10^3$/μL).
    b. a heart rate of 88/min and a $PaCO_2$ of 30 mm Hg.
    c. a temperature of 38.4°C (101.2°F) and confusion.
    d. a respiratory rate of 24/min and a WBC of 3.8 x $10^9$/L (3.8 x $10^3$/μL).

29. An intervention that may prevent GI bacterial and endotoxin translocation in a critically ill client with SIRS is

    a. early enteral feedings.
    b. surgical removal of necrotic tissue.
    c. aggressive, multiple antibiotic therapy.
    d. strict aseptic technique in all procedures.

30. The development of MODS is confirmed in a client who manifests

    a. a urine output of 30 mL/hr, a BUN of 12 mmol/L (33.6 mg/dL), and a WBC of 1.1 x $10^9$/L (1.1 x $10^3$/μL).
    b. upper GI bleeding, Glasgow Coma Scale score of 7, and a hematocrit of 0.25 (25%).
    c. a respiratory rate of 45/min, a $PaCO_2$ of 60, and a chest x-ray with bilateral diffuse patchy infiltrates.
    d. an elevated serum amylase and lipase, a serum creatinine of 200 μmol/L (2.3 mg/dL), and a platelet count of 15 x $10^9$/L (15 x $10^3$/μL).

## CASE STUDY

### SEPTIC SHOCK

### Client Profile

Mr. M. is an 81-year-old man who was brought to the emergency department in an ambulance from a local nursing home. He was found by the nurses on their 6 A.M. rounds to be very confused, restless, and hypotensive.

### Past Health History

Mr. M. is a type 1 diabetic with a history of prostate cancer and congestive heart failure. He has been a resident of the nursing home for three years. He has had an in-dwelling urinary catheter in place for five days because of difficulty voiding. Until today, Mr. M. has been very oriented and cooperative. His current medications are digoxin, hydrochlorothiazide (HydroDiuril), isosorbide (Isordil), and insulin.

### Subjective Data

- Denies any pain or discomfort

### Objective Data

- Neurological: lethargic, confused, easily roused, does not follow commands; moves all extremities in response to stimuli
- Cardiovascular: B/P 80/60, HR 112 and regular, T 40°C (104°F) rectal; heart sounds normal without murmurs or $S_3$, $S_4$; peripheral pulses weak and thready
- Skin: warm, dry, flushed
- Respiratory: RR 34 and shallow; breath sounds audible in all lobes with crackles bilaterally in the bases
- GI/GU: abdomen soft with hypoactive bowel sounds; urinary catheter in place draining scant, purulent urine

In the emergency department, two 16-gauge IVs were inserted and 700 mL of normal saline was given over the first hour. The client was placed on 40% oxygen via face mask. The urinary catheter was removed and cultured and blood cultures were drawn at three intervals. A new catheter was inserted. The client was started on IV antibiotics and was transferred to the ICU with the diagnosis of septic shock due to Gram-negative sepsis.

In the ICU, a pulmonary catheter was inserted in addition to an arterial line.

- ABG results were pH 7.25; $PaO_2$ 60 mm Hg; $PaCO_2$ 28 mm Hg; $HCO_3^-$ 12 mmol/L (12 mEq/L); and $SaO_2$ 82%.
- Hemodynamic pressures taken were right atrial pressure (CVP), PAP, PAWP, cardiac output, and SVR.
- Laboratory results were WBC 21 x $10^9$/L (21 x $10^3$/μL), Na 133 mmol/L (133 mEq/L), K 4.5 mmol/L (4.5 mEq/L), Cl 96 mmol/L (96 mEq/L), glucose 12 mmol/L (216 mg/dL), creatinine 140 μmol/L (1.6 mg/dL), Hb 120 g/L (12 g/dL), Hct 0.36 (36%).

Mr. M.'s blood pressure continued to drop despite administration of several litres of crystalloids. Dopamine was started and titrated up as needed to try to maintain the client's blood pressure, in addition to more fluid administration. Despite all efforts, including intubation and mechanical ventilation, Mr. M. died on the sixth hospital day. The cause was multiple organ dysfunction syndrome due to Gram-negative sepsis.

## Critical Thinking Questions

1. What risk factors for septic shock were present in Mr. M.?

2. What preventive measures could have been taken by the nursing home staff in regard to Mr. M.?

3. What are the major pathophysiological changes associated with sepsis?

4. Discuss the mechanism for hypotension in the client with septic shock.

5. Explain the physiological reasons for the following assessment parameters found in this client.

Decreased LOC

Warm, dry, and flushed skin

Tachycardia

Tachypnea

Fever

Decreased SVR

Increased CO

Oliguria

Hyperglycemia

6. Why was a pulmonary artery catheter indicated for Mr. M.?

7. Analyze the results of the arterial blood gases.

8. Describe the changes in the hemodynamic pressure that would be expected in Mr. M.

9. Explain the rationale for fluid therapy and the use of dopamine.

10. Based on the assessment data provided, write one or more nursing diagnoses. What collaborative problems are present?

1. Respiratory failure can be defined as

   a. the absence of ventilation.
   b. any episode in which part of the airway is obstructed.
   c. inadequate gas exchange to meet the metabolic needs of the body.
   d. an episode of acute hypoxemia caused by a pulmonary dysfunction.

2. Indicate whether the following descriptions are characteristic of hypoxemic respiratory failure (HO) or hypercapnic respiratory failure (HC).

   _____ a. Primary problem is inadequate oxygen transfer

   _____ b. Most often caused by V/Q mismatch and shunt

   _____ c. Referred to as ventilatory failure

   _____ d. Exists when $PaO_2$ is 60 mm Hg or less, even when oxygen is administered at 60%

   _____ e. Risk of inadequate oxygen saturation of hemoglobin exists

   _____ f. The body is unable to compensate for acidemia of increased $PaCO_2$

   _____ g. Primary problem is insufficient carbon dioxide removal

   _____ h. Referred to as oxygenation failure

   _____ i. Results from an imbalance between ventilatory supply and ventilatory demand

3. Identify whether the following statements are true or false. If a statement is false, correct the bold word(s) to make the statement true.

   _____ a. A V/Q ratio of 1:1 (V/Q = 1) reflects an **alveolar ventilation** of 4 to 5 L that is matched by 4 to 5 L of **blood flow** to the lungs each minute.

   _____ b. The V/Q ratio is **1 or greater** when there is less ventilation to an area of the lung than perfusion.

   _____ c. An extreme V/Q imbalance resulting from blood leaving the heart without being exposed to ventilated areas of the lung is known as **a shunt**.

   _____ d. An intrapulmonary shunt occurs when an obstruction impairs the flow of **blood to ventilated areas of the lung**.

   _____ e. In differentiating between a V/Q mismatch and an intrapulmonary shunt, an increase in $PaO_2$ on oxygen administration occurs in the client with **an intrapulmonary shunt**.

   _____ f. Gas transport is slowed in **shunt**, resulting in exertional hypoxemia that is not present at rest.

4. Match the following physiological mechanisms of hypoxemia with their common causes.

_____ a. V/Q mismatch 1 or greater          1. Pulmonary fibrosis

_____ b. V/Q mismatch 1 or less             2. Ventricular septal defect

_____ c. Anatomical shunt                   3. Pulmonary embolism

_____ d. Intrapulmonary shunt               4. Atelectasis

_____ e. Diffusion limitation               5. Pulmonary edema

5. Match the mechanisms of hypoxemic respiratory failure that may occur in the client with pneumonia with the responsible factors.

_____ a. V/Q mismatch          1. Thickening of alveolar-capillary membrane from secretions and fluid accumulation

_____ b. Diffusion limitation

                               2. Consolidation of lung lobules with exudate and alveolar collapse

_____ c. Shunt

_____ d. Alveolar hypoventilation    3. Decreased alveolar ventilation from obstruction of bronchioles and terminal respiratory units

                               4. Pleuritic pain and inflammation

6. Hypercapnic respiratory failure is most likely to occur in the client who has

   a. rapid, deep respirations in response to pneumonia.
   b. slow, shallow respirations as a result of sedative overdose.
   c. large airway resistance as a result of severe bronchospasm.
   d. poorly ventilated areas of the lung due to pulmonary edema.

7. Acute respiratory failure in a client with chronic lung disease would most likely be indicated by arterial blood gas (ABG) results of

   a. $PaO_2$ 52 mm Hg, $PaCO_2$ 56 mm Hg, pH 7.4.
   b. $PaO_2$ 46 mm Hg, $PaCO_2$ 52 mm Hg, pH 7.36.
   c. $PaO_2$ 48 mm Hg, $PaCO_2$ 54 mm Hg, pH 7.38.
   d. $PaO_2$ 50 mm Hg, $PaCO_2$ 54 mm Hg, pH 7.28.

8. Indicate whether the following manifestations are primarily characteristic of hypoxemic (HO) or hypercapnic (HC) respiratory failure.

_____ a. Cyanosis

_____ b. Morning headache

_____ c. Rapid, shallow respirations

_____ d. Metabolic acidosis

_____ e. "Three-word" dyspnea

_____ f. Use of tripod position

_____ g. Respiratory acidosis

9. The nurse detects the early onset of hypoxemia in the client who experiences

   a. restlessness.
   b. hypotension.
   c. central cyanosis.
   d. cardiac arrhythmias.

10. The nurse assesses that a client in respiratory distress is developing respiratory fatigue and the risk of respiratory arrest when the client

    a. has an increased I/E ratio.
    b. cannot breathe unless he is sitting upright.
    c. uses the abdominal muscles during expiration.
    d. has a change in respiratory rate from rapid to slow.

11. A client has a $PaO_2$ of 50 mm Hg and a $PaCO_2$ of 42 mm Hg because of an intrapulmonary shunt. The client is most likely to respond best to

    a. positive pressure ventilation.
    b. oxygen administration at a $FIO_2$ of 100%.
    c. administration of oxygen per nasal cannula at 1 to 3 L/min.
    d. clearance of airway secretions with coughing and suctioning.

12. A client with a massive hemothorax and pneumothorax has absent breath sounds in the right lung. To promote improved V/Q matching, the nurse positions the client

    a. on the left side.
    b. on the right side.
    c. in a reclining chair bed.
    d. supine with the head of the bed elevated.

13. A client in hypercapnic respiratory failure has a nursing diagnosis of ineffective airway clearance related to increasing exhaustion. An appropriate nursing intervention for the client includes

    a. inserting an oral airway.
    b. performing augmented coughing.
    c. teaching the client "huff" coughing.
    d. teaching the client slow pursed-lip breathing.

14. Hemodynamic monitoring is instituted in severe respiratory failure primarily to

    a. detect V/Q mismatches.
    b. evaluate oxygenation and ventilation status.
    c. evaluate cardiac status and blood flow to tissues.
    d. continuously measure the arterial blood pressure.

15. Drug therapy that is indicated for the client in acute respiratory failure includes

    a. sedatives to reduce the work of breathing.
    b. prophylactic antibiotics to prevent respiratory infection.
    c. inhaled corticosteroids to relieve bronchospasm and inflammation.
    d. agents that relieve symptoms and reverse the underlying disease process.

16. In caring for a client in acute respiratory failure, the nurse recognizes that non-invasive positive pressure ventilation (NIPPV) may be indicated for a client who

    a. is comatose and has high oxygen requirements.
    b. has copious secretions that require frequent suctioning.
    c. responds to hourly bronchodilator nebulization treatments.
    d. is alert and cooperative but has increasing respiratory exhaustion.

17. Although acute respiratory distress syndrome (ARDS) may result from direct lung injury or indirect lung injury as a result of systemic inflammatory response syndrome (SIRS), the nurse is aware that ARDS is most likely to occur in the client with a host insult resulting from

    a. septic shock.
    b. oxygen toxicity.
    c. multiple trauma.
    d. prolonged hypotension.

18. Identify the three primary changes that occur in the injury or exudative phase of ARDS.

    a.

    b.

    c.

19. Clients with ARDS who survive the acute phase of lung injury and who progress to the fibrotic stage manifest

    a. chronic pulmonary edema and atelectasis.
    b. resolution of edema and healing of lung tissue.
    c. continued hypoxemia because of diffusion limitation.
    d. increased lung compliance due to breakdown of fibrotic tissue.

20. In caring for the client with ARDS, the most characteristic sign the nurse would expect the client to exhibit is

    a. refractory hypoxemia.
    b. bronchial breath sounds.
    c. progressive hypercapnia.
    d. increased pulmonary artery wedge pressure.

21. The nurse suspects the early stage of ARDS in any seriously ill client who

    a. develops respiratory acidosis.
    b. has diffuse crackles and rhonchi.
    c. exhibits dyspnea and restlessness.
    d. has a decreased $PaO_2$ and an increased $PaCO_2$.

22. A client with ARDS has a nursing diagnosis of risk for infection. To detect the presence of infections commonly associated with ARDS, the nurse monitors

    a. gastric aspirate for pH and blood.
    b. the quality, quantity, and consistency of sputum.
    c. for subcutaneous emphysema of the face, neck, and chest.
    d. the mucous membranes of the oral cavity for open lesions.

23. The best client response to treatment of ARDS occurs when initial management includes

    a. treatment of the underlying condition.
    b. administration of prophylactic antibiotics.
    c. treatment with diuretics and mild fluid restriction.
    d. endotracheal intubation and mechanical ventilation.

24. When mechanical ventilation is used for the client with ARDS, positive end-expiratory pressure (PEEP) is often applied to

    a. prevent alveolar collapse and open up collapsed alveoli.
    b. permit smaller tidal volumes with permissive hypercapnia.
    c. promote complete emptying of the lungs during exhalation.
    d. permit extracorporeal oxygenation and carbon dioxide removal outside the body.

25. The nurse suspects that a client receiving PEEP is experiencing negative effects of this ventilatory manoeuvre upon finding a(n)

    a. increasing $PaO_2$.
    b. decreasing heart rate.
    c. decreasing blood pressure.
    d. increasing central venous pressure (CVP).

26. Prone positioning is considered for a client with ARDS who has not responded to other measures to increase $PaO_2$. The nurse knows that this strategy

    a. increases the mobilization of pulmonary secretions.
    b. decreases the workload of the diaphragm and intercostal muscles.
    c. promotes opening of atelectatic alveoli in the upper portion of the lung.
    d. promotes perfusion of non-atelectatic alveoli in the anterior portion of the lung.

## CASE STUDY

### ACUTE RESPIRATORY FAILURE

### Client Profile

Mrs. C. is a 75-year-old married woman with severe oxygen- and corticosteroid-dependent COPD. She is admitted to the MICU with acute respiratory failure and pneumonia.

### Subjective Data

- Complains of shortness of breath and difficulty breathing

### Objective Data

- ABGs on 2 L oxygen/min: pH 7.3, $PaCO_2$ 55 mm Hg, $PaO_2$ 60 mm Hg, $SaO_2$ 84%
- Awake, alert, and oriented
- Sitting in tripod position and using pursed-lip breathing

### Collaborative Care

- $O_2$ at 2 L/min per NIPPV
- Albuterol (Ventolin, Proventil) nebulization q1h prn
- IV aminophylline
- IV antibiotics
- IV corticosteroids

**Critical Thinking Questions**

1. What type of respiratory failure is Mrs. C. primarily experiencing? Briefly describe how this situation illustrates the concept of acute on chronic respiratory failure.

2. What factors contributed to the development of respiratory failure in Mrs. C.?

3. What are the pathophysiological effects and clinical manifestations of Mrs. C.'s respiratory failure?

4. How do the tripod position and pursed-lip breathing contribute to respiratory function?

5. What is NIPPV? When is it contraindicated?

6. Which of the treatments instituted for Mrs. C. is the most important in returning her to her usual level of respiratory function?

7. Based on the assessment data presented, write one or more appropriate nursing diagnoses. Are there any collaborative problems?

1. Triage the following client situations that may be present in an emergency department as Level I—Resuscitation, Level II—Emergent, Level III—Urgent, Level IV—Less Urgent, or Level V—Non-urgent.

_____ a. A three-year-old child with a temperature of 39.6°C (103.2°F) who looks unwell. He has not had anything to eat or drink in 24 hours. He is flushed and agitated. Vitals: HR 130, BP110, RR 35.

_____ b. A 22-year-old woman with asthma in acute respiratory distress. She is demonstrating increased work of breathing, is speaking in short sentences, and has an $SpO_2$ of 90%.

_____ c. A 32-year-old man who complains of a constant earache with a pain of 4/10 and has stable vital signs.

_____ d. A 50-year-old man with low back pain and spasms. His pain is chronic in nature and he rates the pain as a 4/10.

_____ e. A 32-year-old woman who is unconscious following an automobile accident. Her GCS is 4.

_____ f. A 58-year-old man with midsternal chest pain that radiates to his jaw. He appears diaphoretic and rates the pain as an 8/10.

_____ g. A teenager with an angulated forearm following a sports injury. His vitals are stable and he reports his pain to be an 8/10. His neurovascular assessment reveals no circulatory compromise.

2. The nurse performing a primary survey in the emergency department is assessing

a. the acuity of the client's condition to determine priority of care.
b. the status of airway, breathing, circulation, or presence of deformity.
c. whether the client is responsive enough to provide needed information.
d. whether the resources of the emergency department are adequate to treat the client.

3. Identify two life-threatening conditions that the nurse may identify during each step of the primary survey and one appropriate intervention that may be performed during the assessment.

|  | **Conditions** | **Interventions** |
|---|---|---|
| A |  |  |
| B |  |  |
| C |  |  |
| D |  |  |

4. During the secondary survey of a trauma client in the emergency department, it is important that the nurse obtain details of the incident primarily because

a. the mechanism of injury can indicate specific injuries.
b. important facts may be forgotten when needed later for legal actions.
c. alcohol use associated with many accidents can affect treatment of injuries.
d. many types of accidents or trauma must be reported to government agencies.

5. Identify the five interventions that are performed during the "F" step of the secondary survey.

   a.

   b.

   c.

   d.

   e.

6. Placement of a nasogastric tube is contraindicated during emergency care when the client has a possible

   a. inhalation injury.
   b. basilar skull fracture.
   c. cervical spine fracture.
   d. intra-abdominal bleed.

7. In assessing the emergency client's health history, what information is obtained with the use of the mnemonic AMPLE?

   a. A

   b. M

   c. P

   d. L

   e. E

8. A trauma client has open wounds, and the nurse questions the client regarding her tetanus immunization status. Tetanus immunoglobulin would be administered if the client has

   a. had only three doses of tetanus toxoid.
   b. had fewer than three doses of tetanus toxoid.
   c. not had a dose of tetanus toxoid in the past five years.
   d. not had a dose of tetanus toxoid in the past 10 years.

9. Following the death in the emergency department of a 36-year-old man from a massive head injury, it would be appropriate for the nurse to

   a. ask the family members whether they have ever considered organ donation.
   b. notify an organ procurement agency that a death has occurred that could lead to organ donation.
   c. explain to the family what a generous act it would be to donate the client's organs to another who needs them.
   d. ask the family to check the client's driver's licence to determine whether he had designated approval of donation of his organs in case of death.

10. Match the heat-related emergencies with their characteristics (answers may be used more than once).

    _____  a. Rectal temperature of 40°C (103.6°F)

    _____  b. Treated with rapid cooling methods

    _____  c. Related to salt deficiency following
            heavy work without taking adequate fluids

    _____  d. High risk of mortality and morbidity

    _____  e. Volume and electrolyte depletion

    _____  f. Elevated core temperature without sweating

    _____  g. Associated with prolonged standing and heat
            exposure

    _____  h. Oxygen administration necessary

    _____  i. Causes mild confusion, headache, and dilation
            of pupils

    _____  j. Extremity swelling is only symptom

1. Heat edema

2. Heat cramps

3. Heat syncope

4. Heat exhaustion

5. Heat stroke

11. During rewarming of a client's toes that have suffered deep frostbite, the nurse

    a. applies sterile dressings to blisters.
    b. places the feet in a cool water bath.
    c. ensures that analgesics are administered.
    d. massages the digits to increase circulation.

12. A client is brought to the emergency department following a skiing accident in which he was not found for several hours. He is unconscious and has a slowed respiratory and heart rate. His core temperature is 32°C (89.6°F). During the initial assessment of the client, the nurse should

    a. avoid moving the client as much as possible.
    b. initiate active core rewarming interventions.
    c. monitor the core temperature via the axillary route.
    d. expose the client to check for areas of frostbite and other injuries.

13. A homeless man is brought to the emergency department in severe hypothermia with a temperature of 29.4°C (85°F). On initial assessment, the nurse would expect to find

    a. shivering and lethargy.
    b. fixed and dilated pupils.
    c. respirations of 10 per minute.
    d. hyperactive reflexes.

14. Indicate whether each of the following conditions occur with freshwater near-drowning (F), saltwater near-drowning (S), or both (B).

   _____  a. Hypervolemia

   _____  b. Pulmonary edema

   _____  c. Hemoconcentration

   _____  d. Destruction of surfactant

   _____  e. Hypovolemia

   _____  f. Metabolic acidosis

15. The priority of management of the near-drowning client is

   a. correction of hypoxia.
   b. correction of acidosis.
   c. maintenance of fluid balance.
   d. prevention of cerebral edema.

16. A client is admitted to the emergency department following a snakebite to the dorsal aspect of the hand. A nursing intervention that is appropriate for the client is

   a. application of ice.
   b. elevation of the extremity.
   c. application of a tourniquet.
   d. removal of rings and watches.

17. The ascending paralysis caused by exposure to the dog tick may cause respiratory arrest unless

   a. the tick is removed.
   b. antibiotics are administered.
   c. an antidote for the neurotoxin is administered.
   d. hemodialysis is instituted to remove the neurotoxin.

18. Identify whether the following statements are true or false. If a statement is false, correct the bold word(s) to make the statement true.

   _____  a. The type of bite that carries the highest risk of infection is a **cat** bite.

   _____  b. Rabies vaccination is always indicated when a bite is caused by a **carnivorous wild animal**.

   _____  c. Emergency management of surface exposure to most toxins is **application of topical steroids**.

   _____  d. Treatment of ingested toxic alkali substances includes administration of **activated charcoal**.

   _____  e. A systemic response to a **brown recluse spider** bite may cause hemolysis leading to renal failure and death.

19. For the following ingested poisons, identify all those for which gastric lavage is contraindicated.

_____    a. Aspirin

_____    b. Cyanide

_____    c. Iron

_____    d. Bleach

_____    e. Acetaminophen

_____    f. Drain cleaner

20. Match the following poisons with the related treatment.

_____    a. Acetaminophen                    1. Immediate dilution with milk

_____    b. Acid                             2. Serum alkalization

_____    c. Iron                             3. N-acetylcysteine

_____    d. Tricyclic antidepressants        4. Chelation therapy

21. In the following table, check the columns that apply to each of the biological agents of terrorism.

| Agent | Bacterial | Viral | Person-to-Person Spread | Antibiotic Treatment | Active Vaccine | Passive Vaccine |
|-------|-----------|-------|--------------------------|----------------------|----------------|-----------------|
| Botulism | | | | | | |
| Anthrax | | | | | | |
| Plague | | | | | | |
| Hemorrhagic Fever | | | | | | |
| Tularemia | | | | | | |
| Small pox | | | | | | |

22. Match the following biological agents of terrorism with their characteristics (answers may be used more than once).

| | | |
|---|---|---|
| _____ | a. Ebola is a highly lethal type of this disease | 1. Botulism |
| _____ | b. The septicemic form is the most lethal | 2. Anthrax |
| _____ | c. Toxins cause hemorrhage and destruction of lung tissue | 3. Small pox |
| | | 4. Plague |
| _____ | d. Neurotoxins that cause paralysis and respiratory failure | 5. Tularemia |
| _____ | e. Spread by flea bites | 6. Hemorrhagic fever |
| _____ | f. Hemorrhage of tissues with organ failure | |
| _____ | g. Lesions are pustular vesicles | |
| _____ | h. Skin lesions are most common form | |
| _____ | i. Only agent without preventive or active treatment | |
| _____ | j. Primarily an infection of rabbits | |
| _____ | k. People under the age of 35 are the most vulnerable population | |
| _____ | l. Death may occur within 24 hours of exposure | |

## CASE STUDY

### HEAT STROKE

**Client Profile**

Mr. M., age 72, was taking a short break from nailing new shingles on his roof during the summer when he lost consciousness and collapsed in his yard. He was brought by ambulance to the emergency department, accompanied by his wife.

**Subjective Data**

- Wife states he has been working all week on the roof, even though he has not felt well the last day or two

**Objective Data**

- Vital signs: T 41.4°C (106.6°F), HR 124 and weak and thready, RR 36 and shallow, BP 82/40
- Skin hot, dry, and pale

## Critical Thinking Questions

1. What factors in Mr. M.'s history place him at risk for heat stroke?

2. What laboratory tests would the nurse anticipate to be ordered, and what alterations in these tests would be indications of heat stroke?

3. How would cooling for Mr. M. be carried out?

4. What supportive treatment is indicated for Mr. M.?

5. What should Mrs. M. be told about Mr. M.'s condition?

6. Based on the assessment data presented, write one or more appropriate nursing diagnoses. Are there any collaborative problems?

# ANSWERS TO WORKSHEETS

## CHAPTER I

1. a, c, d, f
2. fear, anxiety, pain, impaired physical mobility of arm, disturbed body image, ineffective role performance, anticipatory grieving
3. c. Rationale: Although evidence-based practice (EBP) uses results of research to improve quality and outcomes of health care, research utilization is not the only component of EBP. Research results are summarized into a single conclusion about the state of practice, and then it is translated into a clinical practice guideline for implementation based on the practitioner's expertise and the client's unique circumstances.
4. c. Rationale: The classification of nursing interventions (NIC) and outcomes (NOC) provides a standardized language that describes outcomes that are responsive to nursing intervention and interventions that are appropriate for nursing diagnoses. The nurse individualizes care for a specific client by selecting outcomes and interventions based on individual client assessment and nursing diagnoses. Nursing diagnosis classified by NANDA is the language that is used to identify client problems that are the specific domain of nursing practice.
5. a. North American Nursing Diagnosis Association (NANDA); b. Nursing Outcomes Classification (NOC); c. Nursing Intervention Classification (NIC)
6. a. 2; b. 3; c. 4; d. 1; e. 2; f. 5; g. 3; h. 2; i. 5; j. 4
7. a. independent: assessment of physical and psychological status, evaluation of response to medications, and dietary teaching
   b. collaborative: communication with physician regarding assessment findings and laboratory results and communication with dietitian about dietary order and client status
   c. dependent: administration of medication
8. a. I; A need is not a nursing diagnosis; b. I; Traction is not a treatable condition; c. I; Dyspnea is a symptom of activity intolerance, not the cause; d. C; e. I; Surgery is a medical pathological situation that cannot be treated by nursing; f. C; g. I; Bowel obstruction is a medical pathological situation; h. I; Cardiac monitoring is equipment, not a nursing diagnosis.
9. a. CP; b. ND; c. ND; d. CP; e. ND; f. ND; g. ND; h. CP; i. ND; j. CP
10. Activity intolerance related to prolonged bed rest as manifested by shortness of breath on exertion, weakness and fatigue, failure of pulse to return to preactivity level after three minutes.
11. a. Life-threatening problems; b. Maslow's hierarchy of needs; c. Client's perception of importance; d. Identification of nursing diagnoses that may be managed simultaneously
12. For anorexia, nursing measures would include mouth care, odour control, presentation of foods, offering of favourite foods, etc. These measures are very different from those for difficulty swallowing, which would include checking gag reflex, positioning, offering small bites of formed foods, avoiding free liquids in the mouth, etc. The differences show how important it is to determine the correct etiology of a nursing diagnosis.
13. a. I; not measurable, behavioural, nor does it ensure he will take medications; b. C; c. I; not measurable, no criteria, no time designation; d. I; not measurable, not behavioural; e. C
14. There may be many correct answers. Examples include the following:
    a. Turn client every two hours using the following schedule: L side → back → R side → L side → back; inspect and document all at-risk areas for blanching and erythema at each position change.
    b. Provide 250 mL (8 oz) of fluids every two hours (even hours) while client is awake (prefers cold liquids); assist client to choose five fresh fruits or vegetables from menu each day.
15. a. The mistake was made during assessment when the nurse did not ask why the client had not taken her medication regularly and the appropriate etiology for the nursing diagnosis was not validated.
    b. The nursing diagnosis should be changed in this case to reflect an etiology of lack of financial resources, and nursing interventions would not be teaching about the medications but rather perhaps consulting with the physician regarding the use of generic medications or a change in prescription and perhaps providing the client with a list of discount drug sources. The client outcome would remain the same.
16. a. More efficient (selection rather than writing); b. Increased availability to all appropriate health-

care providers; c. Maintenance of client anonymity and confidentiality; d. Contributes to evidence-based practice by easy tracking of the effectiveness of nursing interventions

# CHAPTER 2

1. a. 5; b. 4; c. 7; d. 2; e. 9; f. 1; g. 6; h. 10; i. 3; j. 8
2. a. Learned through the processes of language acquisition and socialization; b. Shared by all members of the same cultural group; c. Adapted to specific conditions such as environmental factors; d. Dynamic and ever-changing
3. a. cultural knowledge; b. cultural awareness; c. cultural encounter; d. cultural skills
4. c. Rationale: Cultural competence is demonstrated by an awareness of traditional treatments that people of other cultures may use to treat illness. Southeast Asians and Hispanics may use cupping to treat a variety of disorders, and this procedure leaves bruising on the skin. The client may be reluctant to disclose traditional treatments upon direct questioning, and the nurse should not presume abuse before considering cultural factors. Only in rare instances would a disease leave perfectly round cup-sized bruises on the skin.
5. Examples may include any instances of the following:
   a. Clients may be late for appointments, skip appointments entirely, or delay seeing a healthcare provider because social events are more important.
   b. Lack of health insurance, limited financial resources, or illegal immigrant status may deter clients from using the healthcare system.
   c. Ethnic foods may be high in sodium and fat or low in calcium and protein. If dietary changes required by health problems are not made within the context of the client's normal diet, chances are high the client will not make the changes.
   d. Personal space zones are a strong cultural trait. A client may move closer to the nurse, causing a feeling of discomfort for the nurse, or if the nurse increases the personal space, the client may be offended.
   e. Religious beliefs or practices, faith in folk medicine, or negative experiences with culturally insensitive health care may delay or prevent clients from seeking health care.

6. b. Rationale: Traditional Aboriginal rituals may include healing ceremonies used in addition to conventional therapy to promote a balance of physical, spiritual, and emotional wholeness believed to be necessary for wellness. These rituals may or may not be part of formal religious beliefs and may positively alter the progression of physical illnesses.
7. b. Rationale: In some cultural groups, especially Asian, Hispanic, and Aboriginal, there is an emphasis on interdependence rather than independence. The nurse should be aware that in other cultures decisions for the client may be made by other family members or may be made collectively by the client and his/her family. All of the other options reflect insensitive assumptions that the client should make an autonomous decision.
8. b. Rationale: In the Arabic culture, male–female roles are strictly observed. A female should not be touched by a male other than her husband, nor should she be alone with another male. An Arabic woman would be very uncomfortable being cared for by a male nurse and might be put in the position of having to refuse the care.
9. cancer
10. a. beta-adrenergic blockers; b. atropine; c. antidepressants; d. antidysrhythmics; e. anti-seizure drugs; f. mydriatrics; g. others: analgesics, antianxiety agents
11. b. Rationale: *Susto* is a culture-bound syndrome also known as "fright sickness" that is a traumatic anxiety-depressive state resulting from a frightening experience. *Empacho* causes abdominal pain and cramping from food balls forming in the intestinal tract; ghost sickness causes nightmares, weakness, and a sense of suffocation; and *bilis*, brought on by strong anger, causes headaches, stomach disturbances, and loss of consciousness.
12. a. Rationale: Knowledge of cultural beliefs and behaviours can be used to determine the degree to which the client shares commonalities with a given culture, but the nurse must be careful not to stereotype the client, assuming that all members of a specific culture are alike and share the same values and beliefs. Individual differences always exist within a culture, and just as the nurse is an individual within a culture, so are clients unique individuals.

| 13. | **Aboriginal Client** | **Traditional Hispanic Client** |
|---|---|---|
| **Communication** | comfortable with silence; silence necessary for thinking; avoid direct eye contact and consider it disrespectful | expect eye contact from others but will not return direct gaze; comfortable with close personal space |
| **Illness factors** | family history of diabetes; less tolerance to alcohol; less pupillary dilation with mydriatrics; use of traditional healers | family history of diabetes; cancer of cervix, esophagus, gallbladder, stomach; less pupillary dilation with mydriatrics; intolerance to and side effects from antidepressants; use of traditional healers |
| **Culture-bound syndromes** | ghost sickness | *empacho*, *susto*, *bilis* or *colera*, *nervios* |

# CHAPTER 3

1. Yes. Although some of the information contained in the medical history may be useful to nursing, the medical history focuses on the diagnosis of clients' health problems, whereas the nursing history is used to gather data that will provide a health profile for comprehensive health care, including clients' potential and actual health problems and health promotion.

2. *Subjective:* short of breath; pain in chest upon breathing; coughing makes head hurt; aches all over. *Objective:* respiratory rate of 28; coughing yellow sputum; skin hot and moist; temperature 39°C (102.2°F).

3. Examples: Many answers could be correct. It is helpful to preface the question with the reason it is being asked.
   a. "Many clients taking drugs for hypertension have problems with sexual function. Have you experienced any problems?"
   b. "Alcohol may interact dangerously with drugs you may receive or may cause withdrawal problems in the hospital. Can you describe your recent alcohol intake?"
   c. "It is important to contact and treat others who may have the infection you do. Would you please tell me who you have been sexually intimate with in the last six weeks?"
   d. "Many people today use herbs or supplements for health reasons, but they may cause some interactions with medications. What types of herbs, vitamins, or supplements do you use?"

4. d. Rationale: Data are required regarding the immediate problem, but gathering additional information can be delayed. The client should not receive pain medication before pertinent information related to allergies or the nature of the problem is obtained. Questions that require brief answers do not elicit adequate information for a health profile. A friend or family member may not be present or adequately informed, and the client may not achieve a pain-free state.

5. c. Rationale: When a client describes a feeling, the nurse should ask about the factors surrounding the situation to clarify the etiology of the problem. An incorrect nursing diagnosis may be made if the statement is taken literally and if the meaning is not explored with the client. A sense of being "tired and wrung-out" does not necessarily indicate a need for rest or sleep, and there is no way to know that treatment will relieve the problem.

6. There may be many correct answers. Examples include the following:
   a. "Can you tell me how you are feeling?"
   b. "Describe your relationship with your wife."
   c. "Can you describe your experience with this illness?"
   d. "What is your usual activity during the day?"

7. a. 1; b. 10; c. 10; d. 8; e. 4; f. 4, 6; g. 2, 3; h. 6; i. 6; j. 6; k. 7; l. 5; m. 3, 9; n. 2; o. 4; p. 12; q. 11; r. 2; s. 10; t. 13

8. d. Rationale: Abnormal lung sounds are usually associated with chronic bronchitis, and their absence is a negative finding. Chest pain is a positive finding, and radiation is not expected in all chest pains. Elevated blood pressure in hypertension is a positive finding, and pupils that are equal and react to light and accommodation is a normal finding.

9. a. Rationale: The screening physical examination is performed for health surveillance and health maintenance purposes. A regional examination addressing specific problems would be performed for the other conditions.

10. a. 2; b. 2; c. 3; d. 2; e. 1; f. 4

11. d. Rationale: The usual sequence of physical assessment techniques is inspection, palpation, percussion, and auscultation. However, because palpation and percussion can alter bowel sounds, in abdominal assessment the sequence should be inspection, auscultation, percussion, and palpation.

12. b. Rationale: A nurse should use the same efficient sequence each examination to avoid forgetting a procedure, a step in the sequence, or a body part, but a specific method is not required. Client safety, comfort, and privacy are considerations but not the priorities. The nursing history data should be collected in an interview to avoid prolonging the examination.

13. *Across:* 6. sign in; 7. otitis; 8. atrium; 10. rash; 12. polyp; 14. uvula; 17. side; 19. ocular; 20. smooth; 21. inhale; 22. masses
*Down:* 1. arthro; 2. artery; 3. ossas; 4. in situ; 5. anemia; 9. thud; 11. apsa; 12. ptosis; 13. laughs; 15. venous; 16. little; 18. irsem

# CHAPTER 4

1. a. maintenance of health; b. management of illness; c. appropriate selection and use of treatment options; d. prevention of disease

2. a. adults approach learning as problem solving
   b. adults are independent learners; adults resist learning when conditions are incongruent with their self-concepts
   c. readiness to learn arises from life's changes; adults learn best when the topic is of immediate value
   d. adults approach learning as problem solving; adults see themselves as doers
   e. adults resist learning when conditions are incongruent with their self-concepts
   f. adults see themselves as doers
   g. past experiences are resources for learning

3. a. Rationale: During the action stage of behaviour change, the client may experience relapses, and the behaviour has not become sustained over a period of time. Walking to manage osteoporosis is a recommended lifetime behaviour, and the change is not in the maintenance stage until it is sustained without relapses. In the termination stage, the behaviour is part of the person's lifestyle and no longer considered a change.

4. a. Example: a sudden episode (acute) where the heart muscle (myocardium) is damaged from a lack of blood supply (infarction)
   b. Example: the intravenous (IV) injection of a dye to visually record (gram) the kidneys (pyelo)
   c. Example: damage (pathy) to the retina (retino) of the eye as a complication of diabetes

5. a. Rationale: An empathetic approach to teaching requires that the nurse discover and understand the world of the client and teach according to the client's needs. The other options are important but not directly related to empathy.

6. a. Rationale: According to the Family Support Model, no part of the system is an independent agent because the well-being of the individual depends on support from the family, community resources, and the medical care system. The support provided by the family unit has been shown to affect a client's health outcome, and thus teaching plans often include identified family members. Family members may not be responsible for continued care of the client, and if clients and families have different educational needs, the nurse addresses this in planning teaching.

7. b. Rationale: To promote self-efficacy, it is important that the person is successful in new endeavours to strengthen the belief in his/her ability to manage a situation. To avoid early failure, the nurse should work with the client to present simple concepts related to knowledge and skills the person already has. Motivation and relevance are important factors in adult learning but are more often a result of self-efficacy, not a method of promoting it.

8. a. Use supplementary illustrations and written materials; provide audiotapes or audiovisual presentations with headphones that block environmental noise and promote auditory function.
   b. Support the client during this time, and do not argue about the need for change in behaviour; wait until the client is ready to learn to begin teaching.
   c. Evaluate the medication schedule and change, if possible, to increase alertness; if sedation is the objective of the medication, consider teaching family members or other caregivers.
   d. Provide only brief explanations, and wait to present more detailed instruction until the pain has been controlled.
   e. Use anxiety-reducing interventions such as sitting with the client or listening to clients talk about their feelings and fears to decrease anxiety before attempting to teach; present non-threatening information first and allow time for gradual learning.
   f. Plan role-playing situations to allow clients to rehearse new behaviours; use peer groups to promote learning from those who have been in the same situation.

g. Provide small amounts of information repeated very frequently; if impairment is marked, it will be necessary to teach a caregiver as well as the client.

h. Set goals for teaching that are most important, and refer the client to a community agency for continued teaching and follow-up after discharge.

i. Be sure that educational materials are written at a grade 8 level; use audiovisual materials with simple, lay language.

j. Provide a variety of written educational materials; refer the client to appropriate Internet resources for information.

9. b. Rationale: The nursing diagnosis should specify the exact nature of the knowledge deficit so that the objectives, strategies, implementation, and evaluation relate to the identified problem. The problem is deficient knowledge, and a nursing diagnosis that states that the knowledge deficit is related to a lack of interest is in error. "Risk for cardiac arrhythmias" is a collaborative problem rather than a nursing diagnosis.

10. Example: The client (who) will select foods high in potassium (behaviour) from a given list of common foods (condition) with 90% accuracy (criterion).

11. d. Rationale: The learning objectives should be jointly developed by the client and the nurse, and once these have been identified, the nurse, the client, and the client's family should choose the strategies that are most beneficial to meet the objectives. This approach supports all interventions identified as successful to adult and client education.

12. a. 5;  b. 6;  c. 1;  d. 1;  e. 3;  f. 2;  g. 4;  h. 3; i. 7;  j. 5;  k. 7;  l. 6;  m. 8;  n. 7

13. c. Rationale: If audiovisual and written materials do not help the client meet the learning objectives, they are a waste of time and expense and the nurse should ensure that these materials are accurate and appropriate for each specific client. Audio and visual materials are often supplementary either before or after other presentation of information and do not need to include all the information the client needs to learn in order to be of value. Clients with auditory and visual limitations may find these materials useful because they can adjust volume and size of the images.

14. Example:
Action: This medicine, atorvastatin, keeps the liver from making so much cholesterol.
Uses: The medicine is used to lower cholesterol and fats in the blood. It helps prevent heart attacks and strokes.

Side Effects: Overall, this medicine does not cause many side effects. Stomach upset or intestinal gas may occur. Other effects can include liver and pancreas problems, skin rashes and itching, hair loss, muscle pain, eye changes, and headache. Call your doctor if these problems occur or get worse.
Precautions: Tell your doctor if you get any yellowing of your eyes or skin or have vomiting. Tell your doctor if you have had any liver disease in the past, alcoholism, low blood pressure, bad infections, seizure disorders, diabetes or thyroid problems, physical injuries, or blood imbalances. Drink very little or no alcohol because this can damage your liver and cause more side effects. If you have other effects not listed above, call your doctor.
Interactions: This medicine will interact with many other medicines to cause problems. Give your doctor a list of all medicines that you take. Do not start any new medicine while you are taking atorvastatin without checking with your doctor.

15. a. Direct observation
b. Ask direct question or use a written measurement tool (ask client to write the symptoms)
c. Direct observation with observation of verbal and non-verbal cues
d. Direct observation

16. b. Rationale: A statement that documents what the client does as a result of teaching indicates whether the learning objective has been met and provides the best documentation of client instruction. "Understand" is not a measurable behaviour and does not validate that learning has occurred. The content and strategies of client education are documented in the teaching plan and would not be repeated in charting related to the outcome of instruction.

## CHAPTER 5

1. There are many correct responses. Examples include the following:
a. Older people cannot learn new skills as well as younger people can ("can't teach an old dog new tricks").
b. Most old people are ill.
Also:
• Old people are not (or should not be) sexually active.
• Old people are terrible drivers.
• Forgetfulness is a sign of senility.

2. a. Rationale: The sense of a life well lived and acceptance of death is characteristic of Erikson's ego-integrity, which is in contrast to the despair

that may occur when life review reveals missed opportunities and wrong directions taken. According to Havighurst, if earlier developmental tasks are met, the work of the older adult is adjusting to declining health and social role changes. Peck's developmental tasks for the older adult include transcending the body, and self-esteem is maintained through the use of wisdom and judgement. In Levinson's theory of development, late adulthood is characterized by periods of change and growth toward personal goals and periods of stability to maintain the life structures necessary to pursue the goals.

3. a. 2;  b. 4;  c. 3;  d. 1;  e. 2;  f. 3;  g. 1
4. b. Rationale: Four characteristics that are common to all adult developmental models include development occurring throughout the lifespan; self-identity and growth through developmental tasks; movement through hierarchic stages from simplicity, rigidity, and narrowness to complexity, flexibility, and comprehensiveness; ultimate goal of achieving autonomy, separateness, and independence.
5. a. 6;  b. 4;  c. 1;  d. 7;  e. 3;  f. 8; g. 5;  h. 2
6. There may be other correct responses, but examples include the following:
   a. decreased intestinal villae; decreased digestive enzyme production and secretion; decreased dentine and gingival retraction; increased taste threshold for salt and sugar
   b. decreased force of cardiac contraction; decreased cardiac muscle mass; increased fat and collagen
   c. decreased skeletal muscle mass; increased joint flexion; stiffening of tendons and ligament; decreased cortical and trabecular bone; changes in eye and ear that impair vision and hearing
   d. decreased bladder smooth muscle and elastic tissue; decreased sphincter control
   e. decreased ciliary action; decreased respiratory muscle strength; decreased elastic recoil
   f. decreased collagen and subcutaneous fat; decreased sebaceous gland activity; decreased sensory receptors; increased tissue fluid; increased capillary fragility; decreased pigment cells
   g. decreased vessel elastin and smooth muscle; increased arterial rigidity; thickened ventrical wall
   h. decreased blood flow to colon; decreased intestinal motility; decreased sensation to defecation
7. c. Rationale: Age-associated memory impairment is characterized by a memory lapse or benign forgetfulness that is not the same as a decline in cognitive functioning. Forgetting a name, date, or recent event is not serious, but the other examples indicate abnormal functioning.

8. a. S—sadness (mood); b. C—cholesterol (high); c. A—albumin (low); d. L—loss (or gain of weight); e. E—eating problems; f. S—shopping (and preparation problems)
9. c. Rationale: Older adults tend to underreport symptoms and treat symptoms of illness by altering their level of daily function to compensate for the symptoms. Delirium may cause a decline in functional health status, but other symptoms are more prominent. A decline in functional health is not typical with asymptomatic pathology, nor is it directly related to the development of illness.
10. a. Preventing and managing crisis; carrying out prescribed regimens
    b. Preventing social isolation; attempting to normalize interactions with others
    c. Carrying out prescribed regimens; controlling symptoms
    d. Preventing social isolation; attempting to normalize interactions with others
    e. Preventing and managing crisis; reordering time; adjusting to changes in the course of the disease; attempting to normalize interactions with others
    f. Controlling symptoms; reordering time; adjusting to changes in the course of the disease
    g. Reordering time; preventing and managing crisis
11. d. Rationale: Older adults with an ethnic identity often have disproportionately low incomes and may not be able to afford medications to treat health problems. Although they often live in older urban neighbourhoods with extended families, they are not isolated. Ethnic diets have adequate nutrition, but health could be impaired if money is not available for food.
12. b. Rationale: During an initial contact with an older adult, the nurse should perform a comprehensive nursing assessment that includes a history using a functional health pattern format, physical assessment, assessment of ADLs and IADLs, mental status evaluation, and a social-environmental assessment. If available, a comprehensive interdisciplinary geriatric assessment may then be done to maintain and enhance the functional abilities of the older adult. The older adult and the caregiver should be interviewed separately, and the older adult should identify his/her own needs.
13. a. Rationale: The results of mental status evaluation often determine whether the client is able to manage independent living, a major issue in older adulthood. Other elements of comprehensive

assessment could determine eligibility for special services, determination of frailty, and total service and placement needs.

14. b. Rationale: For the older adult, new learning must relate to the client's actual experience to have meaning. Written instructions should supplement verbal explanations. Repetition is important, but it should not be excessive to the point of demeaning the client. Long-term memory is resistant to aging, and relating information to the client's experience is much more effective than reviewing basic concepts.

15. b. Rationale: An acute confusional state (delirium) is one of the most common consequences of unscheduled surgery because there is not enough time to physically stabilize or emotionally prepare the client. The risk for other surgical complications is also high in the older adult but not necessarily because the surgery is unscheduled.

16. a. Rationale: Exercise for all older adults is important to prevent deconditioning and subsequent functional decline from many different causes. Walkers and canes may improve mobility but can also decrease mobility if they are too difficult for the client to use. Nutrition is important for muscles, but muscle strength is primarily dependent on use. Risk appraisals are usually performed for specific health problems.

17. a. Rationale: When pain is a known complication of a particular condition, the nurse should offer pain medication at regular intervals in addition to assessing pain with verbal and visual pain scales. Older clients may not ask for pain medication because of cognitive impairment, age-related changes, or because they think pain should be endured. A pain diary can be used for chronic pain that interferes with ADLs and functional ability.

18. a. Absorption of enalapril may be more complete because of delayed gastric emptying and slowed gastrointestinal motility. However, less of the drug may be metabolized to active enalaprilat because of decreased liver function. The drug is not highly plasma protein-bound but decreases in serum albumin and total body water may make more active drug available. Decreased kidney function lengthens the half-life of the drug, prolonging its action. Overall, there is likely to be an increased effect of the drugs, with marked hypotension and development of side effects.

b. When digoxin is added to the regimen for the client, consideration must be made not only of the effect of digoxin but also of its possible interaction with enalapril. Digoxin toxicity is much more likely to occur in the older client because of increased absorption due to decreased GI motility and decreased kidney elimination. The half-life of digoxin may be much prolonged beyond the normally long 36 hours. Although digoxin is not highly plasma protein-bound, decreased serum albumin, decreased total body water, and competition between digoxin and enalapril for plasma proteins could increase the free (active) amount of both drugs.

c. The nurse should monitor the client's blood pressure and apical pulse for hypotension, bradycardia, or marked tachycardia before administration of the drugs, and because the digoxin has such a long half-life, vital signs should also be routinely monitored throughout the day. Periodic serum digoxin levels are also advised in the older adult because of the many physiological changes that can affect the drug's pharmacokinetics.

19. a. Emphasize medications that are essential, attempting to reduce medication usage that is not essential for minor symptoms.

b. Use a standard assessment tool to screen medication use that includes OTC medications, eye and ear medications, and alcohol as well as prescription drugs.

c. Monitor medication dosage strength; normally the strength should be 30%–50% less than that for a younger person.

d. Encourage the use of one pharmacy, and work with physicians and pharmacists to establish routine drug profiles on all older adult clients.

20. a. Psychological abuse and physical neglect; b. Caregiver role strain; c. Community caregiver support group; formal support system for respite care

21. The client may not be covered for the following aspects of care: home care, long-term institutionalized care, alternative healthcare providers, rehabilitation services, prescription drugs, nursing/custodial care; b. Adult day care programs

22. a. Rapid client deterioration; b. Caregiver exhaustion; c. Alteration in or loss of family support system

## CHAPTER 6

1. f. Rationale: Community health nurses do not routinely practise in the hospital setting.
2. e. Rationale: All are community health nursing roles.
3. The birth of public health nursing was influenced by twentieth-century scientific breakthroughs, including vaccinations, pasteurization, and the germ theory of disease and antisepsis. It was also influenced by the movement of people from rural areas to cities, which created the need for new attention to sanitation.
4. c.
5. a. Universal access to healthcare services on the basis of need
   b. Focus on the determinants of health as part of a commitment to health equity and social justice
   c. Active individual and community participation in decisions that affect people's health and life
   d. Partnership with other disciplines, communities, and sectors for health (intersectoral approach)
   e. Appropriate use of knowledge, skills, strategies, technology, and resources
   f. Focus on health promotion/illness prevention throughout the life experience from birth to death
6. 1. Socio-economic considerations (e.g., escalating healthcare system costs)
   2. Technology (e.g., digital camera, telemonitoring)
   3. Changing demographics (e.g., aging population)
   4. Nature and prevalence of illness (e.g., increase in rate of chronic disease)
   5. Increasing consumerism (e.g., increasing client involvement in health care)
7. e. Rationale: A home health care nurse may act as a case manager in some home care programs and would therefore do all the activities listed.
8. a. 6; b. 5; c. 4; d. 3; e. 2; f. 1.
9. f. Rationale: Both outpost/rural nurses and home health nurses primarily function in isolation from healthcare team members, must adapt to the surroundings in which care is given, and make independent decisions.
10. a   maintenance and preventive function. Rationale: The goal of care is to maintain the client at his optimal function and prevent deterioration.
    b. long-term care substitution function. Rationale: If the client were not receiving dialysis at home, he would require hospitalization.
    c. acute care substitution function. Rationale: Without the nursing care in the home, the client would need to remain in hospital.
    d. acute care substitution function. Rationale: Without the nursing care in the home, the client would need to be admitted to hospital.
    e. long–term care substitution function. Rationale: If the parents were not caring for the child at home, the child would require long-term care in an institution.
    f. maintenance and preventive function. The goal of care is to maintain the client at her optimal function and prevent deterioration.
11. f. Rationale:  All provinces and territories in Canada have some basic program of free home care, however, if the client's needs exceed the program service limits, the client/family may need to pay for the additional services.
12. d. Rationale: Hospice nursing is within the scope of home health nursing practice and is a philosophy that applies to any life-threatening illness, whether caused by cancer or other diseases such as end-stage renal failure or congestive heart failure.
13. Any of the following are appropriate:
    a. Caregiver role strain
    b. Interrupted family processes
    c. Self-care deficit
    d. Risk for injury
14. "guest in the house and the stranger in the family."
15. 1. Organizational skills
    2. Ability to make independent decisions
    3. Ability to set priorities and respond to problems promptly
    4. Ability to adapt care to fit a variety of circumstances
    5. Case management and time management skills
16. 1. Outline the unique contributions of community health nurses
    2. Serve as quality indicators
    3. Demonstrate the collective and individual practice accountability of community health nurses
17. Through a national credential (Canadian Community Health Nurse—certified) provided by the Canadian Nurses Association upon successful completion of the certification process.
18. It is important that the contribution nursing makes to the health outcomes of clients be measured and recognized.
19. a. Rationale: Client satisfaction and nurses' work life satisfaction have not been tested for their association with outcomes; therefore there is no empirical evidence to include them as nursing-sensitive outcomes.

## CHAPTER 7

1. a. 5, 12; b. 3, 18; c. 4, 8; d. 1, 6; e. 2, 17; f. 1, 11; g. 2, 16; h. 1, 7; i. 4, 19; j. 4, 10; k. 3, 13; l. 2, 9; m. 2, 15; n. 1, 14

2. a. F;  b. F;  c. T;  d. T

3. b. Rationale: Complementary and alternative therapies are harmonious with the values of nursing that include a view of humans as holistic beings, an emphasis on healing and partnership relationships with clients, and a focus on health promotion and illness prevention. CAM is not inexpensive, nor is it without adverse or even validated therapeutic effects.

4. a. Rationale: The basic concept of disease in Chinese medicine is that the opposing phenomena of yin and yang are out of balance, and this imbalance alters the movement of the vital energy of the body, known as Qi, that influences physiological functions of the body. Acupoints are holes in the Qi meridians where the flow of Qi can be influenced but not released. Health phenomena are organized according to the five elements, but these are not directly a cause of illness.

5. b. Rationale: Acupuncture is used to regulate the flow of Qi with the insertion of needles at acupoints, areas where needles may be inserted to unblock obstruction of energy and re-establish the flow of Qi. Counterirritation and inflammation are not consistent with the theory of Qi, and although electrical stimulation may be applied to the needles in electroacupuncture, this procedure releases neuropeptides within the central nervous system.

6. b. Rationale: Complications from acupuncture are rare, but if they occur, they are most often related to infections from the use of contaminated, non-sterile needles. The other complications may occur but are not as frequent as infections or transmission of infection from one client to another.

7. a. meditation; b. relaxation; c. imagery

8. c. Rationale: The ultimate goal of biofeedback is to teach clients to control normally involuntary physiological responses. The process involves measurement of physiological responses to provide information to persons about their neuromuscular and autonomic nervous system activity and demonstrate the effect of stress relaxation behaviours so that clients can control the physiological functions.

9. b. Clinical studies have indicated that acupuncture is clearly effective in treating adult postoperative and chemotherapy-associated nausea and vomiting, as well as post-operative dental pain. Rolfing is used to improve musculoskeletal movement and alignment, aromatherapy uses essential plant oils to promote and maintain overall health, and electromagnetic therapy is useful for relieving pain and promoting tissue healing.

10. a. Rationale: Clients who are sensitive to energy repatterning, such as premature infants, newborns, children, pregnant women, older people, and those in critical, unstable conditions, should avoid therapeutic touch. It has been reported to promote wound healing and sleep and enhance immune function.

11. d. Rationale: Chiropractic therapy holds that structural distortions of the vertebrae can lead to organ dysfunction and pain anywhere in the body, and as such, chiropractic manipulation is used to treat not only musculoskeletal abnormalities but also a variety of health problems, including dysmenorrhea. Generally, chiropractic practice does not include drug therapy.

12. a. Rationale: Although herbal remedies have been shown to provide beneficial effects for a variety of conditions, interactions with prescription drugs have been described. People do not tend to communicate their use of herbal remedies, and herb-drug interactions are often underreported. Herbs, indeed, can be toxic and are contraindicated or should be used with caution in certain persons.

13. b. Rationale: To serve as a resource for clients regarding complementary and alternative therapies, nurses must first develop their own knowledge base. To teach clients about their use, monitor for adverse effects and interactions with conventional therapies, and assist clients to use the therapies knowledgeably and safely, nurses themselves must be informed.

14. *Down:* 1. kava; 2. evening primrose; 4. comfrey; 5. valerian; 7. DHEA; 8. black cohosh; 11. saw palmetto; 13. aloe; 14. ginseng
*Across:* 3. angelica; 6. chamomile; 9. ginseng; 10. bilberry; 12. feverfew; 13. angelica; 15. St. John's wort; 16. ginkgo biloba

## CHAPTER 8

1. a. R—Selye; b. S—Holmes, Rahe, Masuda; c. T—Lazarus and Folkman; d. R—Selye; e. S—Holmes, Rahe, Masuda

2. stage of resistance

3. stage of exhaustion

4. Use Table 8-2 in the text to calculate your personal score and determine your illness risk.

5. b. Rationale: Daily hassles are experiences and conditions of daily living that have been appraised as being harmful or threatening to a

person's well-being. These are counteracted by uplifts, positive everyday experiences. Threat demands and challenge demands are concepts of the stress-as-transaction theory, and the concept of sense of coherence is a personality characteristic or coping style that is a powerful mediator of stress and illness.

6. c. Rationale: An individual with a sense of coherence is likely to perceive the illness experience as structured and predictable and as a challenge

worthy of investment. Information regarding the nature of the illness would be a resource the client would seek to meet the demand of the illness.

7. a. Stimulus: diabetes mellitus
   b. Primary appraisal outcome: stressful demand
   c. Type of demand: harm or loss
   d. Secondary appraisal outcome: using resources to learn about the disease and planning management of the disease

8.

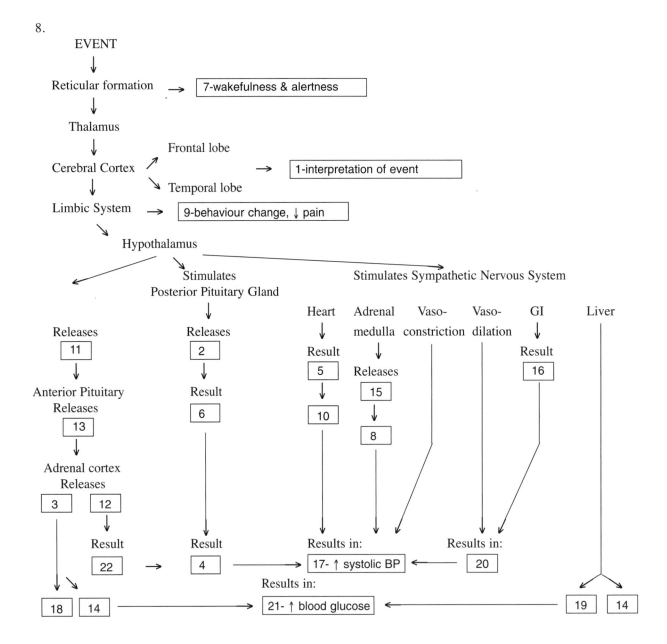

**Word and Phrase List**

1. interpretation of event, fear
2. ↑ ADH
3. cortisol
4. ↑ blood volume
5. ↑ HR and stroke volume
6. ↑ water retention
7. wakefulness and alertness, reabsorption
8. ↑ sympathetic response
9. behaviour change, ↑ pain perception
10. ↑ cardiac output
11. corticotropin-releasing hormone
12. aldosterone
13. ACTH
14. ↑ gluconeogenesis
15. ↑ epinephrine and norepinephrine
16. ↓ digestion
17. ↑ systolic blood pressure
18. ↓ inflammatory response
19. glycogenolysis
20. ↑ blood to vital organs and large muscles
21. ↑ blood glucose
22. ↑ Na and $H_2O$ reabsorption

9. 

| Objective Manifestations: | Subjective Findings: |
|---|---|
| Increased heart rate | Anxiety, fear |
| Increased blood pressure | Decreased perception of pain |
| Cool, clammy skin | |
| Decreased bowel sounds | Verbalization of stress |
| Hyperglycemia | |
| Decreased lymphocytes | Wakefulness, restlessness |
| Decreased eosinophils | |
| Decreased urinary output | |

10. a, c, e, f, g
11. c. Rationale: Allostasis refers to the mechanisms by which the body re-establishes homeostasis in the face of a challenge and includes many of the same physiological responses that occur with any stress. If these allostatic (physiological) responses do not terminate when they are no longer needed, or when stress occurs too frequently, the effects on the body create an allostatic load. Allostatic load is manifested by hypertension, salt and water retention, atherosclerosis, abdominal obesity, and other physical problems.
12. *Problem-focused:*
    - Attending cardiac rehabilitation program
    - Planning dietary changes
    - Starting an exercise program
    - Learning about medications
    *Emotion-focused:*
    - Sharing feelings with spouse or other family members
    - Using meditation
    - Setting aside private time
    - Doing favourite escape activities

13. a. Demands: Assessing the type, number, and duration of demands and prior experience with the demands; a specific assessment guide may be used for particular types of clients.
    b. Response to stress: Noting physiological effects and the presence of diseases of adaptation; also observing behavioural and cognitive responses of the client and significant others
    c. Coping: Assessing the client's evaluation of coping resources and options and evaluating the use and effectiveness of problem-focused and emotion-focused coping efforts
14. c. Rationale: The coping behaviour described is not adaptive, and the client tells the nurse that she does not have the resources to cope with the demands of her illness. There is no evidence that emotional bonds with her family are disrupted, and her behaviour does not match definitions of ineffective denial or impaired adjustment.
15. a. Sleeping regularly seven to eight hours per night
    b. Eating breakfast
    c. Eating regular meals with minimal or no snacking
    d. Eating moderately to maintain an ideal weight
    e. Exercising moderately
    f. Enjoying recreational and relaxing activities with friends
    g. Drinking alcohol in moderation or not at all
    h. Not smoking (best if have never smoked)
    i. Learning to successfully handle life's stressors and hassles

**Case Study**

1. Physiological: fever, pain, anemia, the inflammatory disease itself
   Psychological: no income, the duration and chronicity of the disease, frequent hospital admissions, lack of social support systems
   Effects: Prolonged healing of illness, progression of the inflammatory disease
2. Her refusal to seek support from boyfriend
   Her depression, weakness
   Her experience with the illness and hospitalizations
   Her lack of financial resources
3. Increased weight, hemoglobin and hematocrit, strength
   Decreased body temperature, number of stools
4. One approach may be using a hospital stress rating scale to clarify the client's perception of the situation. The nurse and the client may not rate the stressors the same in intensity. Specific questions may include the following:

"What is the most stressful thing to you about being in the hospital?"

"Can you tell me what having this illness means to you?"

5. Reduce additional stressors, such as sleep deprivation, environmental stimuli

   Set short-term outcomes to achieve success

   Provide pain relief, measures for comfort, rest

   Provide stress-reducing interventions, such as relaxation and guided imagery

6. *Nursing diagnoses:*
   - Ineffective coping related to inadequate resources as manifested by crying, depression
   - Ineffective role performance related to lack of employment
   - Acute pain related to inflammatory process
   - Risk for impaired skin integrity related to frequent stools and emaciation
   - Imbalanced nutrition: less than body requirements related to nausea and frequent watery stools
   - Risk for deficient fluid volume related to frequent watery stools and low-grade fever

   *Collaborative problems:*

   Potential complications: fluid/electrolyte imbalances; intestinal obstruction; fistula/fissure/abscess

# CHAPTER 9

1. c. Rationale: Administering the smallest prescribed analgesic dose when given a choice is not consistent with current pain management guidelines and leads to inadequate pain control. Automatic and uncritical use of the smallest prescribed dose without clear rationale may result in unnecessary suffering, impaired recovery from acute illness, and increased morbidity as a result of respiratory dysfunction, increased heart rate and cardiac workload, and other physical dysfunction. Response to pain is highly variable, therefore careful pain assessment will help the nurse to determine the required dose of pain medication in consultation with the client and the prescribing physician or nurse practitioner (who may order the medication under medical directive in the acute setting).

2. e. Rationale: Initially, this definition raised awareness that the client's self-report is a valid means of pain assessment. However, this definition of pain is too simplistic as many clients need help and support to articulate their experience of pain. The current accepted definition of pain by the International Association for the Study of Pain is "An unpleasant sensory and emotional experience associated with actual or potential tissue or described in terms of such damage."

3. a. physiological—the transmission of nociceptive stimuli to the brain

   b. sensory—how the pain is perceived

   c. affective—the emotions related to the experience of pain

   d. behavioural—the behavioural responses to the pain

   e. cognitive—the beliefs, attitudes, and evaluations about the pain and approaches to pain management

4. a. 3; b. 2; c. 4; d. 4; e. 1; f. 3; g. 4

5. Information carried by large myelinated nerves, such as A-alpha and A-beta fibres, is communicated to the spinal cord faster than information carried by the smaller, slower primary afferent nociceptors (PANs) and may interfere with further transmission of PAN impulses.

6. b. Rationale: Although a peripheral nerve is one cell that carries an impulse directly from the periphery to the dorsal horn of the spinal cord with no synapses, the transmission of the impulse can be interrupted by activation of large fibres (A-beta) with modalties including ice, massage, and TENS. Drugs known as membrane stabilizers or sodium channel inhibitors, such as local anaesthetics and some anticonvulsants can interrupt excitatory nerve fibre neurotransmission at the synapse.

7. c. Rationale: Wide dynamic-range neurons in the dorsal horn of the spinal cord receive input from visceral and somatic structures via nociceptive fibres and A-beta fibres. The message transmitted to the brain from these neurons causes pain to be perceived as originating from the body part innervated by the A-beta fibre rather than from the primary afferent nociceptors. Enlargement of the receptive field of a peripheral neuron with increased response to noxious stimuli is known as *sensitization.*

8. b. Rationale: It is known that the brain is necessary for pain perception, but because it is not clearly understood where in the brain pain is perceived, pain may be perceived even in a comatose client who may not respond behaviourally to noxious stimuli. Any noxious stimulus should be treated as potentially painful.

9. c. Rationale: Modulation is primarily brought about by descending (efferent) fibres that release inhibitory neurotransmitters, such as serotonin, alpha-2 agonists, and opioids. Opioid receptors must be stimulated, not blocked, to change the transmission of nociceptive stimuli, and endorphins are not known to be released during the transduction step of pain.

10. d. Rationale: Limiting or adjusting daily physical activities to express or control pain is an example of the behavioural component of pain. The sensory component is recognition of the sensation as painful, the affective component refers to the emotional responses to pain, and the cognitive component refers to beliefs, attitudes, memories, and meaning attributed to the pain.

11. d. Rationale: Management of neuropathic pain often includes the use of opioids or tricyclic antidepressants to help inhibit pain transmission. Neuropathic pain can be acute, intense, and either short-lived or lingering. Aching and throbbing are more characteristic of nociceptive pain.

12. a. P—pattern: daily pain pattern graph; b. A—area: body outline, pain map; c. I—intensity: pain intensity scale (simple descriptive or 0-10 numeric); d. N—nature: verbal description list, McGill Pain Questionnaire/Brief Pain Inventory

13. a. Always believe the client
    b. Every client has the right to optimal pain management
    c. Base pain management on the client's goals
    d. Use a combination of pharmacological and non-pharmacological approaches to pain management
    e. Use a multidisciplinary approach
    f. Regularly evaluate the effectiveness of pain management strategies.
    g. Prevent, assess for, and manage medication side effects
    h. Always include client and family teaching

14. a. Rationale: Analgesics should be scheduled around the clock for clients with persistent pain to prevent pain from escalating and becoming difficult to relieve. If pain control is not adequate, the analgesic dose may be increased or an adjunctive drug may be added to the treatment plan for breakthrough pain.

15. c. Rationale: Although tolerance to many of the side effects of opioids (nausea, sedation, respiratory depression, pruritus) develops within days, tolerance to opioid-induced constipation does not occur. A bowel regimen that includes a gentle stimulant laxative and a stool softener should be started at the beginning of opioid therapy and continue as long as the drug is taken.

16. PCA use is decreased at night when the client sleeps, and without a continuous infusion of an analgesic, the client is likely to awaken in pain that will require substantial time to bring under control.

17. a. 3; b. 2; c. 1; d. 2; e. 2; f. 4; g. 1; h. 3; i. 2; j. 4

18. b. Rationale: The drug cannot be abruptly discontinued because if physical dependence has occurred, the client may exhibit symptoms of withdrawal such as agitation, anxiety, and flu-like symptoms. A usual practice is to reduce the dose by 50% over the course of one week. Drug tapering should be carried out by the nurse in consultation with the ordering physician, healthcare team, and client.

19. b. Rationale: When a client desires to be stoic about pain, it is important that he or she understands that this is his or her choice, but it is the nurse's responsibility to assess for and address any opioid-related fear, and to explain to the client that (a) pain itself can have harmful physiological effects, and (b) failure to report pain and participate in its control can result in severe unrelieved pain.

**Case Study**

1. Assess the location, quality, and specifics of the pattern of the pain and anything he finds notable about his past pain experiences. Also assess his prior medication use, past experience with opioids, and any addictions.

2. Affective: worried about worsening of disease, afraid of narcotics
   Behavioural: posturing, slow gait, stays in bed with severe pain
   Cognitive: uses emptying mind to block pain

3. The symptoms he has in the mornings are related to the short-acting nature of Percocet and the long interval during the night without an opioid. At this point, a long-acting opioid, such as Oxycontin, should be prescribed for sustained analgesic effect. The Percocet can then be administered as ordered for breakthrough pain.

4. Teach him to evaluate the dose required to control his pain, and see that he knows the range and frequency of his dose.

5. Explain that tolerance and physical dependence are expected with long-term opiate use and should not be confused with addiction. Addiction is a psychological condition characterized by a drive to obtain and take substances for other than their prescribed therapeutic purpose. Fewer than 0.1% of clients receiving analgesics become addicted.

6. Dermal stimulation, such as massage and pressure; additional cognitive and behaviourally based approaches such as relaxation, pacing, and imagery.

7. *Nursing diagnoses:*
   - Persistent pain related to cancer and inadequate pain management
   - Anxiety related to effects of disease process and inadequate pain-relief measures
   - Activity intolerance related to pain, fatigue

   *Collaborative problems:*

   Potential complications on new drug regimen: drug-induced constipation; pruritus; extreme nausea.

## CHAPTER 10

1. a. Rationale: The goals of end-of-life care are to provide comfort and supportive care during the dying process, improve the quality of the remaining life, and help ensure a dignified death. Grieving is a normal process and should be encouraged, but not all clients will progress through all stages of grieving in a systematic way.

2. a. 1) Cheyne-Stokes respiration
     2) noisy, wet-sounding respirations
     3) increased, then slowing respiratory rate
     Also: irregular breathing, terminal gasping
   b. 1) mottling on hands, feet, and legs that progresses to torso
     2) cold, clammy skin
     3) cyanosis on nose, nail beds, knees
     Also: wax-like skin when very near death
   c. 1) slowing of GI tract with accumulation of gas and abdominal distension
     2) loss of sphincter control with incontinence
     3) bowel movement prior to imminent death or at time of death
   d. 1) loss of muscle tone with sagging jaw
     2) difficulty speaking
     3) difficulty swallowing
     Also: gradual loss of ability to move or maintain body position; loss of gag reflex

3. b. Rationale: Hearing is often the last sense to disappear with declining consciousness, and conversations can distress clients even when they appear unresponsive. People should not say anything in front of an unresponsive client that they would not say if the person were alert.

4. a. coma
   b. absent brainstem reflexes
   c. apnea

5. a. Rationale: Photos are a reflection of important people and events in an individual's life and can be an effective method of reviewing one's life experiences. Peacefulness usually comes with healthy grief resolution of an acceptance of the reality of death. Saying goodbyes involves talking with others and verbalizing their feelings of sadness, loss, and forgiveness, while anxiety about unfinished business requires completion of tasks important to the individual.

6. b. Rationale: Bargaining is demonstrated by "if-then" grief behaviour, which is described by Kübler-Ross and corresponds to Rando's confrontation. Avoidance is Rando's description of denial and shock that occur early in the grief process, and Martocchio's anguish, disorganization, and despair corresponds to Kübler-Ross's depression. Reorganization and restoration is Martocchio's acceptance and accommodation phase of grieving.

7. a. 3; b. 6; c. 4; d. 5; e. 1; f. 2

8. a. Rationale: Spiritual distress may surface when an individual is faced with a terminal illness, and it is characterized by verbalization about inner conflicts about beliefs and questioning the meaning of one's own existence. Individuals in spiritual distress may be able to resolve the problem and die peacefully with effective grief work, but referral to spiritual leaders should be of the client's choice.

9. a. living will
   b. Power of Attorney for Personal Care
   c. DNR (Do Not Resuscitate)
   d. advance directives

10. b. Rationale: The Canadian Hospice Palliative Care Association defines palliative care as the combination of active and compassionate therapies intended to comfort and support individuals and families who are living with life-threatening illness. The terms *palliative care* and *hospice* are frequently used interchangeably.

11. b. Rationale: The hospice philosophy is to enhance the remaining time for the person who is terminally ill and provide support for the client and family. Hospice care is usually provided at home, although in-patient care in a free-standing hospice or palliative care unit may be needed for acute symptom management or respite care for families in need of a break. Pain control and client self-determination are important issues for terminally ill clients, not only those referred to a hospice program.

12. d. Rationale: In assisting clients with dying, end-of-life care promotes the grieving process, which involves saying goodbye. Physical care is very important for physical comfort, but assessments should be limited to essential data related to the client's symptoms. Analgesics should be administered for pain, but clients who are sedated cannot participate in the grieving process.

**Case Study**

1. Additional assessment data should include Mr. and Mrs. J.'s reasons for not discussing her illness and impending death with their children, an assessment of their spiritual needs, what decisions, if any, they have made about where and how Mrs. J. prefers to die, and what resources they have used or could use to assist them through the dying process. In addition, assessment and evaluation of their coping skills is necessary. A functional assessment of Mrs. J.'s ADLs should also be made.

2. Maladaptive or dysfunctional grief is demonstrated in this family. Mrs. J. appears to have some degree of acceptance of her impending death but feels rejected by her children. The children may be experiencing fear, guilt, anger, powerlessness, and other emotions that they cope with by withdrawing from the family. Mr. J. is also feeling guilt at wishing the ordeal were over. Healthy grieving is blocked in this family because communication has not occurred.

3. Pain needs to be assessed on an ongoing basis and medications titrated to provide pain relief that is acceptable to Mrs. J. without unnecessary sedation. A short-acting opioid needs to be available for breakthrough pain. Institute complementary therapies to enhance the effect of pain medication. As opioids are increased, constipation and abdominal distension could become a problem, and stool softeners and laxatives will likely need to be used. Although she is underweight, clients tend to take in less food and fluid as death approaches, and maintaining food and fluid intake is not a high priority. Because she spends most of her time in bed and she is very thin, measures to prevent skin breakdown are essential. Oxygen therapy and positioning should be considered as a measure to relieve her shortness of breath.

4. Arrange for family meetings to discuss Mrs. J.'s condition and the feelings of the client and the family. The palliative care nurse or a grief counsellor can help all members of the family express and acknowledge feelings of anger, fear, or guilt. The client and family need to know that the grief reaction is normal, and they should be taught what to expect and how each individual's needs can be met as Mrs. J.'s death approaches.

5. A multidisciplinary team of nurses, physicians, pharmacists, physiotherapists, dietitians, nursing assistants, social workers, clergy, and volunteers is available to this family to provide care and support to the client and family.

6. *Nursing diagnoses:*
   - Compromised family coping related to inadequate coping mechanisms
   - Dysfunctional grieving related to blocked communication and guilt
   - Chronic pain related to ineffective pain management
   - Risk for impaired skin integrity related to immobility and emaciation
   - Risk for constipation related to decreased oral intake and effects of drugs
   - Ineffective breathing pattern related to weakness and disease process
   - Impaired physical mobility related to pain

# CHAPTER 11

1. a. 11; b. 6; c. 9; d. 1; e. 8; f. 2; g. 7; h. 10; i. 3; j. 4; k. 5

2. b. Rationale: Addictive drugs appear to increase the availability of dopamine in the mesolimbic system of the brain through several different methods. Opioids increase the firing rate of dopaminergic neurons, and cocaine decreases the reuptake of dopamine at synapses. Although other neurotransmitters are also increased, it appears that dopamine is responsible for the responses that lead to addiction.

3. a. Rationale: Tolerance results when the prolonged effect of an addictive drug reduces the responsiveness of dopamine receptors in the brain, and to even feel normal, the drug must be taken. To obtain the initial effects of the drug, larger and larger doses must be used.

4. c. Rationale: While all minority groups have a higher incidence of health problems associated with substance abuse, alcohol problems in Aboriginal persons are more than four times that of the general population.

5. **Nicotine/tobacco:**
   a. chronic obstructive pulmonary disease (COPD)
   b. cancers: lung, mouth, esophagus, larynx, stomach, bladder, pancreas
   others: vascular disease: coronary and peripheral; peptic ulcer disease
   **Cocaine and amphetamines:**
   a. cardiac arrhythmias, angina pectoris, myocardial infarction
   b. stroke
   others: pneumonia, nasal septum necrosis or perforation, sinusitis
   **Alcohol:**
   a. cirrhosis of liver
   b. pancreatitis, gastritis
   others: cancers: esophagus, stomach, head and neck, lung

**Cannabis:**
a. bronchitis, chronic sinusitis
b. memory impairment
others: impaired immune function, reproductive dysfunction

6. a. 3;  b. 1;  c. 4;  d. 1;  e. 3;  f. 2;  g. 1;  h. 2; i. 4;  j. 2

7. a. stimulant; sedative-hypnotic
   b. narcotic
   c. hallucinogens
   d. stimulant
   e. sedative-hypnotics
   f. narcotic; sedative-hypnotic

8. d. Rationale: Nicotine replacement contains the same nicotine as that in tobacco but with slower absorption. The nicotine will help prevent withdrawal symptoms as its use is gradually reduced. While the addiction is treated, the carcinogens and gases associated with tobacco smoke are eliminated.

9. a. 2;  b. 3;  c. 4;  d. 1;  e. 3;  f. 4;  g. 3

10. a. Rationale: Headache is a common symptom of caffeine withdrawal and often occurs in heavy caffeine users who are NPO for diagnostic tests and surgery. Nervousness, tremors, anxiety, and bronchial dilation are physiological effects of caffeine.

11. b. Rationale: Of the two patterns of abuse and dependence recognized with sedative-hypnotic drugs, the one most likely in this client is initial prescription use of the drug for treatment of anxiety or insomnia, with the client increasing the dose and frequency of use without medical advice or indication. It is unlikely that this client would have started a pattern with illegal sources.

12. a. gross tremors
    b. seizures
    c. hallucinations
    d. delirium tremens (DTs)

13. c. Rationale: Open-ended questions that indicate that substance use is normal or at least understandable are helpful in eliciting information from clients who are reluctant to disclose substance use.

14. b. Rationale: This behaviour is typical of ineffective denial—the client is unable to admit the impact of the disease/event on life patterns as manifested by minimizing symptoms or events and selectively integrating information and does not meet the definitions or defining characteristics of the other nursing diagnoses.

15. b. Rationale: Smoking is the single most preventable cause of death in this country, and most smokers start by the age of 16. If smoking in preadolescents and adolescents can be prevented, it is unlikely that they will start smoking at a later age. Health problems associated with smoking and future use of other addictive substances would be significantly reduced.

16. a. naloxone (Narcan) is given in case opioids are the cause of the CNS depression
    b. flumazenil (Romazicon) is given in case benzodiazepines are the cause of the CNS depression

17. a. Rationale: The knowledge of when the client last had alcohol intake will help the nurse anticipate the onset of withdrawal symptoms. In clients with alcohol tolerance, the amount of alcohol and the blood alcohol concentration do not reflect impairment as consistently as in the non-drinker. The type of alcohol ingested is not of importance because it is all alcohol in the body.

18. d. Rationale: An extreme autonomic nervous system response may be life-threatening and requires immediate intervention. A quiet room is recommended, but it should be well lit to prevent misinterpretation of the environment and visual hallucinations. Cessation of alcohol intake causes low blood alcohol levels leading to withdrawal symptoms, and fluids should be carefully administered to prevent arrhythmias. Clients should not be restrained if at all possible because injury and exhaustion may occur as clients struggle against restraint.

19. a. Anaesthesia requirements may be decreased as a result of cross-tolerance.
    b. IV alcohol may be used to avoid acute withdrawal and delirium tremens triggered by surgery and the cessation of alcohol consumption.
    c. Post-operative care will require close monitoring for signs of withdrawal and respiratory and cardiac problems.
    d. Increased pain medications may be needed post-operatively if the client is cross-tolerant to opiates.

20. a. Rationale: Because Wernicke's encephalopathy resulting from a thiamine deficiency is a possibility in chronic alcoholism, intravenous thiamine is often administered to intoxicated clients to prevent the development of Korsakoff's psychosis. Thiamine should be given before any glucose solutions because glucose may precipitate Wernicke's encephalopathy. Benzodiazepines may be used for sedation and to minimize withdrawal symptoms but would not be given before thiamine.

21. c. Rationale: This client is demonstrating behaviour characteristic of the precontemplation stage of behaviour change. During this stage, the nurse should help the client increase her awareness of the risks and problems related to alcohol use by

asking the client what she thinks could happen if the behaviour continues, providing evidence of the problem and offering factual information about the risks of the substance use.

22. d. Rationale: The elderly have the highest use of over-the-counter and prescription drugs, and simultaneous use of these drugs with alcohol is a major problem. Illegal drug use is minimal in the elderly except for long-term addicts.

## Case Study

1. Because there is a tendency among substance abusers to take a variety of drugs simultaneously or in a sequence to obtain specific effects, as shown by Mr. C.'s history, he should be assessed for his pattern of abuse. Regular alcohol use in addition to other drug use or the common use of cocaine in combination with heroin or phencyclidine hydrochloride could cause withdrawal symptoms and additional manifestations that would complicate his condition and direct his care. Information about all drugs he uses, including over-the-counter and prescription drugs, is necessary to avoid withdrawal syndromes, acute intoxication, overdose, or drug interactions that may be life-threatening.

2. The nurse should be aware that common behaviours that are likely to influence history taking from Mr. C. include manipulation, denial, avoidance, underreporting or minimizing substance abuse, giving inaccurate information, and inaccurate self-reporting. To obtain reliable information about Mr. C.'s drug abuse patterns, the nurse should first explain that information about his drug use is very important in order to monitor for and prevent serious effects of the drugs while he already very ill. Providing a need for the information and explaining how the information will be used may facilitate more honest responses by Mr. C. The nurse should question him without judgement about his pattern of abuse with open-ended questions, such as "How much or how often do you use alcohol?" or "Can you describe how you use cocaine with other drugs?"

3. Physical effects of drug use that provide clues to drug abuse include collapsed and scarred veins used to inject drugs, nasal septum and mucosa damage, brown or black sputum production, and wound abscesses and cellulitis.

4. Continuous monitoring of Mr. C.'s vital signs, cardiac activity, level of consciousness, respiratory status, temperature, fluid and electrolyte balance, liver function, and renal function is necessary. Complications of cocaine toxicity that may occur and be detected by monitoring include myocardial ischemia or infarction, congestive heart failure, cardiopulmonary arrest, rhabdomyolysis with acute renal failure, stroke, respiratory distress or arrest, seizures, agitated delirium and hallucinations, electrolyte imbalances, and fever. In severe intoxication, the client may progress rapidly through stages of stimulation and depression, which may result in death. Mr. C.'s use of cocaine with alcohol also increases his risk of liver injury and sudden death.

5. Assessment for neurological, cardiovascular, and respiratory problems as described above is a critical nursing intervention in the client with cocaine toxicity. In addition, the nurse should institute seizure precautions, provide airway management, keep open IV lines, administer medications aggressively as prescribed, and employ cardiac life support measures as indicated.
Nursing interventions that are indicated for Mr. C.'s anxiety, nervousness, and irritability include explaining procedures, using short, simple, clear statements in a calm manner; providing a safe, secure environment; decreasing environmental stimuli; reinforcing reality orientation; and encouraging participation in relaxation exercises if possible.

6. Engaging an individual who is addicted to cocaine in treatment is difficult because of the intense craving for the drug and a strong denial that cocaine is addicting or that the individual cannot control it. Motivational interviewing is indicated in even this initial encounter with Mr. C. The nurse should help Mr. C. increase his awareness of risks and problems related to his current behaviour and create doubt about the use of substances. Asking him what he thinks could happen if the behaviour is continued, pointing out the physical symptoms he is experiencing, and offering factual information about the risks of substance abuse are indicated. Often the only motivation for a client with a cocaine addiction to enter a treatment program is family threats, loss of job or professional license, legal action, or major health consequences, but a treatment program is indicated to provide him with new skills and an ability to deal with his addictive behaviour.

7. *Nursing diagnoses:*
   • Ineffective health maintenance
   • Disturbed thought processes
   • Ineffective denial
   • Ineffective coping
   *Collaborative problems:*
   Potential complications: cardiopulmonary arrest, seizures, sudden death, cerebrovascular accident, acute renal failure

# CHAPTER 12

1. a. 3;  b. 1;  c. 4;  d. 5;  e. 2;  f. 6
2. mechanical trauma, heat, microbial, natural substances
3. a. Kupffer cells—fixed; b. alveolar macrophages—fixed; c. microglial cells—fixed; d. monocytes—free; e. histiocytes—free; f. osteoclasts—fixed; g. macrophages—free and fixed
4. Mediators/physiological change:
   a. IL-1 released from mononuclear phagocytic cells and $PGE_2$ synthesis/increases hypothalamic thermostatic set point
   b. histamine, kinins, prostaglandins/vasodilation and hyperemia
   c. histamine, kinins, prostaglandins/increased capillary permeability and fluid shift to tissues
   d. release of chemotactic factors at site of injury/increased release of neutrophils and monocytes from bone marrow
5. d. Rationale: *A shift to the left* is the term that is used to describe the presence of immature, banded nuclei neutrophils in the blood in response to an increased demand for neutrophils during tissue injury. Monocytes are increased in leukocytosis but are mature cells.
6. c. Rationale: Chemotaxis involves the release of chemicals at the site of tissue injury that attract neutrophils and monocytes to the site of injury. The attraction is chemotaxis, and when monocytes move from the blood into tissue, they are transformed into macrophages. The complement system is a pathway of chemical processes that results in cellular lysis, and vasodilation and increased capillary permeability cause the slowing of blood flow at the area.
7. c. Rationale: Eosinophils are white blood cells that are released in large quantities during allergic reactions and are involved in phagocytosis of allergen–antibody complexes. Neutrophils are the first white blood cells to increase in infection, followed by monocytes, which continue in high amounts in chronic infections. T lymphocytes are involved in immunity.
8. d. Rationale: The processes that are stimulated by the complement system include enhanced phagocytosis, increased vascular permeability, chemotaxis, and cellular lysis. Prostaglandins and leukotrienes are released by damaged cells, and body temperature is increased by action of prostaglandins and interleukins. All chemical mediators of inflammation increase the inflammatory response and, as a result, increase pain.
9. a. F, production of prostaglandins; b. T; c. F, cytokines; d. T; e. F, mononuclear phagocytic cells

10. b. Rationale: Labile cells of the skin, lymphoid organs, bone marrow, and mucous membranes divide constantly and regenerate rapidly following injury. Stable cells, such as those in bone, liver, pancreas, and kidney, regenerate only if injured, and permanent cells found in neurons and cardiac muscle do not regenerate when damaged.
11. a. 9;  b. 5;  c. 2;  d. 8;  e. 6;  f. 1;  g. 4;  h. 10; i. 7;  j. 3
12. c. Rationale: The process of healing by secondary intention is essentially the same as primary healing. With the greater defect and gaping wound edges of an open wound, healing and granulation take place from the edges inward and from the bottom of the wound up, resulting in more granulation tissue and a much larger scar. Tertiary healing involves suturing two layers of granulation tissue together and may require debridement of necrotic tissue.
13. keloid formation, contracture, dehiscence, excess granulation tissue, and adhesions
14. methicillin-resistant *Staphylococcus aureus* (MRSA), vancomycin-resistant enterococci (VRE), penicillin-resistant *Streptococcus pneumoniae* (PRSP); hand washing.
15. c. Rationale: One of the most important factors in the development of antibiotic-resistant strains of organisms has been inappropriate use of antibiotics, and clients and their families should be taught to take full courses of prescribed antibiotics without skipping doses, not to request antibiotics for viral infections, not to take antibiotics prophylactically unless specifically prescribed, and not to take leftover antibiotics. Hand washing and avoiding others with infection are general measures to prevent transmission of infections.
16. b. Rationale: There is a 13% increase in metabolism for every degree Centigrade increase, or a 7% increase for every degree Fahrenheit increase in temperature above 100°F (37.8°C). This client has an increase of 1.2 degrees above 100, multiplied by 7% = a total increase of 8.4%. 8.4% of 1800 calories is 151, the amount calories should be increased for the client during the fever. For the Centigrade calculation, find out the amount over 100°F [38.44°C – 37.78°C], which is 0.66°C. Multiply 0.66°C by 0.13 to get 0.0858, or 8.5%; 8.5% of 1800 calories is 153 calories.
17. a. 2;  b. 4;  c. 1;  d. 3;  e. 4;  f. 1;  g. 3;  h. 2; i. 4
18. a. Rationale: Granulation tissue includes proliferating fibroblasts, capillary sprouts, white blood cells, exudate, and ground substance for laying collagen and epithelial tissues. Damage to granulation tissue prolongs healing. All open wounds heal with granulation tissue and must be pro-

tected with a sterile, moist environment. Topical antimicrobials may actually cause tissue damage, and not all open wounds have excessive wound exudate that needs to be removed.

19. d. Rationale: Hand washing is the most important factor in preventing infection transmission and is recommended by the Centers for Disease Control and Health Canada for all types of isolation precautions in healthcare facilities.

20. d. Rationale: Although obesity, hyperglycemia, mental deterioration, malnutrition, old age, and incontinence contribute to development of pressure ulcers, the immobility of the comatose client presents the greatest risk for tissue damage related to pressure.

21. c. Rationale: Relief of pressure on tissues is critical to prevention and treatment of pressure ulcers, and although pressure-reduction devices may relieve some pressure and lift sheets and trapeze bars prevent skin shear, they are no substitute for frequent repositioning of the client.

22. a. 3;  b. 4;  c. 2;  d. 1

**Case Study**

1. pain, redness of leg, edema of leg, fever
2. purulent; yellow wound
3. The WBC count is increased to $18.3 \times 10^9$/L ($18.3 \times 10^3$/µL) from a normal of 4 to $11 \times 10^9$/L (4 to $11 \times 10^3$/µL), indicating a pronounced leukocytosis that would be seen in acute inflammation. Neutrophils are normally 50%–70% of the white cells, and hers are increased to 80%, indicating early response of neutrophils to tissue damage. She also has a "shift to the left" in that normally only 0%–8% of the neutrophils in the blood are immature, banded-nucleus cells, and she has 12% bands. All of these findings are consistent with an acute inflammatory process.
4. History of diabetes, with possible circulatory impairment to lower extremities and altered blood glucose levels; increased weight; inadequate nutrients for healing possible because confined to bed and has no one to help with meals; presence of infection in the wound
5. ASA interferes with the synthesis and release of PGs that are in part responsible for fever and also acts on the heat-regulating centre in the hypothalamus, resulting in peripheral dilation and heat loss. Mild to moderate fevers (up to 39.4°C [103°F]) are not usually harmful and may benefit defence mechanisms, and antipyretics are often only prescribed to control higher temperatures. To prevent acute swings in temperature and cycles of chilling/perspiring, antipyretics should be given regularly at 2- to 4-hour intervals.

6. The wound should be kept moist, with continuous cleansing to remove non-viable tissue and to absorb excessive drainage. Moist gauze or absorption dressings would be the best choice in the wound that is infected.

7. Hand washing—before application of clean gloves and immediately after gloves are removed; Clean gloves—when in contact with infectious material, such as dressings or linens with exudate; Biohazard disposal—of dressings, gloves; CDC/Health Canada Contact Precautions in addition to routine/standard precautions if *Staphylococcus aureus* is methicillin resistant

8. *Nursing diagnoses:*
   - Pain related to inflammation of left leg
   - Hyperthermia related to inflammatory process
   - Risk for deficient fluid volume related to increased metabolic rate
   - Risk for imbalanced nutrition: less than body requirements related to decreased intake of essential nutrients

   *Collaborative problems:*
   Potential complication: septicemia

# CHAPTER 13

1. a. 9; b. 3; c. 7; d. 5; e. 8; f. 10; g. 4; h. 1; i. 2; j. 11; k. 6

2. c. Rationale: Failure of the two chromosomes to separate during meiosis is known as *non-disjunction* and causes an abnormal number of chromosomes, such as in Down syndrome and Turner's syndrome. The result is two copies of the same chromosome, or sometimes a copy of a chromosome is missing. When genetic material is exchanged between the two chromosomes in a cell, *crossing over* occurs, creasing a greater amount of diversity in the genetic makeup of oocytes and sperm.

3.

| | | Mother | |
| --- | --- | --- | --- |
| | | H | H |
| Father | H | HH unaffected | HH unaffected |
| | h | Hh affected | Hh affected |

   a. 50%
   b. 0%
   c. 50%

4.

Mother

|  | P | p |
|---|---|---|
| P | PP<br><br>unaffected | Pp<br><br>carrier |
| P | PP<br><br>unaffected | Pp<br><br>carrier |

(Father, labelled on left side vertically)

a. 50%
b. 50%
c. 0%

5.  c. Rationale: Gene therapy that involves using vectors, or gene carriers, can be done both in and outside the body. A common vector is a modified virus that can deliver genetic material into a cell. With ex vivo therapy, cells are removed from the body, transduced with a vector, and then reinfused back into the body. With in vivo therapy, the altered gene in the virus is directly installed into the body.

6.  a. 3; b. 1; c. 4; d. 1; e. 2; f. 3; g. 2; h. 4

7.  a. bone marrow and thymus gland; b. T lymphocytes, B lymphocytes, macrophages; c. spleen; d. bone marrow; thymus gland

8.  a. Rationale: Both B and T lymphocytes must be sensitized by a processed antigen to activate the immune response. Processing involves the taking up of an antigen by macrophages and expression of the antigen on the macrophage cell membrane. Antigens need not be protein, and a few antigens may but may not combine with larger molecules that are antigenic.

9.  a. Rationale: T cytotoxic cells directly attack antigens on the cell membrane of foreign pathogens and release cytolytic substances that destroy pathogens. CD4 cells (T helper cells) and CD8 cells (T suppressor cells) are involved in the regulation of humoral antibody response and cell-mediated immunity. Natural killer cells are involved in non-specific killing of cells but are not considered T lymphocytes.

10.  c. Rationale: Interferon produces an antiviral effect in cells by reacting with viruses and inducing the formation of an antiviral protein that prevents new viruses from becoming assembled. Most cytokines are immunomodulatory and do not directly affect antigens, and cytokines such as interleukins may stimulate activation of immune cells.

11.  b. Rationale: Production of immunoglobulins by B lymphocytes is the essential component in humoral immunity. Tumour surveillance and production of cytokines are functions of T lymphocytes in cellular immunity, and B lymphocytes do not directly attack antigens.

12.  a. Rationale: B lymphocytes activated by presentation of an antigen differentiate into many plasma cells that secrete immunoglobulins and only a few memory cells that retain recognition of the antigen as foreign. Helper cells are T lymphocytes, and natural killer cells are large granular lymphocytes that are neither B nor T lymphocytes.

13.  a. 4;  b. 5;  c. 4;  d. 3;  e. 2;  f. 1;  g. 5;  h. 1; i. 3

14.  a. immunity against pathogens that survive inside cells; b. fungal infections; c. rejection of foreign tissue; d. contact hypersensitivity reactions; e. tumour surveillance

15.  c. Rationale: Decline of T and B cell activity occurs with advancing age, but circulating autoantibodies increase. Increased autoantibodies are a factor in autoimmune diseases, which increase in persons over the age of 50. T cell reduction is responsible for decreased tumour surveillance, resulting in an increase in cancer, and decreased hypersensitivity, resulting in anergy.

16.  a. 2;  b. 1;  c. 4;  d. 3

17.  a. 2;  b. 1;  c. 1;  d. 4;  e. 3;  f. 1;  g. 4;  h. 2; i. 1;  j. 3;  k. 1;  l. 1;  m. 4

18.  a.  1) Edema and itching at injection site
       2) Rapid, weak pulse
       3) Hypotension
       4) Laryngeal spasm
       5) Dilated pupils
     b.  1) Maintain airway and provide oxygen
       2) Start IV for fluid and medication access
       3) Prepare to administer 5 mL of 1:10,000 epinephrine IV
       4) Position flat with legs elevated
       5) Have diphenhydramine (Benadryl) and aminophylline available

19.  c. Rationale: Allergic individuals have elevated levels of IgE that react with allergens to produce symptoms of allergy. Immunotherapy involves injecting allergen extracts that will stimulate increased IgG that combines more readily with allergens without releasing histamine. The goal is to keep a "blocking" level of IgG high.

20.  d. Rationale: Because there is always a possibility of an anaphylactic reaction when allergens are injected, a healthcare provider, emergency equipment, and essential drugs should always be available whenever injections are given. The allergen should always be administered in an extremity away from a joint so that a tourniquet can be applied for a severe reaction, and sites should be

rotated. The client should be carefully observed for a reaction for 20 minutes after an injection.

21. d. Rationale: Two types of latex allergies can occur: a type IV allergic contact dermatitis that is caused by the chemicals used in the manufacturing process of latex gloves, and a type I allergic reaction that is a response to the natural rubber latex proteins, occurs within minutes of contact with the proteins, and may manifest with reactions ranging from skin redness to full-blown anaphylactic shock. Powder-free gloves and avoidance of oil-based hand creams when wearing gloves help prevent allergic reactions to latex.

22. genetic susceptibility and initiation of autoreactivity (a trigger)

23. c. Rationale: Plasmapheresis is the removal of plasma from the blood and in autoimmune disorders is used to remove pathogenic substances found in plasma, such as autoantibodies, complexes of antibodies and antigens, and inflammatory mediators. Circulating blood cells are not affected by plasmapheresis.

24. b. Rationale: The hereditary association that has been noted between HLA type and immune or autoimmune disorders may make it possible to identify members of a family at greatest risk for developing autoimmune disorders.

25. Histocompatibility refers to tissues that are genetically compatible with each other. Several genes determine what antigens are on the human leukocyte and all nucleated cells and platelets. These genes are grouped together on chromosome 6, are labelled as HLA-A, HLA-B, HLA-C, HLA-D, and HLA-DR, and have many possible alleles. If tissue is transplanted that has different antigens on cell surfaces, the recipient's body recognizes the tissue as foreign, and the immune system responds to destroy the tissue.

26. b. Rationale: At the current time, HLA typing is used to determine paternity and to match tissue for transplantation. As more knowledge is gained, there is a strong possibility that HLA associations with certain diseases can be specified and an individual's risk for disease identified.

27. drug-induced immunosuppression with antineoplastic agents and corticosteroids

28. graft-versus-host disease

29. c. Rationale: Standard immunotherapy involves the use of three different immunosuppressants that act in different ways: a calcineurin inhibitor (cyclosporin, tacrolimus), a corticosteroid, and the antimetabolite mycophenolate mofetil. Although cyclosporin is still used, tacrolimus is the most frequently prescribed calcineurin inhibitor.

**Case Study**

1. IgE is the immunoglobulin involved in most allergic reactions. Chemical mediators that would be active in the client's allergic rhinitis include histamine, serotonin, slow-releasing substance of anaphylaxis (SRS-A), eosinophil chemotactic factor-anaphylaxis (ECF-A), and complement anaphylatoxins.

2. The procedure would involve either the scratch test or prick test technique. Intradermal allergy testing is not used unless these methods do not cause conclusive reactions. A positive result is manifested by a local wheal-and-flare response that occurs within minutes after insertion of the extract and may last for eight to twelve hours.

3. Precautions to prevent or treat severe allergic reactions are important:
   Never leave the client alone during the testing period.
   Always have the following available:
   Emergency equipment (oral airway, laryngoscope, endotracheal tubes, oxygen, tourniquet, IV therapy equipment, cardiac monitor with defibrillator)
   Essential drugs (epinephrine, antihistamines, corticosteroids, and vasopressors)
   Severe local reactions should be treated with removal of the extract and application of anti-inflammatory topical cream to the site.

4. Antihistamines relieve allergic symptoms by competing with histamine for H1 receptor sites and thus blocking the effect of histamine. Action of most antihistamines is not very effective against histamine-induced bronchoconstriction. This client should be taught to take antihistamines on a regular basis since he has perennial allergic rhinitis that is not limited to contact with seasonal allergens. He must also be cautioned about the common side effects of antihistamines: drowsiness and impaired coordination, dry mouth, GI upset, urinary retention, blurred vision, and dizziness.

5. Household dust is controlled with air conditioners and air filtration systems in the home, as well as daily damp dusting and frequent vacuuming with high-filtration vacuum bags.

6. Precautions:
   - Always have the following available:
     - Physician
     - Emergency equipment (oral airway, laryngoscope, endotracheal tubes, oxygen, tourniquet, IV therapy equipment, cardiac monitor with defibrillator)
     - Emergency drugs (epinephrine, antihistamines, corticosteroids, and vasopressors)

- Administer the extract in an extremity away from a joint so that a tourniquet can be applied for a severe reaction.
- Always aspirate for blood before injection of the allergen extract.
- Assess for systemic reactions manifested by pruritus, urticaria, sneezing, laryngeal edema, and hypotension.
- Observe client for systemic reactions for 20 minutes following the injection.

7. *Nursing diagnoses:*
   - Ineffective health maintenance related to insufficient knowledge of medications, methods of decreasing exposure to allergens
   - Risk for injury related to effects of antihistamines

   *Collaborative problems:*
   Potential complication: anaphylaxis

# CHAPTER 14

1. a. Rationale: Sexual contact is the most common method of HIV transmission. The other methods may transmit the virus but not as frequently.
2. a. women; b. vascular access; c. anal intercourse; d. whole blood; e. first two to six months of infection; f. mothers using no therapy; g. needle-stick exposure
3. a. 3;  b. 5;  c. 1;  d. 6;  e. 2;  f. 7;  g. 4
4. a. reverse transcriptase inhibitors: viral RNA is converted to single-strand viral DNA with assistance of the enzyme reverse transcriptase.
   b. protease inhibitors: long strands of viral RNA are cut in the presence of the enzyme protease.
5. c. Rationale: Activated $CD4^+$ T cells are an ideal target for HIV because these cells are attracted to the site of concentrated HIV in the lymph nodes, where they become infected through viral contact with CD4 receptors. $CD4^+$ T cells normally are a major component of the immune system, and their infection renders the immune system ineffective against HIV and other agents. The virus does not stimulate $CD8^+$ T cells, and B lymphocytes are functional early in the disease, as evidenced by positive antibody titres against HIV. Monocytes do ingest infected cells and may become sites of HIV replication and spread the virus to other tissue, but this does not make the immune response ineffective.
6. a. Loss of cellular integrity from HIV budding; b. Syncytial formation may destroy cells that are not infected; c. Destruction of $CD4^+$ T cells by circulating antibodies
7. a. 3;  b. 1;  c. 2;  d. 1;  e. 3;  f. 2;  g. 1;  h. 3; i. 4;  j. 3

8. d. Rationale: AIDS is diagnosed when an individual with HIV infection meets specific criteria, including development of an opportunistic disease such as *Pneumocystis carinii* pneumonia; a $CD4^+$ T cell count of <200/mL; or candidiasis of the bronchi, trachea, lungs, or esophagus. Oral candidiasis may occur in intermediate chronic infection and is not a diagnostic criterion for AIDS. WBC count is not a criterion for AIDS diagnosis.
9. a. 3;  b. 6;  c. 8;  d. 2;  e. 5;  f. 7;  g. 1;  h. 4
10. d. Rationale: Organisms that are nonvirulent or cause limited or localized diseases in an immunocompetent person can cause severe, debilitating, and life-threatening infections in persons with impaired immune function.
11. a. T; b. F, Western blot or immunofluorescence assay (IFA); c. F, $CD4^+$ T cell counts or viral load tests; d. T; e. T
12. d. Rationale: All infants born to HIV-infected mothers will have a positive HIV antibody test because maternal antibodies cross the placental barrier. Within four weeks, detection of HIV in infants is possible with testing for the HIV antigen with the use of HIV DNA PCR, HIV RNA PCR, or viral culture. Only 25% of infants born to untreated HIV-infected women are infected with HIV.
13. b. Rationale: The use of potent combination antiretroviral therapy limits the potential for selection of antiretroviral-resistant HIV variants, the major factor limiting the ability of antiretroviral drugs to inhibit virus replication and delay disease progression. The drugs selected should be ones with which the client has not been previously treated and that are not cross-resistant with antiretroviral agents previously used by the client.
14. c. Rationale: Guidelines for initiating antiretroviral therapy (ART) are currently in a state of flux because of the development of alternative drugs and problems with long-term side effects and compliance with regimens. In the past, ART was always recommended at the time of HIV infection diagnosis, but today new guidelines suggest that treatment can be delayed until higher levels of immune suppression are observed. Whenever treatment is started, an important consideration is the client's readiness to initiate ART because adherence to drug regimens is a critical component of the therapy.
15. b. Rationale: An undetectable viral load in the blood does not mean that the virus is gone—it is still present in lymph nodes and other organs. Transmission to others is still possible, and protective measures must continue to be used.

16. c. Rationale: Pneumococcal, influenza, and hepatitis A and B vaccines should be given as early as possible in HIV infection while there is still immunological function. INH is used for nine to twelve months only if a client has reactive PPD greater than 5 mm, has had a high-risk exposure, or has prior untreated positive PPD. TMP-SMX is initiated when CD4+ T cells are below 200/$\mu$L or when there is a history of PCP, and varicella-zoster immune globulin is indicated only after significant exposure to chicken pox or shingles in clients with no history of disease or a negative VZV antibody test.

17. d. Rationale: After a client has positive HIV-antibody testing and is in early disease, the overriding goal is to keep the viral load as low as possible and to maintain a functioning immune system. The nurse should provide education regarding ways to enhance immune function to prevent the onset of opportunistic diseases in addition to teaching about the spectrum of the infection, options for care, signs and symptoms to watch for, and ways to adhere to treatment regimens.

18. Sexual intercourse:
    Abstain from sexual activity
    Non-contact sexual activities ("outercourse")
    Use of barriers during sexual activity
    Drug use:
    Abstain from drug use
    Do not share equipment
    Use alternative routes to injecting
    Do not have sexual intercourse while under influence of drugs

19. d. Rationale: The nursing diagnosis of risk for impaired skin integrity addresses a nursing problem that occurs as a result of the diarrhea and wasting and is a problem that nursing can treat.

20. d. Rationale: All of the nursing interventions are appropriate for a client with altered thought processes, but the priority is the safety of the client when cognitive and behavioural problems impair the client's ability to maintain a safe environment.

**Case Study**

1. Post-test counselling should include the following:
   Provide resources for medical and emotional support, with immediate assistance.
   Evaluate suicide risk.
   Determine need to test others who have had risky contact with client.
   Discuss retesting to verify results.

Encourage optimism: treatment is available, health habits can improve immune function, client can visit HIV-infected people, and client is infected with HIV but does not have AIDS.

2. Vague symptoms of fatigue, headaches, lymphadenopathy, and night sweats are characteristic of early chronic infection. CD4+ T cell counts are usually >500/mL in early chronic infection. This client experienced what could have been acute retroviral syndrome only two weeks ago, and it would be unlikely that he would be at a later stage than early chronic infection.

3. Additional testing at this visit should include the following:
   CBC
   Another CD4+ T cell count
   Viral load assessment (bDNA or PCR)
   Hepatitis B serology
   PPD skin test by Mantoux method

4. pneumococcal, influenza, and hepatitis A and B vaccines
   INH if PPD is greater than 5 mm reactive or if he has had a high-risk exposure
   nutritional support and education

5. The drug therapy is not curative but has resulted in dramatic improvements in many HIV-infected clients by maintaining immune function and decreasing viral load. It is critical to take the drug combination specifically as prescribed to prevent development of resistance by the virus. If the drugs cannot be taken for any reason, the physician or nurse practitioner should be notified. There are many side effects of the drugs, some of which can be controlled and are not serious but some of which may prevent use of the drugs. It is important to report any changes in his condition or symptoms that develop. He will be closely monitored, and viral loads will be assessed two to four weeks after the therapy is started and periodically after that.

6. Genotype and phenotype testing can be done to test for resistance to antiretroviral drugs. The genotype assay detects drug-resistant viral mutations that are present in the reverse transcriptase and protease genes. The phenotype assay measures the growth of the virus in various concentrations of antiretroviral drugs (similar to bacteria-antibiotic sensitivity tests).

7. *Nursing diagnoses:*
   • Anxiety
   • Fear
   • Ineffective denial
   • Anticipatory grieving
   *Collaborative problems:*
   Potential complications: opportunistic infections; opportunistic malignancies; myelosuppression

# CHAPTER 15

1. a. Rationale: Lung cancer is the leading cause of cancer deaths in Canada. Cancers of the reproductive organs are the second leading cause of cancer deaths.
2. d. Rationale: Malignant cells proliferate indiscriminately and continuously and also lose the characteristic of contact inhibition, allowing growth on top of and in between other cells. Cancer cells do not usually proliferate at a faster rate than normal cells, nor can cell cycles be skipped in proliferation, but malignant proliferation is continuous, unlike in normal cells.
3. a. Rationale: Cancer cells become more fetal and embryonic (undifferentiated) in appearance and function, and some produce new proteins, such as CEA and AFP, on cell membranes that reflect a return to more immature functioning.
4. c. Rationale: The major difference between benign and malignant cells is the ability of malignant tumour cells to invade and metastasize. Benign tumours are more often encapsulated and often grow at the same rate as malignant tumours. Benign tumours may cause death by expansion into normal tissues and organs.
5. a. 4;  b. 1;  c. 2;  d. 6;  e. 3;  f. 5
6. a. T; b. T; c. F, reversible; d. T; e. F, initiation and promotion; f. T; g. F, metalloproteinase enzymes; h. T
7. a. rapid proliferation that causes mechanical pressure, leading to penetration of surrounding tissues
   b. decreased cell-to-cell adhesion, allowing cell movement to exterior of primary tumour and within other organ structures
   c. production of metalloproteinase enzymes capable of destroying the basement membrane of the tumour but also of lymph and blood vessels and other tissues
8. a. 5;  b. 8;  c. 1;  d. 7;  e. 4;  f. 3;  g. 6;  h. 2
9. a. macrophages: stimulate T cells
   b. cytotoxic T cells: stimulate T cells, natural killer cells, B cells, and macrophages
   c. macrophages: augment natural killer cells
   d. cytotoxic T cells: stimulate macrophages
   e. macrophages: hemorrhagic necrosis of tumours
   f. macrophages: stimulate production and function of white blood cells
10. a. embryonal mesoderm—both
    b. meninges—both
    c. meningioma—benign; meningeal sarcoma—malignant
11. a. arose from epithelial tissue of the breast
    b. moderate differentiation as compared with slight differentiation or very abnormal

c. small tumour size, with a small number of lymph nodes involved, with no evidence of distant metastases
12. a. men: annual digital rectal examination for prostate evaluation
    b. men: annual PSA blood test
    c. women: annual Pap test and pelvic examination
    d. women: annual professional breast examination
    e. women: annual mammography
    f. annual fecal occult blood test, or flexible sigmoidoscopy q5yr, or annual fecal occult blood test and flexible sigmoidoscopy q5yr, or double-contrast barium enema every five to ten years, or colonoscopy every 10 years
    g. cancer-related checkup every year
13. b. Rationale: Although other tests may be used in diagnosing cancer, biopsy is the only method by which cells can be determined to be malignant.
14. a. 3;  b. 1;  c. 4;  d. 1;  e. 2;  f. 3;  g. 1;  h. 2
15. c. Rationale: Tissue that is actively proliferating, such as GI mucosa, esophageal and oropharyngeal mucosa, and bone marrow, exhibit early acute responses to radiation therapy. Cartilage, bone, kidney, and nervous tissue, which proliferate slowly, manifest subacute or late responses.
16. b. Rationale: Radiation ionization breaks chemical bonds in DNA, which renders cells incapable of surviving mitosis. This loss of proliferative capacity yields cellular death at the time of division for both normal cells and cancer cells, but cancer cells are more likely to be dividing because of the loss of control of cellular division. Cells are most radiosensitive in the M and G2 phases, but damage in cells that are not in the M phase will be expressed when division occurs. Normal tissues are usually able to recover from radiation damage but not always, and permanent damage may occur.
17. b. Rationale: Brachytherapy is the implantation or insertion of radioactive materials directly into the tumour or in proximity of the tumour and may be curative. The client is a source of radiation, and in addition to implementing the principles of time, distance, and shielding, caregivers should wear film badges to monitor the amount of radiation exposure. Computerized dosimetry and simulation are used in external radiation therapy.
18. a. Rationale: Fatigue associated with radiation therapy may be severe and may be related to changes in cell cycle patterns, accumulation of metabolites from cell destruction, and other side effects of radiation therapy. Alopecia, bone marrow suppression, and skin reactions are local reactions when radiation is directed at specific areas of the body.

19. d. Rationale: Positive response of cancer cells to chemotherapy is most likely in tumours that arise from tissue that has a rapid rate of cellular proliferation, have a small number of cancer cells, are young tumours that have a greater percentage of proliferating cells, are not in a protected anatomical site, and have no resistant tumour cells. A state of optimum health and a positive attitude of the client will also promote chemotherapy success.

20. a. 2; b. 1; c. 4; d. 3; e. 5

21. b. Rationale: One of the major concerns with the IV administration of chemotherapeutic agents is infiltration of drugs into tissue surrounding the infusion site. Many of these drugs are vesicants—drugs that, when infiltrated into the skin, cause severe local breakdown and necrosis. Specific measures to ensure adequate dilution, patency, and early detection of injury are important.

22. a. 4; b. 2; c. 5; d. 1; e. 3

23. a. Rationale: Right atrial catheters are vascular access devices inserted into central veins, which decrease the incidence of extravasation, provide for rapid dilution of chemotherapy, and reduce the need for venipunctures. Most right atrial catheters, except for a Groshong, need to be flushed with heparin to prevent clotting in the tubing. Regional chemotherapy administration delivers the drug directly to the tumour and is the only administration route that can decrease the systemic effects of the drugs.

24. b. Rationale: Clients should always be taught what to expect during a course of chemotherapy, including side effects and expected outcome. Side effects of chemotherapy are serious and may cause death, but it is important that clients are informed what measures can be taken to help them cope with the side effects of therapy. Hair loss related to chemotherapy is usually reversible, and short-term use of wigs, scarves, or turbans can be used during and following chemotherapy until the hair grows back.

25. d. Rationale: Alkylating chemotherapeutic agents and high-dose radiation are most likely to cause secondary resistant malignancies as a late effect of treatment. The other conditions are not known to be later effects of radiation or chemotherapy.

26. b. Rationale: Biological therapies are normal components of the immune system, which have been identified and isolated and are used therapeutically to restore, augment, or modulate host immune system mechanisms to assist in immune activity against cancer cells.

27. a. Rationale: Virtually all biological therapies may cause a flu-like syndrome that includes headache, fever, chills, myalgias, fatigue, and anorexia. The other side effects may be caused by specific agents but not all biological therapies.

28. a. Rationale: The most common cause of morbidity and death in cancer clients is infection. Decreased resistance to infection may be caused by bone marrow depression secondary to therapy or malignant infiltration of the bone marrow by cancer. Nursing measures include good hand-washing techniques, monitoring WBC counts (especially neutrophils), noting even slight temperature elevations, and instituting protective isolation if the client is severely immunosuppressed.

29. b. Rationale: An allogenic bone marrow transplant is one in which bone marrow from an HLA-matched donor is infused into a client who has received high doses of chemotherapy, with or without radiation, to eradicate cancerous cells. In an autologous bone marrow transplant, the client's own bone marrow is removed before therapy. The marrow is treated to remove cancer cells and may be infused right away or frozen and stored for later use. In either case, the new bone marrow will take several weeks to produce new blood cells, and protective isolation is necessary during this time.

30. c. Rationale: Tumour lysis syndrome may occur with chemotherapy and is the result of rapid destruction of large numbers of tumour cells. When the cells are destroyed, fatal biochemical changes can occur, especially hyperuricemia, hyperkalemia, hyperphosphatemia, and hypocalcemia.

31. a. Ability to cope with stressful events in the past
    b. Presence of effective support system
    c. Ability to express feelings and concerns
    d. Older age—usually have greater sense of mortality
    e. Feeling of control
    f. Possibility of cure or control

**Case Study**

1. Chemotherapy-induced bone marrow depression is probably the most relevant factor in his decreased WBC and neutrophil count. Inadequate protein intake would also contribute to impaired recovery of normal blood cells.

2. A temperature of 37. 4°C (99. 4°F) in an immunosuppressed client is a significant finding for infection. He also has warm skin, with some degree of dehydration. His risk of infection is high with a WBC count of 3.2 x $10^9$/L (3.2 x $10^3$/µL) and neutrophils of 0.5 x $10^9$/L (0.5 x $10^3$/µL). The risk for infection increases when neutrophils are less than 1.0 x $10^9$/L (1.0 x $10^3$/µL).

3. Assess for sore throat, chest pain, persistent cough, urinary symptoms, rectal pain, or confusion. Also note catheter site for chemotherapy as a possible source of infection.

4. His nausea, vomiting, and anorexia, as well as any other side effects of chemotherapy; negative attitude also promoted by lack of social support, an inability to cope with stress, and lack of information about expected results of treatment

5. Use antiemetic protocols to control treatment-related nausea and vomiting.
   Offer small, frequent feedings of bland, high-calorie, high-protein foods.
   Use relaxation techniques and distraction when the client is nauseated.
   Offer any fluids or foods the client can tolerate and that may be appealing to him.
   Avoid nagging or being judgemental about food intake.

6. Hand washing, for both staff and client
   Careful sterile technique in caring for IV catheter site
   Avoid visitors with infection

7. *Nursing diagnoses:*
   • Hopelessness related to uncertainty about outcomes and insufficient knowledge about cancer and treatment
   • Imbalanced nutrition: less than body requirements related to decreased oral intake, increased metabolic demands of cancer
   • Deficient fluid volume related to decreased oral fluid intake
   • Risk for infection related to immunosuppression
   *Collaborative problems:*
   Potential complications: septicemia; negative nitrogen balance; myelosuppression

## CHAPTER 16

1. a. F, 1000; b. F, 54 (90 kg x 60%); c. F, hyperkalemia; d. T; e. T; f. F, swell and burst, into; g. F, spaces that normally have little or no fluid; h. T

2. a. 4;  b. 5;  c. 6;  d. 7;  e. 2;  f. 1;  g. 3

3. 301 (2 x 147 + 126/18); increased

4. a. 1, 4; b. 2, 3; c. 1, 4; d. 2, 3

5. a. 1; oncotic pressure; b. 2; osmosis; c. 3; osmosis; d. 4; interstitial hydrostatic pressure; e. 1; plasma hydrostatic pressure; f. 1; tissue oncotic pressure; g. 4; interstitial hydrostatic pressure

6. a. serum osmolality increases as large amount of sodium absorbed
   b. stimulates ADH release from the posterior pituitary, which increases water reabsorption from the kidney, lowering the sodium concentration but increasing vascular volume and hydrostatic pressure, perhaps causing fluid shift into interstitial spaces

7. c. Rationale: Aldosterone is secreted by the adrenal cortex in response to a decrease in plasma volume (loss of water), serum sodium, or renal perfusion. It is also secreted in response to an increase in serum potassium.

8. b. Rationale: The action of aldosterone is to increase sodium reabsorption from the kidney, which retains water in the vasculature, and it also causes potassium excretion. ADH increases the permeability to water in the distal convoluted tubule and collecting duct, causing water retention but not sodium retention.

9. d. Rationale: A major cause of hypernatremia is a water deficit, which can occur in those with a decreased sensitivity to thirst, the major protection against hyperosmolality. All of the other conditions lead to hyponatremia.

10. d. Rationale: As water shifts into and out of cells in response to the osmolality of the blood, the cells that are most sensitive to shrinking or swelling are those of the brain, resulting in neurological symptoms.

11. a. 8;  b. 4;  c. 6;  d. 1;  e. 7;  f. 2;  g. 9;  h. 3; i. 10; j. 6;  k. 1;  l. 5

12. a. hypernatremia, hypokalemia, hypomagnesemia
    b. hyperkalemia, hypocalcemia, hyperphosphatemia, hypermagnesemia
    c. hypokalemia, hyponatremia, hypocalcemia

13. d. Rationale: Because of the osmotic pressure of sodium, water will be excreted with the sodium lost with the diuretic. A change in the relative concentration of sodium will not be seen, but an isotonic fluid loss will occur.

14. c. Rationale: Potassium maintains normal cardiac rhythm, transmission and conduction of nerve impulses, and contraction of muscles. Cardiac cells demonstrate the most clinically significant changes with potassium imbalances because of changes in cardiac conduction. Although paralysis may occur with severe potassium imbalances, cardiac changes are seen earlier and much more commonly.

15. b. Rationale: In a metabolic acidosis, hydrogen ions in the blood are taken into the cell in exchange for potassium ions as a means of buffering excess acids. This results in an increase in serum potassium until the kidneys have time to excrete the excess potassium.

16. d. Rationale: Chvostek's sign is a contraction of facial muscles in response to a tap over the facial nerve. This indicates the neuromuscular irritability of low calcium levels, and intravenous calcium is the treatment to prevent laryngeal spasms and respiratory arrest. Calcitonin is indicated for

treatment of high calcium levels, and loop diuretics may be used to decrease calcium levels. Oral vitamin D supplements are part of the treatment for hypocalcemia but not for impending tetany.

17. c. Rationale: Kidneys are the major route of phosphate excretion, a function that is impaired in renal failure. A reciprocal relationship exists between phosphorus and calcium, and high serum phosphate levels of kidney failure cause a low calcium concentration in the serum.

18. 7.35 to 7.45; 20 to 1

19. hydrogen ion concentration

20. a. 2;  b. 4;  c. 3;  d. 2;  e. 1;  f. 4;  g. 1;  h. 2;  i. 5;  j. 1

21. c. Rationale: The amount of carbon dioxide in the blood directly relates to carbonic acid concentration and subsequently hydrogen ion concentration. The carbon dioxide combines with water in the blood to form carbonic acid, and in cases where carbon dioxide is retained in the blood, acidosis occurs.

22. a. Secretion of small amounts of hydrogen ions into renal tubule
    b. Combining hydrogen ions with ammonia ($NH_3$) to form ammonium ($NH_4$)
    c. Excreting weak acids

23. a. 4;  b. 2;  c. 1;  d. 3
    Respiratory acid–base imbalances are associated with excesses or deficits of carbonic acid. Metabolic acid–base imbalances are associated with excesses or deficits of bicarbonate.

24. a. Kidney conservation of bicarbonate and excretion of hydrogen ions
    b. Deep, rapid respirations (Kussmaul's breathing) to increase $CO_2$ excretion
    c. Decreased respiratory rate and depth to retain carbon dioxide and kidney excretion of bicarbonate

25. a. 4;  b. 3;  c. 2;  d. 1;  e. 4;  f. 3;  g. 3;  h. 2;  i. 1

26. b. Rationale: The anion gap, calculated by subtracting the serum chloride and bicarbonate levels from the serum sodium level should normally be 10–14 mmol/L. The anion gap is increased in metabolic acidosis associated with acid gain (e.g., diabetic acidosis) but remains normal in metabolic acidosis caused by bicarbonate loss (e.g., diarrhea).

27. a. 1. pH >7.45 indicates alkalosis
    2. $PaCO_2$ is low, indicating respiratory alkalosis
    3. $HCO_3^-$ is normal
    4. Respiratory alkalosis matches the pH
    5. Although uncommon, if $HCO_3^-$ was decreased, compensation would be present.
    Interpretation: respiratory alkalosis

b. 1. pH <7.35 indicates acidosis
    2. $PaCO_2$ is low, indicating a respiratory alkalosis
    3. $HCO_3^-$ is low, indicating an metabolic acidosis
    4. Metabolic acidosis matches the pH
    5. The $PaCO_2$ does not match but is moving in the opposite direction, which indicates the lungs are attempting to compensate for the metabolic acidosis.
    Interpretation: metabolic acidosis; partially compensated

c. 1. pH <7.35 indicates acidosis
    2. $PaCO_2$ is high, indicating a respiratory acidosis
    3. $HCO_3^-$ is normal
    4. Respiratory acidosis matches the pH
    5. Normal $HCO_3^-$ is found until the kidneys have time to retain bicarbonate.
    Interpretation: respiratory acidosis

d. 1. pH >7.45 indicates alkalosis
    2. $PaCO_2$ is high, indicating a respiratory acidosis
    3. $HCO_3^-$ is high, indicating a metabolic alkalosis
    4. Metabolic alkalosis matches the pH
    5. The $PaCO_2$ does not match but is moving in the opposite direction, indicating the lungs are attempting to compensate for the alkalosis.
    Interpretation: metabolic alkalosis, partially compensated

e. 1. pH is within normal range but toward alkalosis
    2. $PaCO_2$ is high, indicating a respiratory acidosis
    3. $HCO_3^-$ is high, indicating a metabolic alkalosis
    4. Because the body will not overcompensate, the metabolic alkalosis is a closer match with the pH.
    5. The high $PaCO_2$ indicates the ability of the lungs to compensate for the metabolic alkalosis.
    Interpretation: compensated or chronic metabolic alkalosis indicated by the high $PaCO_2$ and a pH within normal range

f. 1. pH is within normal range but toward acidosis
    2. $PaCO_2$ is high, indicating a respiratory acidosis
    3. $HCO_3^-$ is high, indicating a metabolic alkalosis
    4. Because the body will not overcompensate, the respiratory acidosis is a closer match with the pH.

5. The high $HCO_3^-$ indicates the ability of the kidneys to compensate for the respiratory acidosis.

Interpretation: compensated respiratory acidosis as reflected by high $HCO_3^-$ and pH in normal range

28. b. Rationale: Fluids such as $D_5W$ provide water which produces a movement of water from the extracellular fluid to the intracellular fluid. Although $D_5W$ is physiologically isotonic, the dextrose is rapidly metabolized, leaving free water to shift into cells.

29. d. Rationale: An isotonic solution does not change the osmolality of the blood and does not cause fluid shifts between the extracellular fluid and intracellular fluid. In the case of extracellular fluid loss, an isotonic solution, such as lactated Ringer's solution, is ideal because it stays in the extracellular compartment. A hypertonic solution would pull fluid from the cells into the extracellular compartment, resulting in cellular fluid loss and possible vascular overload.

**Case Study**

1. Status: fluid volume deficit
   Physical assessment: decreased skin turgor; dry mucous membranes; weak pulses, low blood pressure; confusion
   Laboratory findings: elevated BUN; elevated hematocrit
   Status: hypokalemia
   Physical assessment: weakness, confusion; irregular heart rhythm, tachycardia
   Laboratory findings: potassium 2.5 mmol/L (2.5 mEq/L)
   Etiology: diuretic therapy
2. ECG changes are associated with hypokalemia, metabolic alkalosis.
3. Metabolic alkalosis: pH 7.52
   base bicarbonate excess (43 mmol/L [43 mEq/L])
   Etiology: diuretic-induced hypokalemia is the primary factor.
   Compensation: compensation is not complete because the pH is out of normal range, but increased $PaCO_2$ and slow and shallow respirations indicate the attempt by the lungs to increase carbon dioxide to compensate for excess bicarbonate.
4. Less fluid reserve because older adults have less total body fluid; older adults also have decreased thirst sensation
5. Aldosterone would be secreted in response to a hyperkalemia, and in her case its release would be inhibited by the hypokalemia. However, her low blood pressure and extracellular fluid deficit would stimulate secretion of aldosterone to

increase sodium and water retention but cause even more potassium loss.
6. General care: Encourage and assist with oral fluid intake
   Provide skin care with assessment, changes in position, no soap
   Assessments:
   Vital signs q4hr
   I&O; daily weights
   Cardiac monitoring until electrolytes and acid-base normal
   Type and rate of IV fluid and electrolyte replacement
   Lung sounds for signs of fluid overload in cardiac-compromised client
   Daily serum electrolyte and blood gas levels
   Neurological changes
7. *Nursing diagnoses:*
   - Deficient fluid volume related to excessive ECF loss or decreased fluid intake
   - Ineffective health maintenance related to lack of knowledge of drugs and preventive measures
   - Risk for injury related to confusion, muscle weakness
   - Risk for impaired skin integrity related to dehydration
   *Collaborative problems:*
   Potential complications: arrhythmias; hypovolemic shock; hypoxemia

# CHAPTER 17

1. a. diagnosis; b. cosmetic; c. palliation; d. curative; e. curative
2. a. Rationale: Ambulatory surgery is usually less expensive and more convenient, generally involving fewer laboratory tests, fewer preoperative and post-operative medications, less psychological stress, and less susceptibility to hospital-acquired infections. However, the nurse is still responsible for assessing, supporting, and teaching the client undergoing surgery, regardless of where the surgery is performed.
3. a. Rationale: Excessive anxiety and stress can affect surgical recovery, and the nurse's role in psychologically preparing the client for surgery is to assess for potential stressors that could negatively affect surgery. Specific fears should be identified and addressed by the nurse by listening and by explaining planned post-operative care. Falsely reassuring, ignoring her behaviour, and telling her not to be anxious are not therapeutic.
4. a. Dong quai; b. feverfew; c. garlic; d. ginkgo biloba; e. ginseng; f. goldenseal

5. c. Rationale: Risk factors for latex allergies include a history of hay fever and allergies to foods such as avocados, kiwi, bananas, potatoes, peaches, and apricots. When a client identifies such allergies, the client should be further questioned about exposure to latex and specific reactions to allergens.

6. a. Personal or family history of:
   Problems with anaesthesia:
   - Possible malignant hyperthermia
   History of allergies:
   - Possible drug reactions
   Smoking:
   - Perioperative respiratory complications
   Medication/alcohol/drug use:
   - Interaction with anaesthetics
   - Laboratory tests that should be evaluated
   - Impaired liver function
   b. Obesity
   - Predisposed to dehiscence, infection, herniation
   - Need for increased anaesthesia
   Nutritional deficiencies:
   - Impaired healing
   c. Urinary retention:
   - Surgical drugs may increase retention postoperatively.
   Constipation:
   - Surgical drugs and analgesics may slow bowel motility.
   d. Respiratory disease:
   - URI may lead to cancellation of surgery.
   - Increased laryngo/bronchospasm
   - Increased secretions
   Musculoskeletal problems:
   - Mobility restrictions affecting neck will alter intubation and airway management
   - Surgical positioning and post-operative ambulation may be altered.
   e. Use of sleeping medication:
   - Interaction with anaesthetics
   - Need for preoperative sedation
   f. Pain tolerance:
   - Post-operative pain management plan
   Sensory devices:
   - Care of glasses, contacts, hearing aids
   g. Body image:
   - Alterations in self-perception and body image from surgery
   h. Fear and anxiety related to surgery; poor coping skills:
   - Stress management

7. d. Rationale: BUN, serum creatinine, and electrolytes are commonly abnormal in renal disease and should be evaluated before surgery. Other tests are often evaluated in the presence of diabetes, bleeding tendencies, and respiratory or heart disease.

8. a. Rationale: Obesity, as well as spinal, chest, and airway deformities, may compromise respiratory function during and after surgery. Dehydration may require preoperative fluid therapy, and an enlarged liver may indicate hepatic dysfunction that will increase perioperative risk related to glucose control, coagulation, and drug interactions. Weak peripheral pulses may reflect circulatory problems that could affect healing.

9. c. Rationale: All preoperative clients have the right to know what to expect and how to participate effectively in the surgical experience, including information related to preoperative preparation required before surgery. Specific measures such as teaching coughing and deep-breathing techniques and fluid and food restrictions are surgery-specific, and all clients may not receive actual descriptions of the surgical procedure, based on individual need for and response to information.

10. a. Notify the physician because the client needs further explanation of the planned surgery.
    b. Sufficient comprehension

11. c. Rationale: Preoperative checklists are a tool to ensure that the many preparations and precautions performed before surgery have been completed and documented. Client identification, instructions to the family, and administration of preoperative medications are often documented on the checklist that ensures that no details are omitted.

12. b. Rationale: Atropine, an anticholinergic medication, is frequently used preoperatively to decrease oral and respiratory secretions during surgery, and the addition of morphine will help relieve discomfort during the preoperative procedures. Antiemetics decrease nausea and vomiting during and after surgery, and scopolamine and some benzodiazepines induce amnesia. An actual sleep state is rarely induced by preoperative medications unless an anaesthetic agent is administered before the client is transported to the operating room.

13. c. Rationale: One of the major reasons that older adults need increased time preoperatively is the presence of impaired vision and hearing that slows understanding of preoperative instructions and preparation for surgery. Thought processes and cognitive abilities may also be impaired in some older adults. The older adult's decreased adaptation to stress because of physiological changes may increase surgical risks, and overwhelming surgery-related losses may result in ineffective coping that

is not directly related to time needed for preoperative preparation. The involvement of family members in preoperative activities may be appropriate for clients of all ages.

**Case Study**

1. Family—children with cystic fibrosis that require extra care and expense and concern that wife will not be able to manage without him; fear of cancer and the unknown; anemia—contributes to fatigue and ability to cope
2. General preoperative instruction: information related to preoperative routines and preparation, such as food and fluid restrictions, approximate length of surgery and post-operative recovery
   Outpatient instruction: when to arrive and the time of the surgery; how and where to register, what to wear and bring, and the need for a responsible adult for transportation home after the procedure
3. Smoking history increases the risk for postoperative respiratory complications—the earlier the client can stop smoking before surgery, the less the risk
   Mild obesity may contribute to problems with clearance of respiratory secretions and complete expansion of the lungs—should have preoperative instruction about deep-breathing and coughing techniques
   Fear of the diagnosis of cancer can alter adaptation and recovery—nurse can help minimize risk with specific information about the experience and with supportive listening
4. *Nursing diagnoses:*
   - Fear related to possible diagnosis of cancer
   - Interrupted family processes related to family roles shift
   - Ineffective health maintenance related to tobacco use
   *Collaborative problems:*
   Potential complications: hemorrhage; laryngospasm/bronchospasm; pneumonia

# CHAPTER 18

1. b. Rationale: Although all the factors are important to the safety and well-being of the client, the first consideration in the physical environment of the surgical suite is prevention of transmission of infection to the client.
2. b. Rationale: Persons in street clothes or attire other than surgical scrub clothing can interact with personnel of the surgical suite in unrestricted areas, such as the holding area, nursing station, control desk, or locker rooms. Only authorized personnel wearing surgical attire and air covering are allowed in semi-restricted areas, such as corridors, and masks must be worn in restricted areas, such as operating rooms, clean core, and scrub sink areas.
3. a. 2;  b. 1;  c. 4;  d. 2;  e. 2;  f. 1;  g. 3;  h. 2
4. a. Allergy to skin preparation agents, adhesive tapes, or latex; b. Musculoskeletal impairments requiring adaptations in positioning; c. Pain requiring adaptation in moving or procedures; d. Decreased level of consciousness requiring increased safety and protection techniques; e. Vision or hearing impairments requiring adaptations in communication
   Also: Skin conditions requiring special skin preparation and precautions against infection
5. a. Rationale: The most important procedure in admitting a client to the operating room is a specific identification process that ensures that the correct client is undergoing surgery. Verification of the client's understanding of the risks of surgery and a thorough preoperative assessment with history and physical examination are completed preoperatively. Skin preparation is done as part of the surgical procedure.
6. a. Rationale: The protection of the client from injury in the operating room environment is maintained by the circulating nurse by ensuring functioning equipment, preventing falls and injury during transport and transfer, and being with the client during anaesthesia induction.
7. a. Rationale: The mask covering the face is not considered sterile, and if in contact with sterile gloved hands, contaminates the gloves. The gown at chest level and to 5 cm (2 in.) above the elbows is considered sterile, as is the drape placed at the surgical area.

8. c. Rationale: Musculoskeletal deformities can be a risk factor for positioning injuries and require special padding and support on the operating table. Skin lesions and break in sterile technique are risk factors for infection, and electrical or mechanical equipment failure may lead to other types of injury.

9. c. Rationale: The Perioperative Nursing Data Set of outcome statements related to perioperative safety include the client's freedom from any type of injury, including medications. Outcomes related to physiological responses include those of physiological function, such as respiratory function; behavioural responses include knowledge and actions of the client and family, including the consistency of the client's care with the perioperative plan and the client's right to privacy.

10. a. Rationale: Midazolam (Versed) is a rapid, short-acting, sedative-hypnotic benzodiazepine that is used to prevent recall of events under anaesthesia because of its amnestic properties.

11. a. Maintenance anaesthesia—monitor for laryngo/bronchospasm, respiratory depression, and early pain

    b. Dissociative anaesthesia with analgesia and amnesia—monitor for agitation, hallucinations, nightmares

    c. Induction and maintenance of anaesthesia; promote early analgesia—assess for nausea and vomiting, monitor respiratory status

    d. Produce deep muscle relaxation—monitor respiratory muscle movement, airway patency

12. a. 5;  b. 4;  c. 1;  d. 3;  e. 2

13. b. Rationale: During epidural and spinal anaesthesia, a sympathetic nervous system blockade may occur that results in hypotension, bradycardia, and nausea and vomiting. A spinal headache may occur after, not during, spinal anaesthesia, and unconsciousness and seizures are indicative of intravenous absorption overdose. Upward extension of the effect of the anaesthesia results in inadequate respiratory excursion and apnea.

14. b. Rationale: Although malignant hyperthermia can result in cardiac arrest and death, if the client is known or suspected to be at risk for the disorder, appropriate precautions taken by the anaesthesiologist can provide for safe anaesthesia for the client. Because preventive measures are possible if the risk is known, it is critical that preoperative assessment include a careful family history of surgical events.

# CHAPTER 19

1. d. Rationale: Technological advances and shorter-acting anaesthetic agents have made changes in anaesthesia recovery. Ambulatory and outpatients often do not need as much time to recover, and different phases and recovery areas may be used to direct care. A collaborative PACU team should determine the standards for client selection, anaesthetics used, discharge criteria, and client outcomes for fast tracking in a specific institution.

2. c. Rationale: Physiological status of the client is always prioritized with regard to airway, breathing, and circulation, and respiratory adequacy is the first assessment priority of the client on admission to the PACU from the operating room. Following assessment of respiratory function, cardiovascular, neurological, and renal function should be assessed, as well as the surgical site.

3. c. Rationale: The admission of the client to the PACU is a joint effort between the anaesthesiologist, who is responsible for supervising the post-anaesthesia recovery of the client, and the PACU nurse, who provides care during anaesthesia recovery. It involves a verbal report by the anaesthesiologist of the details of the surgical and anaesthetic course, preoperative conditions influencing the surgical and anaesthetic outcome, and PACU treatment plans to ensure client safety and continuity of care.

4. b. Rationale: Even before clients awaken from anaesthesia, their sense of hearing returns, and all activities should be explained by the nurse from the time of admission to the PACU to assist in orientation and decrease confusion.

5. a. Rationale: ECG monitoring is performed on clients to assess initial cardiovascular problems during anaesthesia recovery. Fluid and electrolyte status is an indication of renal function, and determination of ABGs and direct arterial blood pressure monitoring are used only in special cardiovascular or respiratory problems.

6. a. 3;  b. 1;  c. 3;  d. 1;  e. 2;  f. 2;  g. 1;  h. 3

7. d. Rationale: An unconscious or semiconscious client should be placed in a lateral position to protect the airway from obstruction by the tongue. Deep breathing and elevation of the head of the bed are implemented to facilitate gas exchange when the client is responsive. Oxygen administration is often used, but the client must first have a patent airway.

8. c. Rationale: Hypotension with normal pulse and skin assessment is typical of residual vasodilating effects of anaesthesia and requires continued observation. An oxygen saturation of 88% indicates hypoxemia, while a narrowing pulse pressure accompanies hypoperfusion. A urinary output >30 mL/hr is desirable and indicates normal renal function.

9. c. Rationale: A distended bladder may cause both hypertension and emergence delirium. Although hypoxemia is a common cause of emergence delirium, it is associated with hypotension. Delayed awakening may result from neurological injury, and cardiac arrhythmias most often result from specific respiratory, electrolyte, or cardiac problems.

10. a. Rationale: During hypothermia, oxygen demand is increased, and metabolic processes slow down. Oxygen therapy is used to treat the increased demand for oxygen. Anti-arrhythmics and vasodilating drugs would be used only if the hypothermia caused symptomatic cardiac arrhythmias and vasoconstriction. Sedatives and analgesics are not indicated for hypothermia.

11. a. client awake; b. vital signs stable; c. no excess bleeding or drainage; d. no respiratory depression; e. oxygen saturation greater than 90%

12. *Nursing diagnoses:*
- Ineffective airway clearance related to decreased respiratory excursion
- Impaired physical mobility related to decreased muscle strength
- Constipation related to decreased physical activity and impaired GI motility
- Risk for infection related to surgical incision, immobility, and decreased circulation

*Collaborative problems:*

Potential complications:

thromboembolism; paralytic ileus; urinary retention; pneumonia

13. c. Rationale: Incisional pain is often the greatest deterrent to client participation in effective ventilation and ambulation, and adequate and regular analgesic medications should be provided to encourage these activities. Controlled breathing may help the client manage pain but does not promote coughing and deep breathing. Explanations of rationale and use of an incentive spirometer help gain client participation but are more effective if pain is controlled.

14. c. Rationale: Secretion and release of aldosterone and cortisol from the adrenal gland and ADH from the posterior pituitary as a result of the stress response cause fluid retention during the first two to five days post-operatively, and fluid

overload is possible during this time. Aldosterone causes renal potassium loss with possible hypokalemia, and blood coagulation is enhanced by cortisol.

15. a. 1) leg exercises 10 to 12 times every one to two hours
   2) no pillows under knees
b. 1) slow progression to ambulation—elevate head of bed one to two minutes; client to dangle legs, stand by bed
   2) client to sit if becomes faint; if fainting occurs, lower client to floor
c. 1) client to promote normal position for voiding or use bedside commode or ambulate to bathroom
   2) client to run water from faucet; pour warm water over perineum
d. 1) encourage client to expel flatus
   2) reposition in bed frequently; position on right side
e. 1) use sterile technique for wound care; use proper drain management
   2) frequent assessment of wound

16. a. 2; b. 4; c. 1; d. 1; e. 3; f. 4

17. c. Rationale: Dressings over surgical sites are initially removed by the surgeon unless otherwise specified and should not be changed. Some drainage is expected for most surgical wounds, and the drainage should be evaluated and recorded to establish a baseline for continuing assessment.

18. d. Rationale: During the first 24 to 48 post-operative hours, temperature elevations to 38°C (100.4°F) are a result of the inflammatory response to surgical stress. Dehydration and lung congestion or atelectasis in the first two days will cause a temperature elevation above 38°C (100.4°F). Wound infections usually do not become evident until three to five days post-operatively and manifest with temperatures above 38°C (100.4°F).

19. d. Rationale: Before administering all analgesic medications, the nurse should first assess the nature and intensity of the client's pain to determine if the pain is expected, if prior doses of the medication have been effective, and if any undesirable side effects are occurring. The administration of prn analgesic medication is based on the nursing assessment. If possible, pain medication should be in effect during painful activities, but activities may be scheduled around medication administration.

20. c. Rationale: All post-operative clients need discharge instruction regarding what to expect and what self-care can be assumed during recovery.

Diet, activities, follow-up care, symptoms to be reported, and instructions about medications are individualized to the client.

**Case Study**

1. Orienting as client recovers from the sedating medication; promoting voiding; providing oral fluids and intake
2. Syncope is possible because of the effects of the drug and instrumentation of the bladder. The client should be slowly progressed to ambulation by elevating the head of the bed, then to dangling the legs, then to standing at the side of the bed before attempting ambulation.
3. Inability to void is the most likely problem. The client could also have respiratory depression or unstable vital signs because of the effects of the drugs or have complications such as bladder bleeding.

4. By standard discharge criteria for PACUs: stable vital signs, oxygen saturation greater than 90%, awake and oriented, no excessive bleeding or drainage, and no respiratory depression, in addition to the specific criteria ordered for this client
5. An outpatient also needs to be mobile and alert with the ability to provide self-care near the level of preoperative functioning. Post-operative pain, nausea, and vomiting must be controlled, and the client must be accompanied by an adult to drive her home.
6. *Nursing diagnoses:*
   - Impaired urinary elimination related to bladder irritation
   - Risk for infection related to incomplete bladder emptying
   - Risk for injury related to sedation
   - Acute pain related to bladder irritation
   *Collaborative problems:*
   Potential complications: hemorrhage; infection

## CHAPTER 20

1. a. anterior compartment; b. posterior chamber; c. anterior chamber; d. iris; e. cornea; f. pupil; g. lens; h. suspensory ligaments; i. ciliary body; j. sclera; k. choroids; l. retina; m. optic nerve; n. posterior compartment

2. a. zonules; b. aqueous humor; c. vitreous humor; d. cornea; e. ciliary body; f. rods; g. lens; h. cones; i. sclera; j. limbus; k. conjunctiva; l. puncta; m. optic disc; n. choroids; o. canal of Schlemm; p. iris; q. pupil

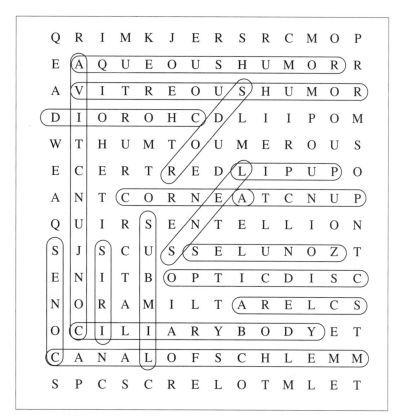

3.  a. F, myopia; b. T; c. F, nearsightedness/myopia; d. T; e. F, tears
4.  a. 2; b. 5; c. 2; d. 3; e. 2; f. 3; g. 6; h. 4; i. 2; j. 4; k. 1
5.  a. Loss of orbital fat; b. Chronic exposure to UV light or other environmental irritants; c. Cholesterol deposits in the peripheral cornea; d. Liquifaction and detachment of vitreous; e. Decreased cones; f. Increased rigidity of iris; g. Deposition of lipids; h. Decreased tear secretion
6.  a. Rationale: The use of corticosteroids has been associated with the development of cataracts and glaucoma. Use of oral hypoglycemic agents alerts the nurse to the presence of diabetes and risk for diabetic retinopathy. Antihistamine and decongestant drugs may cause eye dryness, while β-adrenergic blocking agents may cause additive effects in clients with glaucoma for whom these medications may be prescribed.
7.  a. UV light exposure; age-related eye problems, improper contact lens care, family history of ocular problems or diseases affecting the eye
    b. Deficiencies of zinc, vitamins C and E
    c. Constipation and straining to defecate increases intraocular pressure
    d. Work and leisure activities that increase eye strain, lack of protective eyewear during sports
    e. Lack of sleep
    f. Presence of eye pain
    g. Decreased self-concept and self-image, loss of independence
    h. Loss of roles and responsibilities, occupational eye injuries
    i. Eye medications that may cause fetal abnormalities; change in sexual activity related to self-image
    j. Grief related to loss of vision, emotional stress
    k. Values and beliefs that limit treatment decisions
8.  With the right eye, the client standing at 20 feet from a Snellen chart can read to the 40-foot line on the chart with two or fewer errors, and with the left eye, the client can read only to the 50-foot line on the chart. This client can read at 20 feet what a person with normal vision can read at 40 and 50 feet.
9.  d. Rationale: PERRLA means pupils equal (in size), round, and react to light (pupil constricts when light shines into same eye and also constricts in the opposite eye) and accommodation (pupils constrict with focus on near object). Nystagmus on far lateral gaze is normal but is not part of the assessment of pupil function.
10. a. Confrontation test; b. Cardinal field of gaze; c. Jaeger chart; d. Snellen chart; e. Tono-pen tonometry
11. b. Rationale: A normal yellowish hue to the normally white sclera is found in dark-pigmented persons and the older adult. Infants and some older adults may exhibit a normal blue cast to the sclera because of thin sclera. Iris colour does not affect the colour of the sclera, and inflammatory conditions of the eye may cause dilation of small blood vessels in the normally clear bulbar conjunctiva, reddening the sclera and conjunctiva.
12. b. Rationale: Fluorescein is a dye that is used topically to identify corneal irregularities; irregularities stain a bright green on application of the dye. A tonometer is used to measure intraocular pressure. Corneal reflex testing establishes the function of the trigeminal nerve (CN V) and should not be done in the client who may have a corneal abrasion. Corneal light reflex testing is performed to evaluate eye position.
13. a. 3; b. 7; c. 6; d. 5; e. 1; f. 8; g. 4; h. 2
14. c. Rationale: Although fluorescein dye can be used topically to identify corneal lesions, in angiography the dye is injected intravenously and outlines the vasculature of the retina, locating areas of retinopathy. A mirrored lens is used in gonioscopy to examine the anterior chamber angle, and electroretinography is the measurement of the electrical response of the retina to a flash of light.
15. a. 5; b. 1; c. 4; d. 7; e. 9; f. 6; g. 3; h. 8; i. 2
16. a. increased production and dryness of cerumen, increased hair; b. atrophy of the eardrum; c. decreased cochlear efficiency due to decreased blood supply, decreased hair cells, and decreased neurons
17. d. Rationale: Presbycusis is a sensorineural hearing loss that occurs with aging and is associated with decreased ability to hear high-pitched sounds. Tinnitus is present in some, but not all, presbycusis. A sensation of fullness in the ears is related to a blocked eustachian tube, and difficulty in understanding the meaning of words is associated with a central hearing loss occurring with problems arising from the cochlea to the cerebral cortex.
18. a. Childhood middle ear infections with perforations and scarring of the eardrum lead to conductive hearing impairments in adulthood.
    b. Many medications are ototoxic, causing damage to the auditory nerve. Over-the-counter agents such as ASA and non-steroidal anti-inflammatory agents are potentially ototoxic, as well as prescription diuretics, antibiotics, and chemotherapeutic drugs.
    c. A head injury may damage areas of the brain to which auditory and vestibular stimuli are

transmitted, with a resultant loss of hearing or balance.

d. Some congenital hearing disorders are hereditary, and the age of onset of presbycusis also follows a familial pattern.

e. It is well documented that exposure to loud noises causes damage to the auditory organs and hearing loss. Noise exposure earlier in life also can result in increased hearing loss with age.

f. Persons with hearing loss may withdraw from social relationships because of difficulty with communication. A hearing loss often leaves the client feeling isolated and cut off from valued relationships.

19. a. T; b. F, upward and backward; c. F, the umbo instead of the cone of light; d. T; e. F, left; f. T; g. F, acute otitis media

20. a. SHL; b. CHL; c. CHL; d. SHL; e. CHL; f. SHL

21. a. Rationale: Hearing is most sensitive between 500 and 4000 Hz, and a 40 to 45 dB loss in the frequency between 4000 and 8000 Hz will cause difficulty in distinguishing high-pitched consonants. A 10 dB loss is not significant at 8000 Hz. A hearing aid is rarely recommended for a hearing loss of less than 26 dB, and problems in everyday communication situations occur only when the thresholds are 25 dB or higher.

22. b. Rationale: Irrigation of the external ear with water causes a disturbance in the endolymph that normally results in nystagmus directed opposite the side of instillation. The absence of nystagmus indicates that peripheral or central vestibular functions are impaired. An improvement in hearing would occur only if there were an obstruction of the ear canal, which would not be an indication for caloric testing. Severe pain upon irrigation would not be related to vestibular function.

# CHAPTER 21

1. a. 4; b. 5; c. 2; d. 2; e. 1; f. 1; g. 1; h. 4; i. 3; j. 2; k. 2; l. 1

2. b. Rationale: A soft lens should be moved off the cornea and then gently pinched to release it from the eye. A small suction cup may be used for hard lenses, but cotton balls should not be placed on the lenses. Blinking will not remove soft lenses, and an unconscious client may not have a blink reflex.

3. d. Rationale: The most common correction for absence of the crystalline lens today is surgical replacement with an intraocular lens. In the past, aphakic spectacles or contact lenses were used, but they are heavy and cause marked magnifica-

tion. Photorefractive keratectomy involves the use of a laser to reshape the cornea to correct refractive errors.

4. d. Rationale: A person who is legally blind has some usable vision that will benefit from vision enhancement techniques. A person with total blindness has no light perception and no usable vision, and one with functional blindness has the loss of usable vision but some light perception. Dependency on others from visual impairment is individual and cannot be assumed.

5. a. Address client, not others with the client, in normal conversational tones

b. Face client and make eye contact

c. Introduce self when approaching the client and let client know when leaving

d. Orient to sounds, activities, and physical surroundings

e. Use sighted-guide technique to ambulate and orient client

f. Do not move objects positioned by client without knowledge and consent of client

g. Ask client what help is needed and how to provide it

6. c. Rationale: Emergency management of foreign bodies in the eye includes covering and shielding the eye, with no attempt to treat the injury, until an ophthalmologist can evaluate the injury. Irrigations are performed as emergency management in chemical exposure. Pressure should never be applied because it may further injure the eye.

7. a. 4; b. 5; c. 7; d. 6; e. 1; f. 3; g. 2

8. d. Rationale: All infections of the conjunctiva or cornea are transmittable, and frequent, thorough hand washing is essential to prevent spread from one eye to the other or to other persons. Artificial tears are not normally used in external eye infection. Photophobia is not experienced by all clients with eye infections, and cold compresses are indicated for some infections.

9. d. Rationale: Although cataracts do become worse with time, surgical extraction is considered an elective procedure and is usually performed when clients decide that they want or need to see better for their lifestyle. There are no known measures to prevent cataract development or progression. Surgical extraction is safe, but the client will still need glasses for near vision and for any residual refractive error of the implanted lens.

10. c. Rationale: The lens opacity of cataracts causes a decrease in vision, abnormal colour perception, and glare. Blurred vision, halos around lights, and eye pain are characteristic of glaucoma; light flashes, floaters, and "cobwebs" or "hairnets" in the field of vision followed by a painless, sudden loss of vision are characteristic of detached retina.

11. a. Rationale: Assessment of the visual acuity in the client's unoperated eye enables the nurse to determine how visually compromised the client may be while the operative eye is patched and healing and to plan for assistance until vision improves. The patch on the operative eye is usually removed within 24 hours, and although vision in the eye may be good, it is not unusual for visual acuity to be reduced immediately after surgery. Activities that are thought to increase intraocular pressure, such as bending, coughing, and the Valsalva manoeuvre, are restricted postoperatively.

12. a. vitreous shrinking during aging, pulling and tearing the retina; b. rhegmatogenous; c. laser photocoagulation, cryopexy; d. scleral buckling

13. a. Rationale: Post-operatively the client must position the head so that the bubble is in contact with the retinal break and may have to maintain this position for up to 16 hours a day for five days. The client may go home within a few hours of surgery or may remain in the hospital for several days. No matter the type of repair, reattachment is successful in 90% of retinal detachments. Post-operative pain is expected and is treated with analgesics.

14. b. Rationale: The client with ARDM can benefit from low-vision aids in spite of increasing loss of vision, and it is important to promote a positive outlook by not giving clients the impression that "nothing can be done" for them. Laser treatment may help a few clients with choroidal neovascularization, and photodynamic therapy is indicated for a small percent of clients with wet ARDM, but there is no treatment for the increasing deposit of extracellular debris in the retina.

15. c. Rationale: Verteporfin, the dye used with photodynamic therapy to destroy abnormal blood vessels, is a photosensitizing drug that can be activated by exposure to sunlight or other high-intensity light. Clients must cover all their skin to avoid thermal burns when exposed to sunlight. Blind spots occur with laser photocoagulation used for dry ARMD. Head movements and position are not of concern following this procedure.

16. a. Rationale: In glaucoma, increased intraocular pressure ultimately damages the optic nerve and retina. Deposition of drusen and degeneration of the macula are characteristic of age-related macular degeneration, and aqueous humor clouding and ciliary body paralysis are not specifically related to eye disorders.

17. c. Rationale: Because glaucoma develops slowly and without symptoms, it is important that intraocular pressure be evaluated every two to four years in persons between the ages of 40 and 64 and every one to two years in those over 65 years old. More frequent measurement of intraocular pressure should be done in a client with a family history of glaucoma, a black client, and a client with diabetes or cardiovascular disease. The disease is chronic, but vision impairment is preventable in most cases with treatment.

18. a. POAG; b. PACG; c. PACG; d. PACG; e. POAG; f. PACG; g. POAG; h. POAG; i. POAG; j. PACG

19. a. beta-adrenergic blocking agent that decreases aqueous humor production
    b. adrenergic agonist that decreases production of aqueous humor
    c. cholinergic agent that stimulates iris sphincter contraction leading to miosis and opening of the trabecular network, increasing aqueous outflow
    d. carbonic anhydrase inhibitor that decreases aqueous humor production

20. To remove the prosthesis, pull the lower lid down and toward the cheekbone. To insert the prosthesis, open the upper lid with pressure on the upper bony orbit, place the top of the prosthesis under the upper lid, and pull the lower lid down, slipping the lower edge of the prosthesis under the lower lid with a little pressure on the prosthesis.

21. a. Rationale: Clients receiving ototoxic drugs should be monitored for tinnitus, hearing loss, and vertigo to prevent further damage caused by the drugs. Ears should not be cleaned with anything but a washcloth and finger, and ear protection should be used in any environment with noise levels above 90 dB. Exposure to the rubella virus during the first 16 weeks of pregnancy may cause fetal deafness, and the vaccine should never be given during pregnancy.

22. a. 6; b. 2; c. 3; d. 1; e. 5; f. 4

23. Advanced age; use of three potentially ototoxic drugs (ASA, quinidine, and furosemide)

24. d. Rationale: Antibiotic eardrops for external otitis should be applied without touching the auricle to avoid contaminating the dropper and the solution, and the client should hold the ear upward for several minutes to allow the drops to run down the canal. An ear wick may be placed in the canal to help deliver the drops, but it remains in the ear throughout the course of treatment. The use of lubricating eardrops followed by irrigation is performed for impacted cerumen. "Swimmer's ear" is best prevented by avoiding swimming in contaminated waters; prophylactic antibiotics are not used.

25. a. F, antibiotics; b. F, cholesteatoma; c. T; d. T; e. F, chronic; f. T; g. F, with the head of bed elevated 30 degrees

26. a. Rationale: The Valsalva manoeuvre can be used in serous otitis media to open the eustachian tube and equalize the negative pressure that develops in the middle ear. Measures that prevent an increase in middle ear pressure, such as nose blowing, coughing, or positioning, are not indicated.

27. a. Rationale: Otosclerosis is an autosomal-dominant hereditary disease that causes fixation of the footplate of the stapes, leading to conductive hearing loss. Tuning fork testing in conductive hearing loss would result in a negative Rinne test and lateralization to the poor ear or ear with the greater hearing loss upon Weber testing. During a stapedectomy, the client often reports an immediate improvement in hearing, but the hearing level decreases temporarily postoperatively.

28. b. Rationale: Stimulation of the labyrinth intraoperatively may cause post-operative dizziness, increasing the risk for falls. Nystagmus on lateral gaze may result from perilymph disturbances but does not constitute a risk for injury. A tympanic graft is not performed in a stapedectomy, nor is post-operative tinnitus common.

29. a. vertigo; b. sensorineural hearing loss; c. tinnitus

30. b. Rationale: Nursing care should minimize vertigo by keeping the client in a quiet, dark environment. Movement aggravates the whirling and roaring sensations, and the client should be moved only for essential care. Fluorescent lights or television flickering may also increase vertigo and should be avoided. Side rails should be raised when the client is in bed, but there is no indication for padding.

31. d. Rationale: The benign acoustic neuroma can compress the facial nerve and arteries in the internal auditory canal and may expand into the cranium, but if removed when small, hearing and vestibular function can be preserved. During surgery for a tumour that has expanded into the cranium, preservation of hearing and the facial nerve is reduced.

32. a. C; b. C; c. C; d. C; e. S; f. C; g. S; h. S; i. S; j. C

33. c. Rationale: Initial adjustment to a hearing aid should include voices and household sounds and experimenting with volume in a quiet environment. The next recommended exposure is small parties, the outdoors and, finally, uncontrolled areas, such as shopping areas.

**Case Study**

1. Her race, her family history of glaucoma, and her increasing age place her at a high risk for glaucoma. Black clients are more likely to develop glaucoma, and in every age category should have examinations more often than persons without risk factors because of the increased incidence and more aggressive course of glaucoma in these individuals.

2. To prevent systemic absorption of the drug; Mrs. G. already uses one β-adrenergic blocker (metoprolol) for her hypertension, and systemic absorption of the betaxolol could cause additive effects.

3. The antihistamine comes into question because of its anticholinergic effects. It is allowed because Mrs. G. has open-angle glaucoma with no abnormal angle on gonioscopy. In angle-closure glaucoma the drug is contraindicated because anticholinergic effects of the antihistamine would dilate the pupil, obstructing an already narrowed angle.

4. No, because glaucoma is a chronic disease with no cure. It can be controlled with medication and some surgical interventions but not cured.

5. Alternatives to topical therapy for POAG include a trabeculoplasty that opens outflow channels in the trabecular meshwork, a trabeculectomy in which part of the iris and trabecular meshwork are removed, or cyclocryotherapy in which parts of the ciliary body are destroyed, decreasing production of aqueous humor.

6. Optic disc cupping with the disc becoming wider, deeper, and paler occurs with progression of glaucoma. Visual complaints with increasing damage include increasing peripheral visual field loss with eventual tunnel vision and loss of sight.

7. *Nursing diagnoses:*
   - Anxiety related to potential permanent visual impairment
   - Ineffective health maintenance related to lack of routine assessments for glaucoma
   - Risk for ineffective therapeutic regimen management related to lack of knowledge about disease, treatment, administration of eyedrops, follow-up recommendations

   *Collaborative problems:*
   Potential complications: increased intraocular pressure, blindness

# CHAPTER 22

1. a. hair shaft; b. stratum corneum; c. stratum germinativum; d. melanocyte; e. sebaceous gland; f. eccrine sweat gland; g. apocrine sweat gland; h. blood vessels; i. nerves; j. adipose tissue; k. hair follicle; l. arrector pili muscle; m. connective tissue; n. subcutaneous tissue; o. dermis; p. epidermis

2. a. 5; b. 3; c. 1; d. 6; e. 2; f. 8; g. 1; h. 4; i. 4; j. 7; k. 2

3. a. Decreased subcutaneous fat, decreased elasticity, collagen stiffening, UV exposure, gravity; b. Decreased extracellular fluid, decreased sweat and sebaceous gland activity; c. Increased capillary fragility and permeability; d. Decreased blood supply, increased keratin

4. d. Rationale: A careful medication history is important because many medications cause dermatological side effects and clients also use many over-the-counter preparations to treat skin problems. Freckles are common in childhood and are not related to skin disease. Communicable childhood illnesses are not directly related to skin problems, although varicella viruses may affect the skin in adulthood. Patterns of weight gain and loss are not significant, but the presence of obesity may cause skin problems in overlapping skin areas.

5. a. Poor skin hygiene, excessive or unprotected sun exposure, family history of alopecia, ichthyosis, psoriases, history of skin cancer
   b. Decreased intake of vitamins A, D, E, or C, malnutrition, food allergies, obesity
   c. Incontinence, fluid imbalances
   d. Exposure to carcinogens or chemical irritants
   e. Itching that interferes with sleep
   f. Pain, decreased perception of heat, cold, and touch
   g. Feelings of rejection, prejudice, loss of self-esteem, and impaired body image
   h. Exposure to irritants and allergens, altered relationships with others
   i. Changes in sexual intimacy because of appearance, pain
   j. Skin problems exacerbated by stress
   k. High social value placed on appearance and skin condition with tanning, use of cosmetics

6. d. Rationale: It is necessary for the client to be completely undressed for an examination of the skin. Gowns should be provided and exposure minimized as the skin is inspected generally first, followed by a lesion-specific examination. Skin temperature is best assessed with the back of the hand, and turgor is best assessed with the skin over the sternum.

7. b. Rationale: Discoloured lesions that are caused by intradermal or subcutaneous bleeding do not blanch with pressure, while those caused by inflammation and dilated blood vessels will blanch and refill after palpation. Varicosities are engorged, dilated veins that may empty with pressure applied along the vein.

8. a. Vesicles; b. Discrete, localized to chest and abdomen; c. Colour, size, and configuration

9. a. 9; b. 5; c. 4; d. 7; e. 10; f. 8; g. 1; h. 11; i. 2; j. 6; k. 3

10. d. Rationale: An excoriation is a focal loss of epidermis, does not involve the dermis and, as such, does not scar with healing. Ulcers do penetrate into and through the dermis, and scarring does occur with these deeper lesions. Epidermal and dermal thinning is atrophy of the skin but does not involve a break in skin integrity. Both excoriations and ulcers have a break in skin integrity and may develop crusts or scabs over the lesions.

11. d. Rationale: During assessment of the skin in dark-skinned persons, inspection of skin colour should be done where the epidermis is thin or in areas of least pigmentation. The nailbeds can be used or the mucosa of the eyes or mouth. In black clients, the sclera is normally yellow-tinged and is not a good site for evaluating colour changes. The palms of the hands and soles of the feet are secondary choices to mucosa.

12. d. Rationale: A shave biopsy is done for superficial lesions that can be scraped with a razor blade, removing the full thickness of stratum corneum. Excisional biopsy is done when the entire removal of a lesion is desired. Punch biopsies are done with larger nodules to examine for pathology, as are incisional biopsies.

13. a. Rationale: A culture can be done to distinguish among fungal, bacterial, and viral infections. A Tzanck test is specific for herpesvirus infections, potassium hydroxide slides are specific for fungal infections, and immunofluorescent studies are specific for infections that cause abnormal antibody proteins.

14. a. 9; b. 5; c. 7; d. 8; e. 1; f. 4; g. 3; h. 10; i. 2; j. 6

# CHAPTER 23

1. a. F, ultraviolet B (UVB); b. F, thiazide; c. F, 15; d. T; e. F, B-complex vitamins

2. a. Rationale: Exposure to the sun is the single most important factor in the development of skin cancer and premature aging from loss of elasticity and thinning, wrinkling, and drying of the skin. Radiation exposure and alkaline soaps are less common causes of skin problems, as is indiscriminate self-treatment with over-the-counter skin medications.

3. a. 5; b. 3; c. 5; d. 1; e. 4; f. 1; g. 4; h. 5; i. 2; j. 3

4. A: Asymmetry—one half unlike the other half; B: Border—irregular and poorly circumscribed; C: Colour—varied within lesion; D: Diameter—larger than 6 mm

5. c. Rationale: Because of the high potential for metastasis, wide surgical excision with a margin of normal skin is the initial treatment for malignant melanoma. Mohs' surgery is used for cutaneous malignancies, such as basal or squamous cell carcinomas, where there is concern for preservation of normal tissue. Radiation may be used after excision for malignant melanoma, depending on staging of the disease. Topical nitrogen mustard may be used for treatment of cutaneous T cell lymphoma.

6. a. Chronic disease; b. Obesity; c. Recent antibiotic therapy; d. Recent corticosteroid therapy

7. a. 7; b. 10; c. 6; d. 11; e. 8; f. 14; g. 4; h. 12; i. 1; j. 15; k. 3; l. 9; m. 2; n. 5; o. 13

8. Kaposi's sarcoma, candidiasis, herpes zoster

9. b. Rationale: Urticaria is inflammation and edema in the upper dermis, most commonly caused by histamine released during an antibody–allergen reaction. The best treatment for all types of allergic dermatitis is avoidance of the allergen. Sunlight and warmth would increase the edema and inflammation. Antihistamines may be used for an acute outbreak but not to prevent the dermatitis. Topical γ-benzene hexachloride is used to treat pediculosis.

10. a. Rationale: Pediculosis (head lice and body lice) causes very small, red, non-inflammatory lesions that progress to papular wheal-like lesions and causes severe itching. Lice live on the body as nits (tiny white eggs) that are firmly attached to the hair shaft in head and body lice. Burrows, especially in interdigital webs, are found with scabies.

11. a. Rationale: A lotion is a suspension of insoluble powders in water, which has cooling and drying properties, useful when itching is present.

Creams and ointments have an oil and water base that lubricates and protects skin, while a paste is a mixture of powder and ointment.

12. d. Rationale: Psoralen is absorbed by the lens of the eye, and eyewear that blocks 100% of UV light must be used for 24 hours after taking the medication. Since UVA penetrates glass, the eyewear must also be worn indoors when near a bright window. Psoralen does not affect the accommodative ability of the eye.

13. a. Clean skin; no occlusive dressings
    b. Diagnosis of lesion first; thin layers; massaged in at prescribed frequency
    c. Advise of side effects and risks associated with driving or operating heavy machinery
    d. Avoid sunlight; causes photosensitivity; warn client it will cause painful, eroded dermatitis before healing

14. a. 4; b. 1, 2, 3, 5; c. 1, 3; d. 2, 3, 6; e. 2, 6

15. a. Rationale: Dressings used to treat pruritic lesions should be cool to cause vasoconstriction and to have an anti-inflammatory effect. Water is most commonly used, and it does not need to be sterile. Acetic acid solutions are bacteriocidal and are used to treat skin infections.

16. b. Rationale: Tepid or warm solutions should be used when the purpose is debridement, and saline is a common debridement solution. Baths are appropriate for debridement, but sodium bicarbonate and oatmeal are used for pruritus.

17. a. Vasoconstriction; b. Decrease inflammation and blood flow; c. Decrease vasodilation and stop itch sensation; d. Vasoconstriction and stop itch sensation

18. b. Rationale: Defining characteristics for body image problems include verbalization of self-disgust and reluctance to look at lesions as evidenced in this client. Social isolation is indicated only by evidence of decreased social activities and anxiety by verbalization of anxiety or frustration. Impaired therapeutic regimen management is indicated by evidence of a lack of self-care or understanding of the disease process.

19. a. Rationale: Lichenification is thickening of the skin, caused by chronic scratching or rubbing, and can be prevented by controlling itching. It is not an infection, nor is it contagious, as the other options indicate.

20. b. Rationale: Nursing interventions for nursing diagnoses should address the etiology of the problem. In this case, if appearance causes the anxiety, the nurse should help the client improve appearance. A male client especially may need to be taught skilful use of cosmetics and cover-up techniques to enhance appearance.

21. a. Rationale: Improvement of body image is the most common reason for undergoing cosmetic surgery, with appearance being an important part of confidence and self-assurance. Acne scars, pigmentation problems, and wrinkling can also be treated with cosmetic surgery, but the surgery does not prevent the skin changes associated with aging.

22. a. Face lift; b. Liposuction; c. Dermabrasion; d. Chemical face lift/peel; e. Topical tretinoin

23. a. Rationale: Skin flaps as grafts include moving skin and subcutaneous tissue to another part of the body and are used to cover wounds with poor vascular beds, add padding, and cover wounds over cartilage and bone. Both types of free grafts include just skin, and soft tissue extension involves placement of an expander under the skin, which stretches the skin over time to provide extra skin for covering the desired area.

**Case Study**

1. Mr. J. B. should have cleansed the wound with soap and water and sought medical care for cleaning and suturing. A sterile dressing should have been applied and the arm elevated to reduce edema.

2. *Staphylococcus aureus* and *Streptococcus*

3. That systemic antibiotics will be necessary and that warm, moist packs or dressings should be used to help localize the infection; hospitalization will be necessary if it becomes severe.

4. Gangrene of the extremity; possible septicemia

5. *Nursing diagnoses:*
   - Impaired skin integrity related to trauma
   - Acute pain related to inflammatory process
   - Hyperthermia related to inflammatory process
   *Collaborative problems:*
   Potential complications: gangrene; septicemia

## CHAPTER 24

1. a. 4; b. 1; c. 2; d. 4; e. 1; f. 3; g. 3

2. a. T; b. F, alkaline substances; c. F, chemical; d. T; e. F, electrical burn

3. a. major; b. major; c. moderate uncomplicated; d. major; e. minor (or superficial partial-thickness may not be classified)

4. a. Rationale: Dry, waxy white, leathery, or hard skin is characteristic of full-thickness burns in the emergent phase, and they may turn brown and dry in the acute phase. Deep partial-thickness burns in the emergent phase are red, shiny, and have blisters. Edema may not be as extensive in full-thickness burns because of thrombosed vessels.

5. a. $3\frac{1}{2} + 1 + 7\frac{1}{2} + 2 + 3\frac{1}{2} = 17\frac{1}{2}$
   b. $4\frac{1}{2} + 9 + 4\frac{1}{2} = 18$
   c. No, because edema and inflammation obscure the demarcation of zones of injury
   d. Major

6. d. Rationale: The first intervention is to remove the source and stop the burning process. Airway maintenance would be second, then establishing IV access, followed by assessing for other injuries.

7. a. Fluid loss and formation of edema—usually 24 to 48 hours but may be up to five days; b. Mobilization of fluid and diuresis—weeks to months; c. Burned area covered and wounds healed—weeks to months

8. a. Rationale: With increased capillary permeability, water, sodium, and plasma proteins leave the plasma and move into the interstitial spaces, decreasing serum sodium and albumin. Less sodium is excreted from the kidney because serum levels are low. Serum potassium is elevated because injured cells and hemolyzed RBCs release potassium from cells. An elevated hematocrit is caused by water loss into the interstitium, creating a hemoconcentration. Urine specific gravity increases because of water preservation by the kidneys during hypovolemia.

9. a. Rationale: Although all the selections add to the hypovolemia that occurs in the emergent burn phase, the initial and most pronounced effect is caused by fluid shifts out of the blood vessels as a result of increased capillary permeability.

10. a. Rationale: Burn injury causes widespread impairment of the immune system, with depression of neutrophil activity, decreased T helper cells, and decreased levels of interleukins.

11. c. Rationale: Because of the hypovolemia and relative fluid loss, intense thirst is a common finding in the initially burned client. Severe pain is not common in full-thickness burns, nor is unconsciousness unless there are other factors present. Fever is a sign of infection in later burn phases.

12. d. Rationale: In circumferential burns, circulation to the extremities can be severely impaired, and pulses should be monitored closely for signs of obstruction by edema. Swelling of the arms would be expected, but it becomes dangerous when it occludes vessels. Pain and eschar are also expected.

13. b. Rationale: Clients with major injuries involving burns to the face and neck require intubation within one to two hours after burn injury to prevent the necessity for emergency tracheostomy, which is done if symptoms of upper respiratory obstruction occur. Carbon monoxide poisoning is treated with 100% oxygen, and eschar constriction of the chest is treated with an escharotomy.

14. d. Rationale: Acute tubular necrosis occurs when kidney tubules are mechanically blocked by myoglobin (from muscle cell breakdown) and hemoglobin (from RBC breakdown). Fluid intake at a rate to maintain urinary output at 75 to 100 mL/hr, osmotic diuretics such as mannitol, and sodium bicarbonate to alkalinize the urine help flush the myoglobin and hemoglobin from the circulatory system through the kidneys.

15. To calculate fluid replacement, the client's weight in pounds must be converted to kilograms: 132 lb = 60 kg.
    a. lactated Ringer's; 9600 mL (4 mL x 60 x 40)
    b. 4800, 1015 to 1730; 2400, 1730 to 0130; 2400, 0130 to 0930
    c. serum sodium levels
    d. urine output (30 to 50 mL/hr); VS (BP ≥90 mm Hg, P ≤100, R 16 to 20); alert, oriented to time, place, and person

16. d. Rationale: When the client's wounds are exposed with open method, the staff must wear hats, masks, gowns, and gloves. Sterile water is not necessary in the debridement tank, and topical anti-infective agents should be applied with sterile gloves. Open method of treatment does not use dressings.

17. a. Rationale: Morphine is the drug of choice for pain control, and during the emergent phase, it should be administered IV because GI function is impaired and IM injections will not be absorbed adequately.

18. b. Rationale: The client with large burns often develops paralytic ileus within a few hours, and a nasogastric tube is inserted and connected to low, intermittent suction. After GI function returns, feeding tubes may be used for nutritional supplementation and $H_2$ blockers may be used to prevent Curling's ulcers. Free water is not given to drink because of the potential for water intoxication.

19. c. Rationale: Clients with ear burns are not allowed to use pillows, because of the danger of the burned ear sticking to the pillowcase, and clients with neck burns are not allowed to use pillows, because contractures of the neck can occur.

20. a. hypermetabolic state resulting from increased plasma catacholamines and substrate mobilization
    b. massive catabolism resulting from protein breakdown and increased gluconeogenesis
    c. calories and protein for tissue repair

21. c. Rationale: At the end of the emergent phase, fluid mobilization moves potassium back into the cells and sodium returns to the vascular space, causing hypokalemia and hypernatremia. As diuresis in the acute phase continues, sodium will be lost in the urine and potassium will continue to be low unless replaced. Excessive fluid replacement with 5% dextrose in water without potassium supplementation can cause hyponatremia with hypokalemia. Prolonged hydrotherapy and free oral water intake can cause a decrease in both sodium and potassium.

22. c. Rationale: The limited range of motion in this situation is related to the client's inability or reluctance to exercise the joints because of pain, and the appropriate intervention is to help control the pain so that exercises can be performed. The client is probably never without some pain, and although exercises and enlisting the help of the physiotherapist are important, neither of these interventions addresses the cause.

23. a. Rationale: Early signs of sepsis include an elevated temperature and increased pulse and respiratory rate accompanied by decreased BP and, later, decreased urine output and perhaps paralytic ileus. A burn wound may become locally infected without causing sepsis.

24. a. Dementia; b. Curling's ulcer; c. Stress diabetes

25. a. cultured epithelial autograft; b. eschar (or necrotic tissue), split-thickness grafts; c. aspirating the fluid with a TB syringe or rolling the fluid with a sterile swab to an opening in the peripheral margin of the graft

26. a. Rationale: Midazolam is useful when clients' anticipation of the pain experience increases their pain because it causes a short-term memory loss, and if given before a dressing change, the client will not recall the event. A dosage range of morphine is useful, as is client-controlled analgesia, but seldom will these doses effectively relieve the discomfort of dressing changes. Buprenorphine has an analgesic action but is a narcotic antagonist and so cannot be used with other narcotics.

27. a. Rationale: Pressure garments help keep scars flat and prevent elevation and enlargement above the original burn injury area. Lotions and splinting are used to prevent contractures. Avoidance of sun is necessary for one year to prevent hyperpigmentation and sunburn injury to healed burn areas.

**Case Study**

1. Discharge planning should be initiated at the time of admission, when the client is stabilized. Resuming a functional role in society and accomplishing functional and cosmetic reconstruction are the end goals toward which all care is directed. The nurse should coordinate the discharge process with the whole healthcare team involved with Kim's care—the physician, physio-

therapists and occupational therapists, dietitian, home care nurses, and counsellors.

2. Kim will continue to need a high-calorie, high-protein diet, but not to the same extent as during the acute phase. She should be taught about her diet and also to monitor for unwanted weight gain and to reduce calories as indicated. She may also have a functional disability in feeding herself and may need padded utensils or special assistive devices.

3. Kim will need to continue the splinting and exercise routines diligently until healing is complete—probably for at least a year.

4. Stress that exercise and performance of activities of daily living will decrease the tightness and limitation of movement. Set achievable short-term goals with her that can be measured, or have her identify a few activities she wants most to do that are realistic and work toward success with those. She is receiving a secondary gain from her husband in her dependence and regression, and the nurse should help her husband see the importance of her re-establishing independence and enlist his help in coaching the client with exercises.

5. Provide information and expected outcomes related to the healing of her injuries to both client and husband. Encourage both the client and her husband to participate in the client's care, and have them identify how care can be managed at home. Let them know that it is possible to maintain contact with hospital personnel after discharge to answer questions and give them support.

6. Kim and her family may experience a wide range of emotional responses—fear, anxiety, anger, guilt, or depression—and Kim may be very concerned about her children's reactions to the appearance of her injuries. The nurse should encourage the client's expression of negative feelings and fears while still hospitalized. Arranging for short visits from her children while she is still hospitalized and while the visits can be controlled would be helpful. Preparation of the family can also be enhanced by helping all family members become aware of routines and activities that will need to be continued during rehabilitation.

7. The procedures for dressing changes and graft care should be formally demonstrated to the client and her husband with time for them to practice and return the demonstrations. It is most likely the husband must be involved because she will be unable to manage dressings to her hands. Referral to home care nurses is essential for follow-up and evaluation when the client is discharged to ensure that rehabilitation is continuing.

8. *Nursing diagnoses:*
   - Anticipatory grieving related to impact of injury on appearance, relationships, and lifestyle
   - Anxiety related to appearance
   - Self-care deficit related to inability or unwillingness to participate in self-care
   - Impaired therapeutic regimen management related to insufficient knowledge of wound care, follow-up care
   - Situational low self-esteem related to effects of burn on appearance, increased dependence on others, and disruption of lifestyle and role responsibilities
   - Risk for disuse syndrome related to effects of immobility

   *Collaborative problems:*

   Potential complications: graft rejection/infection; contractures

## CHAPTER 25

1. a. nasal cavity; b. right main-stem bronchi; c. segmental bronchi; d. terminal bronchiole; e. alveolar duct; f. alveoli; g. septa; h. pores of Kohn; i. respiratory bronchiole; j. cilia; k. goblet cell; l. mucus; m. dust particle; n. left main-stem bronchi; o. carina; p. trachea; q. larynx; r. epiglottis; s. pharynx

2. a. right mid-clavicular line; b. right anterior axillary line; c. right upper lobe; d. right middle lobe; e. right lower lobe; f. left lower lobe; g. left upper lobe; h. angle of Louis; i. first rib; j. suprasternal notch; k. trachea; l. larynx; m. thyroid cartilage; n. mid-sternal line; o. vertebral line; p. spinal processes; q. left upper lobe; r. left lower lobe; s. right lower lobe; t. right upper lobe; u. scapular line

3.  a. thoracic cage; b. epiglottis; c. trachea;
    d. carina; e. dead space; f. surfactant; g. alveolar
    sacs; h. compliance; i. larynx; j. turbinates;
    k. angle of Louis; l. parietal pleura; m. phrenic
    nerve; n. cilia; o. visceral; p. empyema

4.  a. F, arterial oxygen saturation, as a percentage;
    b. F, arterial oxygen tension, in mm Hg; c. T;
    d. T; e. F, 65 mm Hg
5.  a. Rationale: When the oxygen–hemoglobin
    curve shifts to the right, blood picks up less oxy-
    gen from the lungs but delivers oxygen more
    readily to the tissues, thus low concentrations of
    oxygen may be given to prevent oxygen toxicity.
    Shifts to the right occur with acidosis, hyperther-
    mia, and increased $PaCO_2$. Alkalosis, hypother-
    mia, and decreases in $PaCO_2$ cause a leftward
    shift of the oxygen–hemoglobin curve, which
    may be treated with higher concentrations of
    oxygen to compensate for decreased oxygen
    unloading in the tissues.
6.  c. Rationale: Normally, an $SaO_2$ of 85% corre-
    lates with a $PaO_2$ of about 60 mm Hg. In a left-
    ward shift of the oxygen–hemoglobin curve,
    oxygen is less readily delivered to the tissues and
    a lower $PaO_2$ is present. In a rightward shift of
    the curve, an $SaO_2$ of 85% would reflect a higher
    $PaO_2$ than normal, about 65 mm Hg. Leftward
    shifts are commonly caused by alkalosis,
    hypothermia, and decreases in $PaCO_2$.

7.  b. Rationale: Normal findings in arterial blood
    gases in the older adult include a decreased $PaO_2$
    and $SaO_2$ but normal pH and $PaCO_2$. A normal
    $PaO_2$ for a 75-year-old client would be deter-
    mined by the following equation:
    $PaO_2$ (mm Hg) = 103.5 – (.42 × age [yr]) or
    103.5 – 31.5 = 72 mm Hg
    Normal $PaO_2$ levels are expected in clients of 60
    years of age or less.
8.  c. Rationale: Normal venous blood gas values
    reflect the normal uptake of oxygen from arterial
    blood and release of carbon dioxide from cells
    into the blood, with a decrease in pH due to
    higher $PvCO_2$ and also much lower $PvO_2$ and
    $SvO_2$. Mixed venous blood gases are used when
    clients are hemodynamically unstable to evaluate
    the amount of oxygen delivered to the tissue and
    the amount of oxygen consumed by the tissues.
9.  c. Rationale: Pulse oximetry is inaccurate if the
    probe is loose, if there is low perfusion, or if
    there is dark skin colour, and before other mea-
    sures are taken, the nurse should check the probe
    site. If the probe is intact at the site and perfusion
    is adequate, an ABG analysis should be done to

verify accuracy, and oxygen may be administered depending on the client's condition and assessment of respiratory and cardiac status.

10. c. Rationale: Poor peripheral perfusion that occurs with hypovolemia or other types of conditions that cause peripheral vasoconstriction will cause inaccurate pulse oximetry, and ABGs may need to be used to monitor oxygenation status and ventilation status in these clients. It would not be affected by fever or anaesthesia and is a method of monitoring arterial oxygen saturation in clients receiving oxygen therapy.

11. a. How the client's $SpO_2$ compares with the expected normal values
    b. Determining the trend and rate of development of the hypoxemia
    c. Assessing for the presence of other signs and symptoms of inadequate oxygenation
    d. What the oxygenation status is with activity or exercise

12. c. Rationale: An $SpO_2$ of 88% and a $PaO_2$ of 55 mm Hg indicate inadequate oxygenation and are the criteria for prescription of continuous oxygen therapy (Table 25-3). These values may be adequate for clients with chronic hypoxemia if no cardiac problems occur but will affect their activity tolerance.

13. c. Rationale: Lowering of the pH of cerebrospinal fluid by the combination of excess $CO_2$ and water to form carbonic acid stimulates chemoreceptors in the medulla to increase respiratory rate and volume to provide elimination of the excess $CO_2$. Peripheral chemoreceptors in the carotid and aortic bodies also respond to increases in $PaCO_2$ to stimulate the respiratory centre. Excess $CO_2$ does not increase the amount of hydrogen ions available in the body but does combine with the hydrogen of water to form an acid.

14. c. Rationale: Ciliary action impaired by smoking and increased mucus production may be caused by the irritants in tobacco smoke, leading to impairment of the mucociliary clearance system. Smoking does not directly affect filtration, the cough reflex, or reflex bronchoconstriction, but it does impair the respiratory defence mechanism provided by alveolar macrophages.

15. a. Decreased functional alveoli, small airway closure earlier in expiration
    b. Decreased elastic recoil and decreased chest wall compliance
    c. Decreased functional cilia, decreased force of cough
    d. Decreased alveolar macrophage activity, decreased IgA

16. a. Smoking history; gradual change in health status; family history of lung disease
    b. Decreased fluid intake; anorexia and weight loss
    c. Constipation; incontinence
    d. Decreased exercise tolerance; dyspnea on rest or exertion; sedentary habits
    e. Sleep apnea; awakening with dyspnea, wheezing, or cough; night sweats
    f. Decreased cognitive function with restlessness, irritability; chest pain or pain with breathing
    g. Inability to maintain lifestyle; altered self-esteem
    h. Loss of roles at work or home; exposure to respiratory toxins at work
    i. Sexual activity altered by respiratory symptoms
    j. Dyspnea-anxiety-dyspnea cycle; poor coping with stress of chronic respiratory problems
    k. Non-compliance with treatment plan; conflict with values

17. a. 1;  b. 2;  c. 3;  d. 2;  e. 1;  f. 2;  g. 4;  h. 4;  i. 1;  j. 1

18. a. Rationale: To assess the extent and symmetry of chest movement, the nurse places the hands over the lower anterior chest wall along the costal margin and moves them inward until the thumbs meet at midline, then asks the client to breathe deeply and observes the movement of the thumbs away from each other. To determine tracheal position, the nurse places the index fingers on either side of the trachea just above the suprasternal notch and gently presses backward. The palms are placed against the chest wall to assess tactile fremitus.

19. b. Rationale: An increased anteroposterior diameter is characteristic of a barrel chest, in which the anteroposterior diameter is about equal to the side-to-side diameter. Normally the anteroposterior diameter should be one third to one half the side-to-side diameter. A prominent protrusion of the sternum is pectus carinatum, and diminished movement of the two sides of the chest indicates decreased chest excursion. Lack of lung expansion due to kyphosis of the spine results in shallow breathing with decreased chest expansion.

20. d. Rationale: Bronchovesicular breath sounds are normal breath sounds when they are heard anteriorly over the main-stem bronchi on either side of the sternum and posteriorly between the scapula. However, if they are heard in the peripheral lung fields, they are considered abnormal breath sounds. Adventitious lungs sounds are crackles, rhonchi, wheezes, and pleural friction rubs.

21. a. 7; b. 6; c. 5; d. 8; e. 1; f. 2; g. 4; h. 3

22. d. Rationale: Because antibody production in response to infection with the TB bacillus may not be sufficient to produce a reaction to TB skin testing immediately after infection, two-step testing is recommended for individuals likely to be tested often, such as healthcare providers. An initial negative skin test should be repeated in one to three weeks, and if the second test is negative, the individual can be considered uninfected. All of the other answers indicate a negative response to skin testing but, as single testing, do not allow for delay in antibody production.

23. c. Rationale: Samples for arterial blood gas must be iced to keep the gases dissolved in the blood, unless the specimen is to be analyzed in less than one minute and taken directly to the laboratory. The syringe used to obtain the specimen is rinsed with heparin before taking the specimen, and pressure is applied to the arterial puncture site for five minutes after obtaining the specimen. Changes in oxygen therapy or interventions should be avoided for 20 minutes before the specimen is drawn because these changes may alter blood gas values.

24. a. Rationale: A pulmonary angiogram involves the injection of an iodine-based radiopaque dye into the pulmonary artery or the right side of the heart, and iodine or shellfish allergies should be assessed before injection. A bronchoscopy requires NPO status for six to twelve hours before the test, and invasive tests, such as bronchoscopy, mediastinoscopy, or biopsies, require informed consent. Nuclear scans use radioactive materials for diagnosis, but the amounts are very small, and no radiation precautions are indicated for the client.

25. c. Rationale: To prevent damage to the lung tissue and to facilitate entry into the pleural cavity, the client having a thoracentesis is seated upright, with the elbows or arms on an overbed table.

26. c. Rationale: The greatest chance for a pneumothorax occurs with a bronchoscopic lung biopsy because of the possibility of lung tissue injury during this procedure. Air could enter the pleural space during a thoracentesis, but this is rare. A ventilation-perfusion scan and positron emission tomography involve injections, but no manipulation of the respiratory tract.

27. d. Rationale: A pulmonary arteriogram outlines the pulmonary vasculature and is useful to diagnose obstructions or pathological conditions of the pulmonary vessels, such as a pulmonary embolus. The tissue changes of TB and cancer of the lung may be diagnosed by chest x-ray, CT, MRI, or PET. Airway obstruction is most often diagnosed with pulmonary function testing.

28. a. 3; b. 7; c. 2; d. 4; e. 5; f. 6; g. 1

## CHAPTER 26

1. a. F, nasal septoplasty; b. T; c. T; d. F, seasonal; e. T

2. a. Rationale: Direct pressure on the entire soft lower portion of the nose for 10 to 15 minutes is indicated for epistaxis, in addition to sitting the client upright, leaning forward, to prevent swallowing of blood. Ice compresses to the nose may be used in addition to having the client suck on an ice cube to constrict the nasal vessels.

3. a. Rationale: After packing of the posterior nasopharynx, some clients experience a decrease in $PaO_2$ and an increase in $PaCO_2$ because of impaired respiration, and the nurse should monitor respiratory rate and rhythm and $SpO_2$. The nares are cleaned and petroleum jelly is applied after the packing is removed. A low-grade fever may be an indication of infection and is not expected, and non-steroidal anti-inflammatory drugs should not be used because their antiplatelet effects may prolong bleeding.

4. b. Rationale: The most important factor in managing allergic rhinitis is identification and avoidance of triggers of the allergic reactions. Immunotherapy may be indicated if specific allergens are identified and cannot be avoided. Drug therapy is an alternative to avoidance of the allergens, but long-term use of decongestants may cause rebound nasal congestion.

5. d. Rationale: Dyspnea and purulent sputum in a client who has a viral URI indicate lower respiratory involvement and a possible secondary bacterial infection. Bacterial infections are indications for antibiotic therapy, but unless symptoms of complications are present, injudicious administration of antibiotics may produce resistant organisms. Elevated temperature, purulent nasal drainage, cough, sore throat, and myalgia are common symptoms of viral rhinitis and influenza.

6. d. Rationale: The influenza vaccine is recommended for individuals at increased risk for influenza-related complications, such as those aged 50 and older, residents of long-term care facilities, adults with chronic diseases, healthcare workers, and providers of care to at-risk persons. It is also recommended for any person wishing to reduce chances of acquiring influenza. Antiviral agents will help reduce the duration and severity of influenza in those at high risk, but immunization is the best control.

7. c. Rationale: Echinacea, goldenseal, and zinc have been shown to be effective stimulants of the immune system, and all three may help reduce symptoms and duration of the common cold. Echinacea and goldenseal should be taken for limited periods, usually only for the duration of the problem. Antibiotics should not be used for a common cold.

8. c. Rationale: Classic antihistamines available without a prescription increase mucus viscosity and promote continued symptoms of sinusitis and should be avoided. Antibiotics should be taken for at least one week after symptoms are relieved, and ASA products may be used to relieve sinus pain or fever. Nasal irrigations with a saline solution may also be used.

9. c. Rationale: Although inadequately treated β-hemolytic streptococcal infections may lead to rheumatic heart disease or glomerulonephritis, antibiotic treatment is not recommended until strep infections are definitely diagnosed with culture or antigen tests. The manifestations of viral and bacterial infections are similar, and appearance is not diagnostic, except when candidiasis is present.

10. c. Rationale: During apneic periods of sleep, severe hypoxemia and hypercapnia stimulate ventilation and awaken the client, perhaps as many as 200 to 400 times a night, resulting in insomnia and excessive daytime sleepiness. Morning headaches also may occur. The degree of mattress firmness and a history of upper respiratory infections are not relevant factors.

11. d. Rationale: Compliance is poor with the use of the nasal BiPAP device, but it is highly effective, and the client should be supported in its use. Emphasizing that it can eliminate the problems of snoring, personality changes, and cardiovascular complications associated with sleep apnea encourage its use. The device should be used every night, and nighttime sedatives are contraindicated to prevent relaxation of pharyngeal muscles that contributes to airway closure. Head-of-bed elevation is not indicated.

12. a. Stridor; b. Use of accessory muscles; c. Suprasternal and intercostal retractions; d. Wheezing
Others: restlessness, tachycardia, cyanosis

13. b. Rationale: With a tracheostomy rather than an endotracheal tube, client comfort is increased because there is no tube in the mouth, and because the tube is more secure, mobility is improved. It is preferable to perform a tracheotomy in the operating room because it requires careful dissection, but it can be per-formed with local anaesthetic in ICU or in an emergency. With a cuff, tracheal pressure necro-sis is as much a risk with a tracheostomy tube as with an endotracheal tube, and infection is also as likely to occur since the defences of the upper airway are bypassed.

14. a. 1; b. 3; c. 1; d. 2; e. 3; f. 2; g. 3

15. c. Rationale: An inner cannula is a second tubing that fits inside of the outer tracheostomy tube and can be removed and cleaned of mucus that has accumulated on the inside of the tube. Many tra-cheostomy tubes today do not have inner cannu-las because if humidification is adequate, accu-mulation of mucus should not occur.

16. a. Keep a replacement tube of equal or smaller size at the bedside for emergency reinsertion.
b. Tracheostomy tapes should not be changed the first 24 hours after insertion.
c. The first tube change is performed by the physician no sooner than seven days after tra-cheostomy.

17. b. Rationale: Cuff pressure should be monitored every eight hours to ensure that an air leak around the cuff does not occur and that the pressure is not too high to allow adequate tracheal capillary per-fusion (Table 26-6). Tracheostomy tubes are not usually changed sooner than seven days after a tracheotomy. Mouth care should be performed a minimum of every eight hours and more often as needed to remove dried secretions. ABGs are not routinely assessed with tracheostomy tube place-ment unless symptoms of respiratory distress con-tinue.

18. b. Rationale: If a tracheostomy tube is dislodged, the nurse should immediately attempt to replace the tube by grasping the retention sutures (if available) and spreading the opening. The obtura-tor is inserted in the replacement tube, water-soluble lubricant is applied to the tip, and the tube is inserted in the stoma at a 45-degree angle to the neck. The obturator is immediately removed to provide an airway. If the tube cannot be reinserted, the physician should be notified, and the client should be assessed for the level of respiratory distress, positioned in semi-Fowler's position, and ventilated with an MRB only if nec-essary until assistance arrives.

19. d. Rationale: If coloured secretions are coughed or suctioned from the trachea after the client has attempted to swallow coloured water, it indicates that swallowing is not functional and aspiration has occurred. Uncoloured water is not discernable as aspirate, and aspiration of small amounts may not cause any respiratory symptoms. The pres-ence of a gag reflex does not ensure that a client

can adequately swallow with a tracheostomy tube in place, and no fluids except clear liquids should be used to assess aspiration risk.

20. b. Rationale: The primary risk factors associated with head and neck cancers are heavy tobacco and alcohol use and family history. Chronic infections are not known to be risk factors, and while oral cancer may cause a change in the fit of dentures, denture use is not a risk factor for oral cancer.

21. a. Rationale: If laryngeal tumours are small, radiation is the treatment of choice because it can be curative and can preserve voice quality. Surgical procedures are used if radiation treatment is not successful or if larger or advanced lesions are present.

22. a. Rationale: With removal of the larynx, the client will not be able to communicate verbally, and it is important to arrange with the client a method of communication before surgery so that post-operative communication can take place. Dry mouth and stomatitis results from radiation therapy. Vigorous coughing is not encouraged immediately post-operatively, and information related to community resources is usually introduced during the post-operative period.

23. a. Rationale: Following a radical neck dissection, drainage tubes are often used to prevent fluid accumulation in the wound, as well as possible pressure on the trachea. A tracheostomy tube is in place, but mechanical ventilation is usually not indicated. The client has placement of a nasogastric tube to suction immediately after surgery, which will later be used to administer tube feedings until swallowing can be accomplished.

24. c. Rationale: A supraglottic laryngectomy involves the removal of the epiglottis and false vocal cords, and the removal of the epiglottis allows food to enter the trachea. Supraglottic swallowing requires performance of the Valsalva manoeuvre before placing food in the mouth and swallowing. The client then coughs to remove food from the top of the vocal cords, swallows again, and then breathes after the food has been removed from the vocal cords.

25. b. Rationale: Suctioning of the tracheostomy with the use of a mirror is a self-care activity that the client is taught before discharge. Voice rehabilitation is usually managed by a speech therapist or speech pathologist, but the nurse should discuss the various types and the advantages and disadvantages of the different options. The laryngectomy stoma should be covered with a shield during showering and covered with light scarves or fabric when aspiration of foreign materials is likely.

26. a. Rationale: The voice prosthesis provides the most normal voice reproduction but requires surgical insertion of the device into a fistula made between the esophagus and the trachea. Esophageal speech involves trapping air in the esophagus and releasing it to form sound, but only 10% of clients can develop fluent speech with this method. The electrolarynx, whether mouth placed or held to the neck, allows for speech with a metallic or robotic sound.

**Case Study**

1. Assessment of respiratory status—rate, depth, and rhythm; observation of surgical site for hemorrhage and edema

2. Elevate the head of the bed to semi-Fowler's position to decrease edema; minimize facial movement; administer analgesics (non-ASA); may have PO fluids when awake, and cold fluids will help decrease swelling

3. His face will become more normal as the swelling decreases; however, there will be an interim period before the swelling entirely subsides.

4. How to clean his nose and nares with cotton swabs and water or hydrogen peroxide and to apply water-soluble jelly to the nares; to report any continued drainage of serosanguinous fluid from nose after 24 hours or any fresh bleeding; pain management techniques that do not use ASA or ASA-containing products for pain relief; to avoid vigorous nose-blowing.

5. *Nursing diagnoses:*
   - Disturbed body image related to post-operative edema and changed facial appearance
   - Acute pain related to incisional edema
   - Risk for ineffective breathing pattern related to presence of packing and nasal edema
   *Collaborative problems:*
   Potential complication: nasal hemorrhage

# CHAPTER 27

1. c. Rationale: Acute bronchitis is the greatest threat to those who have chronic bronchitis, and they often are provided with antibiotics to take at the first symptoms, which include fever, increased productive cough, and exertional dyspnea. Diffuse wheezing may be heard on auscultation but would not usually be noted by the client. Pleuritic pain may also occur, but the cough is productive.

2. a. Aspiration from the nasopharynx or oropharynx; b. Inhalation of microbes in the air; c. hematogenous spread from infections elsewhere in the body

3. c. Rationale: Pneumonia that onsets in the community is usually caused by different microorganisms than pneumonia that develops during hospitalization, and treatment can be empirical—based on observations and experience without knowing the exact cause. In at least half the cases of pneumonia, a causative organism cannot be identified from cultures, and treatment is based on experience.

4. a. 3; b. 2; c. 2; d. 1; e. 2; f. 1; g. 2; h. 2; i. 1; j. 3; k. 1

5. a. Red hepatization; b. Resolution; c. Congestion; d. Grey hepatization

6. d. Rationale: Community-acquired pneumonia usually has an acute onset with fever, chills, productive cough with purulent or bloody sputum, and pleuritic chest pain. A recent loss of consciousness or altered consciousness is common in those pneumonias associated with aspiration, such as anaerobic bacterial pneumonias.

7. d. Rationale: Prompt treatment of pneumonia with appropriate antibiotics is important in treating bacterial and mycoplasma pneumonia, and antibiotics are often administered on the basis of the history, physical examination, and a chest x-ray showing a typical pattern characteristic of a particular organism, without further testing. Sputum and blood cultures take 24 to 72 hours for results, and micro-organisms often cannot be identified with either Gram stains or cultures. Whether the pneumonia is community-acquired or hospital-acquired is more significant than severity of symptoms.

8. c. Rationale: Pneumococcal meningitis is a metastatic complication of pneumococcal pneumonia, as well as infectious pericarditis, arthritis, or endocarditis. Pleurisy, empyema, and pleural effusion may also result from pneumococcal pneumonia, but these conditions are caused by local spread rather than a hematogenous route.

9. a. macrolides; b. sulphamethoxazole (Bactrim); c. vancomycin

10. a. Client with altered consciousness: side-lying position, protect airway, turn and postition q2h
    b. Client with feeding tube: check placement of tube before feeding, residual feeding, keep head of bed up after feedings or continuously with continuous feedings
    c. Client with CNS-depressant drugs: monitor respiration and alertness; avoid oversedation
    d. Client with local anaesthetic to throat: check gag reflex before feeding or offering fluids

    e. Client with difficulty swallowing: cut food in small bites, encourage thorough chewing, provide soft foods, which are easier to swallow than liquids

11. a. Rationale: Secretions are liquefied and more easily removed by coughing when fluid intake is at least 3 L/day. Positioning and oxygen administration may help ineffective breathing patterns and impaired oxygen exchange but are not indicated for retained secretions. Deep breaths are necessary to move mucus from distal airways.

12. b. Rationale: The client with pneumococcal pneumonia is acutely ill with fever and the systemic manifestations of fever, such as chills, thirst, headache, and malaise. Interventions that monitor temperature and aid in lowering body temperature are appropriate. Diarrhea is not associated, nor are disorientation and confusion unless the client is very hypoxemic. Pleuritic pain is a local manifestation of pneumococcal pneumonia, not a systemic manifestation.

13. b. Rationale: The pneumococcal vaccine is good for a lifetime except for immunosuppressed clients, who should receive the vaccine every five to six years. The influenza virus undergoes minor changes each year, and the vaccine should be taken by those at risk for influenza and lower respiratory infections annually in the fall before exposure to the flu virus occurs. Antibiotic therapy is not appropriate for all upper respiratory infections unless secondary bacterial infections develop.

14. a. False; b. False; c. True

15. b. Rationale: Drug-resistant strains of TB have developed because TB clients' compliance to drug therapy has been poor and there has been general decreased vigilance in monitoring and follow-up of TB treatment. Antituberculous drugs are almost exclusively used for TB infections. TB can be effectively diagnosed with sputum cultures. The incidence of TB is at epidemic proportions in clients with HIV, but this does not account for drug-resistant strains of TB.

16. d. Rationale: The tubercular bacilli create a cellular immune response with development of an epithelioid granuloma that is surrounded by lymphocytes. The central portion of the granuloma undergoes necrosis characterized by a cheesy appearance and is named caseous necrosis and eventually heals with fibrosis and calcification.

17. b. Rationale: A client with class 3 TB has clinically active disease, and respiratory isolation is required for active disease until the client has been on drug therapy for at least two weeks or until smears are negative on three consecutive days. A TB infection without clinical evidence of

TB is class 2, class 4 includes clients with a history of TB but without current disease, and class 5 includes those suspected of having TB pending definite diagnosis.

18. b. Rationale: TB usually develops insidiously with fatigue, malaise, low-grade fevers, and night sweats. Chest pain and a productive cough may also occur, but hemoptysis is a late symptom.

19. a. infected with; b. latent; c. 9, 6; d. INH; e. 6; f. positive smear and culture

20. A four-drug regimen consisting of isoniazid, rifampin, pyrazinamide, and either ethambutol or streptomycin

21. d. Rationale: The nurse should notify the public health department if drug compliance is questionable so that follow-up of clients can be made by directly observed treatment (DOT) by a public health nurse or a responsible family member. A client who cannot remember to take the medication usually will not remember to come to the clinic daily or will find it too inconvenient. Additional teaching, or support from others, is not usually effective for this type of client.

22. c. Rationale: Amphotericin B is a toxic drug with many side effects, including hypersensitivity reactions, fever, chills, malaise, nausea and vomiting, and abnormal renal function, but it does not commonly cause immunosuppression. The side effect that would most commonly intensify when a client also receives chemotherapeutic agents would be the nausea and vomiting.

23. d. Rationale: Almost all forms of bronchiectasis are associated with bacterial infections that damage the bronchial walls. The incidence of bronchiectasis has decreased with use of measles and pertussis vaccines and better treatment of lower respiratory tract infections.

24. d. Rationale: Mucus production is increased in bronchiectasis and collects in the dilated, pouched bronchi. A major goal of treatment is to promote drainage and removal of the mucus, primarily through deep breathing, coughing, and postural drainage.

25. b. Rationale: The most common cause of lung abscesses is aspiration of oropharyngeal materials into the lung, especially when oral and dental hygiene are poor. Positioning to protect the airway and prevent aspiration in clients with altered consciousness is an important measure.

26. b. Rationale: Although all of the precautions identified in this question are appropriate in decreasing the risk of occupational lung diseases, using masks and effective ventilation systems to reduce exposure is the most efficient and affects the greatest number of employees.

27. a. Rationale: Smoking is responsible for approximately 80%–90% of cases of lung cancer, and enough cannot be said about its contribution to lung cancer as well as many other diseases. To prevent lung cancer, avoid exposure to cigarette smoke. Chest x-rays and evaluation of cough are diagnostic means once cancer has already developed.

28. b. Rationale: Paraneoplastic syndrome is associated with small-cell lung cancer. Small-cell lung cancer is associated with cigarette smoking and has the poorest prognosis because of high malignancy and early spread. Surgical resection of squamous cell lung cancer and adenocarcinoma is possible if localized, and large-cell tumours are somewhat radiosensitive. Adenocarcinoma is associated with lung scarring and chronic interstitial fibrosis.

29. d. Rationale: Although chest x-rays, lung tomograms, CT scans, MRI, and PET can identify tumours and masses, exact diagnosis of a lung malignancy requires identification of malignant cells either in sputum specimens or biopsies. It is important to note that a negative sputum cytology does not rule out the possibility of cancer, but positive findings can confirm it.

30. a. 3; b. 6; c. 8; d. 7; e. 1; f. 5; g. 2; h. 4

31. d. Rationale: The most successful programs for smoking cessation combine behavioural approaches to alter habits with pharmacological intervention to decrease the physical addiction to nicotine. Other methods may work for some individuals and include hypnosis, education, environmental control, and social support.

32. b. Rationale: Before making any judgements about the client's statement, it is important to explore what meaning he finds in the pain. It may be that he feels it is deserved punishment for smoking, but further information needs to be obtained from the client. Immediate referral to a counsellor negates the nurse's responsibility in helping the client, and there is no indication that he is not dealing effectively with his feelings.

33. a. Open pneumothorax; b. flail chest; c. hemothorax; d. closed pneumothorax; e. tension pneumothorax; f. chylothorax; g. chest tube, water-seal drainage

34. b. Rationale: A tension pneumothorax causes many of the same symptoms as a pneumothorax, but severe respiratory distress from collapse of the entire lung with movement of the mediastinal structures and trachea to the unaffected side are present in a tension pneumothorax. Percussion dullness on the injured site indicates the presence of blood or fluid, and decreased movement and diminished breath sounds are characteristic of a

pneumothorax. Muffled and distant heart sounds indicate a cardiac tamponade.

35. a. Collection of air and fluid from chest cavity with air vented to second chamber
    b. Water-seal chamber allowing escape of air but preventing its re-entry to collection chamber
    c. Suction-control chamber to which water is added to control the amount of suction

36. b. Rationale: The water-seal chamber should bubble intermittently as air leaves the lung with exhalation in a spontaneously breathing client, and continuous bubbling indicates a leak. The water in the suction-control chamber will bubble continuously, and the fluid in the tubing in the water-seal chamber fluctuates with the client's breathing. Water in the suction-control chamber, and perhaps in the water-seal chamber, evaporates and may need to be replaced periodically.

37. d. Rationale: Although stripping or milking chest tubes to promote drainage is somewhat controversial, there is no indication to milk the tubes when there is no bloody drainage, as in a pneumothorax. Tubing should be looped on the bed without any dependent loops to promote drainage, and clients should cough and deep breathe at least every two hours to aid in lung re-expansion. Clamping of chest tubes may cause a tension pneumothorax, but tubes may be clamped momentarily to check for leaks in the system.

38. a. 3;  b. 5;  c. 1;  d. 6;  e. 4;  f. 2

39. d. Rationale: A thoracotomy incision is large and involves cutting into bone, muscle, and cartilage, resulting in significant post-operative pain. The client has difficulty deep breathing and coughing because of the pain, and analgesics should be provided before attempting these activities. Water intake is important to liquefy secretions, but it is not indicated in this case, nor should a client with chest trauma or surgery be placed in the Trendelenburg position because it increases intrathoracic pressure.

40. a. 2;  b. 6;  c. 5;  d. 7;  e. 9;  f. 8;  g. 1;  h. 3; i. 4

41. a. 3;  b. 1;  c. 2;  d. 4

42. b. Rationale: High pressure in the pulmonary arteries increases the workload of the right ventricle and eventually causes right ventricular hypertrophy and dilation, known as cor pulmonale. Eventually decreased left ventricular output may occur because of decreased return to the left atrium, but it is not the primary effect of pulmonary hypertension. Alveolar interstitial edema is pulmonary edema associated with left ventricular failure. Pulmonary hypertension does not cause systemic hypertension.

43. d. Rationale: If possible, the primary management of cor pulmonale is treatment of the underlying pulmonary problem that caused the heart problem. Low-flow oxygen therapy will help prevent hypoxemia and hypercapnia, which causes pulmonary vasoconstriction.

44. c. Rationale: Acute rejection may occur as early as five to seven days after surgery and is manifested by low-grade fever, fatigue, and oxygen desaturation with exertion. Complete remission of symptoms can be accomplished with bolus corticosteroids. CMV and other infections can be fatal but usually occur weeks after surgery and manifest with symptoms of pneumonia. Obliterative bronchiolitis is a late complication of lung transplantation, reflecting chronic rejection.

**Case Study**

1. Low-flow oxygen; vasodilators; calcium channel blocking agents (nifedipine [Adalat], diltiazem [Cardizem]); prostacyclins (epoprostenol [Flolan], bosentan [Tracleer]); diuretics

2. Yes, since she is a medical treatment failure and can be potentially treated with either a lung or heart-lung transplant. She meets additional criteria of being less than 60 years old and a non-smoker.

3. A heart-lung transplant is indicated for the client because she has heart damage from the pulmonary hypertension, although there is evidence that even a single-lung transplant can markedly correct pulmonary hypertension and the resultant cor pulmonale.

4. Ability to cope with the post-operative regimen, which includes the following:
   • Strict adherence to immunosuppressive drugs
   • Continuous monitoring and reporting of manifestations of infection
   • Financial resources for the procedure, drugs, and follow-up care
   • Social/emotional support system, since she is a single mother

5. *Nursing diagnoses:*
   • Activity intolerance related to fatigue secondary to hypoxemia
   • Excess fluid volume related to pump failure
   • Impaired gas exchange related to mechanical failure
   • Ineffective role performance related to inability to perform role responsibilities
   • Anxiety related to breathlessness
   • Risk for impaired skin integrity related to edema
   *Collaborative problems:*
   Potential complications: arrhythmias; hypoxemia

# CHAPTER 28

1. c. Rationale: Obstructive pulmonary diseases are those in which there is increased resistance to airflow as a result of airway obstruction by accumulated secretions, edema, swelling of the inner lumen, bronchospasm, or destruction of lung tissue. In emphysema and chronic bronchitis, the obstruction is relatively constant, but with asthma the obstruction varies. Air trapping and hyperinflation of the lungs are characteristic.

2. a. 3;  b. 5;  c. 1;  d. 4;  e. 6;  f. 7;  g. 2

3. d. Rationale: Respiratory infections are one of the most common precipitating factors of an acute asthma attack. Sensitivity to food and drugs may also precipitate attacks, and exercise-induced asthma probably occurs to some extent in all clients with asthma. Psychological factors can interact with the asthmatic response to worsen the disease, but it is not a psychosomatic disease.

4. a. Rationale: Diminished or absent breath sounds may indicate a significant decrease in air movement resulting from exhaustion and an inability to generate enough muscle force to ventilate and is an ominous sign. The other symptoms are expected in an asthma attack.

5. d. Rationale: Early in an asthma attack an increased respiratory rate and hyperventilation create a respiratory alkalosis with increased pH and decreased $PaCO_2$, accompanied by a hypoxemia. As the attack progresses, pH shifts to normal, then decreases, with ABGs that reflect respiratory acidosis with hypoxemia.

6. c. Rationale: There are no absolute criteria by which a decision is made to intubate and mechanically ventilate a client with status asthmaticus, but as the client becomes more fatigued, more carbon dioxide is retained, and exhaustion of respiratory effort is a major consideration in instituting mechanical ventilation.

7. c. Rationale: Peak expiratory flow rates (PEFRs) normally are up to 600 L/min and in status asthmaticus may be as low as 100 to 150 L/min. An $SaO_2$ of 85% and FEV1 of 85% of predicted are typical of mild to moderate asthma, and a flattened diaphragm may be present in the client with long-standing asthma but does not reflect current bronchoconstriction.

8. a. 2, 3;  b. 1, 6;  c. 1, 6;  d. 2, 8;  e. 1, 7; f. 1, 4;  g. 1, 6;  h. 2, 7;  i. 1, 3;  j. 2, 3; k. 1, 6;  l. 1, 4;  m. 1, 3

9. Correct instructions are: a, b, d, f, g, i, j, k

10. b. Rationale: The client who is in an acute asthma attack is very anxious and fearful. It is important to stay with the client and interact in a calm, unhurried manner. Helping the client breathe with pursed lips will facilitate expiration of trapped air and help the client gain control of breathing.

11. b. Rationale: Initial drug therapy for acute asthma distress involves the use of inhaled salbutamol with a spacer or nebulizer. Other medications may be added if the client does not respond to inhaled β-adrenergic agonists.

12. b. Rationale: Over-the-counter cough medications should not be used to control cough in children with asthma. All of the other responses are appropriate for the client with asthma.

13. a. 3;  b. 3;  c. 3;  d. 3;  e. 1;  f. 4;  g. 2;  h. 3; i. 2;  j. 1

14. a. AAT; b. smoking, inhaled irritants, infection; c. collagen, elastin; d. ATT; e. smoking, hereditary ATT deficiency; f. Smoking

15. b. Rationale: The destruction of the alveolar walls and loss of lung elasticity in emphysema lead to the characteristic air trapping in the alveoli. There is increased lung compliance in emphysema because the lungs can be easily inflated but can deflate only partially.

16. c. Rationale: Chronic bronchitis is characterized by chronic inflammation of the bronchial lining, with edema and increased mucus production. Collapse of small bronchioles on expiration is common in emphysema, and abnormal dilation of the bronchi because of destruction of the elastic and muscular structures is characteristic of bronchiectasis.

17. a. B; b. CB; c. B; d. CB; e. E; f. CB; g. E; h. CB; i. B; j. CB; k. E; l. CB

18. b. Rationale: Constriction of the pulmonary vessels, leading to pulmonary hypertension, is caused by alveolar hypoxia and the acidosis that results from hypercapnia. Polycythemia is a contributing factor in cor pulmonale because it increases the viscosity of blood and the pressure needed to circulate the blood. Long-term low-flow oxygen therapy dilates pulmonary vessels and is used to treat cor pulmonale, and high oxygen administration is not related to cor pulmonale.

19. a. Because of air trapping in the lungs, bronchial collapse on exhalation, and bronchial narrowing, the amount of air that can be exhaled in the first second is decreased.

    b. VC is the maximum volume of air that can be exhaled after maximum inspiration, and the same factors that decrease $FEV_1$ decrease VC.

    c. The residual volume of air left in the lungs after forced expiration is increased because of the air trapping.

    d. Air trapping also increases the total lung capacity, as the lungs become overdistended with air that cannot be exhaled, and also leads to the barrel chest and flattened diaphragm seen in COPD.

20. a. Rationale: Respiratory acidosis with hypercapnia and hypoxemia are characteristic of COPD. Bicarbonate levels are increased in an attempt to buffer the acid load of the increased carbon dioxide. In early stages of COPD, ABGs may be normal or show only slightly decreased $PaO_2$ and a normal $PaCO_2$.

21. d. Rationale: Smoking cessation is the single most important factor in preventing further damage to the lungs in COPD, but prevention of infections that further increase lung damage is also important. The client is very susceptible to infections, and infections make the disease worse, creating a vicious cycle. Bronchodilators, inhaled steroids, and lung volume reduction surgery help control symptoms, but these are symptomatic measures.

22. a. 4;  b. 6;  c. 5;  d. 1;  e. 3;  f. 7;  g. 2

23. a. F, carbon dioxide narcosis; b. T; c. F, nitrogen; d. T; e. T

24. a. Rationale: Liquid oxygen reservoirs will last approximately seven to ten days when used at 2 L/min, and the portable units will hold about six to eight hours of oxygen. Compressed oxygen comes in various tank sizes, but generally it will require weekly deliveries of four to five large tanks to meet a seven- to ten-day supply. Oxygen concentrators or extractors are more expensive; they continuously supply oxygen, but they may need to be kept out of the bedroom because they are noisy and interfere with sleep.

25. c. Rationale: Pursed-lip breathing prolongs exhalation and prevents bronchiolar collapse and air trapping, while diaphragmatic breathing emphasizes the use of the diaphragm to increase maximum inhalation and to slow the respiratory rate. Thoracic breathing is not as effective as diaphragmatic breathing and is the method most naturally used by clients with COPD. Huff coughing is a technique used to increase coughing patterns to remove secretions.

26. b. Rationale: Eating is an effort for clients with COPD, and frequently they do not eat because of fatigue, dyspnea, and difficulty holding their breath while swallowing. Foods that require much chewing cause more exhaustion and should be avoided. A low-carbohydrate diet is indicated if the client has hypercapnia because carbohydrates are metabolized into carbon dioxide. Fluids should be avoided at meals to prevent a full stomach, and cold foods seem to give less of a sense of fullness than hot foods.

27. d. Rationale: The tripod position with an elevated backrest and supported upper extremities to fix the shoulder girdle maximizes respiratory excursion and an effective breathing pattern. Staying with the client and encouraging pursed-lip breathing also helps. Inhaled steroids are not effective for acute exacerbation of COPD. Postural drainage is not tolerated by a client in acute respiratory distress. Oxygen is titrated to an effective rate to avoid carbon dioxide narcosis.

28. c. Rationale: Specific guidelines for sexual activity help preserve energy and prevent dyspnea, and maintenance of sexual activity is important to the healthy psychological well-being of the couple. Open communication between partners is needed so that the modifications can be made with consideration of both partners.

29. c. Rationale: Shortness of breath usually increases during exercise, but the activity is not being overdone if breathing returns to baseline within five minutes after stopping. Bronchodilators can be administered 10 minutes before exercise but should not be administered for at least five minutes after activity to allow recovery. Clients are encouraged to walk 15 to 20 minutes a day with gradual increases, but actual patterns will depend on client tolerance. Dyspnea most frequently limits exercise and is a better indication of exercise tolerance than is heart rate in the client with COPD.

30. c. Rationale: Cystic fibrosis is an autosomal recessive, multisystem disease involving altered function of the exocrine glands of the lungs, pancreas, and sweat glands. Abnormally thick, abundant secretions from mucous glands lead to a chronic, diffuse, obstructive pulmonary disorder in almost all clients, while exocrine pancreatic insufficiency occurs in about 85%–90% of clients with CF.

31. d. Rationale: The major objective of therapy in CF is to promote removal of the secretions, and performance of postural drainage, vibration, and percussion has been the mainstay of treatment. Aerobic exercise also seems to be effective in clearing the airways and is an important part of treatment. Antibiotics are used for early signs of infection, and long courses are necessary, but they are not used prophylactically. Bronchodilators have no long-term benefit. CF is a leading indication for heart-lung transplantation.

32. a. Rationale: The presence of a chronic disease that is present at birth and significantly lowers lifespan affects all relationships and development of those clients who live to young adulthood. Children of a parent with CF will either be carriers of CF or have the disease; many men with CF are sterile, and women have difficulty becoming pregnant. Educational and vocational goals may be met in those who maintain treatment programs and health.

### Case Study

1. Change in the amount and colour of sputum; LLL percussion dullness indicates the consolidation found with pneumonia; the other sounds are typical of COPD; elevated temperature
2. Improve ventilation and promote secretion removal; promote client comfort
3. Decreased macrophage activity in the lungs of clients with chronic bronchitis increases the risk of infection; increased inhaled irritants from dust or agricultural chemicals; infection will almost always cause an exacerbation of COPD
4. Respiratory acidosis: low pH; low $PaO_2$, elevated $PaCO_2$
5. Pulmonary rehabilitation involving bronchial hygiene, exercise conditioning, breathing retraining, and energy conservation; home oxygen therapy; nutrition to increase protein and calories; evaluation of medication administration and instruction if needed
6. *Nursing diagnoses:*
   - Ineffective airway clearance related to expiratory airflow obstruction
   - Ineffective breathing pattern related to increased work of breathing
   - Impaired gas exchange: hypoxemia and hypercapnia related to alveolar hypoventilation
   - Imbalanced nutrition: less than body requirements related to lowered energy level and shortness of breath
   - Hyperthermia related to infectious process

   *Collaborative problems:*

   Potential complications: respiratory acidosis; respiratory failure; cor pulmonale

## CHAPTER 29

1. a. 7;  b. 8;  c. 6;  d. 7;  e. 1;  f. 4;  g. 3;  h. 5; i. 3;  j. 6;  k. 4;  l. 8;  m. 3; n. 2;  o. 5;  p. 3
2. a. neutrophils, basophils, eosinophils; b. erythropoietin; c. iron, vitamin $B_{12}$, folic acid; d. lymphedema; e. liver, spleen, lymph nodes
3. a. 3;  b. 2;  c. 1;  d. 2;  e. 1;  f. 3;  g. 1;  h. 3; i. 2
4. b. Rationale: Plasmin causes clot dissolution by attacking fibrinogen or fibrin, the primary component of a clot. Heparin antagonizes thrombin and is an anticoagulant, not a fibrinolytic. As coagulants, fibrinogen is a precursor of fibrin, and prothrombin is a precursor of thrombin.
5. c. Rationale: During fibrinolysis by plasmin, the fibrin clot is split into smaller molecules known as fibrin split products (FSPs) or fibrin degradation products (FDPs). These molecules contribute to anticoagulation by impairing platelet aggregation, reducing prothrombin, and preventing clot stabilization. Tissue thromboplastin, which is released from injured tissues to activate the extrinsic coagulation pathway, is not affected by these products.
6. c. Rationale: Hemoglobin levels decrease in both women and men after middle age and continue to decline with age, although the actual number of RBCs is not significantly reduced. And although leukocyte reserve may be diminished in old age, normally the total WBC count is not affected, and platelets are unaffected by aging.
7. c. Rationale: A pancytopenia is a reduction in all of the blood cells produced by the bone marrow and indicates bone marrow suppression. The liver, spleen, and lymph nodes may filter excessive blood cells but do not cause pancytopenia.
8. b. Rationale: The parietal cells of the stomach secrete intrinsic factor, a substance necessary for the absorption of cobalamin (vitamin $B_{12}$), and if all or part of the stomach is removed, the lack of intrinsic factor can lead to impaired red cell production and pernicious anemia. Recurring infections indicate decreased WBCs and immune response, and corticosteroid therapy may cause a neutrophilia and lymphopenia. Oral contraceptive use is strongly associated with changes in blood coagulation.

9.  a. family history of hematological disorders;
        alcohol and cigarette use
    b. deficiencies of iron, vitamin B$_{12}$, and folic
        acid; GI bleeding
        petechiae or bruising of the skin
        fever, lymph node swelling
    c. frankly bloody or dark, tarry stools, dark or
        bloody urine
    d. fatigue and weakness, change in ability to per-
        form normal ADLs
    e. fatigue unrelieved by sleep
    f. pain, especially in joints, bones
        paraesthesias, numbness, tingling
        changes in hearing, vision, taste, mental status
    g. altered self-perception because of lymph node
        enlargement, skin changes
    h. home or work exposure to radiation or chemi-
        cals; military history
    i. menstrual history and characteristics of bleed-
        ing
        intrapartum or post-partum bleeding problems
        impotence
    j. lack of support to meet daily needs; methods
        of coping with stress
    k. value conflicts with treatment, especially
        blood products or bone marrow transplants

10. a. Rationale: Superficial lymph nodes are evalu-
    ated by light palpation, but they are not normally
    palpable. It may be normal to find small (<1 cm),
    mobile, firm, non-tender nodes. Deep lymph
    nodes are detected with x-ray.

11. b. Rationale: Petechiae are small, flat, red or red-
    dish-brown pinpoint microhemorrhages that
    occur on the skin when platelet levels are low,
    and when they are numerous, they group, causing
    reddish bruises known as purpura. Jaundice
    occurs when anemias are of a hemolytic origin,
    resulting in accumulation of bile pigments from
    red blood cells. Enlarged, tender lymph nodes are
    associated with infection, and sternal tenderness
    is associated with leukemias.

12. d. Rationale: A smooth, shiny, reddened tongue is
    an indication of iron-deficiency anemia or perni-
    cious anemia that would be reflected by a
    decreased hemoglobin level. The increased WBC
    could be indicative of an infection; the decreased
    neutrophils, of a neutropenia; and the increased
    RBC, of polycythemia.

13. d. Rationale: A platelet count of 80 x 10$^9$/L
    (80 x 10$^3$/µL) is a thrombocytopenia and could
    place the client at risk for bleeding, necessitating
    consideration in nursing care. Chemotherapy may
    cause bone marrow suppression and a depletion
    of all blood cells. The other factors are all within
    normal range.

14. a. iron-deficiency anemia; b. inflammatory condi-
    tions of any kind; c. infection; d. heparin therapy;
    e. hemolysis of red blood cells; f. multiple
    myeloma

15. c. Rationale: A client with O Rh$^+$ blood has no A
    or B antigens on the red cell but does have anti-A
    and anti-B antibodies in the blood and has an Rh
    antigen. AB Rh$^-$ blood has both A and B antigens
    on the red cell but no Rh antigen and no anti-A or
    anti-B antibodies. If the AB Rh$^-$ blood is given to
    the client with O Rh$^+$ blood, the antibodies in the
    client's blood will react with the antigens in the
    donor blood, causing hemolysis of the donor
    cells. There will be no Rh reaction because the
    donor blood has no Rh antigen.

16. a. Rationale: A contrast CT involves the use of an
    iodine-based dye that could cause a reaction if the
    client is sensitive to iodine. Metal implants or
    internal appliances and claustrophobia should be
    determined before magnetic resonance imaging
    (MRI). Prior blood transfusions are not a factor in
    this diagnostic test.

17. d. Rationale: The preferred, and the most easily
    aspirated, sites for bone marrow examination are
    the anterior and posterior iliac crests. Alternative
    sites in adults are the sternum and the scapulae
    because they contain red marrow, but the tibia
    has only yellow marrow in adults.

18. c. Rationale: The aspiration of bone marrow con-
    tents is done with local anaesthesia at the site of
    the puncture, but the aspiration causes a suction
    pain that is quite painful, but very brief. There
    generally is no residual pain following the test.

19. d. Rationale: Lymph node biopsy is usually done
    to determine if malignant cells are present in
    lymph nodes and can be used to diagnose lym-
    phomas as well as metastatic spread from any
    malignant tumour in the body. Leukemias may
    infiltrate lymph nodes, but biopsy of the nodes is
    more commonly used to detect any type of neo-
    plastic cells.

## CHAPTER 30

1.  a. 2, 4;  b. 3, 4;  c. 2, 4;  d. 1, 4;  e. 1, 4;
    f. 3, 4;  g. 1, 6;  h. 1, 6;  i. 1, 5;  j. 3, 4;
    k. 1, 4;  l. 3, 4

2.  b. Rationale: The client's hemoglobin (Hb) level
    indicates a moderate anemia, and at this severity,
    additional findings usually include dyspnea and
    fatigue. Pallor, smooth tongue, and sensitivity to
    cold usually manifest in severe anemia when the
    Hb level is below 60 g/L (6 g/dL).

3.  a. Rationale: Nutritional deficiencies account for
    the majority of anemia seen in older adults, and

the drugs that many older adults use for chronic illness may contribute to anemia. Anemias that are familial usually manifest before older adulthood, and exposure to chemical toxins as a source of anemia is not as common as nutritional deficiencies. Although post-menopausal bleeding can contribute to anemia in a susceptible older woman, it is rarely significant.

4. c. Rationale: Tachycardia occurs in severe anemia as the body compensates for hypoxemia and the low viscosity of the blood contributes to the development of systolic murmurs and bruits. Depression of the CNS is common with fatigue, lethargy, and malaise. Poor skin turgor may be present, but fever is not associated with anemia. The skin and mucous membranes are pale, with a bluish tinge to the sclera.

5. d. Rationale: Clients with any type of anemia have decreased hemoglobin and symptoms of hypoxemia, leading to activity intolerance. Impaired skin integrity and body image disturbance may be appropriate for clients with jaundice from hemolytic anemias, and altered nutrition is indicated when iron, folic acid, or vitamin B intake is deficient.

6. a. 2; b. 7; c. 5; d. 1; e. 8; f. 4; g. 3; h. 1; i. 3; j. 2; k. 3; l. 7; m. 6; n. 5; o. 1; p. 2; q. 4

7. a. The hypoxia resulting from loss of RBCs in chronic blood loss stimulates the kidney to release erythropoietin, stimulating production of RBCs and reticulocytes, but in pernicious anemia, normal reticulocytes are not produced because of the lack of cobalamin.

   b. Sickle cell anemia is a hemolytic anemia involving an accelerated RBC breakdown leading to increased serum bilirubin levels, while acute blood loss results in loss of the RBC and the bile pigments from the body.

   c. The mean corpuscular volume (MCV) is a determination of the relative size of an RBC, and macrocytic anemias, such as folic acid deficiency and cobalamin deficiency, are characterized by the production of large, immature RBCs that would reflect an increased MCV. In iron-deficiency anemia, the MCV is low because of the lack of hemoglobin in the cells.

8. b. Rationale: Constipation is a common side effect of oral iron supplementation, and increased fluids and fibre should be consumed to prevent this effect. Because iron can be bound in the GI tract by food, it should be taken before meals unless gastric side effects of the supplements necessitate its ingestion with food. Black stools are an expected result of oral iron preparations. Taking iron with ascorbic acid or orange juice enhances absorption of the iron, but enteric-coated iron often is ineffective because of unpredictable release of the iron in areas of the GI tract where it can be absorbed.

9. c. Rationale: Parenteral iron is very irritating and can stain the skin, so needles are changed between withdrawing and administering the medication; 0.5 mL of air is left in the syringe to completely clear the solution from the syringe during administration; it is administered Z-track in the large upper outer quadrant of the buttocks; and the site is not massaged after administration.

10. d. Rationale: To replace the body's iron stores, iron supplements should be continued for two to three months after the hemoglobin (Hb) level returns to normal, but if the cause of the iron deficiency is corrected, the supplements do not need to be taken for a lifetime. Milk and milk products are poor sources of dietary iron. Activity should be gradually increased as Hb levels return to normal since aerobic capacity can only be increased when adequate Hb is available.

11. b. Rationale: Pernicious anemia is a type of cobalamin (vitamin $B_{12}$) deficiency that results when parietal cells in the stomach fail to secrete enough intrinsic factor to absorb ingested cobalamin. Extrinsic factor IS cobalamin and may be a factor in some cobalamin deficiencies but not in pernicious anemia.

12. a. Rationale: Neurological manifestations of weakness, paraesthesias of the feet and hands, and impaired thought processes are characteristic of pernicious anemia. Cardiovascular effects are most common with acute blood loss, and aplastic anemias include a leukopenia that leads to decreased immunological responses.

13. a. Rationale: Without cobalamin replacement, individuals with pernicious anemia will die in one to three years, but the disease can be controlled with cobalamin supplements for life. Hematological manifestations can be completely reversed with therapy, but long-standing neuromuscular complications may not be reversed. Since pernicious anemia results from an inability to absorb cobalamin, dietary intake of the vitamin is not a treatment option, nor is a bone marrow transplant.

14. b. Rationale: A common cause of folic acid deficiency is chronic alcohol abuse. Laboratory results in folic acid deficiency include decreased serum folate levels and increased mean corpuscular hemoglobin concentration (MCHC) due to the large cell size. Achlorhydria and macrocytic RBCs are characteristic of pernicious anemia, and increased indirect bilirubin and increased reticulocytes are characteristic of thalassemia and sickle cell anemia.

15. d. Rationale: Because red meats are the primary dietary source of cobalamin, a strict vegetarian is most at risk for cobalamin-deficiency anemia. Meats are also an important source of iron and folic acid, but whole grains, legumes, and green leafy vegetables also supply these nutrients. Thalassemia is not related to dietary deficiencies.

16. d. Rationale: The anemia of aplastic anemia may cause an inflamed, painful tongue; the thrombocytopenia may contribute to blood-filled bullae in the mouth and gingival bleeding; and the leukopenia may lead to stomatitis and oral ulcers and infections.

17. b. Rationale: Hemorrhage from thrombocytopenia and infection from neutropenia are the greatest risks for the client with aplastic anemia. The client will experience fatigue from anemia, but bleeding and infection are the major causes of death in aplastic anemia.

18. a. F, clinical symptoms; b. T; c. F, blood transfusions or iron supplements; d. T; e. F, kidney; f. T

19. b. Rationale: Because red cells are abnormal in sickle cell anemia, the mean RBC survival time is 10 to 15 days (rather than the normal 120 days) because of accelerated RBC breakdown by the liver and spleen. Antibody reactions with RBCs may be seen in other types of hemolytic anemias but are not present in sickle cell anemia.

20. b. Rationale: During a sickle cell crisis, the sickling cells clog small capillaries, and the resulting hemostasis promotes a self-perpetuating cycle of local hypoxia, deoxygenation of more erythrocytes, and more sickling. Administration of oxygen may help control further sickling, but additional oxygen does not reach areas of local hypoxia caused by occluded vessels.

21. d. Rationale: Because pain usually accompanies a sickle cell crisis and may last for four to six days, pain control is an important part of treatment. Rest is indicated to reduce metabolic needs, and fluids and electrolytes are administered to reduce blood viscosity and maintain renal function. Although thrombosis does occur in capillaries, elastic stockings, which primarily affect venous circulation, are not indicated.

22. d. Rationale: The client with sickle cell disease is particularly prone to infection, and infection can precipitate a sickle cell crisis. Clients should seek medical attention quickly to counteract upper respiratory infections because pneumonia is the most common infection of the client with sickle cell disease. Fluids should be increased to decrease blood viscosity, which may precipitate a crisis, and moderate activity is permitted.

23. a. T; b. T; c. F, bleeding; d. F, increased agglutination function of platelets; e. F, petechiae; f. T; g. T; h. F, increased

24. b. Rationale: Thrombus and embolization are the major complications of polycythemia vera because of increased hypervolemia and hyperviscosity. Active or passive leg exercises and ambulation should be implemented to prevent thrombus formation. Hydration therapy is important to decrease blood viscosity, but because the client already has hypervolemia, a careful balance of intake and output must be maintained and fluids are not injudiciously increased.

25. b. Rationale: Corticosteroids are used in initial treatment of ITP because they suppress the phagocytic response of splenic macrophages, decreasing platelet destruction. They also depress autoimmune antibody formation and reduce capillary fragility and bleeding time. All of the other therapies may be used but only in clients who are unresponsive to corticosteroid therapy.

26. c. Rationale: The major complication of thrombocytopenia is hemorrhage, and it may occur in any area of the body. Cerebral hemorrhage may be fatal, and evaluation of mental status for CNS alterations to identify CNS bleeding is very important. Fever is not a common finding in thrombocytopenia. Protection from injury to prevent bleeding is an important nursing intervention, but strict bed rest is not indicated. Oral care is performed very gently with minimum friction and soft swabs.

27. d. Rationale: A prolonged partial thromboplastin time occurs when there is a deficiency of clotting factors, such as factor VIII associated with hemophilia A. Factor IX is deficient in hemophilia B, and prolonged bleeding time and decreased platelet counts are associated with platelet deficiencies.

28. c. Rationale: Although whole blood and fresh frozen plasma contain the clotting factors that are deficient in hemophilia, specific factor concentrates have been developed that are more pure and safer in preventing infection transmission. Thromboplastin is factor III and is not deficient in clients with hemophilia.

29. b. Rationale: During an acute bleeding episode in a joint, it is important to totally rest the involved joint and slow bleeding with application of ice. Drugs that decrease platelet aggregation, such as ASA or NSAIDs, should not be used for pain. As soon as bleeding stops, mobilization of the affected area is encouraged with ROM exercises and physical therapy.

30. a. 5; b. 8; c. 3; d. 6; e. 2; f. 7; g. 1; h. 4

31. d. Rationale: Both recognition of clients who are at risk for DIC and early detection of bleeding, both occult and overt, are primary nursing goals in the care of clients who could develop DIC. Management of the primary problem is important, but it does not necessarily assist in early recognition of acute DIC, and susceptible clients are not treated unless symptoms develop. Although DIC causes microvascular thrombosis, detection is usually made with signs of bleeding.

32. a. Yes—WBC below $4 \times 10^9$/L ($4 \times 10^3$/µL or 4000/µL); b. $0.92 \times 10^9$/L ($0.92 \times 10^3$/µL or 920/µL), obtained by multiplying 2.3 by percentage of neutrophils 40%; c. Yes—neutrophils less than 1 to $1.5 \times 10^9$/L (1 to $1.5 \times 10^3$/µL or 1000 to 1500/µL); d. Moderate—neutropenia of 0.5 to $1 \times 10^9$/L (0.5 to $1 \times 10^3$/µL or 500 to 1000/µL)

33. a. Rationale: An elevated temperature is of most significance in recognizing the presence of an infection in the neutropenic client because there is no leukocytic response, and when the WBC count is depressed, the normal phagocytic mechanisms of infection are impaired, and the classic signs of inflammation may not occur. Cultures are indicated if temperature is elevated but are not used to monitor for infection.

34. d. Rationale: Despite its seeming simplicity, hand washing before, during, and after care of the client with neutropenia is the major method to prevent transmission of harmful pathogens to the client. HEPA filtration and LAF rooms may reduce the number of aerosolized pathogens, but they are expensive, and LAF use is controversial. Antibiotics are administered when febrile episodes occur but are not used prophylactically to prevent development of resistance.

35. a. Rationale: Although myelodysplastic syndromes, like leukemia, are a group of disorders in which hematopoietic stem cells of the bone marrow undergo clonal change and may cause eventual bone marrow failure, the primary difference from leukemias is that myelodysplastic cells have some degree of maturation and the disease progression is slower than in acute leukemias.

36. a. 4; b. 4; c. 1; d. 2; e. 3; f. 2; g. 3; h. 1; i. 3; j. 2; k. 4

37. b. Rationale: Induction therapy is aggressive treatment with chemotherapeutic agents, which often causes the client to become devastatingly ill and predisposed to complications because the bone marrow is even further suppressed by the drugs. Induction therapy is usually administered for 10 days and may be followed by intensification therapy that involves high-dose therapy for several months.

38. c. Rationale: Almost all leukemias cause some degree of hepatosplenomegaly because of infiltration of these organs as well as the bone marrow, lymph nodes, bones, and CNS by excessive white blood cells in the blood.

39. d. Rationale: Whether the donor bone marrow is from a matched donor or taken from the client during a remission for later use, bone marrow transplant always involves the use of combinations of chemotherapy and total body radiation to totally eliminate leukemic cells and the client's bone marrow stem cells before IV infusion of the donor cells. There is a severe pancytopenic period following the transplant, during which the client must be in protective isolation and during which RBC and platelet transfusions may be given.

40. b. Rationale: A client newly diagnosed with leukemia is most likely to respond with anxiety about the effects and outcome of the disease, and the risk of infection from altered WBCs is always present, even if other blood cells are not yet affected by the disease.

41. a. NHL; b. HD; c. B; d. NHL; e. HD; f. NHL; g. HD; h. B; i. HD; j. HD

42. a. Rationale: GM-CSF is a type of colony-stimulating factor that is a naturally produced protein which stimulates proliferation and differentiation of granulocytes and monocytes. It is used to hasten recovery from bone marrow depression after chemotherapy or decrease bone marrow suppression associated with chemotherapy administration. Monoclonal antibodies, such as rituximab and ibritumomab tiuxetan, as well as interferons, may be used to destroy malignant cells of NHL.

43. a. F, determine treatment; b. T; c. F, B cells, bone; d. T

44. d. Rationale: The laboratory results typical in multiple myeloma reflect the excessive production of plasma cells that produce abnormal and excessive amounts of immunoglobulin, known as myeloma protein, and the results of bone destruction by these cells and substances. Bone destruction results in increased serum levels of calcium and uric acid, and excretion of excessive uric acid and myeloma protein can result in kidney damage. Bone marrow damage results in neutropenia, anemia, and thrombocytopenia. A neutrophilic leukocytosis and anemia are seen in Hodgkin's disease.

45. c. Rationale: Splenectomy may be indicated for treatment for ITP, and when the spleen is removed, platelet counts increase significantly in most clients. In any of the disorders in which the spleen removes excessive blood cells, splenectomy will most often increase peripheral RBC, WBC, and platelet counts.

46. a. Rationale: Chills and fever are symptoms of an acute hemolytic or febrile transfusion reaction, and if these develop, the transfusion should be stopped immediately, and saline infused through the IV line to keep the vein open. The physician and blood bank should be notified immediately, the ID tags rechecked, and vital signs and urine output monitored. Mild and transient allergic reactions indicated by itching and hives might permit restarting of the transfusion after treatment with antihistamines. This reaction, however, requires the immediate stopping of the transfusion due to the high fever. Bacterial contamination or an acute hemolytic reaction must be investigated.

47. c. Rationale: Canadian blood safety standards require platelets to be transfused through Y-type blood transfusion sets, which have a built-in filter (170–260 microns). In Canada, platelet bags are not agitated while they are transfusing. They are agitated during storage in the blood bank. Baseline vital signs should be taken before the transfusion is started, after the first 15 minutes, and at the completion of each bag of platelets, and the nurse should closely monitor the client, especially during the first 15 minutes of each bag transfused. Platelets are stored at room temperature and should not be refrigerated. Client identification and ABO compatibility are always checked prior to administration.

48. a. 3; b. 2; c. 1; d. 1; e. 5; f. 2; g. 1; h. 5; i. 3; j. 4

49. a. Rationale: The onset of TRALI is acute, with evidence of pulmonary edema, developing during or within six hours of completion of a transfusion. This reaction is not a fluid overload or other event, but an immune-mediated one involving the passive transfer of white cell antibodies from donor to recipient. This results in the development of pulmonary edema and potentially severe decrease in oxygen in the blood (hypoxemia).

**Case Study**

1. Traumatized placental and uterine tissues that release tissue factor into circulation, initiating the coagulation cascade

2. Venipuncture site bleeding, oozing of blood from other sites; respiratory problems, such as tachypnea, hemoptysis, and orthopnea; hematuria; hematemesis

3. Elevated FSPs; reduced factors V, VII, VIII, X; elevated D-dimers (cross-linked fibrin fragments); prolonged prothrombin and partial thromboplastin times; prolonged thrombin time; reduced fibrinogen, platelets

4. In the bleeding client, therapy is administered on the basis of specific component deficiencies. Platelets are given to correct thrombocytopenia, cryoprecipitate replaces factor VIII and fibrinogen, and fresh-frozen plasma replaces all clotting factors except platelets and provides a source of antithrombin. This client is not manifesting symptoms of thrombosis, so anticoagulation is probably not indicated at this time.
   Treatment of the underlying condition may include a D&C or even a hysterectomy, if necessary, to remove the stimulus of DIC.

5. *Nursing diagnoses:*
   - Ineffective tissue perfusion: cardiopulmonary, cerebral, peripheral, and renal related to blood loss and thrombosis
   - Decreased cardiac output related to fluid volume deficit
   - Risk for impaired tissue integrity related to altered coagulation
   - Anxiety/fear related to disease process and therapy
   *Collaborative problems:*
   Potential complication: hemorrhage; thrombosis; hypovolemia/shock; renal failure

# CHAPTER 31

1. a. mitral valve; b. tricuspid valve; c. ventricular septum; d. cusp; e. chordae tendineae; f. papillary muscle

2. a. aorta; b. superior vena cava; c. aortic semilunar valve; d. right atrium; e. right coronary artery; f. right marginal artery; g. posterior interventricular artery; h. right ventricle; i. left ventricle; j. anterior interventricular artery; k. left marginal artery; l. circumflex artery; m. left atrium; n. left coronary artery; o. pulmonary trunk; p. aorta; q. superior vena cava; r. right atrium; s. small cardiac vein; t. middle cardiac vein; u. right ventricle; v. left ventricle; w. great cardiac vein; x. coronary sinus; y. posterior vein; z. left atrium; aa. pulmonary trunk

3. a. right coronary artery, left anterior descending artery, left circumflex artery; b. right coronary artery; c. diastolic

4. a. 4; b. 7; c. 2; d. 5; e. 8; f. 1; g. 3; h. 6

5. a. 2; b. 4; c. 2; d. 1; e. 4; f. 5; g. 3; h. 3; i. 1

6. a. preload (decreased); CO decreased
   b. preload (decreased); CO decreased
   c. afterload (increased); CO decreased
   d. contractility (increased); CO increased
   e. preload (decreased); CO decreased
   f. preload (decreased); CO decreased

7. a. 2; b. 3; c. 1; d. 2; e. 2; f. 3

8. a. increased heart rate, increased force of contraction, vasoconstriction; b. decreased heart rate; c. stimulation of baroreceptors (in aortic arch and carotid sinus); d. 60, 96 mm Hg

9. a. loss of vascular distensibility and elastic recoil during systole; b. increased collagen and decreased elastin; c. decrease in SA node cells and bundle of His fibres; d. decreased number and function of receptors; e. valvular lipid accumulation and calcification

10. d. Rationale: Recreational or abused drugs, especially stimulants, such as cocaine and methamphetamine, are a growing cause of cardiac arrhythmias and problems associated with tachycardia, and IV injection of abused drugs is a risk factor for inflammatory and infectious conditions of the heart. Streptococcal, but not viral, pharyngitis is a risk factor for rheumatic heart disease. Although calcium is involved in contraction of muscles, calcium supplementation is not a significant factor in heart disease, nor is metastatic cancer.

11. a. hyperlipidemia, hypertension, smoking, obesity, sedentary or stressful lifestyle, history of hereditary or familial cardiovascular disease, diabetes mellitus

b. obesity, high intake of sodium, fat, cholesterol, and triglycerides

c. dependent edema, incontinence or constipation; use of diuretics with increased urinary output

d. lack of aerobic exercise; decreased activity tolerance; symptoms during exercise

e. attacks of shortness of breath interrupting sleep; use of several pillows to sleep

f. chest pain; pain in legs with walking; vertigo, cognitive changes

g. loss of self-esteem resulting from fatigue and decreased activity

h. stress or conflict in roles

i. change in sexual activity caused by shortness of breath or fatigue; impotence

j. high stress, anxiety, denial/anger/hostility as coping mechanisms

k. treatment conflict with value system

12. d. Rationale: Normal reduction in blood pressure in a standing position is up to 15 mm Hg in the systolic pressure and from 3 to 5 mm Hg in the diastolic pressure. Reductions greater than these are abnormal and may be caused by drugs, fluid loss, or pathological conditions.

13. d. Rationale: A palpable vibration of a blood vessel is called a thrill and usually indicates turbulent blood flow through the vessel. A weak, thready pulse has very little pressure and is difficult to palpate. A bruit is an abnormal buzzing or humming sound that may be auscultated over pathological vessels, and a bounding pulse is an extra full, hard pulse that may occur with atherosclerosis or hypervolemia.

14. a. 1; b. 6; c. 4; d. 5; e. 7; f. 2; g. 3; h. 6; i. 6; j. 3

15. a. $S_2$; b. $S_1$; c. $S_2$; d. $S_1$; e. $S_1$; f. $S_1$; g. $S_2$; h. $S_2$; i. $S_1$

16. a. 7; b. 4; c. 9; d. 10; e. 8; f. 2; g. 1; h. 3; i. 6; j. 5

17. c. Rationale: In a Cardiolite scan, technetium-99 Sestimibi is injected at the maximum heart rate on a bicycle or treadmill and used to evaluate blood flow in different parts of the heart. It is taken up in an area of cardiac damage from myocardial infarction, producing hot spots. Simply monitoring electrocardiographic activity during exercise is an exercise stress test, and an echocardiogram uses transducers to bounce sound waves off the heart. Insertion of electrodes into the heart chambers via the venous system to record intracardiac electrical activity is an electrophysiology study.

18. b. Rationale: Holter monitoring involves placing electrodes on the chest, attached to a recorder that will record ECG rhythm for 24 to 48 hours while the client engages in normal daily activities. The recording is later analyzed for cardiac arrhythmias. Frequent, but not continuous, ECGs are serial ECGs. An electrophysiology study is an invasive test that records intracardiac electrical activity in different cardiac structures, and positron emission tomography uses radioisotopes to evaluate myocardial perfusion and metabolic function.

19. c. Rationale: Because there is a significant risk for clotting around the catheter insertion site, causing obstruction of arterial blood flow, it is very important to access circulation to the extremity distal to the site frequently following a cardiac catheterization. Some swelling and pain at the site are expected, but the site is also monitored for bleeding, and a pressure dressing and perhaps a sandbag may be applied. Frequent vital signs and cardiac assessment are also necessary. Identification of iodine sensitivity should be done before the test.

20. a. Rationale: Troponin is a myocardial muscle protein that is released into circulation after injury and is specific to myocardial tissue. Apoproteins are water-soluble proteins that combine with lipids to form lipoproteins and may be associated with cardiac risk but do not indicate cardiac damage. LDH and AST are tissue enzymes that may indicate cardiac damage, but these tests have been replaced by CK-MB and troponin testing.

21. d. Rationale: A risk assessment for coronary artery disease is determined by comparing the total cholesterol to HDL, and a ratio can be calculated by dividing the total cholesterol level by the high-density lipoprotein level. The ratio provides more information than either value alone, and an increased ratio indicates an increased risk. The female client has a ratio of 3.56 compared with the male client's ratio of 6.56.

# CHAPTER 32

1. a. B; increased rate and contractility of the heart (stroke volume) increases CO stimulation of renin production, causing increased SVR and increased CO
   b. B; peripheral arteriole vasoconstriction and increased contractility of the heart
   c. SVR; constriction of selected vascular beds
   d. SVR; vasoconstriction
   e. SVR; arteriole vasoconstriction
   f. CO; increased vascular volume
   g. CO; increased vascular volume

2. The vasoconstriction caused by the $\alpha_1$-adrenergic agent raises the blood pressure, stimulating the baroreceptors. The baroreceptors send impulses to the sympathetic vasomotor centre in the brainstem, which inhibit the sympathetic nervous system, resulting in a decreased heart rate, decreased force of contraction, and vasodilation.

3. Lower blood pressure because of decreased stroke volume and decreased heart rate, both of which decrease cardiac output

4. c. Rationale: Hypertension is diagnosed when the average of two or more resting BP measurements on at least three different occasions reveals an SBP of 140 mm Hg or greater or a DBP of 90 mm Hg or greater. Elevations of either SPB or DBP meet the criteria.

5. b. Rationale: Stage 2 hypertension is moderate hypertension, with BP ranges of 160 to 179/100 to 109. An average BP of 155/88 is stage 1, and the average BPs of 160/110 and 182/106 are stage 3.

6. a. Age—hypertension progresses with increasing age; b. Gender—hypertension is more prevalent in men to age 55, then more in women; c. Race—Blacks have twice the incidence of hypertension of Whites; d. Family history—hypertension is strongly familial.

7. c. Rationale: Secondary hypertension has an underlying cause that can often be treated, in contrast to primary or essential hypertension, which has no single known cause. Isolated systolic hypertension occurs when the systolic BP is consistently elevated over 160 mm Hg, but the diastolic BP remains less than 90 mm Hg, which is more prevalent in the older adult. The only type of hypertension that does not cause target organ damage is pseudohypertension.

8. a. Rationale: Hypertension is often asymptomatic, especially if mild or moderate, and has been called the "silent killer." The absence of symptoms often leads to non-compliance with medical treatment and a lack of concern about the disease in clients. With severe hypertension, symptoms usually occur and may include a morning occipital headache, fatigability, dizziness, palpitations, angina, and dyspnea.

9. b. Rationale: Elevated blood pressure causes the entire inner lining of arterioles to become thickened from hyperplasia of connective tissues in the intima and affects coronary circulation, cerebral circulation, peripheral vessels, and renal and retinal blood vessels. The narrowed vessels lead to ischemia, and ultimately damage, of these organs.

10. b. Rationale: The increased systemic vascular resistance of hypertension directly increases the workload of the heart, and congestive heart failure occurs when the heart can no longer pump effectively against the increased resistance. The heart may be indirectly damaged by atherosclerotic changes in the blood vessels, as are the brain, retina, and kidney.

11. a. Elevated BUN and creatinine may indicate destruction of glomeruli and tubules of the kidney resulting from hypertension.
    b. Serum potassium levels are decreased when hypertension is associated with hyperaldosteronism. Clients who take potassium-wasting diuretics are at risk for hypokalemia and therefore must increase their potassium intake or take supplements of potassium.
    c. Fasting glucose levels are elevated when hypertension is associated with glucose intolerance and insulin resistance.
    d. An increased uric acid level may be caused by diuretics used to treat hypertension.
    e. An elevated LDL indicates an increased risk for atherosclerotic changes in the client with hypertension. Individuals with hypertension are encouraged to exercise, as it helps decrease LDL and increase HDL.

12. a. Dietary modifications to restrict sodium; maintain intake of potassium, calcium, and magnesium; and promote weight reduction if overweight
    b. Moderation or cessation of alcohol intake
    c. Daily moderate-intensity physical activity for at least 30 minutes
    d. Cessation of smoking if a smoker

13. a. Rationale: The recommendation for initial pharmacological management of hypertension is monotherapy with either a diuretic or a beta blocker. Other drugs used for initial monotherapy include calcium channel blockers, ACE inhibitors, α-adrenergic blockers, and the combined α-β–adrenergic blockers. If the BP is not controlled in a few months with monotherapy, the dose of the first-line drug can be increased, a second drug from a different class can be substituted, or a second drug from a different class can be added.

14. a. 4;  b. 5;  c. 8;  d. 6;  e. 2;  f. 7;  g. 1;  h. 3

15. d. Rationale: Hydrochlorothiazide is a thiazide diuretic that causes sodium and potassium loss through the kidney. High-potassium foods should be included in the diet, or potassium supplements used, to prevent hypokalemia. Enalapril and spironolactone may cause hyperkalemia by inhibiting the action of aldosterone, and potassium supplements should not be used by clients taking these drugs. As a combined α-β-blocker, labetalol does not affect potassium levels.

16. b. Rationale: Prazosin is an α-adrenergic blocker that causes dilation of arterioles and veins and causes orthostatic hypotension. The client may feel dizzy, weak, and faint when assuming an upright position after sitting or lying down and should be taught to change positions slowly, avoid standing for long periods of time, do leg exercises to increase venous return, and lie or sit down when dizziness occurs. Direct-acting vasodilators often cause fluid retention, dry mouth occurs with diuretic use and centrally acting α-blockers, and β-blockers may cause bradycardia.

17. c. Rationale: Sexual dysfunction that may occur with many of the antihypertensive drugs, including thiazide and potassium-sparing diuretics and β-blockers, can be a major reason that a male client does not adhere to his treatment regimen. It is helpful for the nurse to raise the subject because sexual problems may be easier for the client to discuss and handle once it has been explained that the drug may be the source of the problem.

18. a. Rationale: Centrally acting α-blockers may cause severe rebound hypertension if the drugs are abruptly discontinued, and clients should be taught about this effect because many are not consistently compliant with drug therapy. Diuretics should be taken early in the day to prevent nocturia, and the profound orthostatic hypotension that occurs with first-dose α-adrenergic blockers can be prevented by taking the initial dose at bedtime. ASA use may decrease the effectiveness of ACE inhibitors.

19. d. Rationale: Correct technique in measuring blood pressure includes taking and averaging two or more readings taken at least two minutes apart. If the first two readings differ by more than 5 mm Hg, additional readings should be obtained. Initially BP measurements should be taken in both arms to detect any differences, and if there is a difference, the arm with the higher reading should be used for all subsequent BP readings. The cuff should be inflated 10 to 20 mm Hg above the point that no brachial pulse is felt in the arm being used, and the pressure should be released at 2 mm Hg per second to provide an accurate reading.

20. c. Rationale: A major problem in the long-term management of the client with hypertension is poor compliance with the prescribed treatment regimen. Before adding or substituting medications because of a poor response to drug therapy, it is important to ensure that clients have been taking their medication as prescribed. Although drug-related causes and progressive renal damage may be responsible for lack of responsiveness to drug therapy, non-adherence to therapy for a variety of reasons is the most common factor.

21. b. Rationale: Hypertensive emergency, a type of hypertensive crisis, is a situation that develops over hours or days in which a client's BP is severely elevated with evidence of acute target organ damage, especially to the central nervous system. The neurological manifestations are often similar to the presentation of a CVA, but it does not show the focal or lateralizing symptoms of CVA. Hypertensive crises are defined by the degree of organ damage and how rapidly the BP must be lowered, not specific BP measurements. A hypertensive urgency is a less severe crisis in which a client's BP becomes severely elevated over days or weeks, but there is no evidence of target organ damage.

22. c. Rationale: Hypertensive crises are treated with IV administration of antihypertensive drugs, including the vasodilators sodium nitroprusside, nitroglycerin, diazoxide, and hydralazine; adrenergic blockers such as phentolamine, labetalol, and methyldopa; and the ACE inhibitor IV enalaprilat. Sodium nitroprusside is the most effective parenteral drug for hypertensive emergencies. Drugs that are used specifically for hypertensive emergencies include sodium nitroprusside, nitroglycerin, and diazoxide.

23. c. Rationale: Initially the treatment goal in hypertensive emergencies is to reduce the MAP by 10%–20% in the first one to two hours, with further gradual reduction over the next 24 hours. Lowering the BP too far or too fast may cause

hypotension in a person whose body has adjusted to hypertension and could cause a stroke, MI, or visual changes. Only when the client has an aortic dissection, angina, or signs of MI does the systolic BP need to be lowered to 100 to 120 mm Hg as quickly as possible.

24. d. Rationale: Hypertensive urgencies are often treated with oral drugs on an outpatient basis, but it is important for the client to be seen by a healthcare professional within 24 hours to evaluate the effectiveness of the treatment. Hourly urine measurements, ECG monitoring, and titration of IV drugs are indicated for hypertensive emergencies.

**Case Study**

1. Increasing age, which leads to loss of elasticity in large arteries from atherosclerosis; more prevalent in women
2. High sodium intake from canned foods; sedentary lifestyle; weight gain
3. Sodium restriction to 2 g/day; decrease fat to no more than 30% of diet; cholesterol intake of less than 200 mg/day; increase high-potassium foods
4. Regular daily aerobic exercise; need for stress management indicated by weight gain in response to husband's death; teaching about pathology, complications, and management of hypertension
5. Because of her low potassium, a potassium-saving diuretic, such as spironolactone, amiloride, or triamterine, could be used. If a stronger diuretic was needed, potassium supplementation would be indicated.
6. *Nursing diagnoses:*
   • Ineffective health maintenance related to increased caloric intake and deficiency of potassium sources
   • Ineffective coping related to use of food as coping mechanism
   *Collaborative problems:*
   Potential complications: cerebrovascular accident; myocardial infarction, renal failure

## CHAPTER 33

1. a. fatty streak, age 15; b. raised fibrous plaque, age 30; c. complicated lesion, over age 30
2. a. F, endothelial injury; b. T; c. T; d. T; e. F, complicated lesion; f. F, older, with chronic ischemia
3. a. elevated serum lipids, modifiable; b. hypertension, modifiable; c. cigarette smoking, modifiable
4. d. Rationale: The White woman has one unmodifiable risk factor (age) and two major modifiable risk factors (hypertension and physical inactivity). Her gender risk is as high as a man's

because of her age. The white man has one unmodifiable risk factor (gender), one major modifiable risk factor (smoking), and one minor modifiable risk factor (stressful lifestyle). The black man has a an unmodifiable risk factor related to age, one major modifiable risk factor (hypertension), and one minor modifiable risk factor (obesity), but black men are at less risk for CAD than are white men of the same age. The Asian woman has only one major modifiable risk factor (hyperlipidemia).

5. a. 3; b. 5; c. 2; d. 1; e. 1; f. 3; g. 1; h. 6; i. 2; j. 4; k. 2
6. a. <5.2 mmol/L (200 mg/dL)
   b. <2.15 mmol/L (190 mg/dL)
   c. <3.4 mmol/L (130 mg/dL)
   d. >0.97 mmol/L (37 mg/dL)
   e. >1.05 mmol/L (40 mg/dL)
7. a. Rationale: Increased exercise without an increase in caloric intake will result in weight loss, reducing the risk associated with obesity, and exercise increases lipid metabolism and increases HDL2, reducing CAD risk. Exercise may also indirectly reduce the risk of CAD by controlling hypertension, promoting glucose metabolism in diabetes, and reducing stress. Although research is needed to determine whether a decline in homocysteine can reduce the risk of heart disease, it appears that dietary modifications will be indicated for risk reduction.
8. d. Rationale: Stress related to a type A behaviour pattern is associated with increased sympathetic nervous system stimulation, increasing heart rate and contractility and thus the workload of the heart. Hypertension also increases the workload of the heart by requiring more force to pump blood through the diseased arterial vasculature. Smoking also increases the workload by causing catecholamine release. Elevated serum lipids and diabetes are associated with causing vascular changes that decrease oxygen supply. It is not known how physical inactivity directly affects CAD, but exercise is known to increase HDL levels and reduce clot formation.
9. a. Rationale: Step 1 dietary changes include decreased intake of saturated fat and cholesterol and the substitution of skim or 1% milk for whole milk. A step 2 diet is used if the client does not show a trend toward lower blood cholesterol within six months of using a step 1 diet. A step 2 diet includes only the very leanest cuts of meats (although red meat can be used) and only one egg yolk per week. Restriction of alcohol and simple sugars is indicated for control of elevated serum triglyceride levels.

10. a. Rationale: Diet therapy is indicated for a client without CAD who has two or more risk factors and an LDL level equal to or greater than 130 mg/dL. When the client's LDL levels are equal to or greater than 160 mg/dL, drug therapy would be added to diet therapy. Exercise is indicated to reduce risk factors throughout treatment.

11. c. Rationale: This client has elevated cholesterol, LDLs, and triglyceride levels, and nicotinic acid is highly effective in lowering both cholesterol and triglyceride levels by interfering with their synthesis. Gemfibrozil primarily affects VLDL and triglyceride levels, lovastatin primarily decreases liver synthesis of LDL and thus cholesterol, and cholestyramine primarily lowers LDL cholesterol and increases HDL levels.

12. a. stable angina
    b. unstable angina, non-ST-segment-elevation myocardial infarction
    c. ST-segment-elevation myocardial infarction

13. a. increased oxygen demand, decreased oxygen supply; b. increased oxygen demand; c. decreased oxygen supply; d. decreased oxygen supply; e. decreased oxygen supply; f. increased oxygen demand; g. increased oxygen demand; h. increased oxygen demand

14. c. Rationale: When the coronary arteries are occluded, contractility ceases after several minutes, depriving the myocardial cells of glucose and oxygen for aerobic metabolism. Anaerobic metabolism begins and lactic acid accumulates, irritating myocardial nerve fibres that then transmit a pain message to the cardiac nerves and upper thoracic posterior roots. The other factors may occur during vessel occlusion but are not the source of pain.

15. d. Rationale: An increased heart rate decreases the time the heart spends in diastole, which is the time of greatest coronary blood flow. Unlike other arteries, coronary arteries are perfused when the myocardium relaxes and blood backflows from the aorta into the sinuses of Valsalva, which have openings to the right and left coronary arteries. Thus the heart has a decreased oxygen supply at a time when there is an increased oxygen demand.

16. c. Rationale: Location and areas of MIs correlate with the coronary arteries and the areas of the heart they normally perfuse. Anterior wall infarctions are usually caused by lesions in the left anterior descending artery; lateral wall infarctions by occlusion of the left circumflex or descending artery; inferior wall infarctions by occlusion of the right coronary artery or left circumflex artery; and posterior wall infarctions by lesions in the left circumflex artery.

17. c. Rationale: At 10 to 14 days after MI, the myocardium is considered to be especially vulnerable to increased stress because of the unstable state of healing at this point, and this is the time that the client is also increasing physical activity. At two to three days, removal of necrotic tissue is taking place by phagocytic cells, and by four to 10 days, the tissue has been cleared and a collagen matrix for scar tissue has been deposited. Healing with scar tissue replacement of the necrotic area is usually complete by six weeks.

18. a. 6;  b. 3;  c. 5;  d. 1;  e. 5;  f. 3;  g. 1;  h. 2; i. 4;  j. 2

19. c. Rationale: Unstable angina is associated with deterioration of a once stable atherosclerotic plaque that ruptures, exposing the intima to blood and stimulating platelet aggregation and local vasoconstriction with thrombus formation. Clients with unstable angina require immediate hospitalization and monitoring because the lesion is at increased risk of complete thrombosis of the lumen with progression to MI. Any type of angina may be associated with severe pain, ECG changes, and arrhythmias, and Prinzmetal's, or variant, angina is characterized by coronary artery spasm.

20. a. Rationale: One of the primary differences between the pain of angina and the pain of an MI is that angina pain is usually relieved by rest or nitroglycerin, which reduces the oxygen demand of the heart, while MI pain is not. Both angina and MI pain can cause a pressure or squeezing sensation; may radiate to the neck, back, arms, fingers, and jaw; and may be precipitated by exertion.

21. b. Rationale: An exercise stress test will reveal ECG changes that indicate impaired coronary circulation when the oxygen demand of the heart is increased. A single ECG is not conclusive for CAD, and negative findings do not rule out CAD. Echocardiograms of various types may identify abnormalities of myocardial wall motion under stress but are indirect measures of CAD. Coronary angiography can detect narrowing of coronary arteries but is an invasive procedure.

22. d. Rationale: The pain of an MI is usually severe, is usually unrelieved by nitroglycerin, rest, or position change, and usually lasts more than the 15 or 20 minutes typical of angina pain. All of the other symptoms may occur with angina as well as an MI.

23. c. Rationale: The most common complication of MI is cardiac arrhythmias, especially ventricular arrhythmias, which may be life-threatening. Continuous cardiac monitoring allows for identification and treatment of arrhythmias that may cause

further deterioration of the cardiovascular status. Measurement of hourly urine output and vital signs is indicated to detect symptoms of the complication of cardiogenic shock, and crackles, dyspnea, and tachycardia may indicate the onset of congestive heart failure.

24. a. 4; b. 5; c. 2; d. 1; e. 3

25. c. Rationale: Creatine kinase, MB band, is a tissue enzyme that is specific to cardiac muscle and is released into the blood when myocardial cells die. CK-MB levels begin to rise about six hours after an acute MI, peak in about 24 hours, and return to normal within two or three days, and this increase can demonstrate the presence of cardiac damage and the approximate extent of the damage. Troponin, a myocardial muscle protein released with myocardial damage, rises as quickly as CK and remains elevated for two weeks. ECG changes often are not apparent immediately after infarct and may be normal when the client seeks medical attention. An enlarged heart determined by x-ray indicates cardiac stress but is not diagnostic of acute MI.

26. c. Rationale: A differentiation is made between myocardial infarcts that have ST-segment elevations on ECG and those that do not. Chest pain that is accompanied by ST-segment elevations is associated with prolonged and complete coronary thrombosis and is treated with reperfusion therapy.

27. a. nitrates; b. nitrates, calcium channel blocking agents; c. antiplatelet aggregation agents, including ASA; d. β-adrenergic blocking agents; e. nitrates, calcium channel blocking agents, β-adrenergic blocking agents; f. β-adrenergic blocking agents, calcium channel blocking agents

28. b. Rationale: A common complication of nitrates is dizziness caused by orthostatic hypotension, so the client should sit or lie down and place the tablet under the tongue. The tablet should be allowed to dissolve under the tongue, and to prevent the tablet from being swallowed, water should not be taken with it. If the pain is not relieved, two more tablets may be taken at five-minute intervals, but if the pain is present after 15 minutes and three tablets, the client should seek medical attention. Headache is also a common complication of nitrates, which usually resolves with continued use of nitrates, and may be controlled with mild analgesics.

29. a. Rationale: The body has a tendency to develop tolerance not only to the side effects of nitrates but also to the antianginal effect. Providing a nitrate-free period of at least eight hours within each 24-hour period for any route of administration is usually effective in preventing develop-

ment of tolerance. Night is the best time to remove the patch unless the client has nocturnal angina. Patches are designed for continuous nitrate therapy and should not be used on a prn basis. The sites should be changed daily to prevent skin irritation and alterations in absorption, but this does not affect tolerance.

30. a. 4; b. 5; c. 2; d. 1; e. 2; f. 3; g. 6; h. 5; i. 3; j. 1

31. d. Rationale: The most common method of coronary artery bypass involves using segments of a resected saphenous vein to carry blood from the aorta to the coronary artery distal to the site of an obstruction. Synthetic grafts are not used as coronary bypass grafts, although they may be used for other vessels. The internal mammary artery may be diverted from its delivery to the chest wall and attached to a coronary artery distal to an obstruction, but it is left attached to its origin from the subclavian artery.

32. b. Rationale: Although the inferior epigastric artery and the gastroepiploic artery are excellent conduits for bypassing obstructed coronary arteries, their use creates the need for a laparotomy, increasing the length of the surgery and chances of wound complications at the harvest site. Cardiopulmonary bypass during the surgery is used for all coronary bypass surgeries except the minimally invasive direct coronary artery bypass graft (MIDCABG).

33. a. Rationale: Because an NSTEMI is an acute coronary syndrome that indicates a transient thrombosis or incomplete coronary artery occlusion, treatment involves intensive drug therapy with antithrombotics and heparin to prevent clot extension, in addition to nitroglycerin IV. Reperfusion therapy using fibrinolytics, CABG, or PCI are used for treatment of STEMI.

34. d. Rationale: Fibrinolytic therapy causes dissolution of the clot and, if given early in the infarct process, can reperfuse the myocardium before cellular death occurs. Treatment with anti-arrhythmic drugs helps prevent development of lethal arrhythmias, and anticoagulant therapy, such as heparin, may be used to prevent formation of new clots following thrombolytic therapy or to prevent extension of established clots. In cases of severe left ventricular dysfunction and cardiogenic shock, an intra-aortic balloon pump may be used to assist ventricular ejection and promote coronary artery perfusion.

35. a. Rationale: Indications that the coronary artery that was occluded is patent and blood flow to the myocardium is re-established following thrombolytic therapy include relief of chest pain, return of ST segment to baseline on the ECG, the pres-

ence of reperfusion arrhythmias, and marked, rapid rise of the CK enzyme within three hours of therapy. If chest pain is unchanged, it is an indication that reperfusion was not successful.

36. a. 4; b. 5; c. 6; d. 2; e. 1; f. 3

37. a. agent of choice in CAD to prevent platelet aggregation around atheroma; administration at the time of unstable angina may prevent progression to MI
b. IV infusion to prevent abrupt closure of intra-coronary stents during placement; may be used in combination with ASA in clients with unstable angina
c. used as anticoagulants in clients with unstable angina undergoing PCI
d. alternative antiplatelet agents for those who cannot use ASA

38. a. Rationale: This client is indicating positive coping with a realization that recovery takes time and that lifestyle changes can be made as needed. The client who is just going to get on with his life is probably in denial about the seriousness of the condition and the changes that need to be made. Nervous questions about the expected duration and effect of the condition indicate the presence of anxiety, as does the statement regarding the healthcare professionals' role in treatment.

39. a. Administer oxygen; b. Take vital signs; c. Arrange for ECG; d. Administer nitroglycerin or narcotic analgesic; e. Perform a physical assessment of the chest; f. Position the client for comfort

40. a. dependence; b. anxiety/fear; c. depression; d. anger; e. denial

41. a. Rationale: Golfing is a moderate-energy activity that expends about 5 METs and is within the 3-to-5 METs activity level desired of a client by the time of discharge from the hospital following MI. Walking at 8 km/hr (5 mph) and mowing the lawn using a push mower are high-energy activities, and cycling at 21 km/hr (13 mph) is an extremely high-energy activity.

42. c. Rationale: Phase III of rehabilitation is the time at which an exercise program, commonly walking, begins. Phase I occurs while the client is in the hospital and includes rest, Phase II includes self-care activities, and Phase IV includes involvement with the community program for continuing physical training and fitness.

43. b. Rationale: Any activity or exercise that causes dyspnea and chest pain should be stopped in the client with CAD. The training target for a healthy 58-year-old is 80% of maximum heart rate, or 132 beats/min, but in a client with cardiac disease undergoing cardiac conditioning, the heart rate should not exceed 20 beats/min over the resting pulse rate. Heart rate, rather than respiratory rate, determines the parameters for exercise.

44. b. Rationale: Resumption of sexual activity is often difficult for clients to approach, and it is reported that most cardiac clients do not resume sexual activity after MI. The nurse can give the client permission to discuss concerns about sexual activity by introducing it as a physical activity when other physical activities are discussed. Physicians may have preferences regarding the timing of resumption of sexual activity, and the nurse should discuss this with the physician and the client, but addressing the client's concerns is a nursing responsibility. Clients should be informed that impotence after MI is common but that it usually disappears after several attempts.

45. d. Rationale: It is not uncommon for a client who experiences chest pain on exertion to have some angina during sexual stimulation or intercourse, and the client should be instructed to use nitro-glycerin prophylactically. Orogenital sex places no undue strain on the heart, and it and positions during intercourse are a matter of individual choice. Foreplay is desirable because it allows a gradual increase in heart rate.

46. c. Rationale: The majority of persons who experience sudden cardiac death as a result of CAD do not have an acute MI but have arrhythmias that cause death, probably as a result of electrical instability of the myocardium. Primary LV out-flow obstruction is a less common cause of sudden cardiac death. Accidental or traumatic causes of cardiac arrest are not considered sudden cardiac death.

47. d. Rationale: An older adult often has altered responses to CAD and MI, resulting in atypical symptoms, and sudden dyspnea and profound weakness should be investigated. Heart rate does not rise as quickly because of decreased respon-siveness to catecholamines, and diaphoresis is often not present. Pain perception is also blunted in older adults, and pain may not be a presenting symptom.

48. a. Rationale: Orthostatic hypotension may cause dizziness and falls in older adults taking antianginal agents that decrease preload, and they should be cautioned to change positions slowly. Exercise programs are indicated for the older adult and may increase performance, endurance, and ability to tolerate stress. A change in lifestyle behaviours may increase quality of life and reduce the risks of CAD even in the older adult. ASA is commonly used in these clients and is not contraindicated.

49. d. Rationale: CAD is a major cause of death in Canadian women, and they have a much higher mortality rate within one year following MI than do men. Recent research indicates that estrogen replacement does not reduce the risk for CAD even though estrogen lowers LDL and raises HDL cholesterol. Smoking carries specific problems for women because smoking has been linked to a decrease in estrogen levels and to early menopause and has been identified as the most powerful contributor to CAD in women under the age of 50. Men have a higher incidence of sudden cardiac death.

**Case Study**

1. Diabetes mellitus; smoking history; obesity; physical inactivity; stress response
2. Mrs. C. appears unmotivated to assume responsibility for her health, and in the absence of symptoms, has not had a desire to make lifestyle changes. First, assist Mrs. C. to clarify her personal values. Then by explaining the risk factors and having her identify her personal vulnerability to various risks, you may help her recognize her susceptibility to CAD. Help her set realistic goals, and allow her to choose which risk factor to change first.
3. Anxiousness with fist clutching; radiation of the burning from epigastric area into the sternum; prior episodes of chest pain with activity, relieved by rest
4. ST segment changes, elevations
5. Procardia is a calcium channel blocker that decreases cardiac oxygen demand by reducing systemic vascular resistance and decreasing myocardial contractility and heart rate. It also increases oxygen supply by dilating coronary arteries.
6. Inform her that she will have continuous cardiac monitoring while she walks on a treadmill with increasing speed and elevation to evaluate the effects of exercise on the blood supply to her heart. Her pulse, respiration, and blood pressure will be measured while she walks and after the test until they return to normal, and the cardiac monitor will be used after the test until any changes return to normal.
7. *Nursing diagnoses:*
   - Acute pain related to ischemic myocardium
   - Anxiety related to possible diagnosis and uncertain future
   - Ineffective denial related to reluctance to receive medical care or change lifestyle
   - Ineffective coping related to lack of effective coping skills

- Imbalanced nutrition: more than body requirements related to intake of calories in excess of calorie expenditure
*Collaborative problems:*
Potential complications: myocardial infarction; cardiac arrhythmias

# CHAPTER 34

1. a. F, diastolic failure; b. T; c. T; d. F, arrhythmias; e. F, reduced
2. a. ↑ CO: increased force of contraction by stretching of cardiac muscle
      Detrimental effect: overstrain the muscle fibres; mitral valve incompetence
   b. ↑ CO: increased contractile force of muscle; Detrimental effect: increased myocardial oxygen need
   c. ↑ CO: increased heart rate and force of contraction; increased preload
      Detrimental effect: increased myocardial oxygen need; overwhelming preload; increased afterload
   d. 1) ↑ CO: increased fluid retention and vasoconstriction to maintain blood pressure
      Detrimental effect: increased preload and afterload
      2) ↑ CO: increased water retention
      Detrimental effect: increased blood volume when already overloaded
3. a. 4; b. 10; c. 12; d. 5; e. 24; f. 7, 8; g. 10; h. 3
4. 2, 14, 16, 22
5. b. Rationale: In left-sided heart failure, blood backs up into the pulmonary veins and capillaries. This increased hydrostatic pressure in the vessels causes fluid to move out of the vessels and into the pulmonary interstitial space. When increased lymphatic flow cannot remove enough fluid from the interstitial space, fluid moves into the alveoli. This results in pulmonary edema and impaired alveolar oxygen and carbon dioxide exchange. Initially the right side of the heart is not involved.
6. a. Rationale: Clinical manifestations of acute left-sided heart failure are those of pulmonary edema, with bubbling crackles; frothy, blood-tinged sputum; severe dyspnea; tachypnea; and orthopnea. Severe tachycardia and cool, clammy skin are present as a result of stimulation of the sympathetic nervous system from hypoxemia. Systemic edema reflected by jugular vein distension, peripheral edema, and hepatosplenomegaly are characteristic of right-sided heart failure.
7. d. Rationale: Paroxysmal nocturnal dyspnea (PND) is awakening from sleep with a feeling of suffocation and a need to sit up to be able to

breathe, and clients learn that sleeping with the upper body elevated on several pillows helps prevent PND. Orthopnea is an inability to breathe effectively when lying down, and nocturia occurs with heart failure as fluid moves back into the vascular system during recumbency, increasing renal blood flow.

8. d. Rationale: Liver damage and failure indicated by increased liver enzyme levels may occur from severe hepatic venous congestion and edema and is considered a major complication of congestive heart failure. Increased weight gain and ascites are symptoms of right-sided failure, and restlessness and confusion are symptoms of the hypoxemia that occurs with heart failure.

9. b. Rationale: Thrombus formation occurs in the heart when the chambers do not contract normally and empty completely. Both atrial fibrillation and very low left ventricular output (LV ejection fraction of <20%) lead to thrombus formation, which is treated with anticoagulants to prevent emboli release into the circulation.

10. a. Rationale: Because congestion of the pulmonary vessels, pulmonary edema, and pulmonary effusions, as well as the degree of cardiac enlargement, can be seen on chest x-ray, it is an important tool to diagnose and monitor the progress of the client in heart failure. Exercise stress testing and cardiac catheterization are more important tests to diagnose coronary artery disease, and although the BUN may be elevated in congestive heart failure, it is a reflection of decreased renal perfusion.

11. a. 20; b. 12, 23; c. 1, 8, 12; d. 4, 24; e. 1, 18, 19, 7, 10, 14; f. 5; g. 1, 5

12. a. 11; b. 4; c. 10; d. 8; e. 6; f. 7; g. 9; h. 1; i. 2; j. 5; k. 3

13. c. Rationale: Hypokalemia is one of the most common causes of digitalis toxicity because low serum potassium levels enhance ectopic pacemaker activity. When a client is receiving potassium-losing diuretics, such as hydrochlorothiazide and furosemide, it is essential to monitor the client's serum potassium levels to prevent digitalis toxicity.

14. a. Rationale: Spironolactone is a potassium-sparing diuretic, and when it is the only diuretic used in the treatment of congestive heart failure, moderate to low levels of potassium should be maintained to prevent development of hyperkalemia. Sodium intake is usually reduced to at least 2400 mg/day in clients with CHF, but salt substitutes cannot be freely used because most contain high concentrations of potassium.

15. d. Rationale: Although all of these drugs may cause hypotension, nitroprusside is a potent dilator of both arteries and veins and may cause such marked hypotension that dobutamine administration may be necessary to maintain the blood pressure during its administration. Milrinone has a positive inotropic effect, in addition to direct arterial dilation, and nitroglycerine primarily dilates veins. Furosemide may cause hypotension because of diuretic-induced intravascular fluid volume depletion.

16. c. Rationale: All foods that are high in sodium should be eliminated in a 2400-mg sodium diet, in addition to the elimination of salt during cooking. Examples include obviously salted snack foods as well as pickles, processed prepared foods, and many sauces and condiments.

17. a. Hypertension: use of medications, diet, and exercise to control
    b. Valvular defects: surgical replacement before CHF occurs; prophylactic antibiotics
    c. Ischemic heart disease: fibrinolytic treatment or PTCA for occlusions
    d. Arrhythmias: anti-arrhythmic agents or pacemakers to control

18. c. Rationale: Successful treatment of congestive heart failure is indicated by absence of symptoms of pulmonary edema and hypoxemia, as shown by clear lung sounds and a normal heart rate. Weight loss and diuresis, and warm skin, less fatigue, and improved level of consciousness may occur without resolution of pulmonary symptoms. Chest pain is not a common finding in congestive heart failure unless coronary artery perfusion is impaired.

19. d. Rationale: A high Fowler's position increases the thoracic capacity, improving ventilation, and sitting with the legs dependent helps pool blood in the extremities and decrease venous return, or preload. Coughing and deep breathing will not clear the lungs of pulmonary edema. I&O and daily weights should be done to monitor the effects of treatment but do not directly address impaired gas exchange. During periods of acute dyspnea, rest is necessary to decrease oxygen demand.

20. d. Rationale: Further teaching is needed if the client believes that a weight gain of 1.5 kg (2 to 3 lb) in two days is an indication for dieting. In a client with congestive heart failure, this type of weight gain reflects fluid retention and is a sign of CHF that should be reported to the healthcare provider.

21. a. H; b. D; c. R; d. D; e. H; f. D; g. D; h. H; i. D; j. H; k. R; l. H

22. b. Rationale: Clients with all types of cardiomyopathy should avoid strenuous activities that increase the workload of the heart and impair ventricular filling. Alcohol is prohibited in

alcohol-induced dilated cardiomyopathy, and the client with hypertrophic cardiomyopathy should increase fluids to prevent dehydration. Intermittent dobutamine infusions may be prescribed for the client with dilated cardiomyopathy.

23. d. Rationale: The 52-year-old woman does not have any contraindications for cardiac transplantation even though she lacks the indication of adequate financial resources. The post-operative transplant regimen is complex and rigorous, and clients who have not been compliant with other treatments or may not have the means to understand the care would not be good candidates. A history of drug or alcohol abuse is usually a contraindication to heart transplantation.

24. b. Rationale: Because of the need for long-term immunosuppressant therapy to prevent rejection, the client with a transplant is at high risk for infection, the leading cause of death in transplant clients. Acute rejection episodes may occur in clients with transplants, but many can be successfully treated with augmented immunosuppressive therapy.

**Case Study**

1. Right-sided failure: jugular vein distension, peripheral edema, hepatomegaly
Left-sided failure: dyspnea, ↓ SpO$_2$, PMI displacement, pulmonary crackles, ↓ BP, S$_3$, S$_4$ heart sounds
Present with both: fatigue, ↑ HR, arrhythmias

2. In dilated CMP the atria and ventricles are enlarged (cardiomegaly) because of dilation rather than hypertrophy, as occurs in congestive heart failure. Decreased contractile function occurs because of degeneration of myocardial fibres rather than of ventricular remodelling.

3. Chest x-ray: cardiomegaly, pulmonary venous hypertension, pleural effusion
ECG: tachycardia and arrythmias of conduction disturbances
Echocardiogram: reveals thin, dilated ventricular walls; low LV ejection fraction
Cardiac catheterization and coronary angiography: normal coronary arteries, thin-walled ventricles
Endomyocardial biopsy: degenerative myocardium

4. Calm, reassuring approach because of his anxiety and critical condition
Explanations of rationales for all diagnostic tests and medications
Administration of oxygen, sit upright with legs out straight or dependent
Provide emotional and physical rest
Constant monitoring of cardiovascular and respiratory function
Start I&O measurements

5. a. atrial fibrillation, increase myocardial strength
b. diuresis to decrease circulating blood volume and preload
c. inotropic effect and dilate vascular smooth muscle to decrease preload and afterload
d. by blocking renin-angiotensin-aldosterone system, reduce afterload by vasodilation and prevent sodium and water retention
e. block sympathetic response to failure and decrease heart rate

6. Although some clients with dilated CMP respond to drug and nutritional therapy, many do not, and heart transplantation is the primary alternative for a good prognosis for survival. However, donor hearts are in short supply, and many clients with dilated CMP die while awaiting heart transplantation. Experimental artificial hearts are the only other alternative for clients who do not respond to conventional therapy.

7. *Nursing diagnoses:*
- Death anxiety related to feeling of dying
- Impaired gas exchange related to increased circulating blood volume
- Ineffective tissue perfusion related to pump failure
- Decreased cardiac output related to altered cardiac rate and rhythm
- Activity intolerance related to imbalance between oxygen supply and demand
- Risk for impaired skin integrity related to edema

*Collaborative problems:*
Potential complications: cardiogenic shock; ventricular arrhythmias; emboli; liver/renal failure, cardiac arrest

## CHAPTER 35

1. a. F, depolarization; b. F, QRS complex; c. F, 80 beats/min; d. T; e. F, negative, positive; f. T; g. F, 40 to 60; h. T; i. F, ectopic foci

2. a. 4;  b. 6;  c. 5;  d. 1;  e. 2;  f. 3

3. d. Rationale: The normal PR interval is 0.12 to 0.20 seconds and reflects the time taken for the impulse to spread through the atria, AV node and bundle of His, the bundle branches, and Purkinje fibres. A PR interval of six small boxes is 0.24 seconds and indicates that the conduction of the impulse from the atria to the Purkinje fibres is delayed.

4. c. Rationale: Electrophysiological testing involves electrical stimulation to various areas of the atrium and ventricle to determine the inducibility of arrhythmias and frequently induces ventricular tachycardia or ventricular fibrillation. The client may have "near-death" experiences and requires emotional support if this occurs.

5. a. 8; b. 7; c. 13; d. 1; e. 3; f. 11; g. 10; h. 6; i. 12; j. 2; k. 4; l. 5; m. 9

6. a. third-degree (total) heart block, pacemaker; b. sinus tachycardia; c. paroxysmal supraventricular tachycardia; d. type I, second-degree heart block; e. ventricular tachycardia, ventricular fibrillation

7. d. Rationale: In the presence of heart disease, a slow SA impulse may allow for escape arrhythmias and premature beats that can lead to further arrhythmias and decreased cardiac output. Asystole refers to total absence of ventricular activity, and SA activity may be present for a short time. Heart block occurs when the impulse from the SA node is not conducted normally to the ventricles, and sinus arrest is a rare complication of sinus bradycardia.

8. d. Rationale: Although many factors may cause a sinus tachycardia, in the client who has had an acute MI, a tachycardia increases myocardial oxygen need in a heart that already has impaired circulation and may lead to increasing angina and further ischemia and necrosis.

9. a. Rationale: A distorted P wave with normal conduction of the impulse through the ventricles is characteristic of a premature atrial contraction. This arrhythmia is frequently associated in a normal heart with emotional stress or the use of caffeine, tobacco, or alcohol. Aerobic conditioning and holding the breath during exertion (Valsalva's manoeuvre) often cause bradycardia. Sedatives rarely may slow heart rate.

10. b. Rationale: When a P wave is absent, there is no SA node impulse, and the impulse is arising elsewhere in the heart. The most common site for impulse formation after the SA node is the AV node, creating a junctional rhythm. Normally junctional rhythm is 40 to 60 beats/min, but in this case it is accelerated, and an accelerated junctional rhythm is most often associated with acute inferior MI, digitalis toxicity, and acute rheumatic fever.

11. a. Rationale: A rhythm pattern that is normal except for a prolonged P-R interval is characteristic of a first-degree heart block. First-degree heart blocks are not treated but are observed for progression to higher degrees of heart block. Defibrillation is used only for ventricular fibrillation, atropine is administered for bradycardias, and pacemakers are used for higher-degree heart blocks.

12. b. Rationale: Symptoms of decreased cardiac output related to cardiac arrhythmias include a sudden drop in blood pressure and symptoms of hypoxemia, such as decreased mentation, chest pain, and dyspnea. Peripheral pulses are weak, and heart rate may be increased or decreased, depending on the type of arrhythmia present.

13. c. Rationale: Premature ventricular contractions in a client with an MI indicate significant ventricular irritability that may lead to ventricular tachycardia or ventricular fibrillation. Antiarrhythmics, such as α-adrenergic blockers, procainamide, aminodarone, or lidocaine, may be used to control the arrythmias. The Valsalva manoeuvre may be used to treat paroxysmal supraventricular tachycardia.

14. a. Rationale: The PVC is an ectopic beat that causes a wide, distorted QRS complex, greater than 0.12 seconds, because the impulse is not conducted normally through the ventricles. Because it is premature, it precedes the P wave and the P wave may be hidden in the QRS complex, or the ventricular impulse may be conducted retrograde and the P wave may be seen following the PVC. Continuous wide QRS complexes with a rate between 110 and 250 are seen in ventricular tachycardia, while sawtoothed P waves are characteristic of atrial flutter.

15. d. Rationale: The most common arrhythmias to occur when the myocardium is reperfused following thrombolytic therapy or angioplasty are PVCs and ventricular tachycardia, and their presence may be an indicator of the success of the therapy.

16. b. Rationale: In a monitored care area where the arrhythmia is identified and a defibrillator is readily available, it should be used immediately, with the initiation of CPR if the initial shock is not successful. IV drugs are rarely successful without defibrillation and CPR because there is no circulation or cardiac output during ventricular fibrillation.

17. c. Rationale: The intent of defibrillation is to apply an electrical current to the heart that will depolarize the cells of the myocardium so that subsequent repolarization of the cells will allow the SA node to resume the role of pacemaker. An artificial pacemaker provides an electrical impulse that stimulates normal myocardial contractions. Cardioversion involves delivery of a shock that is programmed to occur during the QRS complex of the ECG, but this cannot be done during ventricular fibrillation because there is no normal ventricular contraction or QRS complex.

18. a. Rationale: During asystole or pulseless electrical activity, CPR must be initiated immediately to maintain minimal cardiac output and oxygenation, followed by intubation and administration of epinephrine and atropine. Defibrillation is not effective because the myocardial cells are in a state of depolarization.

19. a. Rationale: In preparation for defibrillation, the nurse should apply conductive materials, such as saline pads, electrode gel, or defibrillator gel pads, to the client's chest to decrease electrical impedance and prevent burns. For defibrillation the initial shock is 200 joules, and the synchronizer switch that is used for cardioversion must be turned off. Sedatives may be used before cardioversion if the client is conscious, but the client in ventricular fibrillation is unconscious.

20. a. Rationale: If the cardioverter-defibrillator delivers a shock, the client has experienced a lethal arrhythmia and needs to lie down to allow recovery from the arrythymia. If the client loses consciousness or if there is repetitive firing, 911 should be called.

21. b. Rationale: High-output electrical generators or large magnets, such as those used in MRI, can reprogram pacemakers and should be avoided. Microwave ovens pose no problems to pacemaker function, but the arm should not be raised above the shoulder for one week following placement of the pacemaker. The pacing current of an implanted pacemaker is not felt by the client, but an external pacemaker may cause uncomfortable chest muscle contractions.

22. c. Rationale: This client is manifesting behaviours that are characteristic of a nursing diagnosis of fear related to perceived vulnerability and reliance on a pacemaker, as evidenced by refusal to move or participate in care. It is important for the nurse to teach the client what activity restrictions are necessary to prevent damage to the pacemaker (avoid direct blows to the generator site) and to affirm that the pacemaker can enhance physiological function and the quality of the client's life.

23. c. Rationale: Catheter ablation therapy uses radiofrequency energy to ablate or "burn" accessory pathways or ectopic sites in the atria, AV node, or ventricles that cause tachyarrhythmias.

24. c. Rationale: One of the most common causes of syncope is neurocardiogenic syncope or "vasovagal" syncope. In this type of syncope, there is accentuated adrenergic activity in the upright position, with intense activation of cardiopulmonary receptors resulting in marked bradycardia and hypotension. Normally testing with the upright tilt table causes activation of the renin-angiotensin system and compensation to increase cardiac output and maintain blood pressure when blood pools in the extremities. However, clients with neurocardiogenic syncope experience a marked decrease in blood pressure and heart rate.

25. d. Rationale: Because brain cells start to die within six minutes of anoxia, it is critical that CPR be initiated within four to six minutes of cardiac or pulmonary arrest. Rapid intervention is the most important factor in preventing biological death or the death of brain cells.

26. a. 2; b. 5; c. 8; d. 4; e. 1; f. 3; g. 7; h. 6

27. b. Rationale: Chest compressions are stopped for no more than 10 seconds at the end of the first minute of CPR to determine if the victim has resumed spontaneous breathing and circulation. Four cycles of compressions and ventilations should take one minute.

28. b. Rationale: The most important factor in the successful resuscitation of a person in cardiopulmonary arrest is rapid intervention to prevent death or brain cell death. It is also critical to use correct CPR technique because the best technique provides only about 30% of the normal cardiac output. Absence of underlying cardiac disease is a factor in successful resuscitation but only if resuscitation is rapidly instituted.

29. b. Rationale: Management of a foreign body airway obstruction in a conscious adult who cannot speak requires the administration of abdominal thrusts until the foreign body is expelled or the client loses consciousness. For a client who is sitting in a chair, the abdominal thrusts should be performed with the client in the chair. If the client loses consciousness, she or he should be positioned on the floor with the nurse astride the client to deliver the abdominal thrusts.

30. d. Rationale: It is important to know what cardiac activity is present or absent before administering drugs in a cardiac emergency. Arrhythmia identification with monitoring is essential to determine the guidelines that should be used for definitive treatment of specific cardiac emergencies. Endotracheal intubation does not have to be performed

before drug administration, nor would defibrillation be performed in the absence of ventricular fibrillation.

31. a. third-degree block; b. atrial flutter; c. premature ventricular contraction; bigeminal; d. sinus bradycardia; e. second-degree block; Type I; f. premature atrial contraction; g. second-degree block, Type II; h. sinus tachycardia; i. first-degree block; j. ventricular fibrillation; k. premature ventricular contraction; trigeminal; l. atrial fibrillation; m. premature atrial contraction; n. normal sinus rhythm; o. ventricular tachycardia

**Case Study**

1. The immediate goal of drug therapy is to decrease the rapid ventricular response to the atrial fibrillation because it leads to decreased cardiac output.

2. Cardioversion may be used to convert the fibrillation to a normal sinus rhythm. Cardioversion is administered with an initial dose of 50 joules synchronized with the QRS complex of the ECG, and the client may be sedated before the procedure.

3. Digoxin is used to treat atrial fibrillation because it decreases the ventricular response by increasing the refractory period of the AV node and it also decreases atrial automaticity.
   Diltiazem is indicated for treatment of atrial fibrillation because it inhibits the influx of calcium ions during depolarization of cardiac cells and slows the AV nodal conduction time, decreasing the ventricular response.
   Coumadin is used to prevent thrombus formation, or extension, in the atria where blood pools because of ineffective atrial contraction. If thrombi form in the left atria, arterial embolization may occur.

4. During atrial fibrillation there is total disorganization of atrial electrical activity and no effective atrial contraction. Fibrillatory waves or undulations occur at a rate of 300 to 600 per minute in the atria, and although not all electrical activity is conducted to the ventricles, the ventricular rate is usually 100 to 160 beats/min and irregular.

5. Atrial rhythm is chaotic, and although no definite P wave can be observed, fibrillatory waves can be seen as a jagged, irregular baseline between QRS complexes. The PR interval cannot be measured. The ventricular rhythm is usually irregular, but QRS complexes are usually of normal contour.

6. *Nursing diagnoses:*
   • Decreased cardiac output related to arrhythmia
   • Activity intolerance related to inadequate cardiac output

   • Impaired gas exchange related to increased preload
   • Anxiety related to vulnerability and cardiac disease
   *Collaborative problems:*
   Potential complications: embolism; congestive heart failure; cardiogenic shock

# CHAPTER 36

1. a. Rationale: The primary cause of right-sided infective endocarditis is intravenous drug use, because venous contamination is first carried to the right side of the heart. Left-sided endocarditis is more common in clients with other bacterial infections and underlying heart disease.

2. a. Rationale: Although a CBC will reveal a mild leukocytosis and ESR rates will be elevated in clients with infective endocarditis, these are non-specific findings, and blood cultures are the primary diagnostic tool for infective endocarditis. Transesophageal echocardiograms can identify vegetations on valves but are used when blood cultures are negative, and cardiac catheterizations are used when surgical intervention is being considered.

3. a. 3; b. 5; c. 2; d. 1; e. 4

4. b. Rationale: Drug therapy for clients who develop endocarditis of prosthetic valves is often not successful in eliminating the infection and preventing embolization, and early valve replacement followed by prolonged drug therapy is recommended for these clients.

5. d. Rationale: The dyspnea, crackles, and restlessness the client is manifesting are symptoms of congestive heart failure and decreased cardiac output, which occurs in up to 80% of clients with aortic valve endocarditis as a result of aortic valve incompetence. Vegetative embolization from the aortic valve occurs throughout the arterial system and may affect any body organ. Pulmonary emboli occur in right-sided endocarditis.

6. d. Rationale: The client with outpatient antibiotic therapy requires vigilant home nursing care, and it is most important to determine the adequacy of the home environment for successful management of the client. The client is at risk for life-threatening complications, such as embolization and pulmonary edema, and must be able to access a hospital if needed. Bed rest will not be necessary for the client without heart damage. Avoiding infections and planning diversional activities are indicated for the client but are not most important while he is on outpatient antibiotic therapy.

7. c. Rationale: Prophylactic antibiotic therapy should be initiated before invasive dental, medical, or surgical procedures to prevent recurrence of endocarditis. Continuous antibiotic therapy is indicated only in clients with implanted devices or ongoing invasive procedures. Symptoms of infection should be treated promptly, but antibiotics are not used for exposure to infection.

8. c. Rationale: The stethoscope diaphragm at the left sternal border is the best method to use to hear the high-pitched, grating sound of a pericardial friction rub. The sound does not radiate widely and occurs with the heartbeat.

9. b. Rationale: The client is experiencing a cardiac tamponade that consists of excess fluid in the pericardial sac, which compresses the heart and the adjoining structures, preventing normal filling and cardiac output. Fibrin accumulation, a scarred and thickened pericardium, and adherent pericardial membranes occur in chronic constrictive pericarditis.

10. a. F, expiration; heard throughout the respiratory cycle; b. T; c. F, drop in the client's blood pressure of 30 mm Hg or more from baseline; d. T; e. T

11. d. Rationale: Relief from pericardial pain is often obtained by sitting up and leaning forward. Pain is increased by lying flat. The pain has a sharp, pleuritic quality that changes with respiration, and clients take shallow breaths. Anti-inflammatory medications may also be used to help control pain, but narcotics are not usually indicated.

12. b. Rationale: Viruses are the most common cause of myocarditis in Canada and the United States, and early manifestations of myocarditis are often those of systemic viral infections. Myocarditis may also be associated with systemic inflammatory and metabolic disorders as well as with other micro-organisms, drugs, or toxins. The heart has increased sensitivity to digoxin in myocarditis, and it is used very cautiously, if at all, in treatment of the condition.

13. d. Rationale: A client who has had rheumatic fever is more susceptible to recurrent attacks after another streptococcal infection, and the most common cause of recurrent infection is failure to take continued prophylactic antibiotics following the first episode of rheumatic fever.

14. d. Rationale: Initial attacks of rheumatic fever and the development of rheumatic heart disease can be prevented by adequate treatment of Group A β-hemolytic streptococcal pharyngitis. Because streptococcal infection accounts for only about 20% of acute pharyntitis, cultures should be done to identify the organism and direct antibiotic therapy. Viral infections should not be treated with antibiotics. Prophylactic therapy is indicated in those who have valvular heart disease or have had rheumatic heart disease.

15. a. Rationale: Although it is unproven, the manifestations of ARF appear to be related to an abnormal immunological response to an upper respiratory infection with group A β-hemolytic streptococci, and antibodies produced in response to the streptococcal antigens cross-react with normal body tissues. It is known that streptococci are not demonstrable in lesions of rheumatic fever, and active streptococcal infection is not apparent when rheumatic fever occurs.

16. c. Rationale: Major criteria for the diagnosis of rheumatic fever include evidence of carditis, polyarthritis, chorea (often very late), erythema marginatum, and subcutaneous nodules. Minor criteria include all laboratory findings as well as fever, arthralgia, and a history of previous rheumatic fever.

17. d. Rationale: The mitral valve is most often involved in chronic rheumatic carditis, and the valve becomes thickened and fibrosed, and leaflets may fuse, leading to stenosis or regurgitation. The aortic valve and tricuspid valve are involved less often and the pulmonary valve rarely.

18. a. To eliminate any residual group A β-hemolytic streptococci, prevent spread of infection, prevent recurrent infection
    b. Anti-inflammatory effect to control fever, arthritic and joint manifestations
    c. Anti-inflammatory effect to control fever, inflammation of severe carditis

19. d. Rationale: When carditis is present in the client with rheumatic fever, ambulation is postponed until any symptoms of heart failure are controlled with treatment, and full activity cannot be resumed until anti-inflammatory therapy has been discontinued. In the client without cardiac involvement, ambulation may be permitted as soon as acute symptoms have subsided, and normal activity can be resumed when anti-inflammatory therapy is discontinued.

20. b. Rationale: The dosage of maintenance prophylactic antibiotics is not adequate for protection when the client with rheumatic heart disease undergoes invasive procedures, and additional doses are necessary at this time. Prophylactic therapy following rheumatic fever should continue for life for those who had rheumatic heart disease, for at least five years for those without carditis after the age of 18, or indefinitely for clients with frequent exposure to group A streptococcus.

21. a. F, decreased, hypertrophy; b. F, valvular stenosis; c. F, mitral; d. F, mitral valve prolapse

22. a. 5; b. 6; c. 2; d. 4; e. 8; f. 1; g. 7; h. 3
23. a. 6; b. 8; c. 2; d. 1; e. 3; f. 4; g. 5; h. 7;
    i. 5; j. 1; k. 8; l. 2; m. 3
24. b. Rationale: Because normal blood flow through the heart chambers is impaired in all valvular disorders, prophylactic anticoagulation therapy is used to prevent systemic or pulmonary embolization. Nitrates are contraindicated for the client with aortic stenosis because an adequate preload is necessary to open the stiffened aortic valve. Anti-arrhythmics are used only if arrhythmias occur, and α-adrenergic or β-adrenergic blocking agents may be used to control heart rate as needed.
25. b. Rationale: Arrhythmias frequently cause palpitations, light-headedness, and dizziness, and the client should be carefully attended to prevent falls. Hypervolemia and paroxysmal nocturnal dyspnea (PND) would be apparent in the client with congestive heart failure.
26. d. Rationale: Although the long-term results of percutaneous transluminal balloon valvuloplasty are not known, the procedure poses fewer complications and requires less post-procedural care than does open valve repair or replacement and is used for those clients, of any age, who are poor surgical risks. It has been used for repair of pulmonic, aortic, and mitral stenosis.
27. c. Rationale: Repair of mitral or tricuspid valves has a lower operative mortality rate than does replacement and is becoming the surgical procedure of choice for these valvular diseases. Open repair is more precise than closed repair and requires cardiopulmonary bypass during surgery. All types of valve surgery are palliative, not curative, and clients require lifelong health care. Anticoagulation therapy is used for all valve surgery for at least a period of time postoperatively.
28. c. Rationale: Mechanical prosthetic valves require long-term anticoagulation, and this is a factor in making a decision about the type of valve to use for replacement. Clients who cannot take anticoagulant therapy, such as women of child-bearing age or clients with a risk for hemorrhage, or clients who cannot be compliant with anticoagulation therapy may be candidates for the less durable biological valves.
29. d. Rationale: The greatest risk to a client who has an artificial valve is the development of endocarditis with invasive medical or dental procedures, and before any of these procedures, antibiotic prophylaxis is necessary to prevent infection. Healthcare providers must be informed of the presence of the valve and the anticoagulant therapy, but the most important factor is using antibiotic prophylaxis before invasive procedures.

**Case Study**

1. His age—incidence is higher in older adults; the invasive endoscopic cholecystectomy
2. Mitral valve prolapse
   Degenerative valve lesions:
       Calcification degeneration of a bicuspid aortic valve
       Senile calcification degeneration of a normal aortic valve
3. Stroke symptoms: embolization of vegetations to cerebral circulation with cerebral infarction
   Petechiae: occur as a result of fragmentation and embolization of vegetative lesions
   Systolic, crescendo-decrescendo murmur: aortic valve involvement
   Fever: infection; occurs in 90% of clients with infective endocarditis
4. It provided a route for introduction of bacteria into the bloodstream to trigger the infectious process.
5. Identification of the organism with blood cultures and appropriate IV antibiotic therapy; antipyretics to control fever; rest—with increase in activity after fever abates and if there are no symptoms of congestive heart failure; valve replacement if there is no response to antibiotic therapy
6. Preoperative prophylactic antibiotic therapy
7. *Nursing diagnoses:*
   • Hyperthermia related to infection
   • Impaired physical mobility related to hemiparesis/hemiplegia
   • Decreased cardiac output related to valvular insufficiency
   • Risk for impaired skin integrity related to immobility
   *Collaborative problems:*
   Potential complications: emboli; congestive heart failure

## CHAPTER 37

1. d. Rationale: Regardless of the location, atherosclerosis is responsible for peripheral arterial disease (PAD) and is related to other cardiovascular disease and its risk factors, such as coronary artery disease and carotid artery disease. Venous thrombosis, venous stasis ulcers, and pulmonary embolism are diseases of the veins and are not related to atherosclerosis.
2. a. 2; b. 3; c. 1
3. c. Rationale: Although most abdominal aortic aneurysms are asymptomatic, on physical examination a pulsatile mass in the periumbilical area slightly to the left of the midline may be detected, and bruits may be audible with a stethoscope

placed over the aneurysm. Hoarseness and dysphagia may occur with aneurysms of the ascending aorta and the aortic arch. Severe back pain with flank ecchymosis is usually present on rupture of an abdominal aortic aneurysm, and neurological loss in the lower extremities may occur from pressure of a thoracic aneurysm.

4. a. Rationale: A CT scan is the most accurate test to determine the diameter of the aneurysm and whether a thrombus is present. The other tests may also be used, but the CT yields the most descriptive results.

5. b. Rationale: Increased systolic blood pressure continually puts pressure on the diseased area of the artery, promoting its expansion. Small aneurysms can be treated by decreasing blood pressure, modifying atherosclerosis risk factors, and monitoring the size of the aneurysm. Anticoagulants are used during surgical treatment of aneurysms, but physical activity is not known to increase their size. Calcium intake is not related to calcification in arteries.

6. b. Rationale: Because atherosclerosis is a systemic disease, the client with an AAA is likely to have cardiac, pulmonary, cerebral, and/or lower extremity vascular problems that should be noted and monitored throughout the perioperative period. Post-operatively, the blood pressure is balanced: high enough to keep adequate flow through the artery to prevent thrombosis but low enough to prevent bleeding at the surgical site.

7. a. secular; b. synthetic graft; c. all; d. iliac; e. endovascular graft; f. renal

8. b. Rationale: The blood pressure and peripheral pulses are evaluated every hour in the acute post-operative period to ensure that blood pressure is adequate and that extremities are being perfused. Blood pressure is kept within normal range—if it is too low, thrombosis of the graft may occur, and if it is too high, it may cause leaking or rupture at the suture line. Hypothermia is induced during surgery, but the client is rewarmed as soon as the surgery is completed. Fluid replacement to maintain urine output at 100 mL/hr would increase the blood pressure too much.

9. c. Rationale: During repair of an ascending aortic aneurysm, blood supply to the carotid arteries may be interrupted, leading to neurological complications manifested by a decreased level of consciousness and altered pupil responses to light, as well as changes in facial symmetry, speech, and movement of upper extremities. The thorax is opened for ascending aortic surgery, and shallow breathing, poor cough, and decreasing chest drainage are expected. Often, lower limb pulses are normally decreased or absent for a short period of time following surgery.

10. a. decreased or absent pulses in conjunction with cool, painful extremities below the level of repair; b. cardiac arrhythmias, chest pain; c. absent bowel sounds, abdominal distension, diarrhea, bloody stools; d. increased temperature, WBCs; surgical site inflammation or drainage; e. low urine output, increasing BUN and serum creatinine; f. decreased voluntary movement and sensation

11. c. Rationale: Clients are taught to palpate peripheral pulses to identify changes in their quality or strength, but rate is not a significant factor in peripheral perfusion. The colour and temperature of the extremities are also important for clients to observe. The remaining statements are all true.

12. d. Rationale: The onset of an aortic dissection involving the distal, descending aorta is usually characterized by a sudden, severe, tearing pain in the back, and as it progresses down the aorta, the abdominal organs and lower extremities may begin to show evidence of ischemia. Aortic dissections of the ascending aorta and aortic arch may affect the heart and circulation to the head, with the development of murmurs, ventricular failure, and cerebral ischemia.

13. d. Rationale: Initial treatment for aortic dissection is to lower the BP and myocardial contractility to diminish the pulsatile forces in the aorta. The aorta is fragile after dissection, and surgery is delayed for as long as possible to allow time for blood to clot in the false lumen and for edema to decrease. Anticoagulants would prolong and intensify the bleeding, and blood is administered only if the dissection ruptures.

14. a. Rationale: Relief of pain is an indication that the dissection has stabilized, and it may be treated conservatively for an extended time with drugs that lower the blood pressure and decrease myocardial contractility. Surgery is usually indicated for dissections of the ascending aorta or if complications occur.

15. a. intermittent claudication; b. non-healing ischemic ulcers, gangrene; c. 0.77, mild to moderate; d. rest

16. b. Rationale: Cilostazol (Pletal) is a type II phosphodiesterase inhibitor that inhibits platelet aggregation and increases vasodilation, significantly increasing pain-free walking distance. The other drugs are all antiplatelet agents used not only to prevent thrombus in diseased peripheral arteries but also to decrease the risk of MI, stroke, and other cardiovascular causes of death.

17. a. 4; b. 3; c. 6; d. 5; e. 1; f. 2

18. c. Rationale: Walking exercise increases oxygen extraction in the legs and improves skeletal muscle metabolism. The client with PAD should walk at least 30 minutes a day, preferably twice a day. Exercise should be stopped when pain occurs and resumed when the pain subsides. Elevation of the limbs impairs arterial circulation, so the legs should be kept dependent. Feet should not be soaked because skin breakdown and maceration may occur. Nicotine in all forms causes vasoconstriction and must be eliminated.

19. d. Rationale: Peripheral arterial occlusive disease occurs as a result of atherosclerosis, and the risk factors are the same as for other diseases associated with atherosclerosis, such as coronary artery disease, cerebral vascular disease, and aneurysms. Major risk factors are hypertension, cigarette smoking, and hyperlipidemia. The risk for amputation is high in clients with severe occlusive disease, but it is not the best approach to encourage clients to make lifestyle modifications.

20. a. A; b. V; c. V; d. A; e. A; f. V; g. A; h. V; i. A; j. V; k. V

21. a. Rationale: Diminished blood perfusion to nerve tissue cells produces a neuropathy manifested by loss of both sensation and deep pain, and injuries to the extremity often go unnoticed. It is important to teach the client to protect the feet and detect and prevent injuries to prevent breaks in the skin that can lead to infection and gangrene.

22. c. Rationale: Loss of palpable pulses and numbness and tingling of the extremity are indications of occlusion of the bypass graft and need immediate medical attention. Pain, redness, and serous drainage at the incision site are expected postoperatively, but decreasing ankle-brachial indices may indicate graft obstruction.

23. a. pain; b. pallor; c. pulselessness; d. paraesthesia; e. paralysis; f. poikilothermia

24. a. R; b. B; c. R; d. B; e. R; f. R; g. B; h. R; i. B; j. R

25. a. damage of the endothelium; b. venous stasis; c. hypercoagulability; d. venous stasis; e. hypercoaguability; f. venous stasis

26. a. F, varicose veins; b. F, superficial vein; c.T; d. F, intermittent compression devices

27. d. Rationale: Prevention of emboli formation can be achieved by bed rest and limiting movement of the involved extremity until the clot is stable, inflammation has receded, and anticoagulation is achieved. Elevating the affected limb will promote venous return, but it does not prevent embolization, and dangling the legs promotes venous stasis and further clot formation.

28. a. 3; b. 3; c. 4; d. 2; e. 2; f. 1; g. 1; h. 4; i. 4

29. b. Rationale: Anticoagulant therapy with heparin or Coumadin does not dissolve clots but prevents propagation of the clot, development of new thrombi, and embolization, while lysis of the clot occurs through the action of the body's intrinsic fibrinolytic system or by the administration of fibrinolytic agents.

30. d. Rationale: Exercise programs for clients recovering from DVT should emphasize swimming and wading, which are particularly beneficial because of the gentle, even pressure of the water. Coumadin will not blacken stools; if these occur, they could be signs of GI bleeding. Dark green and leafy vegetables have high amounts of vitamin K and should not be increased during Coumadin therapy, but they do not need to be restricted. The legs must not be massaged because of the risk for dislodging any clots that may be present.

31. a. Rationale: During walking, the muscles of the legs continuously knead the veins, promoting movement of venous blood toward the heart, and walking is the best measure to prevent venous stasis. The other methods will help venous return, but they do not provide the benefit that ambulation does.

32. a. 4; b. 7; c. 1; d. 5; e. 8; f. 3; g. 9; h. 6; i. 2

33. b. Rationale: Although leg elevation, moist dressings, and topical antibiotics are useful in treatment of venous stasis ulcers, the most important factor appears to be extrinsic compression to minimize venous stasis, venous hypertension, and edema. Extrinsic compression methods include compression gradient stockings, elastic bandages, and Unna's boot.

34. a. Rationale: Until the physician is notified and specific orders for IV therapy, oxygen, and medications are received, the client should be placed in a semi-Fowler's position to facilitate breathing, and the nurse should stay with the client to explain the situation and provide emotional support. The legs should not be elevated, because increased venous return will increase right ventricular preload, and pulmonary circulation may be significantly obstructed by the emboli.

35. d. Rationale: Pulmonary angiography, in which a contrast medium is used to visualize the pulmonary vasculature, is the most definitive diagnostic test to locate a pulmonary embolism. Pulmonary angiography is an invasive test, requiring that a catheter inserted into the femoral or antecubital vein be threaded to the pulmonary artery. ECGs and chest x-rays are not specific tools for

diagnosing pulmonary embolism, and a perfusion lung scan is more useful in screening for pulmonary embolism and evaluating the effectiveness of medical management.

**Case Study**

1. Smoking history; history of atherosclerosis with coronary artery disease; age; gender
2. The primary etiology of an AAA is atherosclerotic plaquing that causes degenerative changes in the media lining of the aorta. The changes lead to loss of elasticity, weakening, and eventual dilation of the aorta. Trauma and infections and a possible genetic component are responsible for a small number of AAAs.
3. The severe back pain
   The shock symptoms: BP 88/68 mm Hg; cool, clammy extremities
4. The first priority is to control the bleeding, which will require immediate surgical repair of the aneurysm. Fatal hemorrhage is likely if the bleeding is not controlled.
5. The client will most likely be taken to surgery from the emergency department, and emergency departments are not the most private or supportive environments. It is important for the nurse to provide privacy as much as possible and allow the client and family to be together and ask questions as necessary. The nurse should also provide explanations of the procedures and interventions that are being implemented and be supportive during this critical time.
6. The only effective treatment for AAA is surgery, and the only way to prevent rupture is to surgically repair the aneurysm before it ruptures. Clients with AAAs should have close medical observation to detect increases in aneurysm size because when the aneurysm is twice normal aorta size, there is a high risk for rupture.
7. *Nursing diagnoses:*
   - Acute pain related to compression of internal structures with blood
   - Decreased cardiac output related to hypovolemia
   *Collaborative problems:*
   Potential complications: organ ischemia; hypovolemic shock; myocardial infarction

# CHAPTER 38

1. a. parotid gland; b. submandibular gland; c. pharynx; d. trachea; e. esophagus; f. diaphragm; g. liver; h. hepatic flexure; i. transverse colon; j. ascending colon; k. ileum; l. cecum; m. ileocecal valve; n. vermiform appendix; o. anal canal; p. rectum; q. sigmoid colon; r. descending colon; s. stomach; t. splenic flexure; u. spleen; v. larynx; w. sublingual gland; x. tongue
   *Inset:* a. hepatic duct; b. liver; c. cystic duct; d. gallbladder; e. duodenum; f. pancreas; g. spleen
2. a. muscularis; b. longitudinal layer; c. circular layer; d. oblique layer; e. submucosa; f. mucosa; g. pyloric sphincter; h. duodenal bulb; i. duodenum; j. pylorus; k. rugae; l. serosa; m. body; n. fundus; o. lower esophageal sphincter
3. c. Rationale: The parasympathetic nervous system stimulates activity of the GI tract, increasing motility and secretions and relaxing sphincters to promote movement of contents. A drug that blocks this activity decreases secretions and peristalsis, slows gastric emptying, and contracts sphincters. The enteric nervous system of the GI tract is modulated by sympathetic and parasympathetic influence.
4. d. Rationale: Cholecystokinin is secreted by the duodenal mucosa when fats and amino acids enter the duodenum and stimulates the gallbladder to release bile to emulsify the fats for digestion. The bile is produced by the liver but stored in the gallbladder. Secretin is responsible for stimulating pancreatic bicarbonate secretion, and gastrin increases gastric motility and acid secretion.
5. d. Rationale: The stomach secretes intrinsic factor, necessary for cobalamin (vitamin $B_{12}$) absorption in the intestine. In removal of part or all of the stomach, cobalamin must be supplemented for life.
6. a. F, lower esophageal sphincter; b. T; c. F, parietal cells; d. T; e. F, conjugated (direct); f. T
7. a. 3; b. 5; c. 7; d. 8; e. 10; f. 9; g. 1; h. 4; i. 2; j. 6
8. a. Rationale: Bacteria in the colon synthesize vitamin K, needed for production of prothrombin by the liver; deaminate undigested or non-absorbed proteins, producing ammonia, which is converted to urea by the liver; and reduce bilirubin in the bowel to urobilinogen. A reduction in normal flora bacteria by antibiotic therapy can lead to decreased vitamin K, resulting in decreased prothrombin and coagulation problems, but would result in decreased serum ammonia levels and

decreased serum urobilinogen. Bowel bacteria do not influence protein absorption.

9. c. Rationale: The ampulla of Vater is the site where the pancreatic duct and common bile duct enter the duodenum, and the opening and closing of the ampulla is controlled by the sphincter of Oddi. Because bile from the common bile duct is needed for emulsification of fat to promote digestion and pancreatic enzymes from the pancreas are needed for digestion of all nutrients, a blockage at this point would affect the digestion of all nutrients. Gastric contents pass into the duodenum through the pylorus or pyloric valve.

10. a. Conjugation and excretion of adrenal steroids, including aldosterone; b. Synthesis of albumin; c. Urea formation from ammonia; d. Conjugation of bilirubin to soluble bilirubin excreted in bile; e. Synthesis of prothrombin, fibrinogen, and other clotting factors; f. Synthesis of cholesterol; g. Conjugation and excretion of estrogen (and other gonadal steroids)

11. The bilirubin from hemoglobin is insoluble (unconjugated) and attached to albumin in the blood, removed by the liver and combined with glucuronic acid to become soluble (conjugated), and excreted in bile into the intestine. Bowel bacteria convert some of the bilirubin to urobilinogen; urobilinogen is absorbed into the blood; and a small amount of urobilinogen is excreted by the kidneys in urine, and the rest is removed by the liver and re-excreted in the bile.

12. d. Rationale: There is decreased tone of the lower esophageal sphincter with aging, and regurgitation of gastric contents back into the esophagus occurs, causing heartburn and belching. There is a decrease in hydrochloric acid secretion in aging. Jaundice and intolerance to fatty foods are symptoms of liver or gallbladder disease and are not normal age-related findings.

13. a. Excessive alcohol intake, smoking, exposure to hepatoxins, recent foreign travel
    b. Anorexia and weight loss, excessive weight gain, inadequate diet
    c. Change in bowel patterns, laxative/enema use, decreased fluid/fibre intake

d. Weakness, fatigue, inability to procure and prepare food, inability to feed self
e. Interruption of sleep with gastrointestinal symptoms
f. Changes in taste or smell, use of pain medications, sensory problems that interfere with food preparation or intake
g. Self-esteem and body image problems related to weight, symptoms affecting appearance
h. Loss of employment because of chronic illness, altered relationships with others
i. Anorexia, alcohol intake, decreased acceptance by sexual partner
j. Gastrointestinal problems or symptoms induced by stress, depression
k. Religious dietary restrictions, vegetarianism

14. c. Rationale: A thin white coating of the dorsum (top) of the tongue is normal. A red, slick appearance is characteristic of cobalamin deficiency, and scattered red, smooth areas on the tongue are known as geographical tongue. The uvula should remain in the midline while the client is saying "Ahh."

15. b. Rationale: The pulsation of the aorta in the epigastric area is a normal finding. Bruits indicate abnormal blood flow, the liver is percussed in the right midclavicular line, and a normal spleen cannot be palpated.

16. c. Rationale: The pancreas is located in the left upper quadrant, the liver is in the right upper quadrant, the appendix is in the right lower quadrant, and the gallbladder is in the right upper quadrant.

17. a. Rationale: Borborygmi are loud gurgles (stomach growling) that indicate hyperperistalsis. The bell of the stethoscope is used to detect low-pitched sounds, and normal bowel sounds are relatively high-pitched. The bowel sounds become higher-pitched when the intestines are under tension, as in bowel obstructions. Absent bowel sounds may be reported only when no sounds are heard for five minutes in each quadrant.

18.

| | (1) NPO | (2) Bowel | (3) Consent | (4) Allergy |
|---|---|---|---|---|
| UGI series | X | | | |
| Barium enema | X | X | | |
| IV cholangiography | X | | | X |
| Gallbladder ultrasonography | X | | | |
| Hepatobiliary scintigraphy | X | | | |
| Upper GI endoscopy | X | | X | |
| Colonoscopy | X | X | X | |
| Endoscopic retrograde cholangiopancreatography | X | | X | |

19. a. Rationale: Amylase is released by damaged pancreatic cells into the blood, and an elevation of the enzyme is important in diagnosing acute pancreatitis. Ultrasonography and ERCP are not as specific as the serum amylase for pancreatitis. The serum γ-glutamyl transpeptidase is elevated in liver and biliary tract disease.

20. c. Rationale: The AST level is elevated in liver disease, but it is important to note that it is also elevated in damage to the heart and lungs and is not a specific test for liver function. Measurement of most of the transaminases are non-specific tests unless isoenzyme fractions are determined. Nervous system symptoms of hepatic encaphalopathy are related to elevated ammonia levels.

21. a. 1, 2; b. 6 (signs of peritonitis); c. 1; d. 3; e. 4; f. 5, 6; g. 4; h. 4; i. 2; j. 5

## CHAPTER 39

1. a. protein: 120 g x 4 = 480 cal = 16% of 3000 cal
   fat: 160 g x 9 = 1440 cal = 48% of 3000 cal
   carbohydrate: 270 g x 4 = 1080 cal = 36% of 3000 cal
   b. An average adult requires an estimated 20–35 calories/kg of body weight per day. For a 70-kg adult, this would be between 1400 and 2450 calories per day (70 kg x 20 and 70 kg x 35). This man would require between 1580 and 2765 calories per day (79 kg x 20 and 79 kg x 35).
   c. He will need to alter the quantity and the quality of the foods he is eating. He needs to reduce his intake as he is ingesting at least 235 calories more than is required for a man his size. As well, the high end of the caloric recommendation is for very active people, so if he is less active, he needs to reduce his intake by an even greater amount. He will need to reduce the fat and carbohydrate intake to obtain the recommended 55% CHO and 30% fat recommendation.

2. a. T; b. F, vitamin $B_{12}$ and iron; c. F, fat; d. F, Kwashiorkor

3. d. Rationale: In Canada, where protein intake is high and generally of good quality, protein-calorie malnutrition is most commonly secondary to problems of the gastrointestinal system. In the developing countries, adequate food sources may not exist, the inhabitants may not be well educated about nutritional needs, and economic conditions may prevent purchase of balanced diets.

4. a. Carbohydrate stored in the liver and muscles in the form of glycogen is used and may be quickly depleted.
   b. Protein, primarily the amino acids alanine and glutamine, is converted to glucose for energy, and a negative nitrogen balance occurs.
   c. Body fat is mobilized and is used as the primary source of energy, conserving protein.
   d. Fat stores are usually depleted in four to six weeks, and body proteins are used because they are the only source of energy available.

5. c. Rationale: The sodium-potassium exchange pump uses 20%–50% of all calories ingested.

When energy sources are decreased, the pump fails to function, and sodium is left in the cell, and potassium remains in extracellular fluids. Hyperkalemia, as well as hyponatremia, occurs.

6. a. F, Overweight (BMI = $60/1.5^2$ = 26.66); b. T; c. F, peripheral nervous system; d. T

7. a. calcium channel blockers; b. cholestyramine; c. warfarin; d. phenothiazines and tricyclic antidepressants; e. phenytoin, barbiturates; f. monoamine oxidase inhibitors; g. erythropoietin

8. b. Rationale: In malnutrition, metabolic processes are slowed, leading to increased sensitivity to cold, slowed heart rate and cardiac output, and decreased neurological function. Because of slowed GI motility and absorption, the abdomen becomes distended and protruding.

9. d. Rationale: Malnutrition that results from a decreased intake of food is most common in individuals with severe anorexia that decreases the desire to eat. Infections create a hypermetabolic state that increases nutritional demand. Malabsorption causes loss of nutrients that are ingested. Draining decubitus ulcers are examples of disorders that cause both loss of protein and hypermetabolic states.

10. c. Rationale: Serum transferrin is a protein that is synthesized by the liver and used for iron transport and decreases when there is protein deficiency. An increase in the protein would indicate a more positive nitrogen balance with amino acids available for synthesis. Decreased lymphocytes and serum prealbumin are indicators of protein depletion, and increased serum potassium shows continuing failure of the sodium-potassium pump.

11. d. Rationale: Anthropometric measurements that include mid-upper arm circumference and triceps skinfold measurements are good indicators of lean body mass and skeletal protein reserves and are valuable in evaluating persons who may have acute protein malnutrition. The other measurements do not specifically address muscle mass.

12. a. Rationale: This breakfast provides fat and energy in each of the items. Defatted milk provides fewer calories and less energy. Pancakes and cereal are mostly carbohydrate.

13. c. Rationale: As her BMI is <18.5, she falls in the category of increased risk of developing health problems (Table 39-7). Her low BMI upon admission, in combination with the possible appetite-suppressing effects of the stress of relocating to a long-term care facility, could significantly affect her eating habits and contribute to further weight loss. On the other hand, she may have had difficulties with access to food or food preparation, and the new facility may provide her with this type of instrumental support. If she has been eating alone and now enjoys eating with others, she may benefit from her new surroundings.

14. b. Rationale: Although calorie intake should be decreased in the older adult because of decreased activity and basal metabolic rate, the need for specific nutrients, such as proteins and vitamins, is believed to be unchanged during aging.

15. a. Rationale: Socio-economic conditions frequently have the greatest effect on the nutritional status of the healthy older adult. Limited income and social isolation can result in the "tea and toast" meals of the older adult.

16. a. Rationale: Standard nasogastric tubes are used for tube feedings for short-term feeding problems because prolonged therapy can result in irritation and erosion of the mucosa of the upper GI tract. Gastric reflux and the potential for aspiration can occur with both tubes that deliver fluids into the stomach. Both NG and gastrostomy tubes can become displaced and deprive the client of the sensations associated with eating.

17. a. Position the client with the head of the bed elevated 30 to 45 degrees.
   Following intermittent feedings, keep the head of the bed elevated for 30 to 60 minutes.
   Measure residual feeding to detect retention of solution in the stomach so that the stomach does not become overdistended.
   b. Start tube feedings with small amounts and low concentrations and gradually increase the amount and strength of the solution.
   Refrigerate opened solutions to prevent bacterial growth but warm them to room temperature before administration.
   c. Flush the tube with water before and after feedings and medication administration.
   In continuous feedings, flush the tube with water every four hours.
   d. Verify position before every feeding, or every eight hours with continuous feedings, by checking that the pH of aspirate is less than 5.
   e. Refrigerate opened solutions.
   Do not hang more solution than will infuse in eight hours, and discard any remaining at the end of eight hours.
   Wash equipment for intermittent feedings after each use, and change tubing every 24 hours with continuous feedings.

18. a. Rationale: If the residual stomach contents are more than 200 mL, the next feeding is held for one hour, and then the residual volume is rechecked. The aspirate should be reinstilled because it contains gastric secretions in addition to the feeding that has not passed from the stomach.

19. a. PPN; b. CPN; c. CPN; d. PPN; e. PPN; f. PPN; g. CPN
20. c. Rationale: In malabsorption syndromes, foods that are ingested into the intestinal tract cannot be digested or absorbed, and tube feedings infused into the intestinal tract would also not be absorbed. All of the other conditions may be treated with enteral or parenteral nutrition, depending on the client's needs.
21. a. Refrigerate solutions until 30 minutes before use; dressing change to catheter site per institutional protocol; IV tubing change every 24 hours; antimicrobial filters on the IV line to be changed every 24 hours; solution in one bottle should not infuse more than 24 hours
    b. Start infusions slowly, gradually increasing rate for 24 to 48 hours; check capillary blood glucose levels every four to six hours; provide sliding-scale doses of insulin as prescribed; do not speed up infusion rates or remove infusion from infusion controllers/pumps; visually check the amount infused every 30 minutes to one hour
    c. Securely fasten catheter to IV tubing; if the tubing disconnects from the catheter, place the client in Trendelenburg's position on the left side to trap "air" in right atrium and notify physician; monitor for signs of air embolus
22. a. Rationale: Bacterial growth occurs at room temperature in nutritional solutions; therefore solutions must not be infused longer than 24 hours. Remaining solution should be discarded. Speeding up the solution may cause hyperglycemia and should not be done.
23. a. Rationale: Proper placement of the tip of the central catheter for parenteral nutrition is in the superior vena cava. If the tip is in the right atrium, the hyperosmolar fluid and the catheter tip may cause erosions of the atrial tissue. Repositioning of the catheter is only done by the physician or specially trained nurses.
24. d. Rationale: When peripheral parenteral nutrition is being run concurrently with fat emulsions, the fat emulsion should be connected below the filter through a Y-injection site as close as possible to the injection site. A separate IV site is not necessary, but the fat emulsion should be administered through the special tubing provided by the manufacturer.
25. c. Rationale: Nausea and vomiting and fever occur when lipids are infused quickly. Symptoms of fat emboli include dyspnea, cyanosis, and chest and back pain. Fatty acid deficiency can occur with prolonged TPN that does not contain the essential fatty acids. Allergies to fat emulsions do occur but manifest as allergic reactions with urticaria, angioedema, and perhaps anaphylactic reactions.
26. a. 31 kg/m²; b. obese Class 1; c. increased
27. a. Restrict dietary intake so that it is below energy requirements.
    b. A goal for weight loss must be set, and 0.5 to 1 kg (1 to 2 lb) a week is realistic. A more rapid loss often causes skin and underlying tissue to lose elasticity and become flabby folds of tissue.
    c. Will confirm eating patterns and often point out bad eating habits that can be changed
    d. It is thought that metabolism is temporarily increased by eating, and more calories are used when several small meals a day are ingested.
    e. Alcohol is not permitted because it increases caloric intake and has low nutritional value.
    f. Exercise increases energy expenditure, decreases appetite, and is important in maintaining weight loss.
    g. Such programs de-emphasize the diet and focus on how and when the person eats, help modify eating habits, and may lead to more success in maintaining weight loss over time.
28. a. When reducing diets severely restrict carbohydrates, the body's glycogen stores become depleted within a few days. The glycogen normally binds to water in fat cells, and it is this water loss that causes weight loss in the first few days. Fat is not burned until the glycogen-water pool is depleted.
    b. Daily weighing is not recommended because of the frequent fluctuation from retained water (including urine) and elimination of feces. A weekly weight is a more reliable indicator of weight loss.
    c. Men are able to lose weight more quickly than are women because women have a higher percentage of metabolically less active fat.
    d. Plateau periods during which no weight is lost are normal occurrences during weight reduction and may last for several days to several weeks, but weight loss will resume if the prescribed weight reduction plan is continued.
29. b. Rationale: Medications are used only as adjuncts to diet and exercise programs in the treatment of obesity. Drugs do not cure obesity without changes in food intake and physical activity, and weight gain will occur when the medications are discontinued. The medications used work in a variety of ways to control appetite, but over-the-counter drugs are probably the least effective and most abused of the drugs.
30. a. 3; b. 1; c. 2; d. 2; e. 3; f. 3; g. 1
31. a. F, gynecoid; b. T; c. T

32. d. Rationale: Sedatives can precipitate severe respiratory complications in morbidly obese clients because of pre-existing hypoventilation caused by pressure on the diaphragm and reduced movement of the muscles of the chest wall. Antihypertensive drugs and hypoglycemic agents are often used to treat complications of obesity, and IV solutions do not pose a problem for the obese client.

33. c. Rationale: Special considerations are needed for the care of the morbidly obese client because most hospital units are not prepared with beds, chairs, blood pressure cuffs, and other equipment that will need to be used with the very obese client. Consideration of all aspects of care should be made before implementing care for the client, including extra time and perhaps assistance for positioning, physical assessment, and transferring the client.

34. d. Rationale: If any medication is to be given intramuscularly to the obese client, it is important to use a needle long enough to reach muscle tissue. This requires an extra-long 7.5- to 10-cm (3- to 4-inch) or spinal needle. If a nasogastric tube present following gastric surgery for morbid obesity becomes blocked or needs repositioning, the physician should be notified. Ambulation is usually started in the evening of surgery, and additional help will be needed to support the client. Respiratory function is promoted by keeping the head of the bed elevated at a 30-degree angle.

35. c. Rationale: Fluids and foods high in carbohydrates tend to promote diarrhea and symptoms of the dumping syndrome in clients with gastric bypass surgery. The diet generally should be high in protein and low in carbohydrates, fat, and roughage, and consist of six small feedings a day because of the small stomach size. Liquid diets are likely to be used for a longer time for the client with a gastroplasty.

36. a. A; b. AB; c. A; d. B; e. A; f. AB; g. AB; h. A

37. c. Rationale: The potential life-threatening cardiac complications related to the hypokalemia are the most important considerations in the client's care. The other nursing diagnoses are important considerations in the client's care but do not pose the immediate risk that the hypokalemia does.

**Case Study**

1. BMI and waist circumference
Food intake history
Assessment of each body system

2. The chemotherapy and radiation have greatly increased nutritional need, but food intake is decreased because of side effects of cancer treatment, weakness may lead to inability to procure and prepare food, she lives alone and has no socialization with meals, and she has feelings of hopelessness about treatment for cancer. She may not have access to foods from her native country, which could be a problem if she prefers them. She may not remember details of nutritional requirements or modifications if the written materials she has been given did not take into account her inability to read English.

3. Edema and possible ascites indicated by hypo-albuminemia
Paleness of skin, mucous membranes indicated by her Hg and Hct

4. Liver damage with fatty infiltration
Susceptibility to infection very high because of chemotherapy and radiation immunosuppression in addition to that of malnutrition

5. Foods that are easy to prepare
How to add protein supplement or powdered milk to foods
Decrease fluids with meals so that more calories are consumed
Eat small multiple feedings that are of nutritional value
Provide all instructions with consideration of her literacy level (use photos, diagrams)

6. *Nursing diagnoses:*
- Imbalanced nutrition: less than body requirements related to anorexia and decreased food intake
- Activity intolerance related to fatigue and weakness
- Hopelessness related to belief that cancer therapy is ineffective
- Risk for infection related to decreased host defence mechanisms
*Collaborative problems:*
Potential complications: liver failure; electrolyte imbalance

# CHAPTER 40

1. a. F, parasympathetic nervous system; b. F, labyrinthine stimulation; c. T; d. F, metabolic alkalosis, hydrochloric acid; e. F, projectile vomiting

2. c. Rationale: The loss of gastric hydrochloric acid causes metabolic alkalosis and increase in pH; loss of potassium, sodium, and chloride; and loss of fluid, which increases the hematocrit.

3. a. Rationale: "Coffee-ground" vomitus indicates stomach bleeding where blood has been mixed with gastric acid, changing it to a dark brown colour. Active bleeding in the lower esophagus usually produces bright red blood in vomitus. Yellow-greenish vomitus is characteristic of bile

reflux or an obstruction below the ampulla of Vater, and a fecal odour to the vomitus is characteristic of a bowel obstruction.

4. d. Rationale: The client with severe or persistent vomiting requires intravenous replacement of fluids and electrolytes until able to tolerate oral intake to prevent serious dehydration and electrolyte imbalances. Oral fluids are not given until vomiting has been relieved, and parenteral antiemetics are often not used until a cause of the vomiting can be established. Nasogastric intubation may be indicated in some cases, but fluid and electrolyte replacement is the first priority.

5. c. Rationale: Water is the fluid of choice for rehydration by mouth. Very hot or cold liquids are not usually well tolerated, and although broth and Gatorade have been used for the client with severe vomiting, the substances are high in sodium and should be administered with caution.

6. d. Rationale: Ondansetron (Zofran) is one of several serotonin antagonists that act both centrally and peripherally to reduce vomiting—centrally on the vomiting centre in the brainstem and peripherally by promoting gastric emptying. Dronabinol (Marinol) is an orally active cannabinoid that causes sedation and has a potential for abuse and is used when other therapies are ineffective. Antihistamines used as antiemetics also cause sedation.

7. a. 4; b. 6; c. 2; d. 3; e. 1; f. 5; g. 3; h. 7; i. 4; j. 6; k. 2

8. c. Rationale: A positive history of use of tobacco and alcohol is the most significant etiological factor in oral cancer. Excessive exposure to ultraviolet radiation from the sun is a factor in the development of cancer of the lip. Herpes simplex infections have not been associated with oral cancer, and difficulty swallowing and ear pain are symptoms of advanced oral cancer, not risk factors.

9. b. Rationale: Because surgical treatment of oral cancers involves extensive excision, a tracheostomy is usually performed with the radical dissections. The first goal of care is that the client will have a patent airway. The other goals are appropriate but of lesser priority.

10. b. Rationale: Measures to assess and treat withdrawal from alcohol should be implemented with clients who have heavy use of this substance, because alcohol is a strong risk factor and withdrawal can be life-threatening. Nutritional needs may need to be addressed with tube feedings post-operatively, and pain medications may need to be increased because of cross-tolerance. Counselling about lifestyle changes is not a priority in the early post-operative course.

11. a. fatty foods; b. chocolate; c. alcohol; d. tea, coffee—also peppermint and spearmint

12. d. Rationale: Bethanechol is a cholinergic drug that increases lower esophageal sphincter tone and increases gastric emptying. Alginic acid reacts with sodium bicarbonate to form a viscous solution that acts as a mechanical barrier to reflux. Histamine $H_2$-receptor blockers decrease gastric acid production, and antacids neutralize hydrochloric acid.

13. c. Rationale: The use of blocks to elevate the head of the bed facilitates gastric emptying by gravity and is strongly recommended to prevent night-time reflux. Small meals should be eaten frequently, but clients should not eat at bedtime or lie down for two to three hours after eating. Liquids should be taken between meals to prevent gastric distension with meals. Activities that involve increasing intra-abdominal pressure, such as bending over, lifting, or wearing tight clothing, should be avoided.

14. c. Rationale: Following a fundoplication, it is most important to maintain patency of the nasogastric tube to prevent overdistension of the stomach and pressure on the suture line, and replacement of an obstructed tube can perforate the surgical repair. Monitoring for return of peristalsis and assessment of the abdominal wounds are common post-operative interventions but are not related to disruption of the surgical site. Positioning on the right side is not indicated following surgical repair of a hiatal hernia.

15. c. Rationale: Dysphagia, occurring with meats, then soft foods, and eventually liquids, is the most common symptom of esophageal cancer and is often pronounced by the time the client seeks medical attention. The client frequently has poor nutritional status because of the inability to ingest adequate amounts of food before surgery. Fluid volume deficit could occur, but this is a late finding in comparison with inadequate food intake.

16. b. Rationale: Following esophageal surgery, the client should be positioned in a semi-Fowler's or Fowler's position to prevent reflux and aspiration of gastric sections. Nasogastric drainage is expected to be bloody for eight to twelve hours post-operatively. Abdominal distension is not a major concern following esophageal surgery, and even though the thorax may be opened during the surgery, clear breath sounds should be expected in all areas of the lungs.

17. a. 2; b. 5; c. 3; d. 1; e. 4

18. a. acute; b. autoimmune atrophic; c. laparoscopy; d. *Heliobacter pylori*; e. intrinsic factor; f. $H_2R$ blocker, bismuth

19. a. Rationale: A bland diet with six small meals a day is recommended to help control the symptoms of gastritis. Non-steroidal anti-inflammatory drugs are often as irritating to the stomach as ASA and should not be used in the client with gastritis. Antacids are often used for control of symptoms but have the best neutralizing effect if taken after meals, and alcohol and caffeine should be entirely eliminated because they may precipitate gastritis.

20. a. Arterial blood that has not been in contact with gastric secretions, as in esophageal or oral bleeding
    b. Blood that has been in the stomach for some time and has reacted with gastric secretions
    c. Slow bleeding from an upper gastrointestinal (GI) source when blood passes through the GI tract and is digested
    d. Bleeding that has been of short duration and blood has not passed through the GI tract

21. a. 4;  b. 8;  c. 1;  d. 7;  e. 6;  f. 2;  g. 5;  h. 3

22. a. Rationale: Although all of the interventions may be indicated when a client has upper GI bleeding, the first nursing priority is to perform a physical assessment of the client's condition, with emphasis on blood pressure, pulse, and peripheral perfusion to determine the presence of hypovolemic shock.

23. d. Rationale: Octreotide is a somatostatin analogue that has been shown to reduce upper GI bleeding and inhibit the release of GI hormones such as gastrin, thereby decreasing hydrochloric acid secretions. Ranitidine is a histamine $H_2$-receptor blocker that decreases acid secretion, and omeprazole inhibits the pump necessary for the secretion of hydrochloric acid. Vasopressin has a vasoconstrictive action useful in controlling upper GI bleeding.

24. b. Rationale: All over-the-counter drugs should be avoided because their contents may include drugs that are contraindicated because of the irritating effects on the gastric mucosa. Clients are taught to check suspicious vomitus or stools for occult blood, but all stools do not need to be tested. Antacids cannot be taken with all medications because they prevent the absorption of many drugs. Misoprostol is used to protect the gastric mucosa in clients who must take NSAIDs for other conditions because it inhibits acid secretion stimulated by NSAIDs.

25. a. Rationale: The client's BUN is usually elevated with a significant hemorrhage because blood proteins are subjected to bacterial breakdown in the GI tract. With control of bleeding, the BUN will return to normal. During the early stage of bleeding, the hematocrit is not always a reliable indicator of the amount of blood lost or the amount of blood replaced and may be falsely high or low. A urinary output of 25 mL/hr indicates impaired renal perfusion and hypovolemia, and a urine specific gravity of 1.030 indicates concentrated urine typical of hypovolemia.

26. b. Rationale: Because the client who requires regular administration of NSAIDs, such as naproxen or diclofenac, is at great risk for GI bleeding, substituting the newer NSAID COX-2 inhibitors, such as valdecoxib, may decrease GI side effects. Famotidine and nizatidine are both $H_2$-receptor blockers that could be used to decrease gastric acidity, and misoprostol could be used with the NSAIDS to inhibit acid secretion.

27. a. D; b. G; c. B; d. D; e. B; f. G; g. G; h. D; i. B; j. D; k. G; l. G; m. B; n. D

28. a. 3;  b. 5;  c. 1;  d. 6;  e. 2;  f. 4

29. a. Rationale: The ultimate damage to the tissues of the stomach and duodenum, precipitating ulceration, is acid back-diffusion into the mucosa. The gastric mucosal barrier is protective of the mucosa, but without the acid environment and damage, ulceration does not occur. Ammonia formation by *H. pylori* and release of histamine impair the barrier but are not directly responsible for tissue injury.

30. b. Rationale: Back pain is a common manifestation of ulcers located on the posterior aspect of the duodenum and is important for nurses to keep in mind during assessment of the client because the more typical epigastric burning and pain may not be present. Duodenal ulcers are more often relieved by food than are gastric ulcers, and when epigastric discomfort occurs, it is lower than that of gastric ulcers. Eating stimulates gastric acid production, increasing discomfort for clients with gastric ulcers, while the pain of duodenal ulcers usually occurs several hours after eating.

31. a. Rationale: Fibroptic endoscopy is an important procedure used for locating and diagnosing any disorder of the upper GI tract, including peptic ulcers, gastritis, esophageal disorders, gastric cancer, and bleeding. Endoscopy is the most reliable test because of the ability to directly visualize and biopsy tissue. Serological testing for *H. pylori* and analysis of gastric secretions may help identify precipitating factors related to ulceration.

32. c. Rationale: There is no specific diet used for treatment of peptic ulcers, and clients are encouraged to eat as normally as possible, eliminating foods that cause discomfort or pain. Eating six meals a day prevents the stomach from being totally empty and is also recommended. Caffeine and alcohol should be eliminated from the diet because they are known to cause gastric irritation,

and milk and milk products should be used because milk can neutralize gastric acidity and contains prostaglandins and growth factors protective of the GI mucosa.

33. a. Remove stimulation for HCl acid and pepsin secretion by keeping stomach empty
    b. Stop spillage of gastrointestinal contents into the peritoneal cavity
    c. Remove excess fluids and undigested food from the stomach

34. a. 0800, 1030, 1300, 1600, 1900, 2200; b. 2100; c. 0600, 1100, 1700, 2100

    Sucralfate should be given on an empty stomach, necessitating administration of the midmorning dose of antacids at least 30 minutes before the pre-lunch dose of sucralfate and the bedtime dose of antacids one hour after the sucralfate. Although newer histamine $H_2$-receptor blockers can be given with antacids, administration of cimetidine and ranitidine should be separated from antacids by at least an hour. Sucralfate binds a number of drugs, including cimetidine, but can be given with ranitidine.

35. a. 3; b. 6; c. 4; d. 2; e. 7; f. 3; g. 1; h. 5; i. 3; j. 7; k. 1

36. c. Rationale: Increased vagal stimulation from emotional stress causes hypersecretion of hydrochloric acid, and stress reduction is an important part of the client's management of peptic ulcers, especially duodenal ulcers. If side effects to medications develop, the client should notify the healthcare provider before altering the drug regimen. Although effective treatment will promote pain relief in several days, the treatment regimen should be continued until there is evidence that the ulcer has completely healed. Interchanging brands and preparations of antacids and histamine $H_2$-receptor blockers without checking with healthcare providers may cause harmful side effects, and clients should take only prescribed medications.

37. c. Rationale: Perforation of an ulcer causes sudden, severe abdominal pain that is often referred to the shoulder, accompanied by a rigid, board-like abdomen and other signs of peritonitis. Vomiting of blood indicates hemorrhage of an ulcer, and gastric outlet obstruction is characterized by projectile vomiting of undigested food, hyperactive stomach sounds, and upper abdominal swelling.

38. a. Rationale: If symptoms of gastric outlet obstruction, such as nausea, vomiting, and stomach distension, occur while the client is on NPO status or has a nasogastric tube, the patency of the NG tube should be suspected. A recumbent position should not be used in a client with an

outlet obstruction because it increases abdominal pressure on the stomach, and vital sign and circulatory status assessment are important if hemorrhage or perforation is suspected. Deep breathing and relaxation may help some clients with nausea but not when stomach contents are obstructed from flowing into the small intestine.

39. d. Rationale: Abdominal pain that causes the knees to be drawn up and shallow, grunting respirations in a client with peptic ulcer disease are characteristic of perforation, and the nurse should assess the client's vital signs and abdomen before notifying the physician. Irrigation of the NG tube should not be performed because the additional fluid may be spilled into the peritoneal cavity, and the client should be placed in a position of comfort—usually on the side with the head slightly elevated.

40. a. 3; b. 4; c. 2; d. 1

41. d. Rationale: Because there is no sphincter control of food taken into the stomach following a Billroth procedure, concentrated food and fluid move rapidly into the small intestine, creating a hypertonic environment that pulls fluid from the bowel wall into the lumen of the intestine, reducing plasma volume and distending the bowel. Postprandial hypoglycemia occurs when the concentrated carbohydrate bolus in the small intestine results in hyperglycemia and the release of excessive amounts of insulin into the circulation, resulting in symptoms of hypoglycemia.

42. a. Rationale: Dietary control of dumping syndrome includes small, frequent meals with low carbohydrate content and elimination of fluids with meals. The client should also lie down for 30 to 60 minutes after meals. These measures help delay stomach emptying, preventing the rapid movement of a high-carbohydrate food bolus into the small intestine.

43. d. Rationale: If the client's nasogastric tube becomes obstructed following a gastrectomy with an intestinal anastomosis, gastric secretions may put a strain on the sutured anastomosis and cause serious complications. Because of the danger of perforating the gastric mucosa or disrupting the suture line, the nurse should notify the physician if the tube needs to be repositioned or replaced.

44. a. Rationale: Although no single causative agent of gastric cancer has been identified, it is known that the person with achlorhydria or pernicious anemia is more likely to develop gastric cancer than is the person with normal gastric acid production. Other possible risk factors include alcohol intake; genetics; a diet of smoked, highly salted, or spiced foods; *H. pylori* infection; and chronic irritation. Peptic ulcer disease, smoking,

and acute gastritis are not known to be associated with gastric cancer.

45. d. Rationale: Anorexia with weight loss, nausea, vomiting, and hematemesis, and anemia and melena may occur in clients with either peptic ulcers or gastric cancer, and antacids and anti-secretory agents may also relieve early symptoms of gastric cancer. However, when epigastric pain has been controlled with ingestion of foods, fluids, or antacids for a period of time but becomes worse regardless of interventions, gastric cancer should be suspected.

46. d. Rationale: A total gastrectomy removes the gastric cells responsible for secreting intrinsic factor necessary for absorption of cobalamin, and lifelong intramuscular or intranasal administration of cobalamin is necessary to prevent the development of pernicious anemia. Wound healing is usually impaired in the client with a total gastrectomy performed for gastric cancer because of impaired nutritional status before surgery. Following a total gastrectomy, the client also requires diet modifications as a result of dumping syndrome and postprandial hypoglycemia. Peptic ulcers are not a common finding after total gastrectomy.

47. b. Rationale: Food poisoning caused by *E. coli* is characterized by profuse diarrhea, abdominal cramping, and bloody stools and is most often associated with contaminated beef, especially ground beef. Salmonella contamination most often occurs with poultry, staphylococcal infections occur with milk and salad dressings, and botulism occurs with fish and low-acid canned products.

**Case Study**

1. Infiltration of the gastric wall by a tumour causes epigastric discomfort, while growth of the tumour into the gastric lumen can cause anorexia and weight loss. Release of substances by cancer cells also contribute to anorexia, nausea, and vomiting. Nausea and vomiting may also be caused if the tumour obstructs the gastric outlet. Fatigue and other symptoms of anemia occur because of chronic blood loss as the lesion erodes through the mucosa.

2. Malnutrition is indicated in Mrs. E. by weight loss, decreased hemoglobin and hematocrit, decreased serum albumin, skin changes and discoloration, and her emaciated appearance.

3. Other factors that may contribute to malnutrition in Mrs. E. include the increased metabolic

demands of tumour cells; responses to radiation therapy, such as vomiting, stomatitis, esophagitis, diarrhea, and decreased bone marrow function; and perhaps pernicious anemia resulting from the achlorhydria common with gastric cancer.

4. Malnourished clients do not respond well to radiation therapy, and normal cells do not recover from radiation damage when malnutrition is present. Depletion of protein stores also places Mrs. E. at risk for impaired immune function.

5. A plan for Mrs. E. and her family should include the following:
   - Increasing nutrition with bland, warm, high-calorie, high-protein foods; small, frequent feedings; and nutritional supplements as tolerated
   - Skin care for radiation therapy
   - Anticipatory planning for pain relief and continuing care as she becomes more impaired
   - Discussion of feelings and concerns of Mrs. E. and her family with explanations of realistic expectations of outcome of her condition

6. In responding to Mrs. E., the nurse should provide accurate information in a way that will decrease her stress and promote her decision-making and coping skills. It is important to tell her that while it is unlikely she will recover from her cancer, the radiation treatment can help shrink the tumour mass and improve her nutritional status and promote a feeling of well-being. She should be told that her family and health care providers will help her function effectively as long as possible.

7. *Nursing diagnoses:*
   - Imbalanced nutrition: less than body requirements related to inability to ingest, digest, and absorb nutrients
   - Fatigue related to anemia and effects of radiation therapy
   - Activity intolerance related to generalized weakness
   - Impaired skin integrity related to malnutrition and radiation therapy
   - Risk for ineffective management of therapeutic regimen related to lack of knowledge regarding disease progression

   *Collaborative problems:*

   Potential complications: sepsis related to immunosuppression; negative nitrogen balance; organ failure

# CHAPTER 4I

1. a. 3; b. 1; c. 2; d. 1; e. 3; f. 2; g. 1; h. 1; i. 2

2. d. Rationale: Antiperistaltic agents, such as loperamide and paregoric, should not be used in infectious diarrhea because of the potential of prolonging exposure to the infectious agent. Demulcent agents may be used to coat and protect mucous membranes in these cases. The other options are all appropriate measures to use in cases of infectious diarrhea.

3. d. Rationale: The first interventions to establish bowel regularity include promoting bowel evacuation at a regular time each day, preferably by placing the client on the bedpan, using a bedside commode, or walking the client to the bathroom. To take advantage of the gastrocolic reflex, an appropriate time is 30 minutes after the first meal of the day or at the client's usual individual timing. Perianal pouches are used to protect the skin only when regularity cannot be established, and evacuation suppositories are also used only if other techniques are not successful.

4. All of the following factors indicate potential causes of constipation that are responsive to nursing intervention:

   a. Repeated ignoring of the urge to defecate causes the muscles and mucosa in the rectal area to become insensitive to the presence of feces, and drying of the stool occurs. The urge to defecate is decreased, and stool becomes more difficult to expel.

   b. The misunderstanding that one must have a daily bowel movement may lead to inappropriate laxative use with chronic dilation and loss of tone in the colon/rectum.

   c. Hemorrhoids are the most common complication of chronic constipation, caused by straining to pass hardened stool.

   d. Increased fibre intake without increasing fluids may predispose the client to impaction or obstruction.

5. c. Rationale: Of the foods listed, dried beans contain the highest amount of dietary fibre and are an excellent source of soluble fibre.

6. d. Rationale: Enemas are fast-acting and are beneficial in the immediate treatment of acute constipation but should be limited in their use. Soapsuds enemas should be avoided because they may lead to inflammation of colon mucosa. Stimulant cathartics irritate the entire intestinal tract and lead to cramping, while stool softeners have a prolonged action, taking up to 72 hours for an effect.

7. a. Rationale: The client with an acute abdomen may have significant fluid or blood loss into the abdomen, and evaluation of blood pressure and heart rate should be the first intervention, followed by assessment of the abdomen and the nature of the pain.

8. Surgery is indicated for a, c, d, and f.

9. c. Rationale: Adequately functioning nasogastric suction should prevent nausea and vomiting because stomach contents are continuously being removed. The first interventions in this case are to check the amount and character of the recent drainage, to check the tube for patency, and to check equipment function. Decreased or absent bowel sounds are expected after a laparotomy, and the Jackson-Pratt should only drain fluid from the tissue of the surgical site. Antiemetics may be given if the NG tube is patent because anaesthetic or narcotic agents may cause nausea.

10. d. Rationale: The client is experiencing paralytic ileus, or impaired peristalsis, which almost always occurs as a result of anaesthetic agents and manipulation of the bowel during surgery. Nasogastric tubes help remove gas and secretions from the stomach but do not prevent the impaired motility of the intestines. Passing flatus or having a bowel movement indicates that the bowel has resumed peristaltic activity.

11. a. Rationale: The abdominal pain and distension that occur from the decreased motility of the bowel should be treated with increased ambulation and frequent position changes to increase peristalsis. Assessment of bowel sounds is not an intervention to relieve the pain, and a high Fowler's position will not affect gut function. Narcotics may still be necessary for pain control, though narcotics do not improve pain related to gas.

12. a. Rationale: The client is having symptoms of an acute abdomen and should be evaluated by a physician immediately. The client's age, location of pain, and other symptoms are characteristic of appendicitis. Heat application and laxatives should not be used in clients with undiagnosed abdominal pain because they may cause perforation of the appendix or other complications. Fluids should not be taken until vomiting is controlled, nor should they be taken in the event that surgery may be performed.

13. a. T; b. F, perforation with peritonitis; c. F, McBurney's point; d. T; e. T

14. a. 5; b. 7; c. 6; d. 2; e. 3; f. 8; g. 4; h. 7; i. 1
15. a. B; b. UC; c. CD; d. B; e. UC; f. CD; g. UC; h. B; i. UC; j. B; k. CD; l. B; m. B; n. CD
16. a. decreased hemoglobin, hematocrit; b. hypo-albuminemia; c. decreased Na, K, Mg, Cl, and bicarbonate; d. elevated WBC
17. c. Rationale: Ulcerative colitis and Crohn's disease have many of the same extraintestinal symptoms, including erythema nodosum and arthritis, as well as uveitis, and conjunctivitis. Pyoderma gangrenosum tends to happen more commonly in clients with Crohn's disease. Primary sclerosis cholangitis occurs in those with ulcerative colitis.
18. a. 2; b. 1; c. 3; d. 4; e. 2; f. 5; g. 2; h. 1; i. 1
19. a. Rationale: The initial procedure for a total colectomy and ileal reservoir can include a colectomy, ileal reservoir construction, ileoanal anastomosis, and a temporary loop ileostomy. The ileostomy is closed in the second surgery after healing from the first surgery is complete, about three to six months after the initial surgery. A loop ileostomy is the most common temporary ileostomy, and provides a diverted fecal stream away from the reservoir. A rectal tube to suction is not indicated in any of the surgical procedures for ulcerative colitis. A catheter placed in an ileostomy stoma would be expected following a total proctocolectomy with a continent ileostomy (Kock pouch), a surgical procedure rarely performed, while a permanent ileostomy stoma would be expected following a total proctocolectomy.
20. a. Rationale: Initial output from a newly formed ileostomy may be as high as 1500 to 2000 mL/day, and intake and output must be accurately monitored for fluid and electrolyte imbalance. Ileostomy bags may need to be emptied every three to four hours, but the appliance should not be changed for several days unless there is leakage onto the skin. This terminal ileal stoma is permanent, and the entire colon and rectum have been removed. An eventual return to a normal, presurgical diet is the goal for the client with an ileostomy. Initial restrictions are based on decreased bowel lumen size due to normal postoperative edema; this subsides over four to six weeks.
21. b. Rationale: Elemental diets are enteral feedings that are high in calories and nutrients, lactose-free, fat- and residue-free, and are absorbed in the proximal small intestine, which allows distal bowel rest. High-fat diets are contraindicated in Crohn's disease because of the loss of absorbing mucosa and altered bile salt metabolism and absorption, and lactose found in milk may not be adequately digested because of lactase deficiency.
22. a. Rationale: Signs of malnutrition include pallor from anemia, hair loss, bleeding, cracked gingivae, and muscle weakness, which support a nursing diagnosis that identifies impaired nutrition. Diarrhea may contribute to malnutrition but is not a defining characteristic. Anorectal excoriation and pain relate to problems with skin integrity, and the hypotension relates to problems with fluid deficit.
23. a. 3; b. 4; c. 5; d. 2; e. 6; f. 1
24. d. Rationale: The increased pressure of fluids and secretions retained in the bowel during an obstruction causes an increase in capillary permeability and extravasation of fluids and electrolytes into the peritoneal cavity, resulting in a severe reduction in circulating blood volume and hypovolemic shock. Secretion of intestinal fluids is increased by the distension occurring with bowel obstruction, and persistent copious vomiting occurs with upper small bowel obstruction. Although bleeding can occur from a necrotic strangulation, it is uncommon and a late event.
25. a. F, upper small bowel obstruction; b. T; c. T; d. F, metabolic acidosis; e. F, strangulated; f. F, mechanical obstruction
26. b. Rationale: Mouth care is critical in the client who has a nasogastric tube due to unpleasant taste and odour as well as mouth breathing, and should be done very frequently. The client is NPO with a nasogastric tube and cannot have ice chips. The tube may be checked for patency and irrigated if blockage is suspected. There are no positioning restrictions with nasogastric tubes.
27. c. Rationale: Although all polyps are abnormal growths, the most common type of polyps (hyperplastic) is non-neoplastic as are several other types of polyps. However, adenomatous polyps are characterized by neoplastic changes in the epithelium, and most colorectal cancers appear to arise from these polyps. Only clients with a family history of familial adenomatous polyposis have close to a 100% lifetime risk of developing colorectal cancer.
28. d. Rationale: Cancers of the right side of the colon (ascending) are usually asymptomatic and cannot be felt or visualized with digital examination or sigmoidoscopy. An annual test for occult blood is the best way to screen for tumours in this area of the bowel. Serum carcinoembryonic anti-

gen (CEA) is not specific for colon cancer and is used most effectively in following the progress of a client after surgery for cancer.

29. An abdominal incision is made, and the proximal sigmoid colon is brought through the abdominal wall and formed into a colostomy. The client is repositioned, a perineal incision is made, and the distal sigmoid colon, rectum, and anus are removed through the perineal incision.

30. b. Rationale: A normal new colostomy stoma should appear pale pink to dark red, and have mild to moderate edema. A purplish stoma indicates inadequate blood supply and should be reported. The colostomy will not have any fecal drainage for two to four days, but there may be some earlier mucus or serosanguineous drainage. Bowel sounds this soon after extensive bowel surgery will be diminished or absent.

31. d. Rationale: Sexual dysfunction may result from an abdominal-perineal resection, but the nurse should discuss with the client that different nerve pathways affect erection, ejaculation, and orgasm and that a dysfunction of one does not mean total sexual dysfunction and also that an alteration in sexual activity does not have to alter sexuality. Simple reassurance of desirability and ignoring concerns about sexual function do not help the client regain positive feelings of sexuality.

32. a. liquid to pasty, frequent function, extremely irritating to skin, less odour and gas than colostomy
    b. formed, usually not irritating to skin, function variable—maybe once every one to three days; odiferous gas
    c. liquid to pasty; irregular function several times a day; can be irritating to skin; odiferous gas

33. b. Rationale: A nursing diagnosis of disturbed body image is characterized by clients' comments that express shame or an altered image of themselves because of a change in appearance. Although this client does not yet have the knowledge to care for the colostomy, the primary problem is that the client cannot or will not yet learn because the colostomy is not acceptable to his image of himself.

34. b. Rationale: Following infusion of the fluid into the stoma, the solution and feces will take about 30 to 45 minutes to return, and the client can plan to read or perform other quiet activities during the wait time. Between 500 and 1000 mL of warm tap water should be used; a cone tip on the end of the tubing prevents bowel damage that could occur if a stiff plastic catheter is used; and the fluid should be elevated about 45 to 60 cm (18 to 24 in.) above the stoma, or about shoulder level, to prevent too-rapid infusion of the solution.

35. a. Rationale: The inflammation and infection of diverticula cause small perforations with spread of the inflammation to the surrounding area in the intestines. Abscesses may form, or complete perforation with peritonitis may occur. Systemic antibiotic therapy is often used, but medicated enemas would increase intestinal motility and increase the possibility of perforation, as would the application of heat. Surgery is indicated when it is necessary to drain abscesses or to resect an obstructing inflammatory mass.

36. a. 6; b. 4; c. 1; d. 5; e. 2; f. 3

37. b. Rationale: Scrotal edema is a common and painful complication after an inguinal hernia repair and can be relieved in part by application of ice and elevation of the scrotum with a scrotal support. Heat would increase the edema and the discomfort, and a truss is used to keep unrepaired hernias from protruding. Coughing is discouraged post-operatively because it increases intra-abdominal pressure and stress on the repair site.

38. b. Rationale: The most common type of malabsorption syndrome is lactose intolerance, and it is managed by restricting the intake of milk and milk products. Antibiotics are used in cases of bacterial infections that cause malabsorption, pancreatic enzyme supplementation is used for pancreatic insufficiency, and restriction of gluten is necessary for control of adult celiac disease (non-tropical sprue, celiac sprue, gluten-induced enteropathy).

39. c. Rationale: Short bowel syndrome results from multiple extensive resections of the small bowel. The other conditions primarily affect the large colon, and do not result in short bowel syndrome.

40. a. 5; b. 4; c. 2; d. 1; e. 3

41. d. Rationale: Warm sitz baths provide comfort and cleaning of the area following all anorectal surgery and may be done three or four times a day for one to two weeks. Stool softeners may be ordered for several days post-operatively to help keep stools soft for passage, but laxatives may cause irritation and trauma to the anorectal area and are not used post-operatively. Early passage of a bowel movement, although painful, is encouraged to prevent drying and hardening of stool in the rectum, resulting in an even more painful, difficult bowel movement.

**Case Study**

1. Changes in bowel patterns with alternating constipation and diarrhea; changes in stool calibre with ribbon or pencil stools; rectal bleeding; sensation of incomplete evacuation
2. Assess drains placed to the lower abdomen, including the type and amount of drainage; apply sterile gauze dressings daily to drain insertion sites; assess the incision for suture integrity, approximation of incision edges, and signs and symptoms of wound infection; assess drainage from the wound for amount, colour, and characteristics; pressure-reducing chair cushions for sitting comfort, light peri-pad and mesh pants for perineal wound drainage, changed daily and prn
3. To be able to manage ostomy care independently; to maintain normal skin integrity; adapt to altered body image
4. It appears that Mr. D. is depersonalizing the stoma and, to preserve his body image, is seeing it as something separate from himself with a name and personality of its own.
5. Previous experience with narcotics; inappropriate dosing for weight/narcotic tolerance; anxiety related to diagnosis; new stoma
6. Care of the perineal wound; importance of fluids and diet; care for colostomy, including skin care, odour control, supplies needed, and where to obtain supplies; signs and symptoms of complications to report and when to seek medical care; name and contact for enterostomal therapy; contacts and resource for support; additional education
7. *Nursing diagnoses:*
   • Disturbed body image related to presence of stoma
   • Acute pain related to surgical incisions and inadequate pain-control measures
   • Knowledge deficit regarding temporary dietary restrictions with new stoma

# CHAPTER 42

1. a. obstructive; conjugated (direct)
   b. increased breakdown of RBCs; unconjugated (indirect)
   c. hepatocellular; both conjugated and unconjugated
2. a. 3; b. 5; c. 4; d. 2; e. 3; f. 1; g. 2; h. 1; i. 5; j. 1
3. a. HBsAg, Anti-HBs; b. HBeAg, Anti-HBe; c. HBcAg, Anti-HBc IgM and Anti-HBc IgG
4. a. HBV DNA; b. Anti-HBs; c. Anti-HBc IgG; d. HbsAg; e. Anti-HAV IgM, Anti-HAV IgG; f. Anti-HDV; g. Anti-HCV; h. HVC RNA; i. Recombinant immunoblot assay (RIBA)
5. d. Rationale: The systemic manifestations of rash, angioedema, arthritis, fever, and malaise in viral hepatitis are caused by the activation of the complement system by circulating immune complexes. Liver manifestations include jaundice from hepatic cell damage and cholestasis, as well as anorexia perhaps caused by toxins produced by the damaged liver. Impaired portal circulation usually does not occur in uncomplicated viral hepatitis but would be a liver manifestation.
6. c. Rationale: Pre-icteric symptoms occur before the onset of jaundice and include a variety of gastrointestinal symptoms as well as discomfort and heaviness in the upper right quadrant of the abdomen. Pruritus, dark urine, and light-coloured stools occur with the onset of jaundice in the icteric phase.
7. d. Rationale: Although fulminant hepatitis can occur with hepatitis A and hepatitis C, it is more common in hepatitis B, especially in hepatitis B infection accompanied by infection with HDV.
8. a. hepatitis B vaccine (Recombivax HB or Engerix-B)
   b. hepatitis B immune globulin (HBIg) *and* hepatitis B vaccine
9. d. Rationale: Individuals who have been exposed to hepatitis A through household contact or foodborne outbreaks should be given immune globulin within one to two weeks of exposure to prevent or modify the illness. Hepatitis A vaccine is used to provide pre-exposure immunity to the virus and is indicated for individuals at high risk for hepatitis A exposure. Although hepatitis A can be spread by sexual contact, the risk is higher for transmission with the oral-fecal route.
10. a. Rationale: No specific drugs are effective in treating acute viral hepatitis, although supportive drugs, such as antiemetics, sedatives, or antipruritics, may be used for symptom control. Antiviral agents, such as lamivudine or ribavirin, and α-interferon may be used for treating chronic

hepatitis B or C but are effective in only 20% to 25% of clients.

11. b. Rationale: The client with hepatitis B is infectious for four to six months, and precautions to prevent transmission through percutaneous and sexual contact should be maintained until tests for HbsAg are negative. Close contact does not have to be avoided, but close contacts of the client should be vaccinated. Alcohol should not be used for at least a year, and rest with increasing activity during convalescence is recommended.

12. a. Rationale: Adequate nutrition is especially important in promoting regeneration of liver cells, but the anorexia of viral hepatitis is often severe, requiring creative and innovative nursing interventions. Strict bed rest is not usually required, and the client usually has only minor discomfort with hepatitis. Diversional activities may be required to promote psychological rest but not during periods of fatigue.

13. c. Rationale: Immunosuppressant agents are indicated in hepatitis associated with immune disorders in order to decrease liver damage caused by autoantibodies. Autoimmune hepatitis is similar to viral hepatitis in presenting signs and symptoms and may become chronic and lead to cirrhosis.

14. a. 3;  b. 4;  c. 1;  d. 2;  e. 1;  f. 2;  g. 3

15. a. 5;  b. 3;  c. 6;  d. 3;  e. 7;  f. 8;  g. 2;  h. 4;  i. 3;  j. 1

16. a. Scarring and nodular changes in liver lead to compression of the veins and sinusoids, causing resistance of blood flow through the liver from the portal vein.
    b. Development of collateral channels of circulation in inelastic, fragile esophageal veins.

17. a. liver lymphatics, liver tissue, intestinal vasculature
    b. decreased liver production of albumin
    c. decreased, decreased, decreased
    d. decreased, aldosterone, ADH
    e. peripheral edema
    f. aldosterone
    g. hypoalbuminemia, hypokalemia (from hyperaldosteronism)

18. b. Rationale: Serum bilirubin, both direct and indirect, would be expected to be increased in cirrhosis. Serum albumin and cholesterol are decreased, and liver enzymes, such as AST, ALT, SGPT, and GTT, are elevated.

19. a. Helps promote diuresis and fluid excretion
    b. Increases plasma colloid osmotic pressure and maintains intravascular volume and kidney perfusion
    c. Increases fluid loss through the kidneys and mobilizes peritoneal fluid; spironolactone blocks effects of the excess aldosterone

    d. Decreases intake of fluid-retaining sodium
    e. Temporary measure to relieve impaired respiration or pain of severe ascites
    f. Shunts peritoneal fluid from the abdomen to the venous system, decreasing ascites and improving hemodynamic factors.

20. d. Rationale: Early signs of this neurological condition include euphoria, depression, apathy, irritability, confusion, agitation, drowsiness, and lethargy. Loss of consciousness is usually preceded by asterixis, disorientation, hyperventilation, hypothermia, and alterations in reflexes. Increasing oliguria is a sign of hepatorenal syndrome.

21. a. Reduction of ammonia formation in the bowel by limiting protein intake
    b. Reduction of ammonia formation by decreasing absorption of ammonia from bowel
    c. Reduction of ammonia formation by reducing bacterial flora that produce ammonia
    d. Reduction of ammonia formation by removing red blood cells as a source of protein

22. a. Rationale: Although there are many physical changes in the appearance of the client with cirrhosis, the presence of jaundice and ascites is often the most distressing to the client. Pruritus and decreased sensory perception do not commonly affect body image, and alopecia and periorbital edema are not manifestations of cirrhosis.

23. d. Rationale: The client with advanced, complicated cirrhosis requires a high-calorie, high-carbohydrate diet with protein and sodium restrictions. Fat is not limited unless it promotes early satiety. The tomato sandwich with low-protein bread and salt-free butter best meets these requirements. Rough foods, such as popcorn, may irritate the esophagus and stomach and lead to bleeding. Peanut butter is high in sodium and protein, and canned chicken noodle soup is very high in sodium.

24. d. Rationale: Ascites causes pressure on the diaphragm and reduces lung volume, and clients should be positioned in a semi-Fowler's or Fowler's position to relieve the pressure on the diaphragm. A paracentesis is not performed unless there is severe respiratory distress from the ascites because the fluid rapidly re-accumulates. Coughing and deep breathing should be performed but do not relieve the pressure, nor does oxygen administration.

25. c. Rationale: Bleeding esophageal varices are a medical emergency and involve treatment with IV vasopressin and nitroglycerin, endoscopic sclerotherapy, shunt therapy and, rarely, balloon tamponade, in addition to measures to replace blood loss. During an episode of bleeding, man-

agement of the airway and prevention of aspiration of blood are critical factors. Occult blood as well as fresh blood from the GI tract would be expected and is not tested. Vasopressin and nitroglycerine cause a decreased heart rate. Portal shunting surgery is performed for esophageal varices but not during an acute hemorrhage.

26. d. Rationale: By shunting fluid sequestered in the peritoneum into the venous system, pressure on esophageal veins is decreased, and more volume is returned to the circulation, improving cardiac output and renal perfusion. However, because ammonia is diverted past the liver, hepatic encephalopathy continues. These procedures do not prolong life or promote liver function.

27. c. Rationale: Abstinence from alcohol is very important in alcoholic cirrhosis and may result in improvement if started when liver damage is limited. Although further liver damage may be reduced by rest and nutrition, most changes in the liver cannot be reversed. Exercise does not promote portal circulation, and very moderate exercise is recommended. Acetaminophen should not be used by the client with liver disease because it is potentially hepatotoxic.

28. c. Rationale: Because the prognosis for cancer of the liver is poor, and treatment is largely palliative, supportive nursing care is appropriate. The client exhibits clinical manifestations of liver failure as seen in any client with advanced liver failure. Whether the cancer is primary or metastatic, there is usually a poor response to chemotherapy, and surgery is indicated only in the few clients that have localization of the tumour to one portion of the liver.

29. d. Rationale: Liver transplantation is indicated for clients with cirrhosis, as well as for many adults and children with other irreversible liver diseases. Although physicians make the decisions regarding the client's qualifications for transplant, nurses should be knowledgeable about the indications for transplantation and be able to discuss the client's questions and concerns related to transplantation. Rejection is less of a problem in liver transplantation than in kidney or heart transplantation.

30. a. 2;  b. 5;  c. 3;  d. 1;  e. 4

31. c. Rationale: The predominant symptom of acute pancreatitis is severe, deep abdominal pain that is usually located in the left upper quadrant but may be in the mid-epigastrium. Bowel sounds are decreased or absent, temperature is elevated only slightly, and the client has hypovolemia and may manifest symptoms of shock.

32. b. Rationale: Although serum lipase levels and urinary amylase levels are increased, an increased serum amylase level is the criterion most commonly used to diagnose acute pancreatitis. Renal clearance of amylase that is higher than the clearance of creatinine is also found in acute pancreatitis.

33. c. Rationale: Pancreatic rest and suppression of secretions are promoted by preventing any gastric contents from entering the duodenum, which would stimulate pancreatic activity. Surgery is not indicated for acute pancreatitis but may be used to drain abscesses or cysts. An ERCP pancreatic sphincterotomy may be performed when pancreatitis is related to gallstones. Pancreatic enzymes are necessary in chronic pancreatitis if a deficiency in secretion occurs.

34. b. Rationale: Food and fluid intake stimulates gastric secretions, which in turn will stimulate pancreatic secretions, so clients are always initially on NPO status. Drugs to reduce gastric secretions, such as $H_2$-receptor blockers and proton pump inhibitors, may be used but have not been found to be effective in controlling pancreatic secretion. Antispasmodics may help relieve pain, but antibiotics are not indicated unless infection is present.

35. c. Rationale: Positions that flex the trunk and draw the knees up to the abdomen help relieve the pain of acute pancreatitis, and positioning the client on the side with the head elevated decreases abdominal tension. Diversional techniques are not as helpful as positioning in controlling the pain. The client is usually NPO because food intake increases the pain and inflammation. Bed rest is indicated during the acute attack because of hypovolemia and pain.

36. c. Rationale: Sodium restriction is not indicated for clients recovering from acute pancreatitis, but the stools should be observed for steatorrhea, indicating that fat digestion is impaired, and glucose levels should also be monitored for indication of impaired β-cell function. Alcohol is a primary cause of pancreatitis and should not be used.

37. c. Rationale: Chronic damage to the pancreas causes pancreatic exocrine and endocrine insufficiency, resulting in a deficiency of digestive enzymes and insulin. Malabsorption and diabetes often result. Abstinence from alcohol is necessary in both types of pancreatitis, as is a high-carbohydrate, high-protein, and low-fat diet. Although abdominal pain is a major manifestation of chronic pancreatitis, more commonly a heavy, gnawing feeling occurs.

38. a. Rationale: Pancreatic extracts are given with meals and food so that enzymes are available for digestion of the nutrients. The enzymes should

not be dissolved in water, nor are they available in liquid form. The effectiveness of the enzyme replacement is monitored by observing for steatorrhea.

39. b. Rationale: Major risk factors for pancreatic cancer are believed to be cigarette smoking, high-fat diet, diabetes, and exposure to benzidine and coke. It is not associated with alcohol intake, as pancreatitis is.

40. a. duodenum; b. gallbladder; c. distal stomach; d. distal common bile duct; e. proximal pancreas; f. pancreatic duct to jejunum; g. common bile duct to jejunum; h. stomach to jejunum

41. a. T; b. F, cholesterol; c. T; d. F, cholelithiasis; e. T

42. a, c, d, f, g

43. a. Obstruction of the common duct prevents bile drainage into the duodenum, with congestion of bile in the liver and subsequent absorption into the blood
    b. Absence of bile in the intestines
    c. Soluble bilirubin in the blood excreted into the urine
    d. Absence of bile salts in duodenum, preventing fat emulsion and digestion
    e. Contraction of the inflamed gallbladder and obstructed ducts, stimulated by cholecystokinin when fats enter the duodenum

44. a. Rationale: Ultrasonography is 90% to 95% accurate in detecting gallstones and is a non-invasive procedure. It is especially useful for clients with contrast-medium allergies but is used for the majority of all clients. Liver function tests will be elevated if liver damage has occurred but do not indicate gallbladder disease. IV cholangiography uses radiopaque dye to outline the gallbladder and the ducts.

45. a. Prevent gallbladder stimulation by food or fluids moving into the duodenum.
    b. Meperidine causes less spasm in the bile ducts than do other opiates.
    c. Inflammation of the gallbladder may be caused by bacterial infection or lead to bacterial colonization.
    d. Counteract smooth muscle spasms of the bile ducts.

46. a. 2; b. 1; c. 3; d. 4

47. d. Rationale: Removal of the gallbladder will prevent further stone formation and inflammation of the gallbladder and is the preferred treatment of choice for most clients. The laparoscopic approach is performed about 85% of the time. A cholecystostomy is usually an emergency procedure in which an incision is made into the gall-

bladder to remove stones; a choledocholithotomy is an incision into the common bile duct to remove stones; a cholecystoduodenostomy is an anastomosis between the gallbladder and duodenum to relieve obstruction at the distal common duct.

48. c. Rationale: The laparoscopic cholecystectomy requires four small abdominal incisions to visualize and remove the gallbladder, and the client has small dressings placed over these incisions. The client with an incisional cholecystectomy is usually hospitalized three to five days, while the laparoscopic procedure allows same-day or next-day discharge with return to work in two to three days. A T-tube is placed in the common bile duct after exploration of the duct during an incisional cholecystectomy.

49. c. Rationale: After removal of the gallbladder, bile drains directly from the liver into the duodenum, and a low-fat diet is recommended until adjustment to this change occurs. Most clients tolerate a regular diet with moderate fats but should avoid excessive fats, as large volumes of bile previously stored in the gallbladder are not available, and steatorrhea could occur with a large fat intake.

50. b. Rationale: The high abdominal incision makes the client reluctant to take deep breaths, and adequate pain relief will enable the client to cough, deep breathe, and move about, preventing postoperative complications. Positioning the client on the operative side is more likely to increase pain.

51. a. Rationale: The T-tube drains bile from the common bile duct until swelling from trauma has subsided and bile can freely enter the duodenum. The tube is placed to gravity drainage and should be kept open and free from kinks to prevent bile from backing up into the liver. The tube is not normally irrigated.

52. c. Rationale: Bile-coloured drainage or pus from any incision may indicate an infection and should be reported to the physician immediately. The bandages on the puncture sites should be removed the day after surgery, followed by bathing or showering. Referred shoulder pain is a common and expected problem following laparoscopic procedures, when carbon dioxide used to inflate the abdominal cavity is not readily absorbed by the body. Nausea and vomiting are not expected post-operatively and may indicate damage to other abdominal organs and should be reported to the physician.

**Case Study**

1. Some etiological factor causes injury to pancreatic cells or activation of the pancreatic enzymes in the pancreas rather than in the intestine, and the activated enzymes digest the pancreas itself, a process known as autodigestion. Activated trypsin can digest the protein of the pancreas and activate elastase and phospholipase. Elastase causes hemorrhage by dissolving the elastic fibres of blood vessels, and phospholipase A causes fat necrosis. The pancreas may be merely edematous or become necrotic.

2. alcohol and gallbladder disease

3. The serum and urinary amylase are elevated, indicating release of these enzymes into the blood circulating through the pancreas. The WBC count is high, indicating marked inflammation. The blood glucose level is elevated, indicating impairment of insulin production and release by the β-cells. The decreased calcium indicates hypocalcemia, a sign of severe pancreatitis.

4. Hypocalcemia occurs in part because calcium combines with fatty acids released during fat necrosis of the pancreas. The nurse should observe for symptoms of tetany, such as jerking, irritability, muscular twitching, and positive Chvostek's and Trousseau's signs. Numbness or tingling around the lips and in the fingers is an early indicator of hypocalcemia.

5. The pain is usually located in the upper left quadrant but may be in the mid-epigastric area and frequently radiates to the back. It has a sudden onset and is described as severe, deep, piercing, and continuous. It is aggravated by eating and often begins when the client is recumbent. It is not relieved by vomiting and may be accompanied by flushing, cyanosis, and dyspnea.

6. Hypovolemia, shock, and the local complications of pseudocysts and abscesses

7. Meperidine—for pain relief with minimal stimulation of the pancreatic ducts
Ranitidine—to decrease hydrochloric acid production by the stomach, because the hydrochloric acid stimulates pancreatic activity

8. NPO status and suction with a nasogastric tube prevent gastric contents from entering the duodenum and stimulating pancreatic secretion.

9. *Nursing diagnoses:*
   - Acute pain related to distension of the pancreas and peritoneal irritation
   - Deficient fluid volume related to nausea, vomiting, NG suction, restricted oral intake
   - Impaired oral mucous membrane related to NG tube and NPO status

   - Imbalanced nutrition: less than body requirements related to dietary restrictions, nausea and vomiting, impaired digestion
   *Collaborative problems:*
   Potential complications: hypovolemia/shock; hypocalcemia; hyperglycemia; fluid and electrolyte imbalance

# CHAPTER 43

1. a. adrenal gland; b. right renal artery; c. right renal vein; d. vena cava; e. bladder; f. urethra; g. ureter; h. aorta; i. kidney; j. pyramid; k. papilla; l. renal pelvis; m. ureter; n. cortex; o. medulla; p. major calyx; q. minor calyx; r. fibrous capsule

2. a. 4; b. 1; c. 2; d. 3; e. 1; f. 5; g. 2; h. 5; i. 5; j. 2; k. 5

3. a. T; b. F, regulate the volume and composition of extracellular fluid; c. T; d. F, high, ADH; e. T

4. a. Rationale: Renin is released in response to decreased arterial blood pressure, renal ischemia, ECF, depletion, and other factors affecting blood supply to the kidney. It is the catalyst of the renin-angiotensin-aldosterone system, which raises blood pressure when stimulated. ADH is secreted by the posterior pituitary in response to serum hyperosmolality and low blood volume. Aldosterone is secreted within the renin-angiotensin system only after stimulation by angiotensin II, and kidney prostaglandins lower blood pressure by causing vasodilation.

5. a. Rationale: Erythropoietin is released when the oxygen tension of the renal blood supply is low and stimulates production of red blood cells in the bone marrow. Hypotension causes activation of the renin-angiotensin-aldosterone system, as well as release of ADH. Hyperkalemia stimulates the release of aldosterone from the adrenal cortex, and fluid overload does not directly stimulate factors affecting the kidney.

6. a. ureteropelvic junction and ureterovesical junction; b. ureterovesical; c. 200 to 250; d. 600 to 1000; e. urothelium

7. a. Rationale: The short urethra of women allows for easier ascension and colonization of bacteria in the bladder than occurs in men. Relaxation of pelvic floor muscles may contribute to stress and urge incontinence but is not associated with urinary tract infections. The bladder capacity of men and women is the same, and the muscular support at the rhabdosphincter in men increases the risk for stricture at this point.

8. d. Rationale: The decreased ability to concentrate urine results in an increased volume of dilute urine, which does not maintain the usual diurnal

elimination pattern. A decrease in bladder capacity also contributes to nocturia, but decreased bladder muscle tone results in urinary retention. Decreased renal mass decreases renal reserve, but function is generally adequate under normal circumstances.

9. a. Smoking history, history of exposure to carcinogenic and nephrotoxic chemicals; family history of kidney disease, geographical residence

b. Low fluid intake or loss of fluids, high calcium and purine intake, coffee intake, weight gain secondary to fluid retention

c. Change in appearance and amount of urine, change in urinary patterns, assistance necessary for emptying bladder

d. Change in energy level, sedentary lifestyle, urine leakage during activity

e. Sleep deprivation from nocturia

f. Pain in flank, groin, suprapubic area, dysuria, absence of pain with other urinary symptoms; cognitive impairment affecting continence

g. Decreased self-esteem and body image because of urinary problems

h. Problems maintaining job and social relationships

i. Change in sexual pleasure or performance

j. Withdrawal or ineffective coping with incontinence or urinary problem

k. Any treatment decisions that are affected by value system

10. c. Rationale: To assess for kidney tenderness, the nurse strikes the fist of one hand against the dorsal surface of the other hand, which is placed flat against the posterior CVA margin. The upper abdominal quadrants and costovertebral angles are auscultated for vascular bruits in the renal vessels and aorta, and an empty bladder is not palpable. The kidneys are palpated through the abdomen, with the client supine.

11. a. 8; b. 6; c. 9; d. 10; e. 5; f. 1; g. 2; h. 12; i. 7; j. 11; k. 4; l. 3

12. b. Rationale: Bacteria in warm urine specimens multiple rapidly, and false or unreliable bacterial counts may occur with old urine. Glucose, specific gravity, and white blood cells do not change in urine specimens, but pH becomes more alkaline, RBCs are hemolyzed, and casts may disintegrate.

13. b. Rationale: Cloudiness from a fresh urine specimen, WBC count above 5/hpf, and presence of casts are all indicative of urinary tract infection, and pH is usually elevated because bacteria split the urea in urine into alkaline ammonia. Cloudy, brown urine usually indicates hematuria or the presence of bile, while colourless urine is usually very dilute. Option "a" is normal.

14. a. Rationale: A urine specific gravity of 1.002 is low, indicating dilute urine and the excretion of excess fluid caused by diuretics. Normal urine specific gravity is 1.003 to 1.030. A high specific gravity indicates concentrated urine that would be seen in dehydration.

15. d. Rationale: During a renal arteriogram, a catheter is inserted most commonly at the femoral artery, and following the procedure the client is positioned with the affected leg extended with a pressure dressing applied. Peripheral pulse monitoring is essential to detect the development of thrombi around the insertion site, which may occlude blood supply to the leg. Gross bleeding in the urine is a complication of a renal biopsy. Allergy to the contrast medium should be established before the procedure, but the medium can be nephrotoxic, and renal function should be monitored after the procedure.

16. b. Rationale: The BUN is increased in renal problems but may also be increased when there is rapid or extensive tissue damage from other causes. Serum creatinine is more specific to renal function and does not vary with other tissue damage.

17. d. Rationale: The rate at which creatinine is cleared from the blood and eliminated in the urine approximates the glomerular filtration rate and is the most specific test of renal function. The renal scan is useful in showing the location, size, and shape of the kidney and general blood perfusion.

18. a. Impaired conversion of inactive vitamin D to active vitamin D results in poor calcium absorption from the bowel, resulting in hypocalcemia.

b. Loss of cells that produce erythropoietin results in lack of stimulation of bone marrow to produce red blood cells.

c. This serum creatinine level is high, indicating the loss of tubular secretion (passage of substances from the blood into the tubule) by the kidney.

19. b. Rationale: Bleeding from the kidney following a biopsy is the most serious complication of the procedure, and urine must be examined for both gross and microscopic blood, in addition to vital signs and hematocrit levels being monitored. Following a cystoscopy the client may have burning with urination, and warm stiz baths may be used. Urinary infections are a complication of any procedure requiring instrumentation of the bladder.

20. a. 5; b. 6; c. 8; d. 9; e. 7; f. 4; g. 3; h. 1; i. 6; j. 3; k. 2; l. 3; m. 7

# CHAPTER 44

1. a. 4; b. 6; c. 8; d. 3; e. 1; f. 2; g. 7; h. 5
2. d. Rationale: The older adult woman has the most risk factors for urinary tract infection: age, female, hospitalization, neurogenic bladder, and instrumentation. The younger male has one risk factor: presence of calculi. The pregnant female has three risk factors: female, pregnancy, and possible previous injury. The older male has two risk factors: age and urinary retention.
3. c. Rationale: The usual classic symptoms of UTI are often absent in older adults who tend to experience non-localized abdominal pain rather than dysuria and suprapubic pain. They also may experience cognitive impairment characterized by confusion or decreased level of consciousness.
4. d. Rationale: Unless a client has a history of recurrent UTIs or a complicated UTI, TMP-SMX or nitrofurantoin (Macrodantin) is usually used to empirically treat an initial UTI without a culture and sensitivity or other testing. Asymptomatic bacteriuria does not justify treatment, but symptomatic UTIs should always be treated.
5. b. Rationale: Voiding before and after sexual intercourse helps wash from the urinary tract bacteria that are milked into the urethra from the vagina and perineum during intercourse. The bladder should be emptied at least every two to three hours. Fluid intake should be increased to about 2000 mL/day without caffeine, alcohol, citrus juices, and chocolate drinks because they are potential bladder irritants. Cleaning the urinary meatus with an anti-infective agent after voiding will irritate the meatus, but the perineal area should be wiped from front to back after urination and defecation to prevent fecal contamination of the meatus.
6. c. Rationale: Ascending infections from the bladder to the kidney are prevented by the normal anatomy and physiology of the urinary tract unless a pre-existing condition, such as bladder tumours, prostatic hyperplasia, strictures, or stones, is present. Resistance to antibiotics and failure to take a full prescription of antibiotics for a UTI usually result in relapse or reinfection of lower urinary tract infections.
7. a. Rationale: Systemic symptoms of fever and chills with leukocytosis and nausea and vomiting are more common in pyelonephritis than in cystitis, and local symptoms of bladder involvement may or may not be present. Either client may have a knowledge deficit regarding prevention of recurrence.
8. a. F, chronic; b. T; c. T; d. F, urine culture; e. T

9. d. Rationale: The symptoms of interstitial cystitis imitate those of an infection of the bladder, but the urine is free of infectious agents. Unlike a bladder infection, the pain with interstitial cystitis increases as urine collects in the bladder and is temporarily relieved by urination. Acidic urine is very irritating to the bladder in interstitial cystitis, and the bladder is small, but urinary retention is not common.
10. b. Rationale: Calcium glycerophosphate (Prelief) alkalinizes the urine and can help relieve the irritation from acidic foods. A diet low in acidic foods is recommended, and if a multivitamin is used, high-potency vitamins should be avoided because these products may irritate the bladder. A voiding diary is useful in diagnosis but does not need to be kept indefinitely.
11. d. Rationale: Glomerulonephritis is not an infection but rather an antibody-induced injury to the glomerulus, where either autoantibodies against the glomerular basement membrane directly damage the tissue, or antibodies reacting with non-glomerular antigens are randomly deposited as immune complexes along the glomerular basement membrane. Prior infection by bacteria or viruses may stimulate the antibody production but is not present or active at the time of glomerular damage.
12. a. GFR; b. GBM; c. GBM; d. GFR; e. GFR; f. GFR
13. d. Rationale: An elevated BUN indicates that the kidneys are not clearing nitrogenous wastes from the blood, and protein may be restricted until the kidney recovers. Proteinuria indicates loss of protein from the blood and may indicate a need for increased protein intake. Hypertension is treated with sodium and fluid restriction, diuretics, and antihypertensive drugs. The hematuria is not specifically treated.
14. a. Rationale: Most clients recover completely from APSGN with supportive treatment. Chronic glomerulonephritis that progresses insidiously over years and rapidly progressive glomerulonephritis that results in renal failure within weeks or months occurs in only a few clients with APSGN. In Goodpasture's syndrome, antibodies are present against both the glomerular basement membrane and the alveolar basement membrane of the lungs, and dysfunction of both kidney and lung is present.
15. c. Rationale: The massive proteinuria that results from increased glomerular membrane permeability in nephrotic syndrome leaves the blood without adequate proteins (hypoalbuminemia) to create an oncotic colloidal pressure to hold fluid in the vessels. Without oncotic pressure, fluid moves

618     Answers to Worksheets

into the interstitium, causing severe edema. Hypercoagulability occurs in nephrotic syndrome but is not a factor in edema formation, and glomerular filtration rate is not necessarily affected in nephrotic syndrome.

16. c. Rationale: Both humoral and cellular immune responses are altered in nephrotic syndrome, and infection is a serious complication. Skin integrity is at risk from massive edema, and hypercoagulability increases the risk for thrombosis. The elevated serum cholesterol level characteristic of nephrotic syndrome results from increased hepatic synthesis and not dietary intake.

17. a. proteinuria and nephrotic syndrome; b. HIV-associated nephropathy; c. acute renal failure

18. a. 7;  b. 4;  c. 1;  d. 5;  e. 9;  f. 2;  g. 6;  h. 3; i. 8

19. c. Rationale: Because crystallization of stone constituents can precipitate and unite to form a stone when in supersaturated concentrations, one of the best ways to prevent stones of any type is by drinking adequate fluids to keep the urine dilute and flowing, which is an output of about 1.5 L a day. Sedentary lifestyle is a risk factor for renal stones, but exercise also causes fluid loss and a need for additional fluids. Protein foods high in purine should be restricted only for the small percentage of clients with stones that are uric acid, and although urinary tract infections contribute to stone formation, prophylactic antibiotics are not indicated.

20. a. 3;  b. 5;  c. 2;  d. 1;  e. 3;  f. 4;  g. 5;  h. 1; i. 3;  j. 4

21. c. Rationale: A classic sign of the passage of a calculus down the ureter is intense, colicky back pain that may radiate into the testicles, labia, or groin and may be accompanied by mild shock with cool, moist skin. Stones obstructing a calyx or at the ureteropelvic junction may produce dull costovertebral flank pain, and large bladder stones may cause bladder fullness and lower obstructive symptoms. Many clients with renal stones do not have a history of chronic urinary tract infections.

22. d. Rationale: Currently it is believed that high dietary calcium intake may actually lower the risk for renal stones by reducing the urinary excretion of oxalate, and oxalate-rich foods should be limited to reduce oxalate excretion. Foods high in oxalate include spinach, rhubarb, asparagus, cabbage, and tomatoes in addition to chocolate, coffee, and cocoa. Milk, milk products, dried beans, and dried fruits are high sources of calcium, and organ meats are high in purine, which contributes to uric acid lithiasis.

23. b. Rationale: A high fluid intake maintains a dilute urine, which decreases bacterial concentration in addition to washing stone fragments and expected blood through the urinary system following lithotripsy. Moist heat to the flank may be helpful to relieve muscle spasms during renal colic, and all urine should be strained in clients with renal stones but to collect and identify stone composition.

24. a. T; b. F, antihypertensives; c. F, hypertension; d. F, anticoagulants; e. T

25. b. Rationale: Adult polycystic kidney disease is an inherited autosomal-dominant disorder that often manifests after the client has children, but the children should receive genetic counselling regarding their life choices. The disease progresses slowly, eventually causing progressive renal failure. Hereditary medullary cystic disease causes poor concentration ability of the kidneys, and Alport's syndrome is a hereditary nephritis that is associated with deafness and deformities of the optic lens.

26. a. 2; b. 3; c. 5; d. 1; e. 4

27. a. Rationale: Both cancer of the kidney and cancer of the bladder are associated with smoking. A family history of renal cancer is a risk factor for kidney cancer, and cancer of the bladder has been associated with use of phenacetin-containing analgesics and recurrent upper urinary tract infections.

28. c. Rationale: There are no early characteristic symptoms of cancer of the kidney, and gross hematuria, flank pain, and a palpable mass do not occur until the disease is advanced. The treatment of choice is a radical nephrectomy and can be successful in early disease. Small renal tumours can be detected with CT scans and MRI. The most common sites of metastases are the lungs, liver, and long bones.

29. b. Rationale: Sitz baths following local bladder surgery promote muscle relaxation and reduce urinary retention. Fluids should be increased to dilute blood in the urine and prevent clots. Irritative bladder symptoms most commonly occur with local instillation of chemotherapeutic agents, and urinary catheterization is not usually necessary with laser photocoagulation.

30. a. 2;  b. 1;  c. 1;  d. 4;  e. 2;  f. 1;  g. 5;  h. 3; i. 4;  j. 2;  k. 3;  l. 1

31. a. Stress and urge; increase urethral tone and suppleness
    b. Urge; relaxes bladder tone and increases sphincter tone, decreasing unwanted contractions
    c. Overflow and reflex; relax spastic bladder neck, preventing retention
    d. Stress; increase urethral tone and resistance

32. c. Rationale: Pelvic floor exercises (Kegel exercises) increase the tone of the urethral sphincters and should be done in sets of 10 or more contractions four to five times a day. Frequent bladder emptying is recommended for clients with urge incontinence and an increase in pressure on the bladder for overflow incontinence. Absorptive perineal pads should only be a temporary measure because long-term use discourages continence and can lead to skin problems.

33. c. Rationale: All urinary catheters in hospitalized clients pose a very high risk for infection, especially antibiotic-resistant, nosocomial infections, and scrupulous aseptic technique is essential in the insertion and maintenance of all catheters. Routine irrigations are not performed. Cleaning the insertion site with soap and water should be performed for urethral and suprapubic catheters, but application of antimicrobial ointments is controversial, and site care for other catheters may require special interventions. Turning the client to promote drainage is recommended only for suprapubic catheters.

34. b. Rationale: Output from ureteral catheters must be monitored every one to two hours because an obstruction will cause overdistension of the kidney pelvis and renal damage. The renal pelvis only has a capacity of 3 to 5 mL, and if irrigation is ordered, no more than 5 mL of sterile saline is used. The client with a ureteral catheter is usually kept on bed rest until specific orders for ambulation are given. Suprapubic tubes may be milked to prevent obstruction of the catheter by sediment and clots.

35. b. Rationale: A nephrectomy incision usually is in the flank, just below the diaphragm, and occasionally the twelfth rib is removed. Although the client is reluctant to breathe deeply because of incisional pain, the lungs should be clear. Decreased sounds and shallow respirations are abnormal and would require intervention.

36. a. 2;  b. 3;  c. 1;  d. 4

37. d. Rationale: Urine drains continuously from an ileal conduit, and the drainage bag must be emptied every two to three hours and measured to ensure adequate urinary output. With an ileal conduit, mucus is present in the urine because it is secreted by the ileal segment as a result of the irritating effect of the urine, but the surgery causes paralytic ileus, and the client will be NPO for several days post-operatively. Fitting for a permanent appliance is not done until the stoma shrinks to its normal size in several weeks. Self-catheterization is performed when clients have formation of a continent Kock pouch.

38. b. Rationale: Because the stoma continuously drains urine, a wick formed of a rolled-up 4 x 4 gauze is held against the stoma to absorb the urine while the skin is cleaned and a new appliance is attached. The skin is cleaned with warm water only, because soap and other agents cause drying and irritation, and clean, not sterile, technique is used. The appliance should be left in place as long as possible before it loosens and allows leakage onto the skin, perhaps up to 14 days.

**Case Study**

1. The Jewett-Strong-Marshall classification of bladder cancer identifies the tumour as superficial (CIS, O, A), invasive (B1, B2, C), or metastatic (D1 through D4). The A classification for Mr. G. indicates that the tumour is superficial with submucosal involvement. The TNM grading system indicates the characteristics of the tumour (T), the nodal involvement (N), and the presence of distant metastasis (M). (See Chapter 15 for TNM classification.)

2. The drug will be instilled into the bladder and needs to be retained for about two hours. His position will be changed about every 15 minutes to ensure that the drug comes into maximum contact with all areas of the bladder, especially the dome. He may have irritative symptoms, such as frequency, urgency, and bladder spasms, in addition to hematuria during the weeks of treatment. BCG therapy may cause flu-like symptoms or systemic infection, but the usual side effects of cancer chemotherapy are not experienced with BCG therapy or with intravesical chemotherapy. BCG stimulates the immune system rather than directly destroying cancer cells.

3. Stop smoking—it is the only significant risk factor in his history.

4. Follow-up is essential to evaluate the effectiveness of the treatment and detect any new tumours while they are in a superficial stage.

5. A cystectomy with urinary diversion would be indicated.

6. *Nursing diagnoses:*
   - Anxiety related to unknown outcome
   - Impaired urinary elimination related to effects of treatment
   - Acute pain related to effects of treatment
   - Risk for infection related to effects of treatment
   *Collaborative problem:*
   Potential complication: bladder injury

## CHAPTER 45

1. a. 1;  b. 3;  c. 1;  d. 3;  e. 2;  f. 1;  g. 3;  h. 2;
   i. 3;  j. 1;  k. 2;  l. 1
2. a. renal ischemia; nephrotoxic injury
   b. basement membrane; tubular epithelium
   c. tubular epithelium; tubules
   d. basement membrane
3.

Hypovolemia

↓ Renal blood flow

Renin release

Activation of angiotensin-aldosterone system

Renal artery vasoconstriction

Decreased renal blood flow

Decreased glomerular capillary pressure

↓ GFR          Tubular dysfunction

oliguria

4.

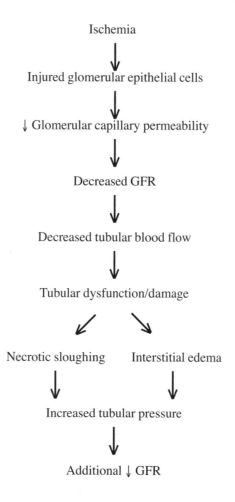

Ischemia

↓

Injured glomerular epithelial cells

↓

↓ Glomerular capillary permeability

↓

Decreased GFR

↓

Decreased tubular blood flow

↓

Tubular dysfunction/damage

↙          ↘

Necrotic sloughing     Interstitial edema

↓          ↓

Increased tubular pressure

↓

Additional ↓ GFR

5. d. Rationale: In prerenal oliguria, the oliguria is caused by a decrease in circulating blood volume, and there is no damage yet to the renal tissue. It can potentially be reversed by correcting the precipitating factor, such as fluid replacement for hypovolemia. Prerenal oliguria is characterized by urine with a high specific gravity and a low sodium concentration, while oliguria of intrarenal failure is characterized by urine with a low specific gravity and a high sodium concentration. Malignant hypertension causes damage to renal tissue and intrarenal oliguria.

6. b. Rationale: A urine specific gravity that is consistently 1.010 and a urine osmolality of about 300 mmol/kg (300 mOsm/kg) is the same specific gravity and osmolality as plasma and indicates that tubules are damaged and not able to concentrate urine. Hematuria is more common with post-renal damage, and tubular damage is associated with a high sodium concentration (>40 mmol/L [40 mEq/L]).

7. a. Rationale: Metabolic acidosis occurs in ARF because the kidneys cannot synthesize ammonia needed to excrete $H^+$, resulting in an increased acid load. Sodium is lost in urine because the kidneys cannot conserve sodium, and impaired

excretion of potassium results in hyperkalemia. Bicarbonate is normally generated and reabsorbed by the functioning kidney to maintain acid–base balance.

8. a. Rationale: The normal BUN/creatinine ratio of 10:1 is increased in renal failure caused by conditions in which there is markedly increased catabolism, or breakdown of tissue, such as in severe injury, infections, fever, or GI bleeding. The BUN is quite high in this case in comparison with the mild elevation of serum creatinine.

9. c. Rationale: The BUN and creatinine levels remain high during the oliguric and diuretic phases of acute renal failure. The recovery phase begins when the glomerular filtration returns to a rate at which BUN and creatinine stabilize and then decrease. Urinary output of 3 to 5 L/day, decreasing sodium and potassium levels, and fluid weight loss are characteristic of the diuretic phase of ARF.

10. d. Rationale: Hyperkalemia is a potentially life-threatening complication of ARF in the oliguric phase. Muscle weakness and abdominal cramping are signs of the neuromuscular impairment that occurs with hyperkalemia, in addition to cardiac conduction abnormalities of peaked T wave, pro-

longed PR interval, prolonged QRS interval, and depressed ST segment. Urine output of 300 mL/day is expected during the oliguric phase, as is the development of peripheral edema.

11. a. F, infection; b. T; c. F, 600; d. F, sodium and potassium serum levels; e. T

12. a. Potassium above 6 mmol/L (6 mEq/L) with cardiac changes; b. Bicarbonate level of 14 mmol/L (14 mEq/L), indicating metabolic acidosis; c. Change in mental status

13. b. Rationale: During acidosis, potassium moves out of the cell in exchange for $H^+$ ions, increasing the serum potassium level. Correction of the acidosis with sodium bicarbonate will help lower the potassium levels. A decrease in pH and the bicarbonate and $PaCO_2$ levels would indicate worsening acidosis.

14. b. Rationale: Stages of chronic kidney disease are based on the glomerular filtration rate and/or the presence of kidney damage over a period of three months. No specific markers of urinary output, azotemia, or urine output classify the degree of chronic kidney disease.

15. c. Rationale: The creatinine clearance test is used to approximate the glomerular filtration rate, and when the GFR is between 30 and 59 mL/min, moderate chronic kidney disease exists.

16. a. Yellowish discoloration; retention of urinary chromogens
   Pallor; anemia of decreased erythropoiesis, folic acid deficiency
   Uremic frost; urea crystallization on skin with very high BUN levels
   Excoriations; Pruritus caused by scratching from calcium-phospate deposition in the skin
   b. Hypertension; sodium retention and fluid overload, increased renin production
   Pericardial friction rub; uremic pericarditis
   Peripheral edema; sodium and fluid retention
   c. Kussmaul's respiration; respiratory compensation of metabolic acidosis
   Dyspnea; pulmonary edema of congestive heart failure and fluid overload
   Pleural friction rub; uremic pleuritis
   d. Mucosal ulcerations; increased ammonia from bacterial breakdown of urea
   Anorexia, nausea, vomiting; irritation of the GI tract from urea
   Diarrhea; hyperkalemia and hypocalcemia
   Urine odour of breath; high urea content of the blood
   e. General CNS depression; high urea content of the blood
   Coma and convulsions; high urea content of the blood

17. a. increased BUN; b. increased creatinine; c. increased glucose; d. decreased RBC; e. increased VLDL; f. increased LDL; g. decreased HDL; h. decreased $T_3$; i. decreased $T_4$; j. decreased fibrinogen; k. decreased factor VIII; l. increased phosphorus; m. decreased calcium; n. increased potassium

18. c. Rationale: The calcium–phosphorus imbalances that occur in chronic kidney disease result in osteomalacia, osteitis fibrosa, and metastatic deposits of calcium phosphate, but pathological fractures are most likely to occur from the osteomalacia resulting from hypocalcemia, which occurs from a deficiency of active vitamin D. Aluminum accumulation is also believed to contribute to the osteomalacia. Osteitis fibrosa involves replacement of calcium in the bone with fibrous tissue and is primarily a result of elevated levels of parathyroid hormone resulting from hypocalcemia.

19. b. Rationale: Conservative management of the client with renal insufficiency with an elevated potassium level would include a dietary potassium restriction of 2–3 g (51–76 mEq), a protein restriction of 0.6–0.8 g/kg (42–56 g for this client), and moderate (2–3 g) restriction of sodium unless there is marked edema or hypertension. Breads and cereals are not allowed in unrestricted amounts, because they contain protein.

20. b. Rationale: The peritoneal membrane is permeable to plasma proteins, amino acids, and polypeptides, and protein may be lost at a rate of 9 to 12 g per day into the dialysate fluid, necessitating an increased amount of protein for the client progressing from renal insufficiency to peritoneal dialysis. Amounts of fats, carbohydrates, and calories are determined by ideal body weight.

21. d. Rationale: A client with chronic kidney disease may have unlimited intake of sugars and starches (unless the client is diabetic), and hard candy is an appropriate snack and may help relieve the metallic and urine taste common in the mouth. Raisins are a high-potassium food, pickled foods have high sodium contents, and ice cream contains protein.

22. a. 3; b. 1; c. 4; d. 2; e. 1; f. 4; g. 2; h. 1

23. a. F, folic acid; b. F, uremia; c. T; d. F, meperidine (Demerol)

24. c. Rationale: The most common causes of chronic kidney disease in Canada are hypertension and diabetes mellitus. The nurse should obtain information on long-term health problems that are related to kidney disease. The other disorders are not closely associated with renal disease.

25. b. Rationale: A daily weight gain of 2 kg (4 lb) indicates fluid retention and in the client with kidney disease could indicate early failure. Proteinuria is not a reliable test for kidney tubular damage and is not performed by the client, and weights are used rather than I&O to evaluate fluid balance. Clients are taught to weigh daily, take daily blood pressures, and be able to identify signs and symptoms of edema, hyperkalemia, and hypocalcemia. Calcium-based phosphate binders should be taken with meals.

26. c. Rationale: A client on hemodialysis will continue to have dietary and fluid restrictions that the machine cannot compensate for, and the client needs additional teaching regarding her therapeutic regimen. The other nursing diagnoses are not supported with defining characteristics.

27. a. HD; b. PD; c. HD; d. PD; e. PD; f. PD; g. HD; h. HD; i. PD

28. d. Rationale: Glucose is added to dialysate fluid to create an osmotic gradient across the membrane in order to remove excess fluid from the blood. The glucose content is so high in peritoneal dialysate that as much as 100 to 150 g per day may be absorbed via the peritoneum, increasing triglyceride levels and creating hyperinsulinism. The dialysate fluid has no potassium so that potassium will diffuse into the dialysate from the blood and usually contains higher calcium to promote its movement into the blood. Dialysate sodium is usually less than or equal to blood to prevent sodium and fluid retention.

29. a. fill, dwell, drain; b. 2; c. automated

30. b. Rationale: Peritonitis is a common complication of peritoneal dialysis and may require catheter removal and termination of dialysis. Infection occurs from contamination of the dialysate or tubing or from progression of exit-site or tunnel infections, and strict sterile technique must be used by health professionals as well as the client to prevent contamination. Too-rapid infusion may cause shoulder pain, and pain may be caused if the catheter tip touches the bowel. Difficulty breathing, atelectasis, and pneumonia may occur from pressure of the fluid on the diaphragm, which may be prevented by elevating the head of the bed and promoting repositioning and deep breathing.

31. a. Rationale: Because the dialysate glucose is absorbed through the peritoneum, diabetics especially have difficulty with blood glucose control and hypertriglyceridemia, which can lead to vascular disease and complicate existing kidney disease.

32. a. 3; b. 2; c. 1; d. 3; e. 1; f. 2

33. d. Rationale: A more permanent, soft, flexible Silastic double-lumen catheter is being used for long-term access when other forms of vascular access have failed. Femoral vein catheters may only remain in place for up to one week and subclavian catheters for one to three weeks. When the vessels of the extremity have already been used for grafts and are needed for additional permanent access, an external access shunt is not used.

34. a. Rationale: While clients are undergoing hemodialysis, they can perform quiet activities that do not require the limb that has the vascular access. Blood pressure is monitored frequently, and the dialyzer monitors dialysis function, but cardiac monitoring is not indicated. The hemodialysis machine continuously circulates both the blood and the dialysate past the semipermeable membrane in the machine. Graft and fistula access involve the insertion of two needles into the site to remove and return blood to the dialyzer.

35. b. Rationale: A patent AV graft creates turbulent blood flow that can be assessed by listening for a bruit or palpated for a thrill as the blood passes through the graft. Assessment of neurovascular status in the extremity distal to the graft site is important to determine that the graft does not impair circulation to the extremity, but neurovascular status does not indicate whether the graft is open.

36. c. Rationale: A complication of hemodialysis, especially in initial treatment, is disequilibrium syndrome, which is caused by too-rapid removal of urea and other solutes from the blood, leaving a high concentration of the solutes in the cerebrospinal fluid and brain. The higher concentration pulls fluid into these areas, causing cerebral edema and the related symptoms. Loss of blood can occur from heparin use and loss into the dialyzer, and hypotension frequently occurs from fluid loss during dialysis, but the symptoms relate to hypovolemia rather than increased intracranial pressure. Muscle cramps result from neuromuscular hypersensitivity not related to disequilibrium syndrome.

37. d. Rationale: Continuous renal replacement therapy is indicated for the client with acute renal failure as an alternative or adjunct to hemodialysis to slowly remove solutes and fluid in the hemodynamically unstable client. It is especially useful for treatment of fluid overload, but hemodialysis is indicated for treatment of hyperkalemia, pericarditis, or other serious effects of uremia.

38. d. Rationale: Extensive vascular disease is a contraindication of renal transplantation, primarily because adequate blood supply is essential to health of the new kidney and circulation of immunosuppressive drugs. Other contraindications include disseminated malignancies, refractory or untreated cardiac disease, chronic respiratory failure, chronic infection, or unresolved psychosocial disorders. Coronary artery disease may be treated with bypass surgery before transplantation, and transplantation can relieve hypertension. Hepatitis B or C infection is not a contraindication.

39. b. Rationale: The best possible match between donor and recipient for transplant includes ABO compatibility, HLA-A, HLA-B, and HLA-DR loci match (six antigens) and a negative antibody cross-match indicating that there are no preformed cytotoxic antibodies to the donated kidney. (See Chapter 13.) Although ABO blood incompatibility and a positive antibody cross-match can be managed in living donor transplants, they complicate the procedure.

40. a. Rationale: Fluid and electrolyte balance is critical in the transplant recipient client, especially because diuresis often begins soon after surgery. Fluid replacement is adjusted hourly, based on kidney function and output. Urine-tinged drainage on the abdominal dressing may indicate leakage from the ureter implanted into the bladder, and the physician should be notified. The donor client has a flank incision where the kidney was removed; the recipient client has an abdominal incision where the kidney was placed in the iliac fossa. The urinary catheter is usually used for two to three days to monitor urine output and kidney function.

41. b. Rationale: Gradual occlusion of the renal blood vessels with signs of increasing renal insufficiency is characteristic of chronic rejection. Recurrence of the original kidney disease may occur, but this is not a rejection problem. Acute rejection occurs when kidney tissue is attacked by T cytotoxic lymphocytes, and hyperacute rejection occurs when the kidney is damaged by immediate attack by preformed antibodies.

42. b. Rationale: Fever, pain at the site, increasing blood pressure with weight gain, and laboratory findings consistent with renal insufficiency are symptoms of acute rejection. The other symptoms may be caused by side effects of immunosuppressant agents.

**Case Study**

1. T cytotoxic lymphocytes recognize the kidney as foreign tissue and attack it, setting in process the inflammatory and complement systems. It usually occurs four days to four weeks after the transplant, but it may occur later, and it is not uncommon to have at least one rejection episode.

2. All of the laboratory results are abnormal, except potassium at high normal, and are typical of renal insufficiency, which occurs during acute rejection:
   - Serum creatinine—decreased excretory function of tubules
   - BUN—decreased ability of the kidney to excrete urea
   - Glucose—insulin resistance occurs in chronic renal failure from unknown cause; may also be increased by corticosteroid therapy
   - Potassium—decreased ability of the kidney to excrete potassium
   - Bicarbonate—impaired generation and reabsorption by the kidney as it is being used to buffer acid load

   Nursing care includes monitoring for central nervous system depression and skin and oral mucus breakdown from high urea; monitoring capillary blood glucose and administering insulin to keep glucose within normal range; and monitoring for increasing weakness and cardiac changes related to hyperkalemia and for symptoms of metabolic acidosis, such as Kussmaul's respiration.

3. Immunosuppressive therapy: designed to reduce proliferation and action of T cytotoxic lymphocytes that are responsible for acute rejection
   - Muromonab-CD3 (Orthoclone OKT3) is a monoclonal antibody that binds to CD3 receptors on lymphocytes and lyses the cells; is given IV to reverse acute rejection
   - Mycophenolate mofetil (Cellcept) is an antimetabolite that inhibits purine synthesis and suppresses proliferation of T and B cells.
   - Methylprednisolone (Solu-Medrol) is a corticosteroid that inhibits cytokine production and T-cell activation.
   - Tacrolimus (Prograf) is a calcineurin inhibitor that prevents production and release of IL-2, IL-4, and $\alpha$-interferon, in addition to inhibiting production of T cytotoxic lymphocytes.

   Supportive therapy: designed to control the symptoms produced by renal insufficiency
   - Furosemide is a loop diuretic that is not influenced by glomerular filtration rate and is used to promote sodium, potassium, and fluid loss through the kidney; helps relieve hypervolemia and hypertension

- Nifedipine is a calcium channel blocker that reduces cardiac output to control blood pressure.
- Sodium bicarbonate helps control the metabolic acidosis of renal insufficiency and replaces that which is not produced or reabsorbed by the kidney.
- Insulin controls the hyperglycemia resulting from insulin resistance.

4. Many side effects may occur from immunosuppressive therapy, but the most common to all is decreased resistance to infection and increased incidence of cancer because of depression of T-cytotoxic lymphocytes.
- Muromonab-CD3 causes fever, tachycardia, infections, headache, vomiting, chills, joint and muscle pain, and diarrhea.
- Mycophenolate mofetil causes gastrointestinal toxicity, leukopenia, and thrombocytopenia.
- As a corticosteroid, methylprednisolone causes cushingoid syndrome, with sodium and water retention, redistribution of fat, muscle weakness with protein wasting, hyperglycemia, and osteoporosis.
- Tacrolimus is nephrotoxic and neurotoxic with headaches, seizures, and tremors; nausea and vomiting; hyperglycemia; hypertension; and hair loss.

5. Increased risk for infections, malignancies; chronic liver disease; increased risk for atherosclerosis with coronary artery disease a major cause of death; joint necrosis from chronic steroid therapy; psychological adjustment—constant fear of rejection and wondering how long the transplant will last; depression if there is failure and a return to dialysis

6. *Nursing diagnoses:*
- Excess fluid volume related to inability of kidney to excrete fluid
- Anticipatory grieving related to threat of loss of kidney
- Disturbed sensory perception related to CNS changes induced by uremic toxins and immunosuppressive drugs
- Risk for infection related to suppressed immune system

*Collaborative problems:*
Potential complications: hypertension; hyperkalemia with cardiac arrhythmias; hyperglycemia; metabolic acidosis

## CHAPTER 46

1. a. hypothalamus; b. pituitary; c. parathyroids; d. thyroid; e. thymus; f. adrenals; g. pancreatic islets; h. ovaries; i. testes
2. a. 3; b. 8; c. 6; d. 1; e. 10; f. 1; g. 3; h. 1; i. 5; j. 1; k. 3; l. 1; m. 7; n. 9; o. 1; p. 2
3. a. T; b. F, growth hormone, $T_3/T_4$ or cortisol; c. T; d. F, false low; e. F, thyroid hormones; f. T; g. F, thyroid gland and adrenal cortex (also gonads); h. T; i. F, steroid hormones
4. a. 3, 2; b. 1, 4; c. 13, 14; d. 6, 5; e. 9, 10; f. 11, 12; g. 8, 7; h. 10, 9; i. 7, 8
5. b. Rationale: ADH release is controlled by the osmolality of the blood, and as the osmolality rises, ADH is released from the posterior pituitary gland and acts on the kidney to cause reabsorption of water from the kidney tubule, resulting in more dilute blood and more concentrated urine. Aldosterone, the major mineralocorticoid, causes sodium reabsorption from the kidney and potassium excretion. Calcium levels are not a factor in serum osmolality.
6. d. Rationale: Parathormone, or parathyroid hormone, is responsible for maintaining adequate serum calcium levels and raises calcium levels by stimulating calcium resorption from the bone, absorption from the intestines, and retention by the kidney. Calcitonin, secreted by the thyroid gland, has the opposite effect. TSH and aldosterone are not involved in calcium balance.
7. d. Rationale: Atrial natriuretic hormone is secreted in response to high blood volume and high serum sodium levels and has an inhibiting effect on ADH and the renin-angiotensin-aldosterone system, effects of which would make the blood volume even higher. Glucagon secretion inhibits insulin secretion, but insulin does not inhibit glucagon. The relationship between cortisol and insulin is indirect—cortisol raises blood glucose levels, and insulin secretion is stimulated by the high glucose levels. Testosterone and estrogen have no reciprocal action, and both are secreted by the body in response to tropic hormones.
8. d. Rationale: Usually insulin and glucagon function in a reciprocal manner, except after a high-protein, carbohydrate-free meal, in which both hormones are secreted. Glucagon increases gluconeogenesis, and insulin causes target tissue to accept the amino acids for protein synthesis.
9. b. Rationale: The mineralocorticoid effects of cortisol causes sodium retention and potassium excretion from the kidney, resulting in hypokalemia. Because water is reabsorbed with the sodium, serum sodium remains normal. In its

effect on glucose and fat metabolism, cortisol causes an elevation in blood glucose, as well as increases in free fatty acids and triglycerides.

10. a. Rationale: Hypokalemia inhibits aldosterone release as well as insulin release. These are the major hormones hypokalemia affects.

11. b. Rationale: Many symptoms of hypothyroidism, such as fatigue, mental impairment, dry skin, and constipation, that would be apparent in younger persons are attributed to general aging in the older adult, thus going unrecognized as a treatable condition.

12. c. Rationale: Assessment of the endocrine system is often difficult because hormones affect every body tissue and system, causing great diversity in the signs and symptoms of endocrine dysfunction. Weight loss, fatigue, and depression are signs that may occur with many different endocrine problems, but goitre, exophthalmos, and the three "polys" are specific findings of endocrine dysfunction.

13. a. Decreased energy level; family history of similar problem
    b. Changes in appetite and weight, difficulty swallowing; changes in hair distribution, colour, and texture; skin changes; hot and cold intolerances
    c. Increased thirst with frequent urination; kidney stones; frequent defecation or constipation
    d. Decrease in previous activity levels; apathy
    e. Sleep disturbances, nightmares, sweating, nocturia, insomnia or excessive sleep
    f. Memory deficits, depression, inability to concentrate; visual disturbances or exophthalmos
    g. Changes in body appearance and self-perception
    h. Changes in ability to maintain usual roles
    i. Menstrual irregularity and infertility; history of large babies; male sexual dysfunction; changes in secondary sex characteristics
    j. perception of stress in life and usefulness of previous coping mechanisms, changes in response to stress
    k. commitment to lifestyle changes, value of health

14. c. Rationale: In the client with thyroid disease, palpation can cause the release of thyroid hormone into circulation, increasing the client's symptoms and potentially causing a thyroid storm. Examination should be deferred to a more experienced clinician if possible. Pressure should not be so great as to damage the cricoid cartilage or laryngeal nerve, and if the thyroid is palpated correctly, the carotid arteries are not compressed.

15. a. parathyroid; b. adrenal; c. thyroid; d. excessive; e. thyroid; f. growth; g. adrenal; h. thyroid

16. a. Rationale: Endocrine disorders related to hormone secretion from glands that are stimulated by tropic hormones can be caused by a malsecretion of the tropic hormone or malsecretion of the target gland. If the problem is in the target gland, it is known as a primary endocrine disorder, and a problem with tropic hormone secretion is known as a secondary endocrine disorder. Serum levels of tropic hormones can illustrate the status of the negative feedback system in relation to target organ hormone levels. If a target organ produces low amounts of hormone, tropic hormones will be increased; if a target organ is overproducing hormones, tropic hormones will be low or undetectable.

17. b. Rationale: Normal secretion and action of insulin will usually result in fasting levels of glucose in two to three hours following carbohydrate ingestion, but to ensure that the level is a fasting level, a minimum of four hours should be allowed. Water may be taken, however, and does not affect the glucose level.

18. a. 4; b. 1; c. 5; d. 8; e. 3; f. 7; g. 6; h. 2

## CHAPTER 47

1. d. Rationale: Insulin is an anabolic hormone, responsible for growth, repair, and storage; it facilitates movement of amino acids into cells, synthesis of protein, storage of glucose as glycogen, and deposition of triglycerides and lipids as fat into adipose tissue. Glucagon is responsible for hepatic glycogenolysis and gluconeogenesis, and fat is used for energy when glucose levels are depleted.

2. a. skeletal muscle, adipose; b. proinsulin c-peptides; c. cortisol and epinephrine; d. type 1

3. a. 2; b. 2; c. 2; d. 1; e. 1; f. 2; g. 1; h. 2; i. 2

4. a. High glucose levels cause loss of glucose in urine with osmotic diuresis; b. Thirst caused by fluid loss of polyuria; c. Cellular starvation from lack of glucose and use of fat and protein for energy

5. d. Rationale: Type 2 diabetes has a strong genetic influence, and offspring of parents who both have type 2 diabetes have a 15% to 45% chance of developing diabetes. While type 1 diabetes is associated with genetic susceptibility related to HLAs, offspring of parents who both have type 1 diabetes have only a 6% to 9% chance of developing the disease. Lower risk factors for type 2 diabetes include obesity, Aboriginal, Hispanic, Asian, South Asia, or African heritage, and age over 55 years.

6. c. Rationale: Insulin resistance syndrome is a cluster of abnormalities that include elevated

insulin levels, hypertension, elevated triglyc-erides and low-density lipoproteins (LDL), and decreased high-density lipoproteins (HDL). These abnormalities greatly increase the risk for cardiovascular disease associated with diabetes, which can be prevented or delayed with weight loss and regular physical activity.

7. d. Rationale: The client has marked hyper-glycemia but has not developed an acidosis, indi-cating that he probably has type 2 diabetes. Type 2 diabetes may be treated with healthy eat-ing and weight loss, oral antihyperglycemic agents, or insulin, depending on the client's response to treatment.

8. c. Rationale: On at least two separate occasions, diabetes is diagnosed with a random plasma glu-cose greater than or equal to 11.1 mmol/L (200 mg/dL), a fasting plasma glucose greater than or equal to 7 mmol/L (126 mg/dL), or a two-hour oral glucose tolerance test over 11.1 mmol/L (200 mg/dL) using a glucose load of 75 gm. Any of the three types of testing may be used, but the fasting plasma glucose test is preferred.

9. c. Rationale: Impaired glucose tolerance exists when a two-hour plasma glucose level is higher than normal but lower than that level diagnostic for diabetes (between 7.8 and 11.1 mmol/L or 140 mg/dL and 200 mg/dL). Impaired fasting glucose exists when fasting glucose levels are greater than the normal of 6.1 mmol/L (110 mg/dL) but less than the 6.9 mmol/L (124 mg/dL) diagnostic of diabetes. Both conditions are risk factors for development of diabetes and cardiovascular disease.

10. c. Rationale: U100 insulin must be used with a U100 syringe, but for those using low doses of insulin, syringes are available that have incre-ments of one unit instead of two units. Errors can be made in dosing if clients switch back and forth between different sizes of syringes. Aspira-tion before injection of the insulin is not recom-mended, nor is the use of alcohol to clean the skin. Because the rate of peak serum concentra-tion varies with the site selected for injection, injections should be rotated within a particular area, such as the abdomen.

11. c. Rationale: A split-mixed dose of insulin requires that the client adhere to a set meal pat-tern to provide glucose for the action of the insulins, and a bedtime snack is usually required when clients take a long-acting insulin late in the day to prevent nocturnal hypoglycemia. Hypo-glycemia is most likely to occur with this dose late in the afternoon and during the night. When premixed formulas are used, flexible dosing based on glucose levels is not recommended.

12. d. Rationale: Lispro is a rapid-acting insulin that has an onset of action of five to fifteen minutes and should be injected at the time of the meal to within 15 minutes of eating. Regular insulin is short-acting with an onset of action in 30 to 60 minutes following administration and should be given 30 to 45 minutes before meals.

13. a. Rationale: When mixing regular with a longer-acting insulin, regular insulin should always be drawn into the syringe first to prevent contamina-tion of the regular insulin vial with longer-acting insulin additives. Air is added to the NPH vial, then air is added to the regular vial, and the regu-lar insulin is withdrawn, bubbles are removed, and the dose of NPH is withdrawn.

14. d. Rationale: Insulin glargine (Lantus), a long-acting insulin that is continuously released with no peak of action, cannot be diluted or mixed with any other insulin or solution. Mixed insulins should be stored needle-up in the refrigerator and warmed before administration. Currently used bottles of insulin can be kept at room tempera-ture.

15. a. Rationale: Insulin pumps provide tight glycemic control by continuous subcutaneous insulin infusion based on the client's basal pro-file, with bolus doses at mealtime at the client's discretion. Intensive insulin therapy consists of several daily insulin injections with dosage based on frequent self-monitoring of blood glucose. Errors in insulin dosing and complications of insulin therapy are still potential risks with inten-sive insulin therapy or insulin pumps.

16. c. Rationale: The client's elevated glucose on arising may be the result of either dawn phenom-enon or Somogyi effect, and the best way to determine whether the client needs more or less insulin is by monitoring the glucose at bedtime, between 2 and 4 A.M., and on arising. If predawn levels are below 4 mmol/L (72 mg/dL), the insulin dose should be reduced, but if the 2-to-4-A.M. blood glucose is high, the insulin should be increased.

17. a. 5; b. 2; c. 1; d. 1; e. 2; f. 4; g. 1; h. 3; i. 3; j. 4; k. 4

18. c. Rationale: If they only have to take a pill for glycemic control, many clients take their diabetes casually and do not consider it the serious condi-tion it is. Hypoglycemic episodes are more pro-longed when they occur as the result of oral anti-hyperglycemic agents but do not occur as often as in clients with insulin use. Blood glucose moni-toring is usually performed bid in clients taking oral agents, and both insulin and OAHAs interact with a variety of other drugs that may alter their actions.

19. a. Rationale: The body requires food at regularly spaced intervals throughout the day, and omission or delay of meals can result in hypoglycemia, especially for the client taking insulin or oral antihyperglycemic agents. Weight loss may be recommended in type 2 diabetes if the individual is overweight, but many clients with type 1 diabetes are thin and require an increase in caloric intake. Less than 10% of total calories should be from saturated fats, and simple sugar should be limited but moderate amounts can be used if counted as a part of total carbohydrate intake.

20. b. Rationale: Maintenance of as near-normal blood glucose levels as possible and achievement of optimal serum lipid levels with dietary modification are believed to be the most important factors in preventing both short-term and long-term complications of diabetes. There is no specific "diabetic diet," and use of dietetic foods is not necessary for diabetes control. Most persons with diabetes eat three meals a day, and some require a bedtime snack for control of nighttime hypoglycemia. A reasonable weight, which may or may not be an ideal body weight, is also a goal of nutritional therapy.

21. b. Rationale: During exercise, a person with diabetes needs both adequate glucose, to prevent exercise-induced hypoglycemia, and adequate insulin because counterregulatory hormones are produced during the stress of exercise and may cause hyperglycemia. Exercise after meals is best, but a 10- to 15-g carbohydrate snack may be taken if exercise is performed before meals or if exercise is prolonged. Blood glucose levels should be monitored before, during, and after exercise to determine the effect of exercise on the levels.

22. c. Rationale: Cleaning the puncture site with alcohol is not necessary and may interfere with test results and lead to drying and splitting of the fingertips. Washing the hands with warm water is adequate cleaning and promotes blood flow to the fingers. Blood flow is also increased by holding the hand down. Punctures on the side of the finger pad are less painful. SMBG should be performed before and after exercise.

23. c. Rationale: Important goals in diabetes education are enabling the client to become the most active participant in care and promoting self-management to the ability of the individual client. Clients who actively manage their diabetes care have better outcomes than those who do not. Management of diabetes includes not only the client but also healthcare providers to teach and support the client. Not all clients with diabetes

are capable of self-management, and family members may be involved in these cases.

24. b. Rationale: The Canadian Diabetes Association recommends that testing for type 2 diabetes with a FPG should be considered in all individuals at the age of 40 and above, and if normal, it should be repeated every three years. Testing for immune markers of type 1 diabetes is not recommended. Testing at a younger age or more frequently should be done for those members of a high-risk ethnic population, including those of Aboriginal, Asian, South Asian, Hispanic, and Afican descents.

25. a. Rationale: During minor illnesses, the client with diabetes should continue drug therapy and food intake. Insulin is important because counter-regulatory hormones may raise blood glucose during the stress of illness, and food or a carbohydrate liquid substitution is important because during illness the body requires extra energy to deal with the stress of the illness. Blood glucose monitoring should be done every four hours, and the health care provider should be notified if the level is more than 14 mmol/L (252 mg/dL) for 24 hours or if fever, ketonuria, or nausea and vomiting occur.

26. c. Rationale: When insulin is insufficient and glucose cannot be used for cellular energy, the body releases and breaks down stored fats and protein to meet energy needs. Free fatty acids from stored triglycerides are released and metabolized in the liver in such large quantities that ketones are formed. Ketones are acidic and alter the pH of the blood, causing acidosis. Osmotic diuresis occurs as a result of loss of both glucose and ketones in the urine.

27. a. 5; b. 6; c. 2; d. 7; e. 4; f. 3; g. 8; h. 1

28. a. Kussmaul's respirations; b. ketonuria; c. sweet, fruity odour to breath; d. decreased arterial pH (acidosis); e. ketonemia

29. c. Rationale: The management of DKA is similar to that of HHNS except that HHNS requires greater fluid replacement because of the severe hyperosmolar state. Bicarbonate is not usually given in DKA to correct acidosis unless the pH is less than 7, because administration of insulin will reverse the abnormal fat metabolism. Total body potassium deficit is high in both conditions, requiring potassium administration, and in both conditions, glucose is added to IV fluids when blood glucose levels fall to 14 mmol/L (252 mg/dL).

30. c. Rationale: During the acute phase of HHNS, polyuria is present because of osmotic diuresis, but as fluid continues to be lost and hypovolemia occurs, decreased renal perfusion with oliguria

and anuria follows. Vital signs will indicate hypovolemia, but CVP will be decreased. Depressed ST segment and T waves on cardiac monitoring are signs of hypokalemia. Rapid, deep breathing is characteristic of a metabolic acidosis and is found in DKA.

31. a. 1;  b. 3;  c. 2;  d. 1;  e. 2;  f. 1;  g. 2;  h. 3

32. b. Rationale: If a client with diabetes is unconscious, immediate treatment for hypoglycemia must be given to prevent brain damage, and 1 mg of glucagon should administered IM or SC. If the unconsciousness has another cause, such as ketosis, the rise in glucose caused by the glucagon is not as dangerous as the low glucose level. Following administration of the glucagon, the client should be transported to a medical facility for further treatment and evaluation. Insulin is contraindicated without knowledge of the client's glucose level, and oral carbohydrate cannot be given when clients are unconscious.

33. a. Rationale: Blood glucose levels of 4.5 to 5 mmol/L (81 to 90 mg/dL) are within the normal range and are desired in the client with diabetes, even following a recent hypoglycemic episode. Hypoglycemia is often caused by a single event, such as skipping a meal or taking too much insulin or vigorous exercise, and once it is corrected, normal control should be maintained.

34. b. Rationale: The development of atherosclerotic vessel disease seems to be promoted by the altered lipid metabolism common to diabetes, and although tight glucose control may help delay the process, it does not prevent it completely. Atherosclerosis in persons with diabetes does respond somewhat to reduction in general risk factors as it does in persons without diabetes, and reduction in fat intake, control of hypertension, abstention from smoking, maintainence of a normal weight, and regular exercise should be carried out by persons with diabetes.

35. a. 3;  b. 1;  c. 2;  d. 1;  e. 4;  f. 1;  g. 4;  h. 2;  i. 1;  j. 3;  k. 2

36. d. Rationale: Complete or partial loss of sensitivity of the feet is common with peripheral neuropathy of diabetes, and diabetics may suffer foot injury and ulceration without ever having pain. Feet must be inspected during daily care for any cuts, blisters, swelling, or reddened areas.

37. a. Rationale: Because the clinical manifestations of long-term complications of diabetes may take 10 to 20 years to develop, and because tight glucose control in the older client is associated with an increased frequency of hypoglycemia, the goals for glycemic control are not as rigid as in the younger population. Treatment is indicated, and insulin may be used if the client does not respond to OAHAs. The client's needs, rather than age, determine the responsibility of others in care.

**Case Study**

1. The hypoglycemia might have been prevented by taking time to eat breakfast and perhaps increasing food intake in anticipation of strenuous exercise. She also should have checked her glucose level before exercising.

2. *Sympathetic response to hypoglycemia:*
Weakness, nervousness, tremor
Vasoconstriction with pallor, numbness, coldness, headache, tachycardia
*Brain neuroglycopenia:*
Confusion, slurred speech, unsteady gait

3. The hypoglycemia should be treated with a fast-acting carbohydrate—125 to 150 mL of fruit juice or regular pop, eight to ten Lifesavers or dextrose/glucose tablets as per directions. Repeat the carbohydrate in 10 to 15 minutes if symptoms are still present or if blood glucose remains below 4 mmol/L (72 mg/dL).
When glucose is greater than 4 mmol/L (72 mg/dL), a regularly scheduled meal or snack of complex carbohydrate and protein should be eaten.
The blood glucose should be checked again about 45 minutes after treatment to ensure that the hypoglycemia does not recur.

4. How to recognize situations that lead to hypoglycemia; review the effects of exercise on glucose levels and the need for both adequate glucose and insulin

5. Monitor her blood glucose before, during, and after exercise; increase dietary intake before exercise; maintain insulin doses; exercise 60 to 90 minutes after meals; carry fast-acting carbohydrates to take at first symptoms

6. *Nursing diagnoses:*
Ineffective therapeutic regimen management related to non-compliance with recommended regimen
*Collaborative problems:*
Potential complications: brain damage, coma, seizures, death

## CHAPTER 48

1. d. Rationale: A normal response to growth hormone (GH) secretion is stimulation of the liver to produce somatomedin C, or insulin-like growth factor-1 (IGF-1), which stimulates growth of bones and soft tissues. The increased levels of somatomedin C normally inhibit growth hormone, but in acromegaly, the pituitary gland secretes GH despite elevated IGF-1 levels. When both GH and IGF-1 levels are increased (IGF-1 levels >300 μg/L [>300 ng/mL]), overproduction of growth hormone is confirmed. GH also causes elevation of blood glucose, and normally GH levels fall during an oral glucose challenge but do not in acromegaly.

2. c. Rationale: The increased production of growth hormone in acromegaly causes an increase in thickness and width of bones and enlargement of soft tissues, resulting in marked changes in facial features, oily and coarse skin, and speech difficulties. Height is not increased in adults with growth hormone excess because the epiphyses of the bones are closed, and infertility is not a common finding because growth hormone is usually

the only pituitary hormone involved in acromegaly.

3. a. Rationale: A transsphenoidal hypophysectomy involves entry into the sella turcica through an incision in the upper lip and gingiva into the floor of the nose and the sphenoid sinuses. Postoperative clear nasal drainage with glucose content indicates CSF leakage from an open connection to the brain, putting the client at risk for meningitis. After surgery, the client is positioned with the head elevated to avoid pressure on the sella turcica, coughing and straining are avoided to prevent increased intracranial pressure and CSF leakage, and although mouth care is required q4h, toothbrushing should not be performed, because injury to the suture line may occur.

4. a. F, lower the levels; b. F, smaller; c. T; d. F, hypersecretion; e. T

5. a. cortisol; b. thyroid; c. vasopressin/ADH analogue; d. growth hormone; e. sex hormones: testosterone; FSH and LH if fertility is desired; estrogen/progesterone if fertility is not an issue

6.

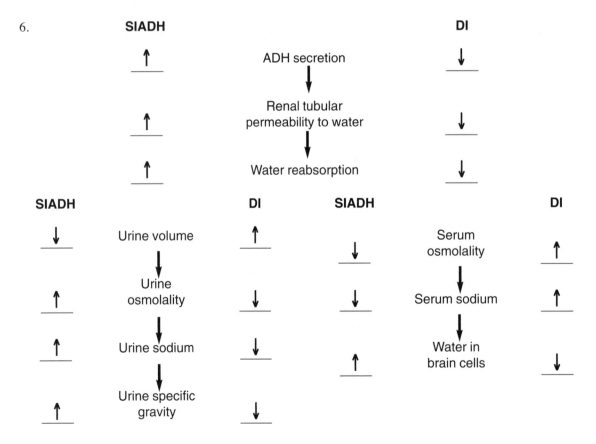

7. a. Rationale: The client with SIADH has marked dilutional hyponatremia and should be monitored for decreased neurological function and convulsions every two hours. ADH release is reduced by keeping the head of the bed flat to increase left atrial filling pressure, and sodium intake is supplemented because of the hyponatremia and sodium loss caused by diuretics. A reduction in blood pressure indicates a reduction in total fluid volume and is an expected outcome of treatment.

8. b. Rationale: The client with SIADH has water retention with hyponatremia, decreased urine output, and concentrated urine with high specific gravity. Improvement in the client's condition is reflected by increased urine output, normalization of serum sodium, and more water in the urine, decreasing the specific gravity.

9. d. Rationale: A client with diabetes insipidus has a deficiency of ADH with excessive loss of water from the kidney, hypovolemia, hypernatremia, and dilute urine with a low specific gravity. When vasopressin is administered, the symptoms are reversed, with water retention, decreased urinary output that increases urine osmolality, and an increase in blood pressure.

10. c. Rationale: Normal urine specific gravity is 1.003 to 1.030, and urine with a specific gravity of 1.002 is very dilute, indicating that there continues to be excessive loss of water and that treatment of diabetes insipidus is inadequate. Headache, weight gain, and oral intake greater than urinary output are signs of volume excess that occur with overmedication. Nasal irritation and nausea may also indicate overdosage.

11. b. Rationale: In nephrogenic diabetes insipidus, the kidney is unable to respond to ADH, so vasopressin or hormone analogues are not effective. Thiazide diuretics slow the glomerular filtration rate in the kidney and produce a decrease in urine output. Low-sodium diets (<3 g/day) are also thought to decrease urine output. Fluids are not restricted, because the client could become easily dehydrated.

12. a. T; b. F, Graves' disease; c.T; d. F, decreased TSH level, 0.35 to 0.95 (35% to 95%); e. F, inhibit, to be avoided

13. d. Rationale: The antibodies present in Graves' disease that attack thyroid tissue cause hyperplasia of the gland and stimulate TSH receptors on the thyroid and activate the production of thyroid hormones, creating hyperthyroidism. The disease is not directly genetic, but individuals appear to have a genetic susceptibility to become sensitized to develop autoimmune antibodies. Goitre formation from insufficient iodine intake is usually associated with hypothyroidism.

14. c. Rationale: A hyperthyroid crisis results in marked manifestations of hyperthyroidism, with severe tachycardia, heart failure, shock, hyperthermia, agitation, nausea, vomiting, diarrhea, delirium, and coma. Although exophthalmos may be present in the client with Graves' disease, it is not a significant factor in hyperthyroid crisis. Hoarseness and laryngeal stridor are characteristic of the tetany of hypoparathyroidism, and lethargy progressing to coma is characteristic of myxedema coma, a complication of hypothyroidism.

15. a. 2;  b. 4;  c. 2;  d. 1;  e. 1;  f. 2;  g. 3;  h. 1; i. 4; j. 2; k. 4

16. a. Risk for injury: corneal ulceration related to inability to close eyelids
    b. Imbalanced nutrition: less than body requirements related to hypermetabolism
    c. Disturbed body image related to change in body appearance
    d. Activity intolerance related to fatigue and dyspnea

17. a. Rationale: To prevent strain on the suture line post-operatively, the head must be manually supported while turning and moving in bed, but range-of-motion exercises for the head and neck are also taught preoperatively to be gradually implemented after surgery. There is no contraindication for coughing and deep breathing, and they should be carried out post-operatively. Tingling around the lips or fingers is a sign of hypocalcemia, which may occur if the parathyroid glands are inadvertently removed during surgery, and should be reported immediately.

18. a. Needed in case airway obstruction occurs because of vocal cord paralysis from recurrent laryngeal nerve damage during surgery or laryneal stridor occurs with tetany
    b. Needed in case hypocalcemia occurs from parathyroid gland removal or damage during surgery, resulting in tetany
    c. In case of airway obstruction, laryngeal stridor or edema around trachea

19. c. Rationale: When a client has had a subtotal thyroidectomy, thyroid replacement therapy is not given because exogenous hormone inhibits pituitary production of TSH and delays or prevents the restoration of thyroid tissue regeneration. However, the client should avoid goitrogens, foods that inhibit thyroid, such as soybeans, turnips, rutabagas, and peanut skins. Regular exercise stimulates the thyroid gland and is encouraged. Salt water gargles are used for dryness and irritation of the mouth and throat following radioactive iodine therapy.

20. a. 4; b. 3; c. 1; d. 5; e. 6; f. 2

21. d. Rationale: Both Graves' disease and Hashimoto's thyroiditis are autoimmune disorders that eventually destroy the thyroid gland, leading to primary hypothyroidism. Thyroid tumours most often result in hyperthyroidism. Secondary hypothyroidism occurs as a result of pituitary failure, and iatrogenic hypothyroidism results from thyroidectomy or radiation of the thyroid gland.

22. a. R/T depression and altered metabolism; AMB excessive sleeping, no relief of somnolence, altered sleep stages

    b. R/T hypometabolism; AMB weight gain, myxedema facies

    c. R/T diminished cerebral blood flow secondary to decreased cardiac output; AMB forgetfulness, memory loss, personality changes, stupor

    d. R/T decreased metabolic rate and mucin deposits in joints; AMB fatigue, weakness, muscular aches and pains

23. d. Rationale: Hypothyroidism affects the heart in many ways, causing cardiomyopathy, coronary atherosclerosis, bradycardia, pericardial effusions, and weakened cardiac contractility. When thyroid replacement therapy is started, myocardial oxygen consumption is increased, and the resultant oxygen demand may cause angina, cardiac arrhythmias, and heart failure. It is important to monitor clients with compromised cardiac status when starting replacement therapy.

24. b. Rationale: Because of the mental sluggishness, inattentiveness, and memory loss that occur with hypothyroidism, it is important to provide written instructions and repeat information when teaching the client. Caloric intake can be increased when drug therapy is started, because of an increased metabolic rate, and replacement therapy must be taken for life. Although most clients return to a normal state with treatment, cardiovascular conditions and psychoses may persist.

25. a. 1; b. 2; c. 1; d. 1; e. 1; f. 2; g. 2; h. 1; i. 2; j. 1

26. b. Rationale: A high fluid intake is indicated in hyperparathyroidism to dilute the hypercalcemia and flush the kidneys so that calcium stone formation is reduced. Seizures are not associated with hyperparathyroidism, but impending tetany of hypoparathyroidism can be noted with Trousseau's phenomenon and Chvostek's sign. The client with hyperparathyroidism is at risk for pathological fractures due to decreased bone density, but mobility is encouraged to promote bone calcification.

27. b. Rationale: Rebreathing in a paper bag promotes carbon dioxide retention in the blood, which lowers pH and creates acidosis. An acidemia enhances the solubility and ionization of calcium, increasing the proportion of total body calcium available in physiologically active form and relieving the symptoms of hypocalcemia. Saline promotes calcium excretion, as does furosemide. Phosphate levels in the blood are reciprocal to calcium, and an increase in phosphate promotes calcium excretion.

28. c. Rationale: The hypocalcemia that results from parathyroid hormone deficiency is controlled with calcium and vitamin D supplementation and possibly oral phosphate binders. Replacement with PTH is not used, because of antibody formation to PTH, the need for parenteral administration, and cost. Milk products, although good sources of calcium, also have high levels of phosphate, which reduce calcium absorption. Whole grains and foods containing oxalic acid also impair calcium absorption.

29. a. Rationale: The effects of glucocorticoid excess include weight gain from accumulation and redistribution of adipose tissue, sodium and water retention, glucose intolerance, protein wasting, loss of bone structure, loss of collagen, and capillary fragility. Clinical manifestations of corticosteroid deficiency include hypotension, dehydration, weight loss, and hyperpigmentation of the skin.

30. c. Rationale: Electrolyte changes that occur in Cushing's syndrome include sodium retention and potassium excretion by the kidney, resulting in a hypokalemia, which may lead to cardiac arrhythmias or arrest. Hypotension, hypoglycemia, and decreased cardiac strength and output are characteristic of adrenal insufficiency.

31. c. Rationale: Although the client with Cushing's syndrome has excess corticosteroids, removal of the glands and the stress of surgery require that high doses of cortisone be administered post-operatively for several days. The nurse should monitor the client post-operatively to detect whether large amounts of hormones were released during surgical manipulation and to ensure that healing is satisfactory.

32. c. Rationale: Vomiting and diarrhea are early indicators of addisonian crisis, and fever indicates an infection, which is causing additional stress for the client. Treatment of a crisis requires immediate glucocorticoid replacement, and IV hydrocortisone, fluids, sodium, and glucose are necessary for 24 hours. Addison's disease is a primary insufficiency of the adrenal gland, and ACTH is not effective, nor would vasopressors be effective with the fluid deficiency of Addison's. Potassium levels are increased in Addison's disease, and KCl would be contraindicated.

33. a. Rationale: Confusion, irritability, disorientation, or depression is often present in the client with Addison's disease, and a positive response to therapy would be indicated by a return to alertness and orientation. Other indications of response to therapy would be a decreased urinary output, decreased serum potassium, and increased serum sodium and glucose. The client with Addison's would be very dehydrated and volume-depleted and would not have pulmonary edema.

34. b. Rationale: A weight reduction in the client with Addison's disease may indicate a fluid loss and a dose of replacement therapy that is too low, rather than too high. Clients with Addison's disease are taught to take two to three times their usual dose of steroids if they become ill, have teeth extracted, or engage in rigorous physical activity and should always have injectable hydrocortisone available if oral doses cannot be taken. Because vomiting and diarrhea are early signs of crisis and because fluid and electrolytes must be replaced, clients should notify their physician if these symptoms occur.

35. a. Sodium and fluid retention because of mineralocorticoid effect; b. GI irritation with increase in secretion of pepsin and hydrochloric acid; c. Corticosteroid-induced osteoporosis; d. Glucose intolerance with hyperglycemia; e. Hypokalemia because of mineralocorticoid effect; f. Inhibition of inflammation and immune response; may reactivate latent TB

36. c. Rationale: Taking corticosteroids on an alternate-day schedule for pharmacological purposes is less likely to suppress ACTH production from the pituitary and may prevent adrenal atrophy. Normal adrenal hormone balance is not maintained during glucocorticoid therapy, because excessive exogenous hormone is used.

37. a. Rationale: Hyperaldosteronism is an excess of aldosterone, which is manifested by sodium and water retention and potassium excretion. Furosemide is a potassium-wasting diuretic that would increase the potassium deficiency. Aminoglutethimide blocks aldosterone synthesis; amiloride is a potassium-sparing diuretic; and spironolactone blocks mineralocorticoid receptors in the kidney, increasing excretion of sodium and water and retention of potassium.

38. b. Rationale: A pheochromocytoma is a catecholamine-producing tumour of the adrenal medulla, which may cause severe, episodic hypertension; severe, pounding headache; and profuse sweating. Monitoring for a dangerously high blood pressure before surgery is critical, as is monitoring for blood pressure fluctuations during medical and surgical treatment.

**Case Study**

1. All of the blood tests are altered because of the effect of glucocorticoids:
   - Elevated glucose—increased gluconeogenesis by liver and induced insulin resistance
   - Elevated WBC—granulocytosis
   - Decreased lymphocytes—lymphocytopenia
   - Increased RBC—polycythemia
   - Decreased K—increased mineralocorticoid effect causing sodium retention and potassium excretion

2. There are several causes of Cushing's syndrome:
   - ACTH-secreting pituitary tumour is the most common cause of endogenous Cushing's syndrome
   - Adrenal tumours
   - Ectopic ACTH production by tumours outside the hypothalamic-pituitary-adrenal axis
   - The pathophysiology of Cushing's syndrome reflects an excess of normal glucocorticoid and mineralocorticoid activity, an exaggeration of normal functions.

3. ACTH levels: high or normal levels of ACTH indicate ACTH-dependent Cushing's or a tumour of the pituitary gland; low or undetectable levels of ACTH indicate an adrenal or ectopic cause.

4. Pituitary cause—transsphenoidal hypophysectomy; adrenal cause—adrenalectomy; ectopic cause—removal if possible

5. A medical adrenalectomy involves treatment with mitotane (Lysodren), a drug that suppresses cortisol production, alters peripheral metabolism of steroids, and decreases plasma and urine steroid levels by actually killing adrenocortical cells.

6. Major nursing responsibilities are included in the following list:
   *Assessment of signs and symptoms of hormone toxicity:*
   - Vital signs q4h
   - Daily weights
   - Glucose monitoring
   - Changes in mental status
   *Assessment for complications:*
   - Signs and symptoms of infection, such as pain or purulent drainage because fever and inflammation may be minimal or absent
   - Signs and symptoms of thromboembolic phenomena, such as chest pain, dyspnea, tachypnea
   - Signs and symptoms of bone pain or limitations in motion, indicating pathological fractures
   - Signs and symptoms of nephrolithiasis from increased calcium excretion

*Preoperative preparation:*
- Instruction about exercises, coughing, and deep breathing
- Explanations about early monitoring for circulatory instability
- Explanations about hormone replacement

7. *Nursing diagnoses:*
- Risk for infection related to suppression of inflammation and immune function
- Risk for injury related to osteoporosis
- Risk for impaired skin integrity related to edema and altered skin fragility
- Disturbed body image related to altered physical appearance

*Collaborative problems:*
Potential complications: thromboembolism; cardiac arrhythmias; pathological fractures; nephrolithiasis; diabetes mellitus; hypertensive crisis

## CHAPTER 49

1. a. ureter; b. urinary bladder; c. ductus deferens; d. corpus cavernosum; e. corpus spongiosum; f. urethra; g. penis; h. glans; i. scrotum; j. testis; k. epididymis; l. anus; m. Cowper's gland; n. rectum; o. prostate gland; p. ejaculatory duct; q. seminal vesicle; r. ureter; s. posterior cul-de-sac; t. cervix; u. fornix of vagina; v. anus; w. vagina; x. labia majora; y. labia minora; z. urethra; aa. clitoris; bb. symphysis pubis; cc. urinary bladder; dd. anterior cul-de-sac; ee. fundus of uterus; ff. round ligament; gg. body (corpus) of uterus; hh. fallopian tube

2. a. prepuce; b. labia minora; c. vagina; d. vestibule; e. perineum; f. anus; g. labia majora; h. urethra; i. clitoris; j. mons pubis; k. pectoralis major muscle; l. alveoli; m. areola; n. nipple

3. a. 3; b. 6; c. 2; d. 7; e. 1; f. 8; g. 4; h. 5

4. a. 4; b. 8; c. 6; d. 7; e. 3; f. 2; g. 1; h. 5

5. a. T; b. F, fallopian tube; c. F, squamocolumnar junction; d. T; e. F, one year

6. a. 2; b. 8; c. 6; d. 1; e. 5; f. 7; g. 4; h. 3; i. 6; j. 8; k. 1; l. 6; m. 5; n. 2

7. a. 2; b. 1; c. 2; d. 1; e. 3; f. 1; g. 1; h. 1

8. a. Rationale: Decreased estrogen levels during menopause lead to atrophy of the vaginal epithelium with vaginal dryness, which may cause dyspareunia. Menopause does cause such changes as atrophy of secondary sex characteristics, vasomotor instability, and increased incidence of osteoporosis, but sexual response is often increased when the threat of pregnancy is eliminated. The use of hormone replacement therapy is controversial, and other methods can be used to reduce the uncomfortable effects of menopause.

9. b. Rationale: Age-related changes in sexual function in males include a need for increased stimulation for an erection, decreased need to ejaculate, and a possible decreased response to sexual stimuli. There is a decreased ability to attain an erection, but it is not related to prostatic changes. A negative social attitude toward sexuality in older adults also affects the sexual activity of people in this age group.

10. c. Rationale: Information related to menstrual history is usually non-threatening and is a good place to begin an interview about reproductive function before asking about more sensitive issues, such as sexual practices, drugs that affect sexual function, or sexually transmitted infections.

11. a. Potential congenital anomalies if rubella occurs during first trimester of pregnancy
    b. Increased sterility in young men with mumps, because of testicular atrophy secondary to orchitis
    c. Impotence and retrograde ejaculation in male with diabetes, in addition to erectile problems from neuropathies
    d. Many may cause impotence in men

12. a. Lack of Pap tests, breast self-examination, prostate examination or testicular self-examination; smoking, alcohol, and caffeine use; family history of breast disease and reproductive cancers
    b. History of anorexia nervosa, decreased calcium intake
    c. Urge and stress incontinence; difficulty in urinating in males; bladder infections
    d. Fatigue and activity intolerance related to menorrhagia
    e. Sleep interruption related to hot flashes and sweating; nocturia
    f. Pelvic pain; dyspareunia
    g. Changes in self-concept related to sexuality and aging
    h. Occupational hazards related to sexual functioning and reproductive capacity; dysfunctional roles and relationships with others
    i. Recent changes in sexual practices; dissatisfaction with sexual expression; reproductive problems that affect sexual satisfactions; changes in menstrual patterns; multiple sexual partners; no protection against sexually transmitted infections
    j. STI effect on sex partners; stress of sexual problems; infertility
    k. Conflict between value system and treatment; abortion issues; infertility issues

13. d. Rationale: The prostate is palpated through the wall of the rectum with a digital rectal examina-

tion. Inguinal hernias are detected by palpating the inguinal ring while the client bears down, and scrotal palpation is done to detect testicular masses or tumours. No specific conditions are indicated by enlargement at the base of the penis.

14. a. Rationale: A decrease in the size of the penis is a normal finding in the older male. Loss of pubic hair is not normal, nor is any enlargement of the breasts. The normally darker colour of the scrotum does not change with aging.

15. d. Rationale: The presence of dimpling or retractions can be observed by having the client put her arms at her sides and over her head, lean forward, and press the hands on the hips. Lying down with the arm over the head flattens the breast for better palpation for lumps or thickness that can be felt with systematic palpation. Compressing the nipple is done to assess for drainage or galactorrhea.

16. d. Rationale: A diamond pubic hair distribution is characteristic of males and is abnormal in females. A small amount of clear vaginal discharge is normal in females, as are episiotomy scars in a woman who has had children. Skene's ducts should be non-palpable.

17. b. Rationale: Pap tests are more accurate if they are performed at mid-cycle or during the secretory phase of the menstrual cycle because there is a greater likelihood that abnormal cells will be detected at this time. Douching should not be done for 24 hours before the examination, but sexual intercourse is not contraindicated.

18. a. 5; b. 4; c. 9; d. 7; e. 3; f. 1; g. 2; h. 8; i. 6

19. b. Rationale: The risk for bleeding is increased following a D&C because the endometrial lining is scraped and injury to the uterus may occur. The nurse should closely assess the amount of bleeding with frequent pad checks the first 24 hours. Infection following D&C is uncommon, and the urinary system is not affected.

20. a. Rationale: A culdoscopy involves insertion of an endoscope through an incision made through the posterior fornix of the cul-de-sac and requires surgical anaesthesia, as does removal of cervical tissue during a conization. A D&C, laparoscopy, and breast biopsy are also operative procedures requiring surgical anaesthesia, but colposcopy, contrast mammography, and endometrial biopsies do not require surgical anaesthesia.

21. a. Rationale: A Huhner test (or Sims-Huhner) involves examination of a mucus sample of the cervix within two to eight hours after intercourse to determine the number and mobility of sperm in the cervical mucus. A semen analysis is a simple examination of semen for the number, mobil-

ity, and structure of sperm. An endometrial biopsy provides a sample of endometrium to evaluate its changes under the influence of progesterone, and a hysterosalpingogram is a contrast x-ray of the uterine cavity and fallopian tubes.

# CHAPTER 50

1. d. Rationale: The importance of performing breast self-examination (BSE) arises from the fact that early detection and treatment of breast cancer are the most significant factors in survival rates, and between BSE and regular mammography, most palpable and non-palpable masses can be identified early enough for successful treatment. Most palpable breast lesions are discovered by women themselves, which is an important tool in early detection, but it must be followed by treatment. The role of BSE in reducing mortality from breast cancer in women under the age of 50 is controversial.

2. a. Ages 20–39: Regular BSE; Annual physical examination by a physician or other health professional; b. Ages 40–49: Regular BSE; physical examination of the breasts by a trained healthcare professional (CBE) every two years; discuss risks and benefits of mammography with a physician; c. Ages 50–69: Regular BSE; (CBE) every two years; mammography every two years; d. Ages 70 or over: Regular BSE; (CBE) every two years; talk to physician about an individualized screening program.

3. c. Rationale: One of the major reasons women do not examine their breasts regularly is because of a lack of confidence in BSE skill, and a teaching program should include allowing time for women to use models to identify problems and perform a return demonstration of the examination on themselves. Fear and denial often interfere with BSE even when women know the perceived risk for cancer is high, know the statistics, and know they should seek medical care if an abnormality is detected.

4. d. Rationale: A definitive diagnosis of breast cancer can be made only by a histological examination of biopsied tissue. A stereotactic core biopsy is as reliable as an open surgical biopsy and has the advantages of decreased length of time for the procedure and recovery and reduced cost. A limitation of fine-needle aspiration is that if negative results are found, more definite biopsy procedures are required.

5. d. Rationale: Most breast lesions are benign, and many mobile cystic lesions change in response to the menstrual cycle, while most malignant tumours do not. Caffeine has been associated

with fibrocystic changes in some women, but research has not established caffeine as a cause of breast pain or cysts. Questions regarding a client's last mammogram or family history are not closely related to the nurse's findings.

6. b. Rationale: Fibrocystic changes make breasts difficult to examine because of fibrotic changes and multiple lumps. A woman with this condition should be familiar with the characteristic changes in her breasts and monitor them closely for new lumps that do not respond in a cyclic manner over one to two weeks. Estrogen antagonizes the condition, and fibrocystic changes are not precancerous.

7. a. 6;  b. 3;  c. 1;  d. 2;  e. 7;  f. 5;  g. 4;  h. 6;  i. 2;  j. 4;  k. 7;  l. 3;  m. 1

8. b. Rationale: After the age of 60, the incidence of breast cancer increases dramatically, and advanced age is the highest risk factor for females. Obesity is a contributing factor for breast cancer, but fibrocystic breast changes are neither a precursor of cancer nor a known risk factor for cancer. Only about 5% to 10% of women with breast cancer may have a BRCA1 or 2 gene, specific genetic abnormalities that contribute to the development of breast cancer.

9. b. Rationale: On palpation, malignant lesions are characteristically hard, irregularly shaped, poorly delineated, non-tender, and non-mobile, and the most common site is the upper outer quadrant of the breast. A fibroademona is firm, defined, and mobile, while fibrocystic lesions are usually large, tender, movable masses found throughout the breast tissue. A painful, immobile mass under a reddened area of skin is most typical of a local abscess.

10. a. Rationale: Axillary lymph node status is one of the most important prognostic factors in primary breast cancer, and the more nodes that are involved, the higher the risk for relapse or metastasis. Aneuploid DNA tumour content indicates that cells have abnormally high or low DNA content in comparison with normal cells and is associated with tumour aggressiveness. Cells in S-phase have a higher risk for recurrence and can produce earlier cancer death. Hormone receptor–negative tumours are usually poorly differentiated histologically, frequently recur, and are usually unresponsive to hormonal therapy.

11. d. Rationale: Even with negative axillary lymph nodes, recurrence occurs in 30% to 35% of clients with breast cancer, illustrating that although most metastases occur through the lymphatic chains, metastasis can occur without invading the axillary nodes. Recurrence may be local or regional, with distant metastases most commonly to bone, lung, brain, and liver.

12. b. Rationale: Either treatment choice is indicated for women with early-stage breast cancer because the 10-year survival rate with lumpectomy with radiation is about the same as that with modified radical mastectomy. Each procedure has advantages and disadvantages that the client must consider in making an informed choice, and the nurse should make that information available to the client to assist in decision making.

13. d. Rationale: Axillary lymph node dissection is almost always performed regardless of the treatment option selected, because of its value in prognosis and decision making regarding adjuvant therapy. A lumpectomy, or breast conservation surgery, is followed by radiation therapy to the entire breast, and the use of chemotherapy or hormone therapy depends on the characteristics of the tumour and evidence of metastases.

14. a. Adjunct to surgery; b. Palliative; c. High-dose brachytherapy; d. Primary; e. Adjunct to surgery; f. High-dose brachytherapy

15. d. Rationale: Because micrometastases have probably occurred even in stage I disease, making breast cancer a systemic disease at the time of diagnosis, and because premenopausal women, especially with hormone receptor–negative tumours, are known to be at higher risk for recurrent or metastatic disease, systemic chemotherapy is recommended even when no evidence of node involvement is found.

16. c. Rationale: Tamoxifen is an anti-estrogen agent that blocks the estrogen-receptor sites of malignant cells and is the usual first choice of treatment in post-menopausal women with hormone receptor–positive tumours, with or without nodal involvement. Tamoxifen reduces the risk for recurrent breast cancer and also that for new primary tumours. The side effects of the drug are minimal and are those commonly associated with decreased estrogen.

17. c. Rationale: As early as in the recovery room following a modified radical mastectomy, the client should start flexing and extending the fingers and wrist of the affected arm with daily increases in activity. Post-operative mastectomy exercises, such as hair care, wall climbing with the fingers, and shoulder rotation and extension, are instituted gradually to prevent disruption of the wound.

18. b. Rationale: Removal of the axillary lymph nodes impairs lymph drainage from the affected arm and predisposes the client to infection of the arm. The arm must be protected from even minor trauma, and blood pressure, venipunctures, and injections should not be done on the arm. The arm should never be dependent, even during

sleep, and should be elevated to promote lymph drainage.

19. c. Rationale: The Reach to Recovery program consists of volunteers who are all women who have had breast cancer and can answer questions about what to expect at home, how to tell people about the surgery, and what prosthetic devices are available. It is a valuable resource for clients who have breast cancer and should be used if available in the community. If a volunteer is not available, the nurse is responsible for assisting the client in the same manner. Although the nurse should stress the importance of wearing a prosthesis, a permanent prosthesis cannot be used until healing is complete and inflammation is resolved.

20. b. Rationale: It is most important for the client planning a mammoplasty that she have a realistic idea about what the surgery can accomplish and about possible complications. Currently surgery cannot restore nipple sensation or erectility, and the breast will not fully resemble its premastectomy appearance, but the outcome is usually more acceptable than the mastectomy scar. The woman's motives for breast reconstruction should not be questioned. There have been allegations of immune-related diseases associated with the use of silicone gel implants only, and these implants are currently off the market in Canada, in response to potential hazards related to silicone leakage.

21. a. Rationale: When an expander is used to stretch the skin and muscle at the mastectomy site, the expander is gradually increased in size by weekly injections of water or saline until the site is large enough to hold an implant. The placement of the expander can be at the time of mastectomy or at a later date. A musculocutaneous flap procedure is a type of reconstruction using the client's own tissue. The nipple of the affected breast is removed at mastectomy, and a new nipple can be reconstructed after breast reconstruction from various normal tissues.

**Case Study**

1. It is likely that micrometastases to distant sites have occurred at the time of the diagnosis of breast cancer even in stage I disease and almost certainly in stage III disease, supporting indications for systemic treatment of the cancer following local surgical treatment. Breast cancer is one of the solid tumours that is most responsive to chemotherapy, and destruction or control of tumour cells that have spread to distant sites is the goal of systemic chemotherapy.

2. a. cyclophosphamide [C]:
   alkylating agent, cell-cycle non-specfic
   *Side effects:* myelosuppression, nausea and vomiting, alopecia, hemorrhagic cystitis
   b. doxorubicin:
   antitumour antibiotic, cell-cycle non-specfic
   *Side effects:* myelosuppression, mucositis, nausea and vomiting, alopecia, cardiotoxicity
   c. 5-fluorouracil:
   antimetabolite, cell-cycle specific
   *Side effects:* myelosuppression, mucositis, nausea and vomiting, alopecia, photosensitivity

3. Teach Mrs. T. to perform the following activities as necessary:
   *Myelosuppression:*
   - Monitor her temperature every day.
   - Report any chilling; sore throat; cough; or rectal, urinary, or chest pain.
   - Keep the venous access catheter site clean and dry.
   - Avoid crowds and anyone with communicable diseases.
   - Wash her hands after toileting and before eating.
   - Report any bleeding, serious bruising, or persistent headaches.
   - Avoid using ASA products.
   - Examine her mouth daily for blood-filled lesions.
   - Guard against bumping and other injury that may cause bleeding.
   *Mucositis:*
   - Examine her mouth daily for bleeding, redness, or ulcers.
   - Use a mouthwash of baking soda or salt water every two hours as needed.
   - Use a soft-bristled toothbrush or sponge-tipped applicators for oral care.
   - Avoid hot, spicy, acidic foods and alcohol and tobacco.
   - Drink water frequently during the day.
   *Nausea and vomiting:*
   - Use antiemetic medications as prescribed.
   - Eat small frequent meals that include bland, lukewarm, high-calorie, high-protein foods, and use liquid nutritional supplements if necessary.
   - Avoid strong odours and sights that increase nausea.
   - Eat and drink slowly.
   - Use gum, tea, or any food that stimulates salivation without causing nausea.
   *Alopecia:*
   - Select a wig and begin to wear it before hair loss begins.

- Wear a scarf or turban to conceal hair loss.
- Use a mild, protein-based shampoo and hair conditioner every four to seven days to avoid drying remaining hair.
- Avoid excessive shampooing, brushing, and combing of hair.
- Avoid use of curling irons, curlers, blow dryers, and hair spray.

4. An estrogen receptor-positive tumour is estrogen-dependent, and estrogen can promote growth of these breast cancer cells. Hormone receptor–positive cells usually are well differentiated, have low proliferative indices, and DNA content equal to that of normal cells. Drugs, such as tamoxifen, that block the estrogen receptor site of malignant cells can cause tumour regression and are widely used to treat recurrent or metastatic cancer that is estrogen–dependent.

5. The nurse should:
   - assist the client to develop a positive but realistic attitude.
   - help her identify sources of support and strength to her.
   - encourage her to verbalize her guilt and anger and fears about her diagnosis and the impact it is having on her life.
   - promote open communication between the client and her husband.
   - provide accurate and complete answers to her questions about her disease.
   - offer information about community resources and local support groups.

6. Fear, denial, and embarrassment are common reasons that women do not perform BSE or have a mammogram, and a lack of practice and skill at breast examination undermines their confidence in performing the examination. Denial was probably a big factor for Mrs. T. in view of the value of her breasts in her relationship with her husband.

7. Teach Mrs. T. that she will need follow-up for the rest of her life at regular intervals. She should expect to have a professional examination every three months for two years, every six months for the next three years, and then annually thereafter. She should be taught to perform breast self-examination of both breasts every month and informed that recurrence of breast cancer is likely.

8. *Nursing diagnoses:*
   - Ineffective therapeutic regimen management related to lack of compliance and information regarding breast cancer surveillance
   - Ineffective coping related to reported feelings of guilt and perceived expectations of husband
   - Impaired physical mobility related to decreased arm and shoulder mobility

*Collaborative problems:*
Potential complications: vascular access catheter displacement or infection; hyperuricemia; bleeding; septicemia; tumour recurrence

## CHAPTER 51

1. c. Rationale: Although there are many factors that relate to the current STI rates, one major factor is the high use of oral contraceptives, long-acting parenteral contraceptives, and IUDs for contraception. The condom, both male and female, provides a barrier to micro-organisms causing STIs and is the only contraceptive device that is prophylactic in regard to STIs. Oral contraceptives provide a more favourable environment for growth of organisms that cause STIs, and while IUDs and parenteral long-acting contraceptives, such as Norplant and Depo-Provera, are not known to increase risk for STIs, they do not provide protection against the diseases.

2. a. 3;  b. 4;  c. 1;  d. 5;  e. 2

3. d. Rationale: An established diagnosis of gonorrhea is treated with both ceftriaxone and doxycycline or tetracycline—ceftriaxone for resistant strains of *N. gonorrhoeae* and doxycycline because of the high frequency of chlamydial infections co-existing with gonorrhea. Gram-stain smears are not useful in diagnosing gonorrhea in women because the female GU tract normally harbours a large number of organisms that resemble *N. gonorrhoeae*, and cultures must be performed to diagnose the disease in women. Penicillin G is used to treat syphilis, and although gonorrhea may lead to PID, its diagnosis would not necessarily indicate the client had PID.

4. a. Rationale: Upward extension of gonorrhea or chlamydia commonly causes salpingitis and pelvic inflammatory disease, which can cause adhesions and fibrous scarring, leading to tubal abnormalities and tubal pregnancies and infertility. Disseminated gonococcal infection is rare, and endocarditis and aneurysms are associated with syphilis.

5. a. S;  b. T;  c. T;  d. P;  e. T;  f. S;  g. L;  h. T; i. S;  j. T

6. c. Rationale: Many other diseases or conditions may cause false-positive tests on non-treponemal VDRL or RPR tests, and additional testing is needed before a diagnosis is confirmed or treatment administered. Positive results on these tests should be confirmed by specific treponemal tests, such as the FTA-ABS test or the MHA test, to rule out other causes. Analysis of CSF is used to diagnose asymptomatic neurosyphilis.

7. d. Rationale: The risk factors of drug abuse and sexual promiscuity are found in clients with both syphilis and HIV infection, and persons at highest risk for acquiring syphilis are also at high risk for acquiring HIV. Syphilitic lesions on the genitals enhance HIV transmission. Also, HIV-infected clients with syphilis appear to be at greatest risk for CNS involvement and may require more intensive treatment with penicillin to prevent this HIV complication.

8. b. Rationale: Although chlamydial infections may cause cervicitis and urethritis in women, it is more common for symptoms to be absent or minor in most infected women. The absence of symptoms necessitates screening of asymptomatic individuals at risk with non-culture tests, such as direct fluorescent antibody (DFA), or enzyme immunoassay (EIA) tests to identify and treat the disease.

9. b. Rationale: Notification and treatment of sex partners are necessary to prevent recurrence and the ping-pong effect of passing STIs between partners. Tetracycline is prescribed qid for seven to ten days, and although alcohol may cause more urinary irritation in the client with chlamydia, it will not interfere with treatment.

10. c. Rationale: Gonorrhea and chlamydia have very similar symptoms in males, and chlamydial infections in men are diagnosed by excluding gonorrhea. When Gram-stain smears and cultures for *N. gonorrhoeae* are negative, a diagnosis of NGU-*Chlamydia* infection is made.

11. a. F, oral or genital lesions; b. T; c. F, decrease recurrences of; d. F, sexual contact should be avoided; e. T

12. d. Rationale: The human papillomavirus is responsible for causing genital warts, which manifest as discrete single or multiple white to grey warts that may coalesce to form large cauliflower-like masses on the vulva, vagina, cervix, and perianal area. Purulent vaginal discharge is associated with gonorrhea or chlamydia, painful perineal vesicles and ulcerations are characteristic of genital herpes, and a chancre of syphilis is a painless indurated lesion on the vulva, vagina, lips, or mouth.

13. a. Rationale: There is a strong association of genital warts to the development of dysplasia and neoplasia of the genital tract, especially when lesions involve the cervix, introitus, and perianal and intra-anal mucosa of women or the penis and perianal and anal mucosa of men. Regular Pap smears in women are critical in detecting early malignancies of the cervix. Oral acyclovir is used to treat HSV-2, but topical use has no value in treating sexually transmitted viral infections.

Sexual partners of clients with HPV should be examined and treated, but because treatment does not destroy the virus, condoms should always be used during sexual activity. Genital warts often grow more rapidly during pregnancy, but pregnancy is not contraindicated.

14. c. Rationale: Although gonorrhea and syphilis are on the increase in Canada, the most common reportable communicable infections in Canada are chlamydial infections, with an estimated 56,000 cases reported annually. Because genital warts infection is not a reportable infection in most provinces and territories, its incidence is difficult to determine, but, to get an idea of how widespread the infection is, approximately 50 million North Americans are currently infected with HPV.

15. a. Treatment with parenteral penicillin will cure both the mother and fetus; b. Erythromycin or silver nitrate required to the eyes of all newborns; c. C-section if mother has active lesions; d. Erythromycin treatment during pregnancy; Caesarean section if active at labour; e. May be spread to newborn by direct contact; Cesarean section not routine unless massive warts block the birth canal

16. a. Rationale: Although sexual abstinence is the most certain method of avoiding all sexually transmitted infections, it is not usually a feasible alternative, and a condom with spermicidal jelly is the next best protection. STIs may be spread through oral-anal intercourse. Conscientious hand washing and voiding after intercourse are positive hygienic measures that will help prevent secondary infections but will not prevent STIs.

17. a. Rationale: STIs that can be treated with a single dose or short course of antibiotic therapy often lead to a casual attitude about the outcome of the infection, which leads to non-compliance with instructions and delays in treatment. This is particularly true of infections that initially show few distressing or uncomfortable symptoms, such as syphilis.

### Case Study

1. The nurse should tell Jack that he must tell his fiancée the truth about the sexual encounter and that it is most important for her to be evaluated for the infection. She may have the infection without symptoms, yet be at risk for development of PID and infertility as a result of the gonorrhea. The nurse may offer a counselling referral, if necessary, for them to work through problems in their relationship.

2. Females often do not have any symptoms, but she could have a vaginal discharge, dysuria, urinary frequency, or changes in her menstrual patterns.

3. In Jack, diagnosis can be confirmed by a positive Gram-stain smear of urethral drainage; in Ann, a positive culture of cervical secretions or of the urethra, anus, or oropharynx is necessary for confirmation of diagnosis.

4. Support and counselling may be needed from the nurse, and the couple should be assisted to verbalize their feelings and concerns. Active listening with a non-judgemental attitude is important. Referral for professional counselling may be indicated.

5. Ceftriaxone IM in a single dose and doxycycline bid or tetracycline qid for seven to ten days is the recommended treatment for gonorrhea with a possible concurrent chlamydial infection. Because chlamydial infections are closely associated with gonococcal infections, both infections are usually treated concurrently even without diagnostic evidence.

6. Men: prostatitis, urethral strictures, and sterility from orchitis or epididymitis
Women: PID, Bartholin's abscess, ectopic pregnancy, infertility from tubal stricture
Both men and women may develop disseminated gonococcal infection.

7. *Nursing diagnoses:*
   - Anxiety related to impact of condition on relationships and disease outcomes
   - Disturbed body image related to symptoms associated with gonorrhea
   - Risk for infection related to failure to practice precautionary measures
   *Collaborative problems:*
   Potential complication: infertility

## CHAPTER 52

1. a. Rationale: The initial visit of a couple seeking assistance with infertility includes a history and physical for both partners, testing for medical problems and STIs, a cervical Pap test, possible semen analysis, and instruction for at-home ovulation testing. Possible future testing options and cost are also discussed. If the couple decides to continue with treatment, further visits will include more intensive evaluation, including post-coital testing, hysterosalpingography, pelvic ultrasonography, and midluteal progesterone/prolactin levels.

2. b. Rationale: To determine the time of ovulation by body temperature, the woman must take and graph her temperature on awakening before any activity, noting any illness or variation in normal patterns. The increase in estrogen as ovulation approaches causes a temperature drop. When ovulation occurs, progesterone is produced and causes a sharp rise in temperature. Using basal body temperature to dictate the timing of sexual intercourse for conception is stressful and may decrease sexual performance and also the possibility of pregnancy. Anovulation can be detected, but it is primarily treated with hormone agents.

3. d. Rationale: Infertility and treatment of infertility frequently result in great emotional and financial stress for a couple, and participation in a support group for infertile couples, as well as individual therapy, are recommended. Many infertile couples cannot be successfully treated, and the cause of infertility can be female, male, or combined. Although the cost of treatment of infertility can be high, expenses should be realistically explained at each step of the treatment so that couples can make realistic decisions and plans.

4. c. Rationale: In the presence of a confirmed pregnancy, uterine cramping with vaginal bleeding is the most important sign of spontaneous abortion. Other conditions causing vaginal bleeding, such as an incompetent cervix, do not usually cause cramping. There is no evidence that any medical treatment improves the outcome for spontaneous abortion. Blood loss can be significant, and the loss of the pregnancy may cause prolonged grieving. D&C is usually performed after the abortion to minimize blood loss and reduce the chance of infection.

5. d. Rationale: PMS is diagnosed when other possible causes for symptoms have been eliminated and is based on a symptom diary that indicates the same symptoms during the luteal phase for two or three consecutive menstrual cycles. Oral contraceptives may be used to control the symptoms of PMS by suppressing ovulation, and although progesterone may also relieve the symptoms of PMS, its effectiveness is not associated with the diagnosis of PMS. There are no laboratory findings that account for the premenstrual symptoms.

6. c. Rationale: Limitation of salt, refined sugar, and caffeine in the diet has been shown to decrease the PMS symptoms of abdominal bloating, increased appetite, and irritability. Exercise is encouraged because it increases release of endorphins, elevating mood, and also has a tranquilizing effect on muscular tension. Estrogen is not used during the luteal phase, but progesterone may be tried. Vitamin $B_6$ and foods high in tryptophan may promote serotonin production, which improves symptoms.

7. c. Rationale: The release of excess prostaglandin $F_2$ alpha ($PGF_2$ alpha) from the endometrium at the time of menstruation or increased sensitivity

to the prostaglandin is responsible for symptoms of primary dysmenorrhea, and drugs that inhibit prostaglandin production and release, such as NSAIDs, are effective in many clients with primary dysmenorrhea. Oral contraceptives are also used for primary dysmenorrhea to suppress ovulation and the associated production of prostaglandins.

8. a. 3; b. 1; c. 3; d. 4; e. 2; f. 4; g. 1

9. c. Rationale: When ovulation does not occur, estrogen continues to be unopposed by progesterone, and excessive build-up of the endometrium occurs. To prevent the risk of endometrial cancer by the buildup of the endometrium or to prevent menorrhagia from an unstable endometrium, progesterone or birth control pills are prescribed to ensure that the client's endometrial lining will be shed at least four to six times a year. Balloon therapy to treat menorrhagia is contraindicated in women desiring future fertility.

10. b. Rationale: Ectopic pregnancy is a life-threatening condition, and if the fallopian tube ruptures, profuse bleeding can lead to hypovolemic shock. All of the interventions are indicated, but the priority should be monitoring the vital signs and pain for evidence of bleeding.

11. a. F, post-menopausal; b. F, estrogen (FSH levels rise); c. T; d. T; e. T

12. *Benefits:*
- Supression of distressing vasomotor symptoms such as hot flashes
- Prevention of osteoporosis and related fractures by retarding bone loss
- Prevention of atrophic to the genitourinary tissues
- Prevention of colorectal cancer

*Risks:*
- Endometrial cancer
- Breast cancer
- Cardiovascular events such as CHD, stroke, and thrombolytic events
- Hyperlipidemia

13. d. Rationale: Regular aerobic, weight-bearing exercises will help prevent both osteoporosis and cardiovascular disease and should be maintained by all post-menopausal women, regardless of hormone therapy status. The diet should be high in complex carbohydrates and vitamin B complex. Calcium intake for women not using HRT should be 1500 mg daily with adequate vitamin D. Vitamin E may be used to decrease the intensity of hot flashes, but this is not a serious menopausal symptom.

14. c. Rationale: Phytoestrogens from plant sources have been shown to be effective in reducing menopausal symptoms. Soy, black cohosh, and dong quai may all decrease hot flashes and improve cardiovascular health, but soy products have almost no ill effects and appear to be very effective in many women. Valerian is used for a tranquilizing effect.

15. b. Rationale: Sexual assault is an act of violence, and the first priority of care for the client should be assessment and treatment of serious injuries involving extragenital areas, such as fractures, subdural hematomas, cerebral concussions, and intra-abdominal injuries. All of the other options are correct, but treatment for shock and urgent medical injuries is the first priority.

16. a. Rationale: Specific informed consent must be obtained from the sexual assault victim before any examination can be made or rape data collected. Following consent the client is advised not to wash, eat, drink, or urinate before the examination so that evidence can be collected for medicolegal use. Prophylaxis for STIs, hepatitis B, and tetanus is administered following examination, and follow-up testing for pregnancy and HIV is done in several weeks.

17. a. 2; b. 1; c. 1; d. 4; e. 3; f. 1; g. 2; h. 1; i. 4

18. a. Rationale: *Gardnerella vaginalis* infection is a bacterial vaginosis that is sexually transmitted, and almost always both partners are infected. Successful treatment of the condition requires oral treatment with metronidazole (Flagyl) or clindamycin (Cleocin) for both partners. Minipads may be used to contain vaginal secretions, but they do not prevent reinfection.

19. b. Rationale: Sexual activity with multiple partners increases the risk for PID, and there is often a history of an acute infection of the lower genital tract caused by gonococcal or chlamydial microorganisms. The only significant contraceptive issue related to PID is that condom use will help prevent sexually transmitted infections that may lead to PID.

20. b. Rationale: Bed rest in the semi-Fowler position promotes drainage of the pelvic cavity by gravity and may prevent the development of abscesses high in the abdomen. Coitus, douching, and tampon use should be avoided to prevent spreading infection upward from the vagina, although frequent perineal care should be done to remove infectious drainage.

21. b. Rationale: The risk for infertility following PID is high, and the nurse should allow time for the client to express her feelings, clarify her concerns, and begin problem solving with regard to the outcomes of the disease. Responses that do not allow for discussion of feelings and concerns

or that tell the client how she should feel or what she should worry about are not therapeutic.

22. a. F, endometriosis; b. F, endometriosis and uterine leiomyoma; c. T; d. T; e. F, pseudomenopause; f. F, metrorrhagia; g. T

23. b. Rationale: A stage O Pap smear indicates cancer in situ that is confined to the epithelial layer of the cervix and requires treatment. While the Bethesda system reports non-malignant changes in cervical cells, the international classification of clinical stages of cervical cancer always identifies malignant cells. Stage 0 is the least invasive, and stage IVB indicates spread to distant organs.

24. c. Rationale: Conization (an excision of a cone-shaped section of the cervix) and laser treatment both are effective in locally removing or destroying malignant cells of the cervix and preserve fertility. Radiation treatments frequently impair ovarian and uterine function and lead to sterility. A subtotal hysterectomy would be contraindicated in treatment of cervical cancer because the cervix would be left intact in this procedure.

25. b. Rationale: Post-menopausal vaginal bleeding is the first sign of endometrial cancer, and when it occurs, a sample of endometrial tissue must be taken to exclude cancer. An endometrial biopsy can be done as an office procedure and is indicated in this case. Abdominal x-rays and Pap tests are not reliable tests for endometrial cancer, and laser treatment of the cervix is indicated only for cervical dysplasia.

26. b. Rationale: Treatment of ovarian cancer is determined by staging from the results of laparoscopy with multiple biopsies of the ovaries and other tissue throughout the pelvis and lower abdomen. Although diagnosis of ovarian tumours may be made by ultrasonography or CT scan, the treatment of ovarian cancer depends on the staging of the tumour. The client's desire for fertility is not a consideration because of the high mortality rate associated with ovarian cancer.

27. a. E;  b. O;  c. C;  d. C;  e. V;  f. E;  g. C;  h. O; i. C;  j. O

28. a. Rationale: Early signs of cancer of the vulva include pruritus, soreness of vulva, unusual odour, and discharge or bleeding of the vulva, with edema of the vulva and lymphadenopathy occurring as the disease progresses. Labial lesions and excoriation more commonly occur with infections, and nodules are more often cysts or lipomas.

29. c. Rationale: A total hysterectomy involves the removal of the uterus and the cervix, but the fallopian tubes and ovaries are left intact. Although menstruation is terminated, normal ovarian production of estrogen continues. A panhysterectomy is the procedure in which the uterus and cervix as well as the tubes and ovaries are removed.

30. b. Rationale: Lower leg pain, especially on extension or with dorsiflexion, is a sign of thrombophlebitis, which is a common complication of hysterectomy or other pelvic surgery and requires immediate medical attention. Abdominal distension with gas pains and depression are expected complications that are treated symptomatically, and interventions may be necessary if clients do not void for eight hours following removal of an indwelling catheter.

31. c. Rationale: A pelvic exenteration is the most radical gynecological surgery and results in removal of the uterus, ovaries, fallopian tubes, vagina, bladder, urethra, and pelvic lymph nodes and, in some situations, also the descending colon, rectum, and anal canal. There are urinary and fecal diversions on the abdominal wall, the absence of a vagina, and the onset of menopausal symptoms, all of which result in severe altered body structure.

32. d. Rationale: To prevent displacement of the intrauterine implant, the client is maintained on absolute bed rest with turning from side to side. Bowel elimination is discouraged during the treatment by cleaning the colon before implantation, and urinary elimination is maintained by an indwelling catheter. Because the client is radioactive, any one nurse should not spend more than 30 minutes daily with the client, and visitors are restricted to less than three hours a day at a minimum of 180 cm (6 feet) from the client.

33. a. Rationale: Kegel exercises help strengthen muscular support of the perineum, pelvic floor, and bladder and are beneficial for problems with pelvic support and stress incontinence. The muscles that should be exercised are those affected by trying to stop a flow of urine.

34. a. 5;  b. 3;  c. 2;  d. 1;  e. 4

35. a. Rationale: An anterior colporrhaphy involves repair of a cystocele, and an indwelling urinary catheter is left in place for several days postoperatively while healing occurs. Bowel function should not be altered and is maintained with a low-residue diet and a stool softener if necessary.

## Case Study

1. The gonococcus spreads directly along the endometrium to the tubes and into the peritoneum, resulting in salpingitis, pelvic peritonitis, or tubo-ovarian abscesses.

2. Clinical manifestations include crampy or continuous bilateral lower abdominal pain that is increased with movement or ambulation; irregular menstrual bleeding and vaginal discharge that is yellow, green, or brownish with a foul odour;

dyspareunia; fever; and chills, with possible nausea and vomiting.

3. Outpatient management would include oral antibiotics, increased fluid intake, good nutrition, restriction of activities, and rest with the head elevated. She should also be instructed to avoid intercourse and douching.

4. Chronic PID is less acute, with increased cramps with menses, irregular bleeding, and moderate pain with intercourse.

5. Elevating the head of the bed promotes drainage of the pelvic cavity by gravity and may prevent the development of abscesses high in the abdomen. Application of heat with heating pads or sitz baths may help localize the infection.

6. Clarify the possible course and outcomes of the disease with the client. Although early treatment may help prevent complications, it is realistic that sterility often results from PID because of adhesions and strictures of the fallopian tubes, and she is at increased risk for ectopic pregnancies. Discuss and listen to her concerns about her future child-bearing ability.

7. *Nursing diagnoses:*
   - Ineffective health maintenance related to lack of protective measures against STIs
   - Anxiety related to outcome of disease on reproductive status
   - Risk for impaired skin integrity related to vaginal drainage
   *Collaborative problems:*
   Potential complications: peritonitis; septic shock; thromboembolism

## CHAPTER 53

1. d. Rationale: Hyperplasia is an increase in the number of cells, and in BPH it is thought that the enlargement caused by the increase in new cells results from endocrine changes associated with aging. Hypertrophy refers to an increase in the size of existing cells. The hyperplasia is not considered a tumour, nor does BPH predispose to cancer of the prostate.

2. c. Rationale: Classic symptoms of uncomplicated BPH are those associated with urinary obstruction and include diminished calibre and force of the urinary stream, hesitancy, dribbling at the end of urination, and a feeling of incomplete bladder emptying because of urinary retention. Irritative symptoms, including nocturia, dysuria, urgency, or hematuria, occur if infection results from urinary retention.

3. c. Rationale: Urinary flow meters are used to measure the urinary flow rate, which is decreased in vesicle neck obstruction. Cystourethroscopy

may also evaluate the degree of obstruction, but a cystometrogram measures bladder tone, post-voiding catheterization measures residual urine, and a rectal ultrasound may determine the size and configuration of the prostate gland.

4. a. Rationale: Finasteride results in suppression of androgen formation by inhibiting the formation of the testosterone metabolite dihydroxytestosterone, the principle prostatic androgen, and results in a decrease in the size of the prostate gland. α-adrenergic blockers are used to cause smooth muscle relaxation in the treatment of BPH, but drugs affecting bladder tone are not indicated.

5. c. Rationale: Placement of stainless steel stents in the prostatic urethra hold back the walls of the prostate to allow for the unobstructed flow of urine in clients with BPH and is done under local anaesthetic on an outpatient basis. Temporary incontinence may result from the procedure.

6. a. 3; b. 5; c. 1; d. 6; e. 1; f. 2; g. 1; h. 4; i. 5; j. 3; k. 2; l. 4

7. d. Rationale: The prostate gland can be easily palpated by rectal examination, and enlargement of the gland is detected early if yearly examinations are performed. If symptoms of prostatic hyperplasia are present, further diagnostic testing, including a UA, PSA, and cystoscopy, may be indicated.

8. b. Rationale: Because of injury to the internal urinary sphincter, there is usually some degree of retrograde ejaculation following any prostate surgery. The semen is ejaculated into the bladder and is eliminated with the next voiding. It is not harmful but may affect fertility because of a smaller amount or absence of normal ejaculate. Urinary incontinence may occur with a prostatectomy but not in all cases, and a vasectomy performed at the time of a prostatectomy does not affect erectile function. Long-term use of a urinary catheter depends on the client and is not a routine procedure.

9. d. Rationale: Bleeding and blood clots from the bladder are expected after prostatectomy, and continuous irrigation is used to keep clots from obstructing the urinary tract. The rate of the irrigation may be increased to keep the clots from forming if ordered, but the nurse should also check the vital signs because hemorrhage is the most common complication of prostatectomy. The traction on the catheter applies pressure to the operative site to control bleeding and should only be relieved with specific orders. The catheter does not need to be manually irrigated unless there are signs the catheter is obstructed, and clamping the drainage tube is contraindicated because it would cause distension of the bladder.

10. b. Rationale: Bladder spasms often occur after a TURP or suprapubic prostatectomy and are caused by bladder irritation, presence of the catheter, or clots leading to obstruction of the catheter. The nurse should first check for the presence of clots obstructing the catheter or tubing and then may administer a B&O suppository if ordered. The client should not try to void around the catheter because this will increase the spasms. The flow rate on the irrigation fluid may be decreased if orders permit because fast-flowing, cold fluid may also contribute to spasms.

11. c. Rationale: Activities that increase intra-abdominal pressure should be avoided until the surgeon approves these activities at a follow-up visit. Stool softeners and high-fibre diets may be used to promote bowel elimination, but enemas should not be used, because they increase intra-abdominal pressure and may initiate bleeding. Because a TURP does not remove the entire prostate gland, the client needs annual prostatic examinations to screen for cancer of the prostate. Fluid intake should be high, but caffeine and alcohol should not be used because they have a diuretic effect and increase bladder distension.

12. a. Hard, with asymmetric enlargement with areas of induration or nodules
    b. Prostate-specific antigen (PSA) higher than that usually seen in BPH; increased prostatic acid phosphatase (PAP), especially with metastasis; elevated alkaline phosphatase in advanced disease
    c. Pelvic or perineal pain, pain of metastasis, fatigue, malaise

13. c. Rationale: A prostatectomy performed with a perineal approach has the highest incidence of residual damage to the nerves needed for erection, and clients should be aware of this complication. Urinary incontinence also frequently occurs after radical prostatectomy. Wound infection is a possibility with a perineal approach because of the proximity of the wound to the anus but can be prevented with frequent perineal care. Loss of libido and gynecomastia are effects of anti-androgen drugs.

14. a. T; b. F, luteinizing hormone-releasing hormone (LHRH) agonists (such as leuprolide [Lupron] or goserelin [Zoladex]) and androgen receptor blockers; c. F, serum PSA measurements; d. T; e. T; f. F, acute bacterial prostatitis; g. T

15. a. 4; b. 8; c. 6; d. 10; e. 12; f. 11; g. 9; h. 1; i. 3; j. 2; k. 7; l. 5

16. b. Rationale: Alpha-fetoprotein (AFP) and human chorionic gonadotropin (HCG) are glycoproteins that may be elevated in testicular cancer. If they are elevated before surgical treatment, the levels are noted, and if response to therapy is positive, the levels will decrease. PSA and PAP are used for screening of prostatic cancer; tumour necrosis factor (TNF) is a normal cytokine responsible for tumour surveillance and destruction; cross-reactive protein (CRP) is found in inflammatory conditions and widespread malignancies; carcino-embryonic antigen (CEA) is a tumour marker for cancers of the gastrointestinal system; and anti-nuclear antibody (ANA) is found most frequently in autoimmune disorders.

17. d. Rationale: Testicular tumours most often present on the testis as a lump or nodule that is very firm, is non-tender, and cannot be transillumi-nated. There may also be scrotal swelling and a feeling of heaviness. All of the other options are normal findings.

18. c. Rationale: Until sperm distal to the anasto-motic site are ejaculated or absorbed by the body, the semen will contain sperm, and alternative contraceptive methods must be used. When a post-operative semen examination reveals no sperm, the client is considered sterile. Following vasectomy there is rarely noticeable difference in the amount of ejaculate because ejaculate is primarily seminal fluid. Vasectomy does not affect testicular production of sperm or hormones, nor does it cause erectile dysfunction.

19. a. Rationale: Only a small percentage of erectile dysfunction is caused by psychological factors, and before treatment for erectile dysfunction is initiated, the cause must be determined so that appropriate treatment can be planned. In the case of the 80% to 90% of erectile dysfunction that is of physiological causes, interventions are directed at correcting or eliminating the cause or restoring function by medical means. New invasive or experimental treatments are not widely used and should be limited to research centres, and clients with systemic diseases can be treated with medical means if the cause cannot be eliminated.

20. There are many appropriate answers for this question, including these examples:
    a. Depression, stress, fear of failure, fatigue, anti-androgens decrease libido
    b. Atherosclerosis, antihypertensive drugs, diabetes
    c. Peripheral neuropathies, sympathectomy, spinal cord injuries/tumours, multiple sclerosis
    d. Antiandrogens, estrogen, thyroid, testosterone deficiency, pituitary tumours

21. a. 3; b. 1; c. 5; d. 2; e. 4; f. 5; g. 1; h. 3

**Case Study**

1. Testicular tumours develop either from the cellular components of the testis (very rare and usually benign) or from the embryonal precursors (germinal tumours that are almost always malignant). Risk factors include age between 15 and 35, a history of cryptorchidism, family history of testicular cancer, orchitis, HIV infection, maternal exposure to DES, and testicular cancer in the contralateral testis.

2. The primary difference on testicular examination between a spermatocele and a testicular cancer is that spermatocele will transilluminate, whereas cancer cannot be transilluminated.

3. About 95% of clients with testicular cancer that is found in early stages obtain a complete remission. He has no back pain or gynecomastia, which would indicate metastatic disease. His prognosis is positive, but he will need careful monitoring to detect any relapse early.

4. Alpha-fetoprotein (AFP) and human chorionic gonadotropin (HCG) are frequently elevated in testicular cancer and should be noted before treatment. If these markers are elevated before treatment and then decrease after treatment, it indicates a positive response to treatment. The levels of AFP and HCG are monitored during long-term follow-up to detect any relapse of the tumour.

5. Initiate conversation with him about his concerns, and allow him to talk about them. It is important to discuss the option of sperm banking before his surgery in case he later wants to have children.

6. The orchiectomy and lymph node resection will most likely be followed with radiation of the remaining lymph nodes and/or a single or multiple chemotherapy regimen. Germ-cell tumours are very sensitive to systemic chemotherapy, and its use is recommended. All of these processes will cause sterility, but the surgery and additional treatment should not alter his sexual function.

7. *Nursing diagnoses:*
   - Anxiety related to effects of surgery
   - Fear related to outcome of disease process and prognosis
   
   No preoperative collaborative problems

# CHAPTER 54

1. a. Golgi apparatus; b. mitochondrion; c. nucleolus; d. nucleus; e. Nissl bodies; f. gemmule; g. axon hillock; h. axon; i. Schwann cell; j. myelin sheath; k. collateral axon; l. node of Ranvier; m. telodendria; n. synaptic knobs; o. neuron cell body; p. dendrites

2. a. posterior horn; b. central canal; c. anterior horn; d. anterior corticospinal tract; e. anterior spinothalamic tract; f. lateral spinothalamic tract; g. anterior spinocerebellar tract; h. lateral corticospinal tract; i. posterior spinocerebellar tract; j. posterolateral tract of Lissauer; k. fasciculus cuneatus; l. fasciculus gracilis

3. *Across:* 3. clefts; 6. synapse; 9. oligodendroglia; 11. myelin; 12. nucleus; 14. potential; 15. pia; 16. pons; 17. LOC; 18. neuron
   *Down:* 1. node of Ranvier; 2. astrocyte; 3. CSF; 4. LE; 5. Schwann cell; 7. axon; 8. regeneration; 10. dendrite; 13. limbic; 14. pain; 15. PO; 16. PO

4. a. F, ependymal cells; b. T; c. F, out of the cell; into the cell; d. F, inhibitory; e. T

5. b. Rationale: The fasciculus gracilis and fasciculus cuneatus tracts carry information and transmit impulses concerned with touch, deep pressure, vibration, position sense, and kinesthesia. Spinothalamic tracts carry pain and temperature sensations; the spinocerebellar tracts carry subconscious information about muscle tension and body position; and descending corticobulbar tracts carry impulses responsible for voluntary impulses from the cortex to the cranial nerves.

6. a. Rationale: The cell bodies of lower motor neurons that send impulses to skeletal muscles in the arms, legs, and trunk are located in the anterior horn of the spinal cord, and lesions generally cause weakness or paralysis and decreased muscle tone. Upper motor neurons include the brainstem and cerebral cortex motor neurons that influence skeletal muscle movement, and lesions at this point cause weakness and paralysis with hyperreflexia and spasticity.

7. a. 8; b. 10; c. 7; d. 1; e. 11; f. 2; g. 12; h. 4; i. 3; j. 5; k. 9; l. 6

8. d. Rationale: Some cranial nerves are only efferent motor nerves (e.g., III, IV, VI, VII, XI, XII), some are only afferent sensory nerves (e.g., I, II, VIII), and some have both motor and sensory functions (e.g., V, IX, X), but spinal nerves always have both sensory and motor fibres. Both cranial and spinal nerves occur in pairs, and while most cell bodies of cranial nerves are located in the brain, the primary cell bodies of CN I, II, and XI are located outside of the brain.

9. a. S; b. S; c. P; d. P; e. S; f. P; g. S; h. P; i. P; j. P; k. P

10. b. Rationale: The circle of Willis is a vascular circle formed by the basilar artery and the internal carotid arteries and may act as an anastomotic pathway when occlusion of a major artery on one side of the brain occurs. The middle cerebral arteries supply the outer portions of the frontal, parietal, and superior temporal lobes, but the circle of Willis may accommodate for plaquing in this artery.

11. a. 6; b. 4; c. 9; d. 7; e. 1; f. 8; g. 2; h. 5; i. 3

12. c. Rationale: A decrease in sensory receptors caused by degenerative changes leads to diminished sense of touch, temperature, and peripheral vibrations in the older adult. Reflexes are decreased but not normally absent, and intelligence does not decrease, although there may be some loss of memory. Hypothalamic modifications lead to increased frequency of spontaneous awakening with interrupted sleep and insomnia.

13. a. Avoid suggesting symptoms.
    b. The onset and cause of illness are especially important aspects of the nursing history.
    c. The mental status must be accurately assessed to ensure that the reported history is factual.

14. c. Rationale: Headaches are a common symptom of neurological problems, and the use of ASA may impair coagulation and lead to gastric bleeding. Fainting or a brief loss of consciousness that can be attributed to vasomotor events is not indicative of neurological impairment, and there is no relationship between kidney stones or gallbladder disease and neurological problems.

15. a. Uncontrolled hypertension, lack of appropriate helmet use, family history of neurological problems
    b. Difficulty chewing and swallowing, vitamin B deficiency
    c. Bowel or bladder incontinence, constipation
    d. Problems in mobility, strength, and coordination; history of falling
    e. Sleep disturbances from pain or immobility; insomnia, frequently awakening
    f. Sensory changes, dizziness; cognitive changes; language difficulties
    g. Decreased self-worth and body image; unkempt physical appearance and hygiene
    h. Changes in roles at work or in family from neurological problems
    i. Decreased sexual desire, stimulation, function, or response
    j. Sense of being overwhelmed, inadequate coping patterns
    k. Religious or cultural beliefs that interfere or assist with planned treatment

16. a. Rationale: During the nursing history the nurse should be assessing mental functioning to determine whether the history is factual and whether the client can remember historical events, assessments that are included in the determination of mental status. Because much of the area covered in the mental status examination is assessed during the history, it does not need to be evaluated further.

17. a. 7; b. 4; c. 8; d. 9; e. 3, 6; f. 12; g. 2, 6, 10; h. 13; i. 11; j. 11; k. 1; l. 5

18. a. Rationale: The primary purposes of the nursing neurological examination are to determine the effects of neurological dysfunction on daily living and the client's and the family's ability to cope with neurological deficits. The examination should be viewed in terms of functional disabilities, rather than dysfunction, of component parts of the nervous system, and findings of the examination should be used to plan appropriate care for deficits in self-care and in activities of daily living.

19. a. 6; b. 8; c. 5; d. 9; e. 10; f. 1; g. 4; h. 7; i. 2; j. 3

20. b. Rationale: The normal response of the triceps reflex is extension of the arm or visible contraction of the triceps. The normal response of the biceps reflex is flexion of the arm at the elbow, while the presence of the brachioradialis reflex is seen with flexion and supination at the elbow.

21. b. Rationale: Deep tendon grading is as follows: 0/5 = absent; 1/5 = weak response; 2/5 = normal response; 3/5 = exaggerated response; 4/5 = hyperreflexia with clonus.

22. d. Rationale: To facilitate insertion of the spinal needle between the third and fourth lumbar vertebrae, the client should round the spine by flexing the knees, hips, and neck while in a lateral position. Sitting on the edge of the bed and bending only the spine does not separate the vertebrae as efficiently. Stimulants are withheld for eight hours before an EEG, and sedation is used for more invasive tests, such as myelography and angiography.

23. a. Rationale: A spinal headache, which may be caused by loss of CSF at the puncture site, is common following a lumbar puncture or a myelogram, and nuchal rigidity may also occur as a result of meningeal irritation. The client is not in danger of paralysis with a lumbar puncture, nor does hemorrhage from the site occur. Contrast media are not used with a lumbar puncture.

24. b. Rationale: Following a myelography (and a lumbar puncture) the client is positioned flat in bed for several hours to avoid a spinal headache, and fluids are encouraged to help in the excretion of the contrast medium. Pain at the insertion site is rare, and the most common complaint after a myelography is a headache.

25. b. Rationale: Cerebral angiography involves the injection of contrast media through a catheter inserted into the femoral or brachial artery and passed into the base of a carotid or vertebral artery and is performed when vascular lesions or tumours are suspected. Allergic reactions to the contrast medium may occur, and vascular spasms or dislodgement of plaques is possible. Neurological and vital signs must be monitored every 15 to 30 minutes for two hours, every hour for the next six hours, and then every two hours for 24 hours following the test. Electroencephalograms and transcranial Doppler sonography are not invasive studies.

26. d. Rationale: Normal glucose levels in cerebrospinal fluid are 2.5 to 4.2 mmol/L (45 to 75 mg/dL). All types of organisms consume glucose, and decreased glucose reflects bacterial activity. Increased levels are associated with diabetes. The other values are all normal.

## CHAPTER 55

1. a. Slightly decreased production, displacement into spinal canal; b. Collapse of veins and dural sinuses, increased venous outflow, and decreased blood flow; c. Distension of dura, slight compression of tissue

2. a. 0 to 15
   b. 50, ischemic; 150, constricted
   c. 70–100 mm Hg
   56 mm Hg: MAP = DBP + 1/3 (SBP-DBP) = 52 + 18 = 70
   CPP = MAP – ICP = 70 – 14 = 56
   d. 45 mm Hg: MAP = DBP + 1/3 (SBP-DBP) = 64 + 15 = 79
   CPP = MAP – ICP = 79 – 34 = 45
   e. 50; 30

3. b. Rationale: Compliance is the expansibility of the brain, and as volume and pressure increase, compliance is lowered, and elastance increases. Elastance is the inverse of compliance and represents the brain's stiffness and ability to accommodate changes in volume. Elastance increases as volume in the brain increases. With high elastance, or stiffness, large increases in pressure occur with only small increases in volume, and with high compliance, small increases in volume are accommodated.

4. a. D; b. I; c. D; d. D; e. I

5. a. 2; b. 1; c. 2; d. 1; e. 3

6. a. CO; b. CO; c. CB; d. CO; e. CB

7. c. Rationale: One of the most sensitive signs of increased intracranial pressure is a decreasing LOC. A decrease in LOC will occur before changes in vital signs, ocular signs, or projectile vomiting occur.

8. c. Rationale: Cushing's triad consists of three vital sign measures that reflect ICP and its effect on the medulla, the hypothalamus, the pons, and the thalamus. Because these structures are very deep, Cushing's triad is usually a late sign of ICP. The signs include an increasing systolic blood pressure with a widening pulse pressure, a bradycardia with a full and bounding pulse, and irregular respirations.

9. c. Rationale: The dural structures that separate the two hemispheres and the cerebral hemispheres from the cerebellum influence the patterns of cerebral herniation. A cingulated herniation occurs where there is lateral displacement of brain tissue beneath the falx cerebri.

10. a. Rationale: An intraventricular catheter is a fluid-coupled system that can provide direct access for micro-organisms to enter the ventricles of the brain, and aseptic technique is a very high nursing priority to decrease the risk for infection. Constant monitoring of ICP wave forms is not usually necessary, and removal of CSF for sampling or to maintain normal ICP is done only when specifically ordered.

11. a. T; b. F, cardiac; c. T; d. T

12. a. 3; b. 5; c. 4; d. 1; e. 6; f. 2

13. d. Rationale: A client with increased intracranial pressure is in a hypermetabolic and hypercatabolic state and needs adequate glucose to maintain fuel for the brain and other nutrients to meet metabolic needs. Malnutrition promotes cerebral edema, and if a client cannot take oral nutrition, other means of providing nutrition should be used, such as tube feedings or total parenteral nutrition. Glucose alone is not adequate to meet nutritional requirements, and 5% dextrose solutions may increase cerebral edema by lowering serum osmolarity. A fluid restriction to reduce cerebral edema must be balanced against a hypovolemia that could decrease cerebral perfusion, and it is a controversial therapy.

14. a. to speak; b. obey commands; c. open eyes to verbal or painful stimuli

15. b. Rationale: No opening of eyes = 1; incomprehensible words = 2; flexion withdrawal = 4; total = 7

16. d. Rationale: Of the body functions that should be assessed in an unconscious client, cardiopulmonary status is the most vital function and gives priorities to the ABCs.

17. c. Rationale: One of the functions of CN III, the oculomotor nerve, is pupillary constriction, and testing for pupillary constriction is important to

identify clients at risk for brainstem herniation caused by increased intracranial pressure. The corneal reflex is used to assess the functions of CN V and VII, and the oculocephalic reflex tests all cranial nerves involved with eye movement. Nystagmus is commonly associated with specific lesions or chemical toxicities and is not a definitive sign of ICP.

18. a. Rationale: Nursing care activities that increase intracranial pressure include hip and neck flexion, suctioning, clustering care activities, and noxious stimuli and should be avoided or performed as little as possible in the client with increased ICP. Lowering the $PaCO_2$ below 20 mm Hg can cause ischemia and worsening of ICP, and if hyperventilation is used, the $PaCO_2$ should be maintained at 30 to 35 mm Hg.

19. d. Rationale: Elevation of the head of the bed is indicated in the client with increased intracranial pressure to promote venous drainage from the head and decrease vascular congestion unless the elevation contributes to decreased cerebral perfusion. Decreased cerebral perfusion is indicated by a decreasing level of consciousness, and the client should be positioned so that ICP is lowered while still maintaining the CPP. Ptosis of the eyelid, unexpected vomiting, and decreased motor functions are signs of ICP.

20. c. Rationale: A $PaO_2$ of 50 mm Hg reflects a hypoxemia that may lead to further decreased cerebral perfusion and hypoxia and must be corrected. The pH and $SaO_2$ are within normal range, and a $PaCO_2$ of 30 mm Hg reflects an acceptable value for the client with moderate hyperventilation.

21. b. Rationale: Pituitary gland secretion may be affected by increased ICP, and observation for pituitary disturbances is important. A decreased urinary output with an increased specific gravity reflects water retention that is characteristic of SIADH. SIADH results in a dilutional hyponatremia, which may contribute to increased cerebral edema, changes in LOC, seizures, and coma. Diabetes insipidus is reflected by increased urinary output and a dilute urine indicated by a decreased urine specific gravity and may result in severe dehydration and decreased cerebral circulation.

22. c. Rationale: If reflex posturing occurs during ROM or positioning of the client, these activities should be done less frequently until the client's condition stabilizes because posturing can cause increases in ICP. Neither restraints nor CNS depressants would be indicated.

23. a. 4; b. 9; c. 1; d. 7; e. 6; f. 10; g. 3; h. 8; i. 12; j. 11; k. 2; l. 5

24. c. Rationale: Testing clear drainage for CSF in nasal or ear drainage may be done with a Dextrostik or Tes-Tape strip, but if blood is present, the glucose in the blood will produce an unreliable result. To test bloody drainage, the nurse should test the fluid for a "halo" or "ring" that occurs when a yellowish ring encircles blood dripped onto a white pad or towel.

25. d. Rationale: An arterial epidural hematoma is the most acute neurological emergency, and typical symptoms include unconsciousness at the scene, with a brief lucid interval followed by a decrease in LOC. An acute subdural hematoma manifests signs within 48 hours of an injury, while a chronic subdural hematoma develops over weeks or months.

26. d. Rationale: A craniotomy is indicated when there is a depressed fracture and fractures with loose fragments in order to elevate the depressed bone and remove free fragments. A craniotomy is also indicated in cases of acute subdural and epidural hematomas in order to remove the blood and control the bleeding. Burr holes may be used in an extreme emergency for rapid decompression, but with a depressed fracture, surgery would be the treatment of choice.

27. a. Rationale: In addition to monitoring for a patent airway during emergency care of the client with a head injury, the nurse must always assume that a client with a head injury may have a cervical spine injury. Maintaining cervical spine precautions in all assessment and treatment activities with the client is essential to prevent additional neurological damage.

28. c. Rationale: Residual mental and emotional changes of brain trauma with personality changes are often the most incapacitating problems following head injury and are common in those clients who have been comatose for more than six hours. Families must be prepared for changes in the client's behaviour in order to avoid family-client friction and maintain family functioning, and professional assistance may be required. There is no indication he will be dependent on others for care, but it is likely he will not return to pre-trauma status.

29. a. F, all; b. F, occipital; c. F, glioblastoma multiforme; d. T; e. T

30. b. Rationale: Frontal lobe tumours often lead to loss of emotional control, confusion, memory loss, disorientation, and personality changes that are very disturbing and frightening to the family. Physical symptoms, such as blindness, disturbances in sensation and perception, and even seizures, that occur with other tumours are more likely to be understood and accepted by the family.

31. a. 4;  b. 6;  c. 1;  d. 5;  e. 2;  f. 3
32. a. Rationale: To prevent undue concern and anxiety about hair loss and post-operative self-esteem disturbances, a client undergoing cranial surgery should be informed preoperatively that the head is usually shaved in surgery while the client is anaesthetized and that methods can be used after the dressings are removed post-operatively to disguise the hair loss. In the immediate post-operative period the client is very ill, and the focus is on maintaining neurological function, but preoperatively the nurse should anticipate the client's post-operative need for self-esteem and maintenance of appearance.
33. d. Rationale: A craniectomy involves the removal of a bone flap, and post-operatively the client should not be positioned on the operative side, but the client with an anterior or middle fossae incision will have a midline incision and have the head of the bed elevated 30 to 45 degrees. If the incision is in the posterior fossa, the client is usually kept flat or at a slight elevation with avoidance of neck flexion.
34. d. Rationale: The primary goal after cranial surgery is prevention of increased ICP, and interventions to prevent ICP and infection post-operatively are nursing priorities. The residual deficits, rehabilitation potential, and ultimate function of the client depend on the reason for surgery, the post-operative course, and the client's general state of health.
35. a. M; b. E; c. E; d. M; e. E; f. M; g. M; h. E; i. M
36. d. Rationale: Meningitis is often secondary to an upper respiratory infection or middle ear infection, where organisms gain entry to the CNS. Epidemic encephalitis is transmitted by ticks and mosquitoes, and non-epidemic encephalitis may occur as a complication of measles, chicken pox, or mumps. Encephalitis caused by the herpes simplex virus carries a high fatality rate.
37. b. Rationale: High fever, severe headache, nuchal rigidity, and positive Brudzinski's and Kernig's signs are such classic symptoms of meningitis that they are usually considered diagnostic for meningitis. Other symptoms, such as papilledema, generalized seizures, hemiparesis, and decreased LOC, may occur as complications of increased intracranial pressure and cranial nerve dysfunction.
38. a. Rationale: Because rapid diagnosis and treatment are crucial in meningitis, diagnosis is made based on history and physical examination, and antibiotic therapy with penicillins or cephalosporins is started after the collection of CSF and blood cultures, even before the diagnosis is con-firmed with positive cultures. Few drugs are available to treat encephalitis, but the antiviral agent vidarabine (Vira-A) is used in the treatment of herpes simplex encephalitis.
39. a. Increased seizures; b. Increased ICP; c. Dehydration; d. Direct neurological damage
40. c. Rationale: The symptoms of brain abscess closely resemble those of meningitis and encephalitis, including fever, headache, and increased ICP, except that the client also usually has some focal symptoms that reflect the local area of the abscess.

**Case Study**

1. The temperature elevation and nuchal rigidity in the presence of increased intracranial pressure and decreasing level of consciousness indicate that Steven has developed a meningeal infection.
2. The risks for meningitis after head injury and surgery include penetrations into the intracranial cavity with the compound fracture that involves a depressed skull fracture with scalp lacerations with a communicating pathway to the intracranial cavity and the incisions necessary for craniotomy for hematoma evacuation. Post-operative drains, invasive monitoring, environmental pathogens, and impaired immune response, also contribute to the development of meningitis.
3. Acute inflammation and infection of the pia mater and the arachnoid membrane cause nuchal rigidity, a sign of meningeal irritation, and fever. The inflammatory response increases CSF production with an increase in pressure, and as the purulent secretion produced by microbial infection spreads to other areas of the brain, cerebral edema and increased ICP occur. Increased ICP is thought to be a result of swelling around the dura, increased CSF volume, and endotoxins produced by the bacteria.
4. Priority interventions include reduction of fever, reduction of ICP, maintaining antibiotic schedule to keep therapeutic levels, maintaining fluid balance, protection from injury if seizures occur, and minimizing environmental stimuli.
5. Access to the meninges could have occurred from facial and cranial fractures and the surgical incisions.
6. *Nursing diagnoses:*
   * Ineffective cerebral tissue perfusion related to cerebral tissue swelling
   * Hyperthermia related to infection and abnormal temperature regulation
   * Risk for ineffective breathing pattern related to decreased LOC and immobility

- Risk for injury related to potential for seizures
- Imbalanced nutrition: less than body requirements related to hypermetabolism and inability to ingest food and fluids
- Risk for impaired skin integrity related to immobility

*Collaborative problems:*

Potential complications: increased intracranial pressure; seizures; hydrocephalus; disseminated intravascular coagulation; brain herniation

## CHAPTER 56

1. c. Rationale: The highest risk factors for thrombotic stroke are hypertension and diabetes. Factors such as obesity, diet high in saturated fats and cholesterol, physical inactivity, cigarette smoking, and excessive alcohol use are also risk factors but carry less risk than hypertension.

2. c. Rationale: The communication between cerebral arteries in the circle of Willis provides a collateral circulation, which may maintain circulation to an area of the brain if its original blood supply is obstructed. All areas of the brain require constant blood supply, and atherosclerotic plaques are not readily reversed. Neurological deficits can result from ischemia caused by many factors.

3. d. Rationale: A TIA is a temporary focal loss of neurological function caused by ischemia of an area of the brain, usually lasting only three hours. TIAs may be due to microemboli from heart disease or carotid or cerebral thrombi and are a warning of progressive disease. Evaluation is necessary to determine the cause of the neurological deficit and provide prophylactic treatment if possible.

4. a. 2; b. 3; c. 3; d. 1; e. 4; f. 3; g. 4; h. 1; i. 2; j. 4; k. 1; l. 4; m. 2

5. c. Rationale: When cerebral infarction occurs, the ischemic cascade causes an inflammatory response that leads to edema and extension of tissue damage. In ischemic strokes, symptoms may progress in the first 72 hours as infarction and cerebral edema increase. Repositioning and passive range of motion should be started the first day to prevent complications, but aggressive rehabilitation is not started until the client's condition is stable.

6. c. Rationale: Clinical manifestations of altered neurological function differ, depending primarily on the specific cerebral artery involved and the area of the brain that is perfused by the artery. The degree of impairment depends on rapidity of onset, the size of the lesion, and the presence of collateral circulation.

7. a. L; b. R; c. R; d. R; e. L; f. R

8. a. T; b. F, expressive aphasia; c. T; d. F, fluent dysphasia; e. F, spasticity

9. a. Rationale: A CT scan is the most commonly used diagnostic test to determine the size and location of the lesion and to differentiate a thrombotic stroke from a hemorrhagic stroke. A PET will show the metabolic activity of the brain and provides a depiction of the extent of tissue damage after a stroke. Lumbar punctures are not performed routinely because of the chance of increased intracranial pressure causing herniation. Cerebral arteriograms are invasive and may dislodge an embolism or cause further hemorrhage and are performed only when no other test can provide the needed information.

10. c. Rationale: An endarterectomy is a removal of an atherosclerotic plaque, and a plaque in the carotid artery may impair circulation enough to cause a stroke. A carotid endarterectomy is performed to prevent a CVA, as are most other surgical procedures. An extracranial–intracranial bypass involves cranial surgery to bypass a sclerotic intracranial artery. Percutaneous transluminal angioplasty uses a balloon to compress stenotic areas in the carotid and vertebrobasilar arteries and often includes inserting a stent to hold the artery open.

11. c. Rationale: The administration of antiplatelet agents, such as ASA, dipyridamole (Persantine), and ticlopidine (Ticlid), reduces the incidence of stroke in those at risk. Anticoagulants are also used for prevention of embolic strokes but increase the risk for hemorrhage. Diuretics are not indicated for stroke prevention, other than for their role in controlling blood pressure, and antilipemic agents have not been found to have a significant effect on stroke prevention. The calcium channel blocker nimodipine is used in clients with subarachnoid hemorrhage to decrease the effects of vasospasm and minimize tissue damage.

12. d. Rationale: The first priority in acute management of the client with a stroke is preservation of life. Because the client with a stroke may be unconscious or have a reduced gag reflex, it is most important to maintain a patent airway for the client and provide oxygen if respiratory effort is impaired. IV fluid replacement, treatment with osmotic diuretics, and perhaps hypothermia may be used for further treatment.

13. b. Rationale: Surgical management with clipping of an aneurysm or wrapping or reinforcing the aneurysm to decrease rebleeding and vasospasm is an option for a stroke caused by rupture of a cerebral aneurysm. Hyperventilation therapy would increase vasodilation and the potential for hemorrhage. Thrombolytic therapy would be absolutely

contraindicated, and if a vessel is patent, osmotic diuretics may leak into tissue, pulling fluid out of the vessel and increasing edema.

14. a. Rationale: The body responds to the vasospasm and decreased circulation to the brain that occurs with a stroke by increasing the blood pressure, frequently resulting in hypertension. The other options are important cardiovascular factors to assess, but they do not result from impaired cerebral blood flow.

15. a. Self-care deficit; b. Unilateral neglect; c. Impaired swallowing; d. Risk for aspiration *Also:* Impaired urinary elimination; risk for impaired skin integrity; ineffective airway clearance; impaired physical mobility

16. d. Rationale: Active ROM should be initiated on the unaffected side as soon as possible, and passive ROM of the affected side should be started on the first day. Having the client actively exercise the unaffected side provides the client with active and passive ROM as needed. Use of footboards is controversial because they stimulate plantar flexion. The unaffected arm should be supported, but immobilization may precipitate a painful shoulder–hand syndrome. The client should be positioned with each joint higher than the joint proximal to it to prevent dependent edema.

17. a. Rationale: The presence of homonymous hemianopsia in a client with right-hemisphere brain damage causes a loss of vision in the left field. Early in the care of the client, objects should be placed on the right side of the client in the field of vision, and the nurse should approach the client from the right side. Later in treatment, clients should be taught to turn the head and scan the environment and should be approached from the affected side to encourage head turning. Eye patches are used if clients have diplopia (double vision).

18. a. Rationale: The first step in providing oral feedings for a client with a stroke is ensuring that the client has an intact gag reflex because feedings will not be provided if the gag reflex is impaired. Then the nurse should evaluate the client's ability to swallow ice chips or ice water after placing the client in an upright position.

19. c. Rationale: Soft foods that provide enough texture, flavour, and bulk to stimulate swallowing should be used for the client with dysphagia. Thin liquids are difficult to swallow, and clients may not be able to control them in the mouth. Pureed foods are often too bland and too smooth, and milk products should be avoided because they tend to increase the viscosity of mucus and increase salivation.

20. c. Rationale: In most clients with a stroke confined to one hemisphere, the urinary reflex arc remains intact, a partial sensation of bladder filling remains, and the client maintains partial voluntary control over urination. Initially the client may experience frequency, urgency, and incontinence, but the use of indwelling catheters impairs bladder training. The nurse should first assess the client's urinary patterns to determine whether there is reflex emptying, retention, or mobility problems that interfere with elimination. Fluids should be maintained at 2000 mL/day, and urinals or bedpans should be offered q2h. Incontinence pads may lead to the client's acceptance of urinary incontinence.

21. b. Rationale: During rehabilitation the client with aphasia needs frequent, meaningful verbal stimulation that has relevance for him. Conversation by the nurse and family should address activities of daily living that are familiar to the client. Gestures, pictures, and simple statements are more appropriate in the acute phase, when clients may be overwhelmed by verbal stimuli. Flash cards are often perceived by the client as childish and meaningless.

22. c. Rationale: Unilateral neglect, or neglect syndrome, occurs when the client with a stroke is unaware of the affected side of the body and puts the client at risk for injury. During the acute phase the affected side is cared for by the nurse with positioning and support, but during rehabilitation the client is taught to consciously care for and attend to the affected side of the body to protect it from injury. Clients may be positioned on the affected side for up to 30 minutes.

23. c. Rationale: Clients with left-brain damage from stroke often experience emotional lability, inappropriate emotional responses, mood swings, and uncontrolled tears or laughter that are out of context with the situation. The behaviour is upsetting and embarrassing to both the client and the family, and the client should be distracted to minimize its presence. Clients with right-brain damage often have impulsive, rapid behaviour that requires supervision and direction.

24. d. Rationale: The client and family need accurate and complete information about the effects of the stroke in order to problem solve and make plans for chronic care of the client. It is uncommon for clients with major strokes to return completely to prestroke function, behaviours, and role, and both the client and family will grieve these losses. The client's specific needs for care must be identified, and rehabilitation efforts should be continued at home. Family therapy and support groups may be helpful for some clients and families.

**Case Study**

1. A CT scan or MRI would be able to determine the size and location of a lesion and differentiate between an infarction and a hemorrhage. A lumbar puncture would not be indicated because of the chance that hemorrhage had increased intracranial pressure. Other tests that might be used when hemorrhage is evident include intra-arterial angiography, digital subtraction angiography, and transcranial Doppler sonography.

2. Unconsciousness, GCS score of 5, and wide pulse pressure with a decrease in pulse and respiration all indicate increased intracranial pressure.

3. The loss of consciousness is associated with a poor prognosis for recovery, and the family should be told that her condition is very guarded.

4. The highest priorities for interventions are those that support her life processes: airway and respiratory function with oxygen administration, fluid management without overloading the vascular system, and measures that decrease intracranial pressure.

5. Anything that impairs clotting is contraindicated in a hemorrhagic stroke: anticoagulants, antiplatelet agents, thrombolytic therapy. Hyperosmolar diuretics are also contraindicated because they may escape from an injured vessel, causing increased edema in brain tissue.

6. Hypothermia and barbiturate therapy may be used, but these treatments have not proved effective. Surgery is the only other option, and clipping of an aneurysm may be performed, or the aneurysm may be wrapped or reinforced with muscle.

7. *Nursing diagnoses:*
   - Ineffective cerebral tissue perfusion related to hemorrhage
   - Ineffective airway clearance related to unconsciousness
   - Self-care deficit related to altered mental state
   - Risk for injury related to inability to monitor personal safety
   - Risk for infection related to immobility
   *Collaborative problems:*
   Potential complications: increased intracranial pressure; brain herniation; seizures

# CHAPTER 57

1. a. 3; b. 1; c. 2; d. 1; e. 3; f. 1; g. 3; h. 3; i. 2; j. 3; k. 2; l. 2

2. d. Rationale: The primary way to diagnose and differentiate between functional headaches is with a careful history of the headaches, requiring assessment of specific details related to the headache. EMGs may reveal contraction of the neck, scalp, or facial muscles in tension-type headaches, but this is not seen in all clients. CT scans and cerebral angiography are used to rule out organic causes of the headaches.

3. d. Rationale: Both migraine headaches and cluster headaches appear to be related to vasodilation of cranial vessels, and drugs that have a vasopressor action, especially sumatriptan, are useful in treatment of migraine and cluster headaches. Methysergide is an ergot alkaloid that blocks serotonin receptors in the central and peripheral nervous systems and is used for treatment of migraine headaches and prevention of cluster headaches. β-blockers and tricyclic antidepressants are used prophylactically for migraine headaches but are not effective for cluster headaches.

4. a. Rationale: When the anxiety is related to a lack of knowledge about the etiology and treatment of a headache, helping the client to identify stressful lifestyles and other precipitating factors and ways of avoiding them is an appropriate nursing intervention for the anxiety. Interventions that teach alternative therapies to supplement drug therapy also give the client some control over pain and are appropriate teaching regarding treatment of the headache. The other interventions may help reduce anxiety generally, but they do not address the etiological factor of the anxiety.

5. a. Rationale: Projectile vomiting is characteristic of brain tumours and other causes of increased intracranial pressure and is not associated with functional headaches. Nausea with vomiting may be present with migraine headaches, however, in addition to visual disturbances, weakness and paralysis, and paraesthesias and confusion.

6. d. Rationale: Generalized seizures have bilateral synchronous epileptic discharge affecting the entire brain at the onset of the seizure, preventing any warning or aura. Loss of consciousness is also characteristic, but many partial seizures also include a loss of consciousness. Partial seizures begin in one side of the brain but may spread to involve the entire brain. Partial seizures that start with a local focus and spread to the entire brain, causing a secondary generalized seizure, are associated with a transient residual neurological deficit post-ictally known as Todd's paralysis.

7. a. 2; b. 4; c. 7; d. 1; e. 3; f. 6; g. 1; h. 5; i. 2; j. 7; k. 7; l. 1; m. 7; n. 4

8. a. F, kindling; b. T; c. T; d. F, client history and description of seizure; e. F, first time or status; f. T

9. c. Rationale: A seizure is a paroxysmal, uncontrolled discharge of neurons in the brain, which interrupts normal function, but the factor that

causes the abnormal firing is not clear. Seizures may be precipitated by many factors, and although scar tissue may stimulate seizures, it is not the usual cause of seizures. Epilepsy is established only by a pattern of spontaneous, recurring seizures.

10. b. Rationale: Most clients with seizure disorders maintain seizure control with medications, but if surgery is considered, three requirements must be met: the diagnosis of epilepsy must be confirmed, there must have been an adequate trial with drug therapy without satisfactory results, and the electroclinical syndrome must be defined. The focal point must be localized, but the presence of scar tissue is not required.

11. d. Rationale: Serum levels of antiseizure drugs are monitored regularly to maintain therapeutic levels of the drug, above which clients are likely to experience toxic effects and below which seizures are likely to occur. EEGs have limited value in diagnosis of seizures and even less in monitoring seizure control.

12. c. Rationale: If antiseizure drugs are discontinued abruptly, seizures can be precipitated, and clients should never just stop their medication. Missed doses should be made up if the omission is remembered within 24 hours, and clients should not adjust medications without professional guidance because this, too, can increase seizure frequency and may cause status epilepticus. If side effects occur, the physician should be notified and drug regimens evaluated. Antiseizure drugs have numerous interactions with other drugs, and the use of other medications should be evaluated by healthcare professionals.

13. a. Rationale: Maintaining an airway during a seizure is important and may involve turning the client to the side, supporting and protecting the head, or loosening constrictive clothing. Oral airways should not be inserted during the seizure, and restraining a client during a seizure may cause injury. Suctioning and oxygen administration may be required after the seizure has ended.

14. b. Rationale: In the post-ictal phase of generalized tonic-clonic seizures, clients are usually very tired and may sleep for several hours, and the nurse should allow the client to sleep as long as necessary. Suctioning is performed only if it is needed, and decreased level of consciousness is not a problem post-ictally unless a head injury has occurred during the seizure.

15. b. Rationale: One of the most common complications of a seizure disorder is the effect it has on the client's lifestyle. This is because of the social stigma attached to seizures, causing clients to hide their diagnosis and to prefer not to be identified as having epilepsy. Job discrimination is a serious problem for people with seizure disorders, but minimizing the effect of the condition is not the client's responsibility—he or she should seek the protection already granted by law, applying to the Canadian Human Rights Commission if necessary. In addition, clients need to identify their disease to employers in case of medical emergencies. Medication regimens usually require only once- or twice-daily dosing, and the major restrictions of lifestyle usually involve driving and high-risk environments.

16. a. 3; b. 5; c. 4; d. 2; e. 1

17. b. Rationale: Most clients with MS have remissions and exacerbations of neurological dysfunction that eventually cause progressive loss of motor, sensory, and cerebellar functions. Intellectual function generally remains intact, but clients may experience anger, depression, or euphoria. A few people have chronic progressive deterioration, and some may experience only occasional and mild symptoms for several years after onset.

18. c. Rationale: Motor and sensory dysfunctions, including paraesthesias as well as patchy blindness, blurred vision, and hearing loss, are the most common manifestations of MS. Bowel and bladder dysfunctions and ataxia also occur, but excessive involuntary movements, tremors, and memory loss are not seen in MS.

19. d. Rationale: There is no specific diagnostic test for MS, and a diagnosis is made primarily by history and clinical manifestations. In later MS, CT and MRI may detect sclerotic plaques. Some clients have elevations of oligoclonal immunoglobulin G, lymphocytes, and monocytes in cerebrospinal fluid, but these findings do not establish a diagnosis of MS.

20. b. Rationale: Mitoxantrone (Novantrone) is an immunosuppressant drug that reduces both B and T lymphocytes and impairs antigen presentation. It is similar to other immunosuppressants in that it increases the risk for infection, but it cannot be used for more than two to three years because it causes cardiac toxicity. It is administered IV monthly.

21. c. Rationale: The main goal in care of the client with MS is to keep the client active and maximally functional, promoting self-care as much as possible to maintain independence. Assistive devices encourage independence while preserving the client's energy. No care that clients can do for themselves should be performed by others. Involvement of the family in the client's care and maintenance of social interactions are also important but are not the priority in care.

22. b. Rationale: Corticosteroids used in treating acute exacerbations should not be abruptly stopped by the client because adrenal insufficiency may result, and prescribed tapering doses should be followed. Infections may cause exacerbations of symptoms and should be avoided, and high-protein diets with vitamin supplements are advocated. Long-term planning for increasing disability is also important.

23. a. Tremor: impaired handwriting and hand activities
    b. Rigidity: muscle soreness and pain; slowness of movement
    c. Bradykinesia: lack of blinking, arm swinging while walking, and facial expression; shuffling gait; difficulty initiating movement

24. b. Rationale: Although clinical manifestations are characteristic in Parkinson's disease, there are no laboratory or diagnostic tests specific for the condition. A diagnosis is made when there are at least two of the three signs of the classic triad, and it is confirmed with a positive response to antiparkinsonian medication. Essential tremors increase during voluntary movement, while the tremors of Parkinson's disease are more prominent at rest.

25. c. Rationale: The bradykinesia of Parkinson's disease prevents automatic movements, and such activities as beginning to walk, rising from a chair, or even swallowing saliva cannot be executed unless they are consciously willed. Handwriting is affected by the tremor and results in the writing trailing off at the end of words. Specific limb weakness and muscle spasms are not characteristic of Parkinson's disease.

26. c. Rationale: Peripheral dopamine does not cross the blood–brain barrier, but its precursor, levodopa, is able to enter the brain, where it is converted to dopamine, increasing the supply that is deficient in Parkinson's disease. Other drugs used to treat Parkinson's disease include bromocriptine, which stimulates dopamine receptors in the basal ganglia, and amantadine, which is believed to promote the release of dopamine from brain neurons. Carbidopa is an agent that is usually administered with levodopa to prevent the levodopa from being metabolized in peripheral tissues before it can reach the brain.

27. a. Rationale: Speech and swallowing in the client with Parkinson's disease can be facilitated by massaging the client's facial and neck muscles to reduce the rigidity that makes chewing, swallowing, and talking difficult for the client. An upright position and suctioning if secretions are present are necessary to prevent aspiration during eating.

28. c. Rationale: The shuffling gait of Parkinson's disease causes the client to be off balance and at risk for falling. Teaching the client to use a wide stance with the feet apart, to lift the toes when walking, and to look ahead helps promote a more balanced gait. Use of an elevated toilet seat and rocking from side to side will enable a client to initiate movement. Canes and walkers are difficult for clients with Parkinson's disease to manoeuvre and may make the client more prone to injury.

29. b. Rationale: The reduction of acetylcholine (ACh) effect in myasthenia gravis (MG) is treated with acetylcholinesterase inhibitors, which prolong the action of ACh at the neuromuscular synapse, but too much of these drugs causes a cholinergic crisis with symptoms very similar to those of MG. To determine whether the client's manifestations are due to a deficiency of ACh or too much anticholinesterase drug, the anticholinesterase drug edrophonium chloride (Tensilon) is administered. If the client is in cholinergic crisis, the client's symptoms will become worse, but if the client is in a myasthenic crisis, the client will improve.

30. c. Rationale: The client in myasthenic crisis has severe weakness and fatigability of all skeletal muscles, affecting the client's ability to swallow, talk, move, and breathe, but the priority of nursing care is monitoring and maintaining adequate ventilation.

31. c. Rationale: Restless legs syndrome that is not related to other pathological processes, such as diabetes mellitus or rheumatic disorders, may be caused by an alteration in dopaminergic transmission in the basal ganglia because dopaminergic agents, such as those used for parkinsonism, are effective in managing sensory and motor symptoms. Polysomnography studies during sleep are the only tests that have diagnostic value, and although exercise should be encouraged, excessive leg exercise does not have an effect on the symptoms.

32. b. Rationale: In ALS there is gradual degeneration of motor neurons with extreme muscle wasting from lack of stimulation and use. However, cognitive function is not impaired, and clients feel trapped in a dying body. Chorea manifested by writhing, involuntary movements is characteristic of Huntington's disease. As an autosomal dominant genetic disease, Huntington's disease also has a 50% chance of being passed to each offspring.

33. c. Rationale: Many chronic neurological diseases involve progressive deterioration in physical or mental capabilities and have no cure, with devas-

tating results for clients and families. Healthcare providers can only attempt to alleviate physical symptoms, prevent complications, and assist clients in maximizing function and self-care abilities as long as possible.

**Case Study**

1. The cause of MS is unknown, although research findings suggest MS is related to infectious (viral), immunological, and genetic factors. T cells are activated by some unknown factor, and these T cells migrate to the CNS and cause a disruption in the blood–brain barrier. Subsequent antigen–antibody reaction within the CNS results in activation of the inflammatory response, and through multiple mechanisms, destruction of the myelin of axons occurs. There is loss of myelin, disappearance of oligodendrocytes, and proliferation of astrocytes. These changes result in characteristic plaque formation, or sclerosis, scattered through the CNS and loss of nerve impulse transmission.

2. The role of precipitating factors, such as exposure to pathogenic agents, in the etiology of MS is controversial. It is possible that their association with MS is random and that there is no cause-and-effect relationship. Possible precipitating factors include emotional stress, excessive fatigue, pregnancy, and a poorer state of health. In Ms. S.'s case, it is possible that the viral neuritis was a precipitating factor.

3. Because there is no definitive diagnostic test for MS, diagnosis is based primarily on history and clinical manifestations. Although MRI can detect sclerotic plaques, a "wait-and-see" approach is often taken with non-specific, transient symptoms such as those Ms. S. originally experienced.

4. Client education should focus on preventing exacerbations or worsening of the disease. Building general resistance to illness, including avoiding fatigue, stress, extremes of heat and cold, and exposure to infection, are important measures in maintaining general health. Vigorous and early treatment of infection is critical if it does occur. It is important to teach the client to (1) achieve a good balance of exercise and rest, (2) eat nutritious and well-balanced meals, and (3) avoid the hazards of immobility (contractures and pressure sores). Clients should know their treatment regimens, the side effects of medications and how to watch for them, and drug interactions with over-the-counter medications. The client should consult a health care provider before taking non-prescription medications.

5. Because there is no cure for MS, treatment is aimed at slowing the disease process and providing symptomatic relief. The disease process is treated with drugs, and the symptoms are controlled with a variety of medications and other forms of therapy. Corticosteroids are helpful in treating acute exacerbations of the disease, probably by reducing edema and acute inflammation at the site of demyelination. Immunosuppressive drugs, such as azathioprine (Imuran), cyclosporine (Sandimmune), and cyclophosphamide (Cytoxan), have been shown to produce some beneficial effects in clients with severe and relapsing MS. A new immunosuppressant drug, mitoxantrone (Novantrone), reduces both B and T lymphocytes. However, the potential benefits of these drugs in clients with MS need to be counterbalanced against the potentially serious side effects. Immunomodulator drugs, such as interferon β-1b (Betaseron), interferon β-1a (Avonex), and glatiramer acetate (Copaxone), have been effective in reducing frequency and severity of exacerbations, but all of these agents must be administered parenterally. Physical therapy and speech therapy may also help improve neurological function.

6. *Nursing diagnoses:*
   - Ineffective role performance
   - Anxiety
   - Disturbed sensory perception: visual
   - Risk for impaired parenting
   *Collaborative problems:*
   Potential complication: blindness

# CHAPTER 58

1. a. Rationale: Conditions that decrease the CNS production of acetylcholine are believed to be a critical factor in the development of delirium. Clients with Parkinson's disease are treated with anticholinergics to help balance the deficiency of dopamine characteristic of Parkinson's disease, and these anticholinergics decrease the acetylcholine in the brain. It is true that delirium and Parkinson's disease are seen in older people, but the relationship is more specific than just age.

2. d. Rationale: Cytokines, such as interferons and interleukins, that are increased during infection, inflammation, and cancer, and even treatment of various disorders with cytokines, are believed to be related to the development of delirium.

3. a. age; b. infection (cytokines); c. hypoxemia (lung disease); d. ICU hospitalization (change in environment, sensory overload); e. pre-existing dementia; f. dehydration; g. hyperthermia

4. d. Rationale: Delirium is an acute problem that usually has a rapid onset in response to a precipitating event, especially when the client has underlying health problems, such as heart disease and sensory limitations. In the absence of prior cognitive impairment, a sudden onset of confusion, disorientation, and agitation is usually delirium. Delirium may manifest with both hypo- and hyperactive symptoms.

5. c. Rationale: Care of the client with delirium is focused on identifying and eliminating precipitating factors if possible. Treatment of underlying medical conditions, changing environmental conditions, and discontinuing medications that induce delirium are important. Drug therapy is reserved for those clients with severe agitation, because the drugs themselves may worsen delirium.

6. a. DL; b. DM; c. DL; d. DL; e. DM; f. DL; g. DM; h. DM; i. DL; j. DM

7. a. T; b. F, vascular; c. T; d. T; e. F, amyloid-β protein

8. a. Rationale: Depression is often associated with Alzheimer's disease, especially early in the disease when the client has awareness of the diagnosis and the progression of the disease. When dementia and depression occur together, intellectual deterioration may be more extreme. Depression is treatable, and use of antidepressants often improves cognitive function.

9. c. Rationale: The only definitive diagnosis of Alzheimer's disease can be made on examination of brain tissue on autopsy, but a clinical diagnosis is made when all other possible causes of dementia have been eliminated. Client's with Alzheimer's disease may have amyloid-β proteins in the blood, brain atrophy, or isoprostanes in the urine, but these findings are not exclusive to those with Alzheimer's disease.

10. c. Rationale: The Mini-Mental State Examination is a tool to document the degree of cognitive impairment and can be used to determine a baseline from which changes over time can be evaluated. It does not evaluate mood or thought processes but can detect dementia and delirium and differentiate these from psychiatric mental illness. A score of 30 indicates full cognitive function.

11. b. Rationale: Because there is no cure for AD, collaborative management is aimed at improving or controlling decline in cognition and controlling the undesirable manifestations that the client may exhibit. Anticholinesterase agents help increase acetylcholine in the brain, but a variety of other drugs are also used to control behaviour. Memory enhancement techniques have little or no effect in clients with Alzheimer's disease, especially as the disease progresses. Clients with Alzheimer's disease have limited ability to communicate health symptoms and problems, leading to lack of professional attention for acute and other chronic illnesses.

12. a. 3, 10; b. 4, 9; c. 1, 8; d. 6, 8; e. 5, 9; f. 7, 11; g. 3, 8; h. 2, 10; i. 5, 9; j. 1, 8; k. 2, 10

13. c. Rationale: Adhering to a regular, consistent daily schedule helps the client avoid confusion and anxiety and is important both during hospitalization and at home. Clocks and calendars may be useful in early Alzheimer's disease, but they have little meaning to a client as the disease progresses. Questioning the client about activities and events they cannot remember is threatening and may cause severe anxiety. Maintaining a safe environment for the client is important but does not change the disturbed thought processes.

14. b. Rationale: Caregiver role strain is characterized by such symptoms of stress as inability to sleep, make decisions, or concentrate and is frequently seen in family members who are responsible for the care of the client with Alzheimer's disease. Assessment of the caregiver may reveal a need for assistance to increase coping skills, effectively use community resources, or maintain social relationships. Eventually the demands on a caregiver exceed the resources, and the person with Alzheimer's disease may be placed in an institutional setting.

15. a. Rationale: Adult day care is an option to provide respite for caregivers and a protective environment for the client during the early and middle stages of AD. The respite from the demands of care allows the caregiver to maintain social contacts and perform normal tasks of living and be more responsive to the client's needs. Visits by home care nurses involve the caregiver and cannot provide adequate respite. Institutional placement is not always an acceptable option at earlier stages of AD, nor is hospitalization an acceptable form of respite care.

**Case Study**

1. The pathophysiology of Alzheimer's disease includes cellular changes with neurofibrillary tangles with altered tau proteins and neuritic plaques containing amyloid-β protein in the cerebral cortex and hippocampus. Excessive loss of cholinergic neurons is also present, and other neurotransmitters, such as serotonin and norepinephrine, are also lost over time.

2. Alzheimer's disease is diagnosed by exclusion. When all other possible causes of mental impair-

ment and persistence of dementia are ruled out, the diagnosis of Alzheimer's remains. Brain atrophy and enlarged ventricles seen in some clients with Alzheimer's disease are also seen in normal people and in other conditions. Only on autopsy can Alzheimer's disease be confirmed by the presence of neurofibrillary tangles in brain tissue.

3. All functions of mental capacity and ability to care for oneself are lost as the disease progresses. There will be deterioration of personal hygiene and all activities of daily living, progression of psychotic symptoms now evidenced by his hallucinations, loss of long-term memory and recognition of his family, and loss of communication.

4. Assess what she is doing now to manage his care. Teach her about the expected progression of the disease, and assist her in planning respite care or arranging for home health assistants. Help her identify problem areas. Encourage her to keep Mr. D. awake and busy during the day so that he will sleep better at night, and so will she.

5. Community resources may include Alzheimer's support groups, adult day care, home health assistants and home nursing, and various forms of assisted living and long-term care facilities.

6. *Nursing diagnoses:*
   - Risk for injury related to impaired judgement, nighttime wandering
   - Risk for other-directed violence related to misinterpretation of environmental stimuli
   - Disturbed thought processes related to effects of dementia
   - Wandering related to cognitive impairment
   - Disturbed sleep pattern related to circadian asynchrony

   *Collaborative problems:*
   Potential complication: psychosis

7. Nursing diagnoses:
   - Anxiety related to erratic behavioural patterns and cognitive decline of husband
   - Altered health maintenance related to fatigue and chronic stress
   - Caregiver role strain related to grieving the family member's illness
   - Risk for other-directed violence (client abuse) related to ineffective coping

   *Collaborative problems:*
   Potential complication: depression

## CHAPTER 59

1. a. T; b. F, Bell's palsy; c. F, corticosteroids; d. F, Bell's palsy; e. T; f. T

2. a. Rationale: The pain of trigeminal neuralgia is excruciating, and it may occur in clusters that continue for hours. The condition is considered benign with no major effects except the pain. Corneal exposure is a problem in Bell's palsy, or it may occur following surgery for treatment of trigeminal neuralgia. Maintenance of nutrition is important but not urgent, because chewing may trigger trigeminal neuralgia and clients avoid eating. Except during an attack, there is no change in facial appearance in a client with trigeminal neuralgia, and body image is more disturbed in response to the paralysis typical of Bell's palsy.

3. a. Rationale: Although percutaneous radiofrequency rhizotomy and microvascular decompression provide the greatest relief of pain, glycerol rhizotomy causes less sensory loss and fewer sensory aberrations with significant pain relief. The suboccipital craniotomy and microvascular decompression require a cranial incision and carry the highest risk for complications.

4. c. Rationale: Because attacks of trigeminal neuralgia may be precipitated by hot or cold air movement on the face, jarring movements, or talking, the environment should be of moderate temperature and free of drafts, and clients should not be expected to converse during the acute period. Clients often prefer to carry out their own care because they are afraid someone else may inadvertently injure them or precipitate an attack. The nurse should stress that oral hygiene be performed because clients often avoid it, but residual food in the mouth after eating occurs more frequently with Bell's palsy.

5. a. Rationale: The most serious complication of Guillain-Barré syndrome is respiratory failure, and it is essential that vital capacity and ABGs are monitored to detect involvement of the nerves that affect respiration. Corticosteroids may be used in treatment but do not appear to have an effect on the prognosis or duration of the disease. Rather, plasmapheresis or administration of high-dose immunoglobulin does result in shortening recovery time. The peripheral nerves of both the sympathetic and parasympathetic nervous systems are involved in the disease and may lead to orthostatic hypotension, hypertension, and abnormal vagal responses affecting the heart. Guillain-Barré syndrome may affect the lower brainstem and CNs VII, VI, III, XII, V, and X, affecting facial, eye, and swallowing functions.

6. c. Rationale: As nerve involvement ascends, it is very frightening for the client, but more than 85% of clients with Guillain-Barré syndrome recover completely with care. Clients also recover if ventilatory support is provided during respiratory failure, although 5% to 10% of clients die from

respiratory failure or cardiac arrhythmias. Guillain-Barré syndrome affects only peripheral nerves and does not affect the brain.

7. a. 3; b. 1; c. 2; d. 1; e. 2; f. 3; g. 2; h. 1; i. 2; j. 3; k. 1

8. d. Rationale: Spinal cord injuries are highest in young men between the ages of 15 and 30 and those who are impulsive or risk takers in daily living. Other risk factors include alcohol and drug abuse as well as participation in sports and occupational exposure to trauma or violence.

9. b. Rationale: Tetraplegia with motor and sensory loss is characteristic of a complete cord injury at the level of C8, with paraplegia with motor and sensory loss at the level of T1. A hemiplegia occurs with central (brain) lesions affecting motor and sensory function, and any partial loss of function is associated with incomplete spinal cord lesions.

10. a. 5; b. 4; c. 1; d. 3; e. 2

11. c. Rationale: The primary injury of the spinal cord rarely affects the entire cord, but the pathophysiology of secondary injury may result in damage that is the same as mechanical severance of the cord. Complete cord dissolution occurs through autodestruction of the cord by hemorrhage, edema, and the presence of metabolites and norepinephrine, resulting in anoxia and infarction of the cord. Edema secondary to the inflammatory response may increase the damage as it extends above and below the injury site.

12. c. Rationale: Spinal shock occurs in about half of all people with acute spinal cord injury. In spinal shock, the entire cord below the level of the lesion fails to function, resulting in a flaccid paralysis and hypomotility of most processes without any reflex activity. Return of reflex activity signals the end of spinal shock. Sympathetic function is impaired below the level of the injury because sympathetic nerves leave the spinal cord at the thoracic and lumbar areas, and cranial parasympathetic nerves predominate in control over respirations, heart, and all vessels and organs below the injury. Neurogenic shock results from loss of vascular tone caused by the injury and is manifested by hypotension, peripheral vasodilation, and decreased cardiac output. Rehabilitation activities are not contraindicated during spinal shock and should be instituted if the client's cardiopulmonary status is stable.

13. b. Rationale: Until the edema and necrosis at the site of the injury are resolved in 72 hours to one week after the injury, it is not possible to determine how much cord damage is present from the initial injury, how much secondary injury occurred, or how much the cord was damaged by edema that extended above the level of the original injury. The return of reflexes signals only the end of spinal shock, and the reflexes may be inappropriate and excessive, causing spasms that complicate rehabilitation.

14. a. Above T5; b. Above C4; c. Below C4; d. Above L3

15. b. Rationale: Care of the client during the acute phase, when the influence of the sympathetic nervous system is decreased, includes monitoring for bradycardia, which can compromise cardiac output and lead to hypoxemia because of the effect of the vagus nerve on the heart and vessels. Anything that causes vagal stimulation may cause cardiac arrest, and cardiovascular instability is a major complication of unopposed vagal stimulation. Return of reflexes, effects of sensory deprivation, and fluctuations in body temperature should also be monitored, but they do not have the priority that cardiovascular status does.

16. a. 7; b. 3; c. 9; d. 7; e. 1; f. 6

17. d. Rationale: Although surgical treatment of spinal cord injuries often depends on the preference of the physician, surgery is usually indicated when there is continued compression of the cord by extrinsic forces or when there is evidence of cord compression. Other indications may include progressive neurological deficit, compound fracture of the vertebra, bony fragments, and penetrating wounds of the cord.

18. a. Rationale: The need for a patent airway is the first priority for any injured client, and a high cervical injury may decrease gag reflex and ability to maintain an airway, as well as the ability to breathe. Maintaining cervical stability is then a consideration, along with assessing for other injuries and the client's neurological status.

19. c. Rationale: Cervical injuries usually require skeletal traction with the use of Crutchfield, Vinke, or other types of skull tongs to immobilize the cervical vertebrae, even if fracture has not occurred. Hard cervical collars are used for minor injuries or for stabilization during emergency transport of the client. Sandbags are also used temporarily to stabilize the neck during insertion of tongs or during diagnostic testing immediately following the injury. Special turning or kinetic beds may be used to turn and mobilize clients who are in cervical traction.

20. d. Rationale: Early, large-dose methylprednisolone is standard treatment for spinal cord injuries because it has been found to improve blood flow and reduce edema in the spinal cord following injury. Tirilazad (Freedox) has the same use as methylprednisolone with perhaps fewer adverse effects. Other vasoactive drugs for

spinal cord damage are currently being studied. Dopamine and IV fluids are used to maintain blood pressure during the initial stage of injury.

21. b. Rationale: Because pneumonia and atelectasis are potential problems related to ineffective coughing and the loss of intercostal and abdominal muscle function, the nurse should frequently monitor the client for breath sounds and respiratory function to determine whether secretions are being retained or whether there is progression of respiratory impairment. Suctioning is not indicated unless lung sounds indicate retained secretions, and the prone position, although used for positioning clients with spinal cord injuries, can compromise respiratory function. Intubation and mechanical ventilation are used if the client becomes exhausted from laboured breathing or if ABGs deteriorate.

22. c. Rationale: During the first two to three days after a spinal cord injury, paralytic ileus may occur, and nasogastric suction must be used to remove secretions and gas from the gastrointestinal tract until peristalsis resumes. IV fluids are used to maintain fluid balance but do not specifically relate to paralytic ileus. Tube feedings would be used only for clients who had difficulty swallowing and not until peristalsis returned, and TPN would be used only if the paralytic ileus were unusually prolonged.

23. a. Rationale: During the acute phase of spinal cord injury, the bladder is hypotonic, causing urinary retention with the risk for reflux into the kidney or rupture of the bladder. An indwelling catheter is used to keep the bladder empty and closely monitor urinary output. Intermittent catheterization and/or other urinary drainage methods may be used in long-term bladder management. Use of incontinent pads is inappropriate because the bladder fails to empty.

24. b. Rationale: In one week following a spinal cord injury, there may be a resolution of the edema of the injury and an end to spinal shock. When spinal shock ends, reflex movement and spasms will occur, which may be mistaken for return of function, but with the resolution of edema, some normal function may also occur. It is important when movement occurs to determine whether the movement is voluntary and can be consciously controlled, which would indicate some return of function.

25. b. Rationale: Manifestations of autonomic dysreflexia include severe hypertension, bradycardia, headache, blurred vision, and flushing and diaphoresis above the level of the lesion, and it is a life-threatening situation. At the first indication, the nurse should check the client's blood pressure, raise the head of the bed to 45 degrees, check for the stimulus that is causing the reaction (usually a distended bladder or rectum), and notify the physician if it is apparent that the problem is autonomic dysreflexia.

26. d. Rationale: A neurogenic bladder is any type of bladder dysfunction related to abnormal or absent bladder innervation and occurs not only with spinal cord injury but also with many other conditions as well. To determine what function the bladder has, diagnostic evaluation must be performed with cystometrograms and perhaps an IV pyelogram and urine culture before appropriate interventions can be instituted. The bladder may have various degrees of flaccidity or spasticity.

27. d. Rationale: Intermittent catheterization five to six times a day is the recommended method of bladder management for the client with a spinal cord injury because it more closely mimics normal emptying and has less potential for infection. The client and family should be taught the procedure using clean technique, and if the client has use of the arms, self-catheterization should be performed. Indwelling catheterization is used during the acute phase to prevent overdistension of the bladder, and suprapubic indwelling catheters and surgical urinary diversions are used if urinary complications occur.

28. d. Rationale: Most clients with a complete lower motor neuron lesion are unable to have either psychogenic or reflexogenic erections, and alternative methods of obtaining sexual satisfaction may be suggested. Clients with incomplete lower motor neuron lesions have the highest possibility of successful psychogenic erections with ejaculation, while clients with incomplete upper motor neuron lesions are more likely to experience reflexogenic erections with ejaculation. Clients with complete upper motor neuron lesions usually only have reflex sexual function with rare ejaculation.

29. a. Rationale: Working through the grief process is a lifelong process that is triggered by new experiences, such as marriage, child rearing, employment, or illness, which the client must adjust to throughout life within the context of his or her disability. The goal of recovery is related to adjustment, rather than acceptance, and many clients do not experience all components of the grief process. During the anger phase, clients should be allowed outbursts, and the nurse should use humour to displace some of the client's anger.

30. b. Rationale: Most metastatic tumours are extradural lesions that may be successfully removed surgically. Most tumours of the spinal cord are slow growing, do not cause autodestruc-

tion and, with the exception of intradural-intramedullary tumours, can be removed with complete functional restoration. Radiation is used to treat metastatic tumours that are sensitive to radiation and that have caused only minor neurological deficits in the client; radiation also is used as adjuvant therapy to surgery for intramedullary tumours.

**Case Study**

1. Susan is experiencing central cord syndrome of the cervical cord, in which there is compression on anterior horn cells. It usually occurs as a result of hyperextension.
2. The cell bodies of lower motor neurons, which send axons to innervate the skeletal muscles of arms, trunk, and legs, are located in the anterior horn of the spinal cord. The cervical segments of the spinal cord contain the lower motor neurons for the arms, and a cervical injury that affects the anterior horn will affect the arms to a greater extent than the legs.
3. Injury to the cord may occur without fracture of the vertebrae, with traumatic twisting or stretching of the cord. The response to the trauma includes secondary injury leading to edema, hemorrhage, and ischemia of the cord, impairing function.
4. Methylprednisolone has been found to improve blood flow and reduce edema in the spinal cord, with the effects of reduction of post-traumatic spinal cord ischemia, improvement of energy balance, restoration of extracellular calcium, improvement of nerve impulse condition, and repression of the release of free fatty acids from spinal cord tissues.
5. Shock and denial are common first reactions to the loss of function with spinal cord injuries, fol-

lowed by anger and depression. During the acute phase, Susan will probably have unrealistic expectations concerning her recovery, sleep a lot, and withdraw. As she progresses she will become angry and refuse to discuss her limitations. Altered body image will be a big problem because she will see herself as different from her peers, an important developmental issue during adolescence.
6. Intensive rehabilitation that focuses on refined retraining of physiological function of her limbs should be planned and will involve much physiotherapy over time. She should be mobilized as quickly as appropriate to prevent hazards of immobility and to encourage her in her progress.
7. *Nursing diagnoses:*
   • Impaired physical mobility related to spinal cord injury and prescribed bed rest
   • Risk for disuse syndrome related to immobilization
   • Self-care deficit: feeding, bathing/hygiene, and grooming related to upper extremity weakness
   • Risk for injury related to sensory deficit and lack of self-protective abilities
   *Collaborative problems:*
   Potential complications: progression of lesion; hypoventilation; spinal shock

## CHAPTER 60

1. a. epiphysis; b. metaphysis; c. diaphysis; d. periosteum; e. compact bone; f. bone marrow; g. medullary cavity; h. epiphyseal growth plate; i. cancellous bone; j. articular cartilage
2. a. periosteum; b. canaliculi; c. haversian canal; d. blood vessels; e. haversian system (osteon)
3. a. joint cavity; b. bursa; c. articular cartilage; d. periosteum; e. joint capsule; f. nerve; g. blood vessel; h. synovial membrane; i. bone

4. a. haversian; b. sarcomere; c. epiphysis; d. osteo-
   cyte; e. tendon; f. periosteum; g. synovium;
   h. isometric; i. calcium; j. canaliculi; k. osteoclast; l. atrophy; m. actin; n. bursae; o. osteoblast;
   p. cartilage; q. ligament; r. fascia; s. hyaline;
   t. striated

5. a. 1; b. 1, 2, 3; c. 1, 2, 3; d. 4; e. 1, 2, 3; f. 1;
   g. 1, 2, 3

6. d. Rationale: Loss of water from discs between
   vertebrae, vertebral disc compression, and narrowing of intervertebral spaces all contribute to a
   loss of height in the older adult. Although bone
   density decreases and cartilage is lost from joints,
   these do not affect the long bones or the height of
   the person.

7. c. Rationale: Cartilage disruption and overgrowth
   of bone around joint margins that occur with
   aging result in joint stiffness and pain that most
   often affect physical mobility. Changes in the
   bones lead to decreased bone mass and the possibility of fractures. Fatigue and a high risk for
   impaired skin integrity are not directly related to
   changes in the musculoskeletal system that are
   associated with aging.

8. a. Rationale: Corticosteroids cause protein catabolism with skeletal muscle wasting and
   increased osteoclast activity with loss of bone
   mass, which can have a marked detrimental
   effect on mobility and activity. Potassium-
   depleting diuretics may cause hypokalemia,
   which is associated with muscle weakness and
   cramps. Oral hypoglycemic drugs and NSAIDs
   are not known to have an effect on the musculoskeletal system.

9. a. History of musculoskeletal injuries, poor use
   of body mechanics or excessive muscular
   stress, family history of joint and bone disease
   b. Presence of obesity, inadequate calcium, vitamin D or C, or protein intake
   c. Inability to physically access toilet; constipation
   d. Limitation of movement; pain, weakness,
   crepitus; extremes of occupational activity—
   sedentary or heavy use of body
   e. Pain interfering with sleep; frequent position
   changes
   f. Musculoskeletal pain; pain management measures
   g. Loss of body image or self-worth, caused by
   musculoskeletal deformity
   h. Change in work and family roles and responsibilities, caused by immobility or pain
   i. Decreased sexual activity and satisfaction
   because of pain, deformity
   j. Decreased coping ability related to effect of
   musculoskeletal problems

10. c. Rationale: Muscle strength is graded on a scale of 0 to 5, with 0 = no detection of muscle strength and 5 = active movement against full resistance (normal). Active movement against gravity and some resistance = 4.

11. b. Rationale: There is no indication to measure the length of limbs during assessment unless a gait disturbance or limb-length discrepancy is noted, and then the limb should be measured between two bony prominences and compared with the measurement of the opposite extremity. Muscle mass measurement and joint movement may affect gait, but differences in limb length will always affect gait. Palpating for crepitus will identify friction between bones, usually at joints.

12. c. Rationale: A goniometer is a protractor device that measures the angle of joints and can be used to determine specific degrees of joint range of motion. It is used when a specific musculoskeletal problem has been identified that affects ROM.

13. a. 10; b. 7; c. 9; d. 1; e. 6; f. 8; g. 5; h. 4; i. 2; j. 3

14. a. Standard x-ray; b. Arthrocentesis; c. Discography; d. Dual-energy x-ray absorptiometry (DEXA); e. Electromyogram; f. Creatine kinase

15. a. Rheumatoid factor (RF); b. Erythrocyte sedimentation rate (ESR); c. Antinuclear antibody (ANA)

## CHAPTER 61

1. d. Rationale: Musculoskeletal problems in the older adult can be prevented with appropriate strategies, especially exercise. Almost all older adults have some degree of decreased muscle strength, joint stiffness, and pain with motion. The use of mild anti-inflammatory agents decreases inflammation and pain and can help the client maintain activity and prevent further deconditioning. Stair walking can create enough stress on fragile bones to cause a hip fracture, and use of ramps may help prevent falls. Walkers and canes should be used as necessary to decrease stress on joints so that activity can be maintained.

2. c. Rationale: Warm-up exercises "pre-lengthen" potentially strained tissues by avoiding the quick stretch often encountered in sports and also increase the temperature of muscle, resulting in increased speed of cell metabolism, increased speed of nerve impulses, and improved oxygenation of muscle fibres. Stretching is also thought to improve kinesthetic awareness, lessening the chance of uncoordinated movement. Taping or wrapping joints may actually predispose a person to injury, and muscle strength is not a key factor in soft-tissue injuries.

3. a. 8; b. 10; c. 6; d. 2; e. 9; f. 1; g. 3; h. 7; i. 4; j. 5

4. b. Rationale: Application of cold, compression, and elevation is indicated to prevent edema resulting from sprain and strain injury. Muscle spasms are usually treated with heat applications and massage, and repetitive strain injuries require cessation of the precipitating activity and physiotherapy. Dislocations or subluxations require immediate reduction and immobilization to prevent vascular impairment and bone cell death.

5. a. Rationale: Immobilization of a joint after the acute damage leads to muscle shortening, atrophy, and possible contractures. Gentle, progressive exercise is indicated to promote circulation and healing and increase muscle strength and function. Immobilization and rest, alternating use of heat and cold, and administration of anti-inflammatory drugs are indicated for management of acute soft tissue injury.

6. a. 4; b. 8; c. 5; d. 6; e. 1; f. 9; g. 2; h. 7; i. 10; j. 3

7. a. 3; b. 5; c. 1; d. 6; e. 2; f. 6; g. 2; h. 4; i. 6; j. 2; k. 5

8. b. Rationale: Deformity is the cardinal sign of fracture but may not be apparent in all fractures. Other supporting signs include edema and swelling, pain and tenderness, muscle spasm, ecchymosis, loss of function, and crepitation.

9. a. Rationale: A malunion occurs when the bone heals in the expected time but in an unsatisfactory position, possibly resulting in deformity or dysfunction. Non-union occurs when the fracture fails to heal properly despite treatment, and delayed union is healing of the fracture at a slower rate than expected. The loss of bone substances as a result of immobilization occurs in post-traumatic osteoporosis.

10. a. F, reduction; b. T; c. F, infection; d. F, skin; e. F, foot of the bed; f. T

11. d. Rationale: The suspension of the extremity provided by the use of a Thomas splint and Pearson attachment in balanced suspension traction allows the client to raise the body off the bed with the support of a trapeze and the unaffected leg. The client is not allowed to turn from side to side, but care is enhanced by upward elevation of the body. Because the other forms of skeletal and skin traction do not suspend the affected limbs, this movement is not possible.

12. a. Rationale: Basic maintenance of traction requires that weights hang free and consist of the prescribed amount of weight, ropes are intact and ride in the pulleys, knots are secure, and pulley clamps are firmly fastened to the bedframe. The client should be in direct alignment with the trac-

tion and should exercise the unaffected limb as much as possible to prevent complications of immobility.

13. d. Rationale: Complaints of abdominal pain or pressure, nausea, and vomiting are signs of cast syndrome that occur when body casts are applied too tightly, causing compression of the superior mesenteric artery against the duodenum. The cast may need to be split or removed, and the physician should be notified. Elevation is not indicated for a spica cast, and the client with a spica cast should not be placed in the prone position during the initial drying stage, because the cast is so large and heavy it may break. A cast should never be covered with a blanket because heat builds up in the cast and may increase edema.

14. b. Rationale: Infection is the greatest risk with an open fracture, and all open fractures are considered contaminated. Tetanus prevention is always indicated if the client has not been immunized or does not have current boosters. Prophylactic antibiotics are often used in management of open fractures, but recent antibiotic therapy is not relevant, nor are previous injuries to the site.

15. d. Rationale: Pulses distal to the injury should be checked before and after splinting to assess for nerve or vascular damage and documented to avoid doubts about whether a problem discovered later was missed during the original examination or was caused by the treatment. Elevation of the limb and application of ice should be instituted after the extremity is splinted.

16. b. Rationale: Neurological assessment includes evaluation of motor and sensory function and, in the upper extremity, includes abduction and adduction of the fingers, opposition of the fingers, and suppination and pronation of the hands. It would also include sensory perception in the fingers. Evaluation of the feet would occur in lower extremity injuries. Assessment of colour, temperature, capillary refill, peripheral pulses, and edema evaluates vascular status.

17. b. Rationale: A client with any type of cast should exercise the joints above and below the cast frequently, and moving the fingers frequently will improve circulation and help prevent edema. Unlike plaster casts, thermoplastic resin or fibreglass casts are relatively waterproof and, if they become wet, can be dried with a hair dryer on low setting. Tape petals are used on plaster casts to protect the edges from breaking and crumbling but are not necessary for synthetic casts. After the cast is applied, the extremity should be elevated at about the level of the heart to promote venous return, and ice may be used to prevent edema.

18. a. Rationale: A swing-to gait is a three-point gait in which the client places the crutches ahead of the unaffected leg and swings up to the level of the crutches, keeping weight off the affected leg. It is safer than a swing-through gait because it provides better balance and stability. Two-point and four-point gaits are used when at least partial weight bearing is allowed on the limb.

19. c. Rationale: Progressive pain that is distal to the injury and is unrelieved by usual analgesics is the earliest sign of compartment syndrome. Paralysis and absence of peripheral pulses will eventually occur if it is not treated, but these are late signs that often appear after permanent damage has occurred. The overlying skin may appear normal because the surface vessels are not occluded.

20. a. Paraesthesia; b. Pain; c. Pressure; d. Pallor; e. Paralysis; f. Pulselessness

21. a. Rationale: Soft tissue edema in the area of the injury may cause an increase of pressure within the closed spaces of the tissue compartments formed by the non-elastic fascia, creating a compartment syndrome. If symptoms occur, it may be necessary to surgically incise the fascia, a procedure known as a fasciotomy. Amputation is usually necessary only if the limb becomes septic because of untreated compartment syndrome.

22. a. Rationale: Initial manifestations of fat embolism usually occur 12 to 72 hours after injury and are associated with fractures of long bones and multiple fractures related to pelvic injuries, including fractures of the femur, tibia, ribs, and pelvis.

23. d. Rationale: Clients with fractures are at risk for both fat embolism and pulmonary embolism from peripheral thromboses, but there is a difference in the time of occurrence, with fat embolism occurring shortly after the injury and thrombotic embolism occurring several days after immobilization. They both may cause pulmonary symptoms of chest pain, tachypnea, dyspnea, apprehension, tachycardia, and cyanosis, but fat embolism may cause petechiae located around the neck, anterior chest wall, axilla, buccal membrane of the mouth, and conjunctiva of the eye, which differentiate it from thrombotic embolism.

24. a. 2; b. 3; c. 1; d. 7; e. 4; f. 2; g. 6; h. 5; i. 7; j. 1; k. 6; l. 3; m. 5; n. 4; o. 6

25. a. F, intracapsular; b. T; c. F, intracapsular; d. T; e. T

26. d. Rationale: The classic signs of a hip fracture are shortening of the leg and external rotation accompanied by severe pain at the fracture site. The client may not be able to move the hip or the knee, but movement in the ankle and toes is not affected.

27. c. Rationale: Although surgical repair is the preferred method of managing intracapsular and extracapsular hip fractures, initially clients may be treated with skin traction, such as Buck's extension or Russell's traction, to temporarily immobilize the limb and relieve the painful muscle spasms before surgery is performed. Prolonged traction would be required to reduce the fracture or immobilize it for healing, creating a very high risk for complications of immobility.

28. a. Rationale: Because the fracture site is internally fixed with pins or plates, the fracture site is stable, and the client is moved from the bed to the chair on the first post-operative day, with ambulation beginning on the first or second post-operative day, without weight bearing on the affected leg. Weight bearing on the affected extremity is usually restricted for three to five months until adequate healing is evident on x-ray. The client may be positioned on either side of the body following internal fixation, and abductor pillows are used for clients who have total hip replacements.

29. d. Rationale: Clients with hip prostheses must avoid extreme flexion, adduction, or internal rotation for at least six weeks to prevent dislocation of the prosthesis. Gradual weight bearing on the limb is allowed, and ambulation should be encouraged.

30. c. Rationale: The low-bulk, high-carbohydrate liquid diet and intake of air through a straw required during mandibular fixation often lead to constipation and flatus, which may be relieved with bulk-forming laxatives, prune juice, or ambulation. Wires or rubber bands should be cut only in the case of cardiac or respiratory arrest, and clients should be taught to clear their mouth of vomitus or secretions. The mouth should be thoroughly cleaned with water, saline, or alkaline mouthwashes or with the use of a Water Pik as necessary to remove food debris. Hard candy should not be held in the mouth.

31. b. Rationale: Clients with peripheral vascular disease often have extensive arterial impairment that necessitates removal of a limb much higher than is indicated by external signs of ischemia, in order for healing to occur. Preoperative arteriography and transcutaneous Doppler studies help determine the point at which blood supply is adequate for healing. As much limb as possible is preserved to enhance rehabilitation. Amputation does not alter the underlying vascular disease.

32. b. Rationale: The disruption in body image caused by an amputation often causes a client to go through psychological stages of grieving, and the client should be allowed to go through a period of depression as a normal consequence of the amputation. The grieving process is not ineffective coping or impaired adjustment but a normal process of adjusting to loss.

33. b. Rationale: Phantom sensation or phantom pain may occur following amputation, especially if pain was present in the affected limb preoperatively. The pain is a real sensation to the client and should be treated with analgesics and other pain interventions. As recovery and ambulation progress, phantom limb sensation usually subsides.

34. b. Rationale: An immediate prosthetic fitting involves the application of a rigid plastic bandage with a prosthetic pylon and ankle–foot assembly. Because the device covers the residual limb, the surgical site cannot be directly seen, and post-operative hemorrhage is not apparent on dressings, requiring vigilant assessment of vital signs for signs of bleeding. Elevation of the residual limb with an immediate prosthetic fitting is not necessary because the device itself prevents edema formation. Exercises to the leg are not performed in the immediate post-operative period, in order to prevent disruption of ligatures and the suture line.

35. a. Rationale: Flexion contractures, especially of the hip, may be debilitating and delay rehabilitation of the client with a leg amputation. To prevent hip flexion, the client should avoid sitting in a chair with the hips flexed or having pillows under the surgical extremity for prolonged periods, and the client should lie on the abdomen for 30 minutes three to four times a day to extend the hip.

36. a. Rationale: Skin breakdown on the residual limb can prevent the use of a prosthesis, and the limb should be inspected every day for signs of irritation or pressure areas. No substances except water and mild soap should be used on the residual limb, and ROM exercises are not necessary when the client is using a prosthesis. A residual limb shrinker is an elastic stocking that is used to mould the limb in preparation for prosthesis use, but a cotton residual limb sock is worn with the prosthesis.

37. a. 3; b. 4; c. 5; d. 1; e. 2

38. d. Rationale: Physical therapy is initiated one day post-operatively with ambulation and weight bearing with a walker for a client with a cemented prosthesis and non-weight bearing on the operative side for an uncemented prosthesis. In addition, the client is turned to both sides and back with support of the operative leg and sits in the chair at least twice a day.

39. b. Rationale: Following a total hip arthroplasty, extremes of internal rotation, adduction, and 90-degree flexion of the hip must be avoided for four to six weeks post-operatively to prevent dislocation of the prosthesis. During hospitalization an abduction pillow is placed between the legs to maintain abduction, and the leg is extended.

40. b. Rationale: Continuous passive motion machines are frequently used following knee surgery to promote earlier joint mobility, and because joint dislocation is not a problem with knee replacements, early exercise with straight leg raises and gentle ROM is also encouraged post-operatively.

41. b. Rationale: Neurovascular checks of the fingers following surgery of the hands are essential to detect compromised vascular and neurological function due to trauma or edema. Post-operatively the hands are elevated with a bulky dressing in place, and when the dressing is removed, a guided splinting program is started. Exercises are performed three to four times a day when the splints are removed and the client is discharged. Before surgery, it must be made clear to the client that the goal of the surgery is to restore function related to grasp, pinch, stability, and strength, and the hands will not necessarily have good cosmetic appearance.

**Case Study**

1. The knee and ankle should be immobilized with the splint. Unless the joints above and below the site are immobilized, the affected area is unstable.

2. A thorough neurovascular assessment consists of a peripheral vascular assessment (colour, temperature, capillary refill, peripheral pulses, and edema) and a peripheral neurological assessment (sensation, motor function, and pain). Both extremities are compared to obtain an accurate assessment.

3. The wound should be cleaned with extensive irrigation with normal saline, and if the wound is highly contaminated, surgical debridement may be necessary. Tetanus immunization is required if a dose of tetanus toxoid has not been given in the past five years, or if the client has had fewer than three doses of toxoid, tetanus immunoglobulin should be administered. Bleeding should be controlled with sterile dressings.

4. Measures to relieve pain include elevating the limb and applying ice to decrease swelling, administering analgesics, and keeping the limb immobilized.

5. It will take about 20 weeks for complete healing of the fracture, but ossification should take place in two to three weeks. At that time the limb can be casted, and he can be mobile with crutches with no weight bearing on the affected limb. Weight bearing will be restricted for six to twelve weeks, depending on the rate of healing. His return to work will depend on how he is able to perform his responsibilities on crutches.

6. Mrs. A. should be called and informed of her husband's accident, and she should be told that Mr. A. is alert and oriented but that he has a fractured leg and will require hospitalization. Care should be taken not to panic her and to reassure her that he is stable.

7. *Nursing diagnoses:*
   - Acute pain related to edema and muscle spasms
   - Risk for peripheral neurovascular dysfunction related to edema
   - Risk for infection related to disruption of skin integrity and presence of environmental pathogens
   - Anxiety related to unknown outcome and restrictions
   *Collaborative problems:*
   Potential complications: fat embolism; compartment syndrome; infection; malunion or non-union

# CHAPTER 62

1. c. Rationale: Chronic infection of the bone leads to formation of scar tissue from the granulation tissue. This avascular scar tissue provides an ideal site for continued micro-organism growth and is impenetrable to antibiotics. Surgical debridement is often necessary to remove the poorly vascularized tissue and dead bone and instill antibiotics directly to the area. Involucrum is new bone laid down at the infection site, which seals off areas of sequestra. Antibiotics can be effective during acute osteomyelitis, and prevention of chronic osteomyelitis requires early antibiotic treatment. Bone and skin grafting may be necessary following surgical removal of infection if destruction is extensive.

2. b. Rationale: The client with osteomyelitis is at risk for pathological fractures at the site of the infection because of weakened, devitalized bone, and careful handling of the extremity is necessary. Range-of-motion exercises should be limited because of the possibility of spread of infection, and edema is not a common finding in osteomyelitis. Careful handling of dressings is necessary to prevent the spread of infection to others.

3. c. Rationale: Because large doses of appropriate antibiotics are necessary in treatment of acute osteomyelitis, it is important to identify the causative micro-organism. The definitive way to determine the causative agent is by bone biopsy or biopsy of the soft tissue surrounding the site. The other tests may help establish the diagnosis but do not identify the causative agent.

4. d. Rationale: Activities such as exercise or heat application, which increase circulation and serve as stimuli for the spread of infection, should be avoided by clients with acute osteomyelitis. Oral or IV antibiotic therapy is continued at home for four to eight weeks, and weight bearing is contraindicated to prevent pathological fractures.

5. b. Rationale: One of the most common adverse effects of prolonged and high-dose antibiotic therapy is overgrowth of *Candida albicans* in the oral cavity and genitourinary tract. These infections are manifested by whitish-yellow, curdlike lesions of the mucosa. A dry, cracked, furrowed tongue is characteristic of severe dehydration, vesicles are characteristic of herpes simplex infections, and mouth and lip ulcers are characteristic of aphthous somatitis, or canker sores.

6. a. 4; b. 1; c. 3; d. 2; e. 1; f. 2; g. 3

7. b. Rationale: Promotion of muscle activity is important in any client with muscular dystrophy, but when the disease has progressed to cardiomyopathy and/or respiratory failure, activity must be balanced with oxygen supply. At this stage of the disease, care should be taken to prevent skin or respiratory complications. The client should be encouraged to perform as much self-care and exercise as energy allows, but this will be limited.

8. a. T; b. F, mechanical strain of paravertebral muscles; c. T; d. F, herniated lumbar intervertebral disk; e. T

9. a. Rationale: Proper daily exercise is an important part of the prevention of back injury, with the goal of maintaining mobility and strength in the back. Good postures are also paramount. Clients should sit with the hips higher than the knees and should sleep in a side-lying position, with knees and hips bent, or on the back, with a device to flex the hips and knees. Although some occupations, such as those requiring prolonged driving and heavy, repetitive lifting, pose a high risk for acute back pain, most jobs require body use. Good body mechanics with proper transfer and turning techniques are necessary in all activities.

10. b. Rationale: Clients with chronic back pain may develop sick role behaviour because of the duration of health problems, poor self-esteem, and inability to adjust to the chronic pain condition, and the nurse should encourage activity within the client's limitation to maintain physical mobility and independence in order to prevent assumption of this behaviour. Coping is improved if the client understands the nature of the pain and can make lifestyle adjustments for the pain. Pain control may require use of NSAIDs and other methods.

11. d. Rationale: During acute back pain, the head of the bed should be kept elevated 20 to 30 degrees and the knees slightly flexed to prevent strain on the back muscles. Exercise of the legs increases pain and should be avoided, and neurovascular, not neurological, assessment of the legs is indicated. This is not an appropriate time to assess body mechanics, because frequently the client cannot even stand upright.

12. b. Rationale: Urinary incontinence following spinal surgery may indicate nerve damage and should be reported to the physician. Paralytic ileus is common following surgery and is often expected immediately post operation. Pain at the graft site, usually the iliac crest or the fibula, often is more severe than pain from the fused area, and although movement and sensation of the arms and legs should not be more impaired than before surgery, they often are not relieved immediately after surgery.

13. c. Rationale: After spinal surgery, clients are logrolled to maintain straight alignment of the spine at all times, requiring the client to be turned with a pillow between the legs and moving the body as a unit. The head of the bed is usually kept flat, and the legs are extended.

14. a. 4; b. 7; c. 5; d. 2; e. 3; f. 1; g. 2; h. 5; i. 1; j. 6

15. c. Rationale: Poorly fitted shoes selected for fashion rather than comfort are the primary factor in the development of foot problems. A few congenital problems predispose to foot problems, and poor hygiene in clients with peripheral vascular disease may lead to foot infections, but these factors are in the minority in comparison with the effect of ill-fitting shoes.

16. a. 3; b. 1; c. 2; d. 1; e. 3; f. 2; g. 2

17. d. Rationale: Risk factors for osteoporosis include female gender, white and Asian race, prolonged immobility, insufficient calcium intake, smoking and alcoholism, and estrogen deficiency. Decreased risk is associated with physical activity, especially stress on bones, and fluoride and vitamin D intake.

18. a. Increased calcium intake and vitamin D; b. Weight-bearing exercise; c. Post-menopausal estrogen replacement therapy

**Case Study**

1. Risk factors for back pain in Mr. Brown include excess body weight, cigarette smoking, and a job that requires heavy lifting and prolonged periods of sitting.

2. Preoperative preparation includes teaching about the restrictions on positioning and movement required following surgery, measures for pain control, and assessments that will be carried out post-operatively. The nurse should ensure that Mr. Brown has received information about the procedure from the surgeon and understands the benefits and risks of the surgery.

3. Mr. Brown will probably be restricted to flat bed rest for at least the first 24 hours to avoid straining the surgical area. Pillows may be used under the thigh of each leg to prevent strain on the back muscles. When turning is allowed, he must be turned with the help of several personnel to avoid changing the alignment of the spine, or log-rolled. Depending on the surgeon's preference, ambulation will usually begin by the second postoperative day, again keeping the spine in alignment.

4. These post-operative assessments should be carried out by the nurse q2–4h during the first 24 to 48 hours:
   - Sensation: in all extremities in all appropriate dermatomes
   - Movement: of all extremities
   - Muscle strength: note any weakness of the extremities
   - Wound: assess dressing for drainage and note amount, colour, characteristics; clear or light yellow drainage should be tested for the presence of glucose, which would indicate spinal fluid leakage
   - Pain: document location, nature, and intensity of pain; evaluate pain after administration of analgesia
   - Bowel activity: assess bowel sounds, passage of flatus, and abdomen; paralytic ileus is common for several days
   - Urinary function: incontinence or retention may indicate nerve damage and should be reported. Intermittent catheterization may be required for bladder emptying, especially until Mr. Brown is allowed to stand to void.

5. Discharge instructions include teaching Mr. Brown to report any persistent limb weakness, abnormal sensations, or pain to the healthcare provider. He should be instructed to avoid standing or sitting for prolonged periods of time. Walking, lying down, and shifting weight from one foot to another should be encouraged. Twisting of the spine is harmful, and he should be taught to think through any activity before bending, lifting, or stooping. A firm mattress or bed board should be used at home. To prevent further back problems, weight loss and smoking cessation should be encouraged. He should be taught correct body mechanics and to do strengthening back exercises after recovery from the surgery (Tables 62-6 and 62-7).

6. *Nursing diagnoses:*
   - Acute pain related to nerve root compression, muscle spasms, and surgical incision
   - Impaired physical mobility related to pain
   - Ineffective therapeutic regimen management related to lack of knowledge regarding posture, exercises, body mechanics, and weight reduction

   *Collaborative problems:*
   Potential complication: paralysis

# CHAPTER 63

1. d. Rationale: Cartilage destruction in the joints affects 90% of people by the age of 40, and when the destruction becomes symptomatic, osteoarthritis is said to be present. Because degenerative changes cause symptoms in only about 60% of those over the age of 65, joint pain and functional disability should not be considered a normal finding in aging persons. Osteoarthritis is not a systemic disease, and although degenerative changes can be accelerated by excessive use of or stress on a joint, many people with joint pain have no history of previous joint stress or injury.

2. a. 3; b. 5; c. 6; d. 1; e. 4; f. 2

3. a. F, Heberden's; b. F, bone surfaces rubbing together; c. T; d. F, acetaminophen; e. T

4. b. Rationale: Principles of joint protection and energy conservation are critical in being able to maintain functional mobility in the client with osteoarthritis, and clients should be helped to find ways to perform activities and tasks with less stress. Range-of-motion, isotonic, and isometric exercises of the affected joints should be balanced with joint rest and protection, but during an acute flare of joint inflammation, the joints should be rested. If a joint is painful, it should be used only to the point of pain, and masking the pain with analgesics may lead to greater joint injury.

5. c. Rationale: Common side effects of NSAIDs include GI irritation and bleeding, dizziness, rash, headache, and tinnitus. Oral lesions and blood dyscrasias are common in clients receiving immunosuppressive agents and disease-modifying agents. Fluid retention, hypertension, and bruising from capillary fragility are frequently seen in clients using systemic corticosteroids.

6. b. Rationale: There are promising results from the use of glucosamine and chondroitin sulphate in the treatment of arthritis, and overall, these substances have few side effects. The one identified contraindication to the use of glucosamine is diabetes mellitus because glucosamine may enhance the effects of hypoglycemic drugs.

7. a. Rationale: An effective alternative is the combination drug diclofenac sodium (Voltaren) and misoprostol (Cytotec), known as Arthrotec. Misoprostol is a protective agent for the NSAID diclofenac. COX2 inhibitors such as celecoxib (Celebrex) and meloxicam (Mobicox) have a safety warning because of cardiovascular events, and are not suitable alternatives unless the cardiac status of the client is known.

8. d. Rationale: In rheumatoid arthritis (RA), autoantibodies known as rheumatoid factors are formed against abnormal IgG, which is stimulated by an unknown factor. When the autoantibodies and the abnormal IgG combine, they form immune complexes that are deposited in the joints, blood vessels, and pleura and cause activation of complement with a resulting inflammatory response. The joint and systemic manifestations of RA are a result of the action of inflammatory mediators and cells. Some clients with RA have a prevalence of the HLA-DR4 antigen, but it does not directly cause damage.

9. a. R; b. O; c. O; d. B; e. R; f. B; g. R; h. O; i. B; j. O; k. R

10. a. 3; b. 6; c. 2; d. 1; e. 4; f. 5; g. 7

11. c. Rationale: A client with moderate RA has no joint deformities but may have limited joint mobility, adjacent muscle atrophy, and inflammation of the joints. Synovial hypertrophy and thickening of the joint capsule may cause spindle-shaped fingers. Splenomegaly may be found with RA, and crepitus on movement and Heberden's nodes are associated with osteoarthritis.

12. c. Rationale: The inflammatory reactions of RA cause an elevation in cross-reactive protein (CRP), a finding that is useful in monitoring the response to therapy. The WBC count may be increased in response to inflammation and is also elevated in synovial fluid. Anemia, rather than polycythemia, is common, and normal IgG levels are not affected.

13. c. Rationale: Because older adults are more likely to take many drugs, the use of multidrug therapy in RA is particularly problematic because of the increased likelihood of untoward drug interactions and toxicity. Rheumatic disorders do occur in older adults but usually in milder form. Interpretation of laboratory values in older adults is more difficult in diagnosing RA because of age-related serological changes, but the disease can be diagnosed. Older adults are not less compliant with drug regimens but may need help with complex regimens.

14. b. Rationale: Most clients with RA experience morning stiffness, and morning activities should be scheduled later in the day after the stiffness subsides. A warm shower in the morning and time to become more mobile before activity are advised. Management of RA includes daily exercises for the affected joints and protection of joints with devices and movements that prevent joint stress. Splinting should be done during an acute flare to rest the joint and prevent further damage.

15. b. Rationale: Pacing activities and alternating rest with activity are important in maintaining self-care and independence of the client with RA, in addition to preventing deconditioning and a negative attitude. The nurse should not carry out activities for clients that they can do for themselves but should support and assist clients as necessary.

16. d. Rationale: An unusually high frequency of HLA-B27 is found in clients with ankylosing spondylitis, psoriatic arthritis, and Reiter's syndrome, and these diseases have a predilection for involvement of the spine, peripheral joints, and periarticular structures, as well as an absence of rheumatoid factor and autoantibodies.

17. d. Rationale: Kyphosis and involvement of costovertebral joints in ankylosing spondylitis lead to a bent-over posture and a decrease in chest expansion, manifestations that are managed with chest expansion and deep-breathing exercises. Postural training emphasizes avoiding forward flexion during any activities, and the client should sleep on the back without the use of pillows.

18. a. 6; b. 4; c. 1; d. 2; e. 3; f. 5; g. 6; h. 1; i. 3; j. 5; k. 4; l. 2

19. d. Rationale: The diagnosis of gout is established by finding monosodium urate monohydrate crystals in the synovial fluid of an inflamed joint or tophus. Hyperuricemia and elevated urine uric acid are not diagnostic for gout, because they may be related to a variety of drugs or may exist as a totally asymptomatic abnormality in the general population. Although there is a familial predisposition to hyperuricemia, both environmental and genetic factors contribute to gout.

20. b. Rationale: Colchicine has an anti-inflammatory action specific for gout and is the treatment of choice during an acute attack, often producing dramatic pain relief in 24 to 48 hours. It may also be used prophylactically to reduce the frequency

of attacks. Probenecid is a uricosuric drug that is used to control hyperuricemia by increasing the excretion of uric acid through the kidney, and allopurinol is also used to control hyperuricemia by blocking production of uric acid. ASA inactivates the effect of uricosuric drugs and should not be used when clients are taking probenecid and other uricosuric drugs.

21. b. Rationale: During therapy with probenecid or allopurinol, the client must have periodic determination of blood uric acid levels to evaluate the effectiveness of the therapy and to ensure that levels are kept low enough to prevent future attacks of gout. Clients should not alter their doses of medications without medical direction, and the drugs used for control of gout are not useful in the treatment of an acute attack. With the use of medications, strict dietary restrictions of alcohol and high-purine foods are usually not necessary. When the client is taking probenecid, urine output should be maintained at 2–3 L to prevent urate from precipitating in the urinary tract and causing kidney stones.

22. a. Rationale: In systemic lupus erythematosus (SLE), autoantibodies are produced against nuclear antigens, cytoplasmic antigens, and blood cell surface antigens, and the clinical manifestations of SLE depend on which cell types or organs are involved. Overproduction of collagen is characteristic of systemic sclerosis, and abnormal IgG reactions with autoantibodies is characteristic of rheumatoid arthritis.

23. a. Cutaneous vascular lesions on sun-exposed skin with classic butterfly rash on face; b. Polyarthralgia and polyarthritis; c. Arrythmias; d. Restrictive lung disease with cough, tachypnea and pleurisy; e. Proteinuria resulting from nephritis; f. Seizures, peripheral neuropathy; g. Anemia, leukopenia, and thrombocytopenia

24. b. Rationale: Clients with SLE often find that one of the most difficult facets of the disease is its extreme variability in severity and progression. There is no characteristic pattern of progressive organ involvement, nor can one predict which systems may become affected. SLE is now associated with a normal lifespan, but clients must be helped to adjust to the unknown course of the disease.

25. c. Rationale: Efficacy of treatment with corticosteroids or immunosuppressive drugs is best monitored by serial serum complement levels and anti-DNA, both of which will decrease as the drugs have an effect. A reduction in ESR is not as specific, and the client with SLE often has a chronic anemia that is not affected by drug therapy.

26. a. Rationale: Acute exacerbations of SLE may be precipitated by overexposure to ultraviolet light, physical and emotional stress, fatigue, and infection or surgery. The major concern in planning a pregnancy is that exacerbations are also common following delivery, and there are increased risks for the mother and fetus during pregnancy. Although SLE has an identified genetic association with HLA-DR2 and HLA-DR3, genetic counselling is not usually recommended. Dietary recommendations include small, frequent meals and adequate iron intake. Although non-pharmacological methods of pain control are encouraged, the use of NSAIDs is often necessary to help control inflammation and pain.

27. a. Rationale: Skin lesions of SLE include discoid lesions and diffuse maculopapular rashes, and it is important to keep the skin clean and dry to prevent infection. Unprescribed ointments, lotions, or cosmetics often exacerbate existing conditions and should not be used.

28. d. Rationale: Systemic sclerosis is a disorder of connective tissue that causes skin thickening and tightening, resulting in expressionless facial features, puckering of the mouth, and a small oral orifice. It also causes symmetric, painless swelling or thickening of the skin of the fingers and hands. It does not cause the swan-neck or ulnar drift deformities seen in RA or SLE, and low back pain and spinal stiffness are associated with ankylosing spondylitis.

29. d. Rationale: One of the most common and early manifestations of CREST syndrome is Raynaud's phenomenon, which causes paroxysmal vasospasms of the digits with diminished blood flow to the fingers and toes on exposure to cold, followed by cyanosis and then erythema on rewarming. The hands and feet must be protected from cold exposure and possible burns or cuts that might heal slowly, and smoking is contraindicated. Ultraviolet light sensitivity is not a factor in systemic sclerosis, nor is fluid intake. Cardiovascular involvement may occur, but it does not require client monitoring.

30. c. Rationale: Dermatomyositis produces symmetric weakness of striated muscle, and weak neck and pharyngeal muscles may produce dysphagia. Deglutition impairment contributes to death from dermatomyositis and requires special attention during mealtime to prevent aspiration. Muscle tenderness or pain is uncommon, as is joint involvement. During an acute attack the client is so weak that bed rest is needed, and passive ROM is usually required.

31. b. Rationale: The diagnosis of dermatomyositis in older men is frequently associated with concurrent malignant disease, and a careful search for possible malignant lesions should be made. The disease is more common in the fifth and sixth decades of life and can be diagnosed with serum muscle enzymes.

32. b. Rationale: People with FMS typically experience non-restorative sleep, morning stiffness, irritable bowel syndrome, and anxiety in addition to the widespread, non-articular musculoskeletal pain and fatigue. FMS is non-degenerative, non-progressive, and non-inflammatory. Neither muscle weakness nor muscle spasms are associated with the disease, although there may be tics in the muscle at the tender points.

33. d. Rationale: Two criteria for the diagnosis of FMS are that (1) pain is experienced in 11 of the 18 tender points on palpation and (2) the client has a history of widespread pain for at least three months. The other findings may also be present but are not diagnostic for FMS.

34. c. Rationale: The pain and related symptoms of FMS cause significant stress, and anxiety is a common finding. Stress management is an important part of the treatment and may include any of the commonly used relaxation strategies as well as psychological counselling.

35. a. Unexplained, persistent, or relapsing chronic fatigue that is of new and definite onset
    b. Fatigue is not due to ongoing exertion.
    c. Fatigue is not substantially alleviated by rest.
    d. Fatigue results in substantial reduction in occupational, educational, social, or personal activities.

**Case Study**

1. Mrs. M. should be told that rheumatoid arthritis is a disease that affects all of her body, even though her joints are primarily affected at this time. She needs to know that it is not known what causes RA but that antibodies are formed which react with substances, causing inflammation and damage to a variety of organs. Joint changes include inflammation of the lining of the joints and eventual filling of the joint with bone, completely immobilizing the joint and causing deformities similar to those she is developing in her hands. She should be told that the fatigue and low-grade fever she has are part of the disease and that with disease control these symptoms will improve.

2. The painful, stiff hands and feet, the fatigue, the low-grade fever, and the ulnar drift deviation are all manifestations of RA.

3. Methotrexate is a chemotherapeutic agent that has an anti-inflammatory effect but causes bone marrow suppression and hepatotoxicity. Its dosage in RA is much smaller than that used for cancer therapy, and side effects are not as common. When used in RA, it frequently reduces clinical symptoms in days to weeks with few, if any, adverse effects. Teaching Mrs. M. about methotrexate is an important nursing responsibility. Periodic blood chemistry and hematology tests must be done, the client should take a daily supplement of folic acid, and the client should report signs of anemia or any infection. Methotrexate is teratogenic, and Mrs. M. should be informed that contraception must be used during and three months after treatment.

4. Protection of her joints will be enhanced if she can maintain a normal weight, avoid tasks that cause pain, use assistive devices to prevent joint stress, and avoid forceful, repetitive movements. She should plan regularly scheduled rest periods alternated with activity throughout the day and should develop organizing and pacing techniques that spread tasks through the day or the week. Suggesting that she take a warm shower or bath in the morning to relieve her morning stiffness may be helpful. Exercise regimens will be prescribed for Mrs. M., and she should be encouraged to follow the regimens daily.

5. Because of the chronicity and disability associated with arthritis, clients are often vulnerable to claims of unproven remedies. The nurse should recognize that the copper bracelet will do no harm but may be a waste of money for Mrs. M. It is important to encourage her to recognize that regular, proven methods of treatment used on a consistent basis are the best way to control her condition. The more she is taught about the disease and its management, the more compliant she will be with treatment regimens.

6. Additional sources of information and sharing are available from the Arthritis Foundation and should be suggested to Mrs. M.

7. *Nursing diagnoses:*
   • Acute and chronic pain related to joint inflammation
   • Impaired physical mobility related to joint pain, stiffness, and deformity
   • Fatigue related to disease activity
   • Ineffective therapeutic regimen management related to use of unproven remedies
   • Risk for infection related to altered immune function
   *Collaborative problems:*
   Potential complication: bone marrow suppression

## CHAPTER 64

1. d. Rationale: One of the primary characteristics of critical care nurses that is different from those of generalist medical-surgical nurses is the use of advanced technology to accurately measure physiological parameters and manage life-threatening complications. All nursing addresses human responses to health problems and requires knowledge of physiology, pathophysiology, pharmacology, and psychological support to the client and family. Diagnosis and treatment of life-threatening diseases are roles of medicine.

2. a. Physiologically unstable; b. Risk for serious complications; c. Risk for serious complications; d. Intensive nursing support

3. a. Rationale: When anxiety in the ICU client is related to the environment that has unfamiliar equipment, high noise and light levels, and an intense pace of activity, which leads to sensory overload, the nurse should eliminate as much of this source of stress as possible by muting phones, limiting overhead paging, setting alarms appropriate to the client's condition, and eliminating unnecessary alarms. Flexible visiting schedules for family members and providing as much autonomy in decisions about care as possible are indicated when impaired communication and loss of control contribute to the anxiety. Use of sedation to reduce anxiety should be carefully evaluated and implemented when nursing measures are not effective.

4. c. Rationale: The family of the critically ill client is very important in the recovery and well-being of the client, and the extent to which the family is involved and supported affects the client's clinical course. Although the cost of planning and providing critical care is a concern to families, it is not the major reason that family members are included in the client's care. Family members may be responsible for making decisions about the client's care only when the client is unable to make personal decisions. Most families have questions regarding the client's quality of care because of anxiety and lack of information about the client's condition.

5. a. Decreased; b. Increased; c. Decrease; d. Increase; e. Increased; f. Increases

6. d. Rationale: Cardiac output is dependent on heart rate and stroke volume, and stroke volume is determined by preload, afterload, and contractility. If cardiac output is decreased and heart rate is unchanged, stroke volume is the variable factor. If the preload determined by PAOP and the afterload determined by SVR are unchanged, the factor that is changed is contractility of the myocardium.

7. b. Rationale: Referencing hemodynamic monitoring equipment means positioning the monitoring equipment so that the zero reference point is at the vertical level of the left atrium of the heart. The port of the stopcock nearest the transducer is placed at the phlebostatic axis, the external landmark of the left atrium. The phlebostatic axis is the intersection of two planes: a horizontal line midchest, halfway between the outermost anterior and posterior surfaces, transecting a vertical line through the fourth intercostal space at the sternum.

8. a. T; b. F, pulmonary artery; c. F, left ventricle; d. T; e. T

9. c. Rationale: During insertion of a pulmonary artery catheter, it is necessary to monitor the ECG continuously because of the risk for arrhythmias, particularly when the catheter reaches the right ventricle. It is the physician's responsibility to obtain informed consent regarding the catheter insertion. During the catheter insertion the client is placed supine with the head of the bed flat. An Allen test to confirm adequate ulnar artery perfusion is performed before insertion of an arterial catheter in the radial artery for arterial pressure monitoring.

10. a. Slowly inflate the pulmonary artery catheter balloon with 1.0 to 1.5 mL of air while observing the pressure tracing, and measure the PAOP at the end of expiration, limiting the balloon inflation to less than four respiratory cycles.
    b. Rapidly inject the prescribed amount and temperature of solution into the right atrial lumen of the pulmonary artery catheter, and read the computer display of the cardiac output.

11. a. MAP—75 mm Hg (90 + 136/3)
    PAP—26 mm Hg (20 + 1/3 of 18)
    SV—25.8 mL/beat (3.2 x 1000/124)
    SVR—1625 dyne sec/cm$^5$ (75 – 10 x 80/3.2)
    b. All of the changes in the hemodynamic parameters are characteristic findings in the client with heart failure: increased pulmonary congestion and pressures; increased pressure in the left atrium and ventricle; increased systemic vascular resistance; and decreased stroke volume, cardiac output, and systemic blood pressure.

12. b. Rationale: The normal mixed venous oxygen saturation of 60%–80% becomes decreased with decreased arterial oxygenation, low cardiac output, low hemoglobin, or increased oxygen consumption. With normal cardiac output, arterial oxygenation, and hemoglobin, the factor that is

responsible for decreased $SvO_2$ is increased oxygen consumption, which can result from increased metabolic rate, pain, movement, or fever.

13. d. Rationale: When a pulmonary artery pressure tracing indicates a wedged wave form when the balloon is deflated, this indicates that the catheter has advanced and has become spontaneously wedged. If the catheter is not repositioned immediately, a pulmonary infarction or a rupture of a pulmonary artery may occur. If the catheter is becoming occluded, the pressure tracing becomes blunted, and pulmonary edema and increased pulmonary congestion increase the pulmonary artery wave form. Balloon leaks that are found when injected air does not flow back into the syringe do not alter wave forms.

14. c. Rationale: The counterpulsation of the intra-aortic balloon pump increases diastolic arterial pressure, forcing blood back into the coronary arteries and main branches of the aortic arch, increasing coronary artery perfusion pressure and blood flow to the myocardium. The balloon pump also causes a drop in aortic pressure just before systole, decreasing afterload and myocardial oxygen consumption. These effects make the IABP valuable in treating unstable angina, acute myocardial infarction, and a variety of surgical heart situations. Its use is contraindicated in incompetent aortic valves, dissecting aortic aneurysms, and generalized peripheral vascular disease.

15. a. F, afterload; b. T; c. F, diastolic

16. c. Rationale: Because the IABP is inserted into the femoral artery and advanced to the descending thoracic aorta, compromised distal extremity circulation is common and requires that the cannulated extremity be extended at all times. Repositioning the client is limited to side-lying or supine positions with the head of the bed elevated no more than 30 to 45 degrees. Assessment for bleeding is important because the IABP may cause platelet destruction, and occlusive dressings are used to prevent site infection.

17. d. Rationale: Weaning from the IABP involves reducing the pumping to every second or third heart beat or gradually decreasing the augmentation pressure until the IABP catheter is removed. The pumping and infusion flow are continued to reduce the risk for thrombus formation around the catheter until it is removed.

18. b. Rationale: Ventricular assist devices are temporary devices that can partially or totally support circulation until the heart recovers and can be weaned from cardiopulmonary bypass or a donor heart can be obtained. The devices currently available do not permanently support circulation, and many clients die while awaiting a donor heart.

19. c. Rationale: A nasal endotracheal tube is longer and smaller in diameter than an oral endotracheal tube, creating more airway resistance and increasing the work of breathing. Suctioning and secretion removal are also more difficult with a nasal endotracheal tube, and they are more subject to kinking than are oral tubes. Oral tubes require a bite block to stop the client from biting the tube and may cause more laryngeal damage because of their larger size.

20. b. Rationale: An alert client should be informed of the sensations likely to be experienced during endotracheal intubation, in order to help prevent anxiety and panic when feelings of suffocation are experienced. The client may be asked to extrude the tongue during nasal intubation. The client is positioned with the mouth, pharynx, and trachea in direct alignment, with the head extended in the "sniffing position," but the head must not hang over the edge of the bed. Talking is not possible during intubation or while the tube is in place because the tube splits the vocal cords.

21. d. Rationale: The first action by the nurse following endotracheal intubation is to auscultate the chest to confirm bilateral breath sounds and observe to confirm bilateral chest expansion. If this evidence is present, the tube is secured and connected to an $O_2$ source. Then the placement is confirmed immediately with x-ray, and the tube is marked where it exits the mouth. Then the client should be suctioned as needed.

22. c. Rationale: The minimal occluding volume (MOV) involves adding air to the endotracheal tube cuff until no leak is heard at peak inspiratory pressure but ensures that minimal pressure is applied to the tracheal wall to prevent pressure necrosis of the trachea. The minimal occluding volume should apply between 20 and 25 mm Hg pressure on the trachea to prevent injury. The cuff does not secure the tube in place but rather prevents escape of ventilating gases through the upper airway.

23. a. eight, between 20 and 25 mm Hg; b. suctioning; bag-valve mask (BVM); c. half; d. 100, 120; e. 10; f. hyperoxygenates (or hyperventilates)

24. c. Rationale: Suctioning an endotracheal tube is performed when adventitious sounds over the trachea and/or bronchi confirm the presence of secretions that can be removed by suctioning. Visible secretions in the ET tube, respiratory distress, suspected aspiration, increase in peak airway pressures, and changes in oxygen status are

other indications. Peripheral crackles are not an indication for suctioning, and suctioning as a means of inducing a cough is not recommended, because of the complications associated with suctioning.

25. d. Rationale: If serious arrhythmias occur during suctioning, the suctioning should be stopped, and the client should be slowly ventilated via MRB with 100% oxygen until the arrhythmia subsides. Clients with bradycardia should not be suctioned excessively. Ventilation of the client with slow, small-volume breaths using the MRB is performed when severe coughing results from suctioning.

26. a. Use two nurses—one to hold the tube while it is untaped or the holder is loosened and another to perform care.
    b. After completion of care, confirm the presence of bilateral breath sounds to ensure that the position of the tube was not changed.

27. c. Rationale: Because the client with an ET tube cannot protect the airway from aspiration and cannot swallow, the cuff should always be inflated and the head of the bed elevated while the client is receiving tube feedings or mouth care is being performed. Clients with ET tubes cannot phonate, and clearing the ventilatory tubing of condensed water is important to prevent respiratory infection. The mouth and oropharynx should be suctioned with a Yankauer or tonsil suction to remove accumulated secretions that cannot be swallowed.

28. a. Rationale: The nurse should carefully observe the client for respiratory distress and laryngospasm following extubation, which may indicate a need for immediate reintubation. The tube and the oropharynx are suctioned before removal of the tube, and the client is encouraged to cough after the tube is removed. ABGs are not routinely assessed after tube removal, but $SpO_2$ may be monitored.

29. d. Rationale: A maximal inspiratory pressure of $-15$ cm $H_2O$ indicates that the client does not have enough negative inspiratory force, or muscular strength, to promote effective ventilation and is an indication for mechanical ventilation. Other indications for mechanical ventilation include $PaCO_2$ greater than 55 mm Hg, tidal volume less than 5 mL/kg, and resting minute ventilation greater than 10 L/min.

30. a. N; b. P; c. B; d. N; e. N; f. B; g. P; h. N
31. a. 2; b. 1; c. 2; d. 2; e. 1
32. a. CPAP—continuous positive airway pressure; b. SIMV—synchronized intermittent mandatory ventilation; c. CMV—controlled mechanical ventilation; d. PSV—pressure support ventilation; e. ACV—assist-control ventilation; f. PEEP—positive end-expiratory pressure; g. HFV—high-frequency ventilation; h. PC/IRV—pressure-controlled/inverse-ratio ventilation

33. c. Rationale: Positive pressure ventilation, especially with end-expiratory pressure, increases intrathoracic pressure with compression of thoracic vessels, resulting in decreased venous return to the heart, decreased left ventricular end-diastolic volume (preload), decreased cardiac output, and lowered blood pressure. None of the other factors are related to increased intrathoracic pressure.

34. d. Rationale: Decreased cardiac output associated with positive pressure ventilation and PEEP results in decreased renal perfusion, release of renin, and increased aldosterone secretion, which causes sodium and water retention. ADH may be released because of stress, but ADH is responsible only for water retention, and increased intrathoracic pressure decreases, not increases, the release of atrial natriuretic factor, causing sodium retention. There is decreased, not increased, insensible water loss via the airway during mechanical ventilation.

35. b. Rationale: The ABGs reflect a trend toward respiratory alkalosis, and although the $PaCO_2$ is within normal limits, if a client with COPD is ventilated with a return to a normal $PaCO_2$, the client will develop an alkalosis because of chronically retained bicarbonate. The client is being overventilated, and the rate or volume of respirations should be decreased to maintain the $PaCO_2$ at the client's normal value. PEEP is generally contraindicated or used with extreme caution in clients with COPD, and these clients usually do better with a short inspiratory and longer expiratory time.

36. c. Rationale: Neuromuscular blocking agents produce a paralysis that facilitates ventilation, but they do not sedate the client. It is important for the nurse to remember that the client can hear, see, think, and feel and should be addressed and given explanations accordingly. Communication with the client is possible, especially from the nurse, but visitors for an anxious and agitated client should provide a calming, restful effect on the client.

37. a. Anemia resulting in poor $O_2$ transport; b. Decreased respiratory strength; c. Delayed weaning; d. Decreased resistance to infection; e. Decreased recovery

38. b. Rationale: A leaking cuff can lower the tidal volume delivered by the ventilator, resulting in

hypoventilation. Other causes are low Tv or respiratory rates, an SIMV rate that is too low, presence of lung secretions, or obstruction. A decreased $PaCO_2$ and increased pH indicate a respiratory alkalosis from hyperventilation, and cardiac arrhythmias can occur with either hyper- or hypoventilation.

39. b. Rationale: A variety of ventilator weaning methods are used, but all should provide for weaning trials with adequate rest between weaning trials to prevent respiratory muscle fatigue. Weaning is usually carried out during the day, with the client ventilated at night until there is sufficient spontaneous ventilation without excess fatigue. In all methods, clients usually require a 10% increase in $FIO_2$ to maintain arterial oxygen tension. If the client becomes hypoxemic, ventilator support is indicated.

40. c. Rationale: Care of a ventilator-dependent client in the home usually requires extensive nursing care and financial and time commitments. The nurse should ensure that family members understand the potential sacrifices they may have to make and the impact that home mechanical ventilation will have over time, before final decisions and arrangements are made.

**Case Study**

1. The best indicators to use to monitor Mr. V.'s hemodynamic status are the values determined from the pulmonary artery catheter, the urinary output, and the blood pressure, because infectious processes are altering his level of consciousness, skin temperature, and other vital signs that may commonly be used to monitor hemodynamic status. Of the hemodynamic parameters, it is most important to monitor CO, SVR, and $SVO_2$ because these parameters are the most out of range and suggest septic shock.

2. PEEP is used for Mr. V. to increase his oxygenation because his $PaO_2$ is decreased, but it can increase intrathoracic pressure, suppressing venous return and increasing intracranial pressure.

3. Mr. V.'s MAP is 64 mm Hg (46 + 1/3 of 54). The MAP necessary to promote tissue and cerebral perfusion and yet not increase ICP would be a MAP that maintains a CPP of 70 mm Hg. With an intracranial pressure of 22 mm Hg, MAP needs to be 92 mm Hg to maintain cerebral perfusion, yet not increase ICP. (CPP = MAP – ICP, or 70 = 92 – 22.) His current MAP results in a cerebral perfusion pressure of 42, which is inadequate to maintain cerebral perfusion.

4. Fluid therapy would include rapid administration of 0.9% sodium chloride, colloids, or both to expand vascular volume and maintain tissue perfusion, with monitoring of PAP, PAOP, and CO to evaluate fluid replacement. Lactated Ringer's is contraindicated because of the client's elevated lactate levels. Antibiotics specific for cryptococcal infections, such as fluconazole (Diflucan), should be initiated immediately, and a broad-spectrum antibiotic, such as an aminoglycoside, is indicated for bacterial prophylaxis. Vasopressor agents, such as norepinephrine (Levophed), dopamine (Intropin), or phenylephrine (Neo-Synephrine), are indicated to promote vasoconstriction and increase systemic vascular resistance. After fluid therapy has been initiated, an osmotic diuretic, such as mannitol, may be used to pull water out of the brain tissue and decrease intracranial pressure. ASA or other antipyretics should be given to control his temperature because increased temperature increases metabolic rate and oxygen need. Sodium bicarbonate is not indicated to correct the client's acidosis unless the pH is below 7.20.

5. Gastrointestinal ischemia may cause translocation of bowel bacteria into the systemic circulation, creating a source of further infection and sepsis. Early institution of enteral tube feedings may help promote perfusion of the gastrointestinal tract and prevent bacterial translocation.

6. *Subjective assessment findings:*
Seizures reflect the cerebral irritation caused by the inflammation of the meninges and the increased intracranial pressure.
*Objective assessment findings:*
   - Increased intracranial pressure is responsible for the GCS score of 6 and is reflected by the ICP of 22 mm Hg.
   - The infectious process of the meningitis is reflected by the increased body temperature and the WBC count of $18.5 \times 10^9$/L ($18.5 \times 10^3$/μL).
   - The response of the sympathetic nervous system to the inflammation and sepsis is seen in the elevated blood glucose level.
   - Most of the other findings reflect the development of septic shock, systemic inflammatory response syndrome (SIRS), and possible development of multiple organ dysfunction syndrome (MODS).
   - Shock is evident from the lowered blood pressure, metabolic acidosis, markedly reduced systemic vascular resistance (SVR), and decreased urinary output resulting from poor renal perfusion.

- Septic shock is characterized by activation of mediators that cause widespread vasodilation and increased capillary permeability, resulting in decreased systemic vascular resistance (SVR) and high cardiac output (CO) because of the decreased peripheral resistance. The vasodilation causes the skin to be warm and dry. Septic shock also results in poor oxygen utilization, resulting in elevated mixed venous oxygen saturation ($SVO_2$). All of these processes are reflected in the assessment findings in this client.
- The ABGs and increased lactate indicate the metabolic acidosis resulting from anaerobic metabolism of cells. The $PaCO_2$ and $HCO_3^-$ are low, and the respiratory rate is increased, indicating the body's attempt to compensate for the metabolic acidosis by using bicarbonate to buffer lactic acid and by hyperventilation to blow off extra carbon dioxide.
- The decreased urinary output and decreased arterial oxygenation may reflect not only poor perfusion to the kidneys and lungs but also initial organ damage and development of MODS.

7. *Nursing diagnoses:*
- Ineffective cerebral tissue perfusion related to cerebral tissue swelling
- Ineffective peripheral tissue perfusion related to deficit in capillary blood supply
- Ineffective protection related to neurosensory alterations
- Hyperthermia related to inflammatory process
- Ineffective airway clearance related to unconsciousness and presence of artificial airway
- Risk for injury related to endotracheal intubation, mechanical ventilation, seizure activity, and environmental hazards
- Risk for aspiration related to presence of artificial airway
- Imbalanced nutrition: less than body requirements related to increased caloric demands and inability to take nourishment orally
- Risk for decreased cardiac output related to impeded venous return by PEEP

*Collaborative problems:*
Potential complications: ARDS; DIC; organ ischemia—neurological, renal, GI, respiratory; pneumothorax or pneumomediastinum; MODS

# CHAPTER 65

1. d. Rationale: Although all of the factors may be present, regardless of the cause, the end result is inadequate supply of oxygen and nutrients to body cells from inadequate tissue perfusion.
2. a. 2;  b. 1;  c. 1;  d. 2;  e. 2
3. a. 2;  b. 3;  c. 5;  d. 1;  e. 2;  f. 1;  g. 5;  h. 4;  i. 3;  j. 5;  k. 1;  l. 5;  m. 5; n. 2
4. a. F, hypovolemic; b. T; c. T; d. T; e. F, absolute hypovolemia; f. T
5. a. decreased capillary hydrostatic pressure; b. α-adrenergic stimulation; c. β-adrenergic stimulation, increased heart strength and rate; d. renin release; e. aldosterone secretion; f. increased venous return to heart, increased blood pressure; g. increased serum osmolality, release of ADH; h. renal water reabsorption
6. a. Increased heart rate (β-adrenergic stimulation); b. Cool, pale skin (α-adrenergic stimulation); c. Thirst (with fluid shift to intravascular space); d. Decreased urinary output (ADH and aldosterone); e. Fluctuating blood pressure; f. Decreased bowel sounds (α-adrenergic stimulation); Others: abdominal distension, edema (sodium retention)
7. a. Rationale: When sepsis is the cause of shock, the endotoxins stimulate a cascade of inflammatory responses that start with release of TNF and IL-1, which stimulate other inflammatory mediators that increase neutrophil and platelet aggregation and adhesion to the endothelium. There is an increase in coagulation and inflammation and fibrinolysis, and platelet-activating factor causes formation of microthrombi and vessel obstruction. The process does not occur in other types of shock until late stages.
8. a. Renin-angiotensin activation causes arteriolar constriction, decreasing perfusion.
   b. Vasoconstriction of the pulmonary arterioles decreases the blood flow to pulmonary capillaries, and a ventilation–perfusion mismatch occurs. Areas of the lung that are oxygenated are not perfused by blood, because of the decreased blood flow, resulting in additional hypoxemia and decreased oxygen for cells.
   c. Capillary permeability and profound vasoconstriction cause increased hydrostatic pressure with shift of fluid to interstitial spaces and decreased circulating blood volume.
   d. Decreased myocardial perfusion occurs as the heart fails, leading to arrhythmias and myocardial ischemia, further decreasing cardiac output and oxygen delivery to cells.

9. d. Rationale: During both the compensated and progressive stages of shock, the sympathetic nervous system is activated in an attempt to maintain cardiac output and systemic vascular resistance, and clinical manifestations reflect the effects of this stimulation. In the refractory or irreversible stage of shock, the sympathetic nervous system can no longer compensate to maintain homeostasis, and a loss of vasomotor tone affects perfusion to all vital organs, causing increasing cellular hypoxia, metabolic acidosis, and cellular death.

10. c. Rationale: In every type of shock there is a deficiency of oxygen to the cells, and high-flow oxygen therapy is indicated. Vasopressor therapy may be indicated in some cases but only after fluid replacement has been established. Fluid therapy is not indicated for cardiogenic shock, and not all clients require intubation and ventilation.

11. b. Rationale: In early compensated shock, activation of the renin-angiotensin system stimulates the release of aldosterone, which causes sodium reabsorption and potassium excretion by the kidney, elevating serum sodium levels and decreasing serum potassium levels. Blood glucose levels are elevated during the compensated stage of shock in response to catecholamine stimulation of the liver, which releases its glycogen stores in the form of glucose. Metabolic acidosis does not occur until the progressive stage of shock, when compensatory mechanisms become ineffective and anaerobic cellular metabolism causes lactic acid production.

12. b. Rationale: In late irreversible shock, progressive cellular destruction causes an elevation of liver enzymes and other laboratory findings that indicate organ damage. Metabolic acidosis is usually severe as cells continue anaerobic metabolism, and the respiratory alkalosis that may occur in the progressive stage has failed to compensate for the acidosis. Urine specific gravity becomes fixed or increased as the kidneys fail, and hemoglobin and hematocrit are usually increased in a client with burns as fluid leaves the vascular space.

13. a. Rationale: Lactated Ringer's solution may increase lactate levels, which a damaged liver cannot convert to bicarbonate, and may intensify the metabolic lactic acidosis that occurs in progressive shock, necessitating careful attention to the client's acid–base balance. Sodium and potassium levels as well as hemoglobin and hematocrit levels should be monitored in all clients receiving fluid replacement therapy.

14. 45 mL/hr. Adequate fluid replacement is indicated by a urinary output of 0.5 mL/kg/hr.

15. b. Rationale: When large amounts of crystalloid fluids are given to critically ill clients to maintain vascular volume, about two-thirds of the volume will diffuse out of the vascular space into the interstitial space, causing systemic edema. Increased vascular volume from the fluids will increase CO, PAWP, and urinary output.

16. a. Rationale: A decreased mixed venous oxygen saturation ($SvO_2$) indicates that the client has used the venous oxygen reserve and is at greater risk for anaerobic metabolism. The $SvO_2$ decreases when more oxygen is used by the cells, as in activity or hypermetabolism. All of the other values indicate an improvement in the client's condition.

17. d. Rationale: As a vasopressor, norepinephrine may cause severe vasoconstriction, which would further decrease tissue perfusion, especially if fluid replacement is inadequate. Vasopressors generally cause hypertension, reflex bradycardia, and decreased urine output because of decreased renal blood flow; they do not directly affect acid-base balance.

18. b. Rationale: Vasoactive drugs are those that can either dilate or constrict blood vessels, and both are used in various stages of shock treatment. When using either vasodilators or vasoconstrictors, it is important to maintain a MAP of at least 60 mm Hg so that adequate perfusion is maintained.

19. a. Restore coronary artery blood flow with thrombolytic therapy, angioplasty, emergency revascularization; increase cardiac output with inotropic agents; reduce workload by dilating coronary arteries, decreasing preload and afterload; use circulatory assist devices, such as an intra-aortic balloon pump
    b. Fluid and blood replacement, control of bleeding with pressure, surgery
    c. Fluid resuscitation, antimicrobial agents, inotropic agents with vasopressors
    d. Epinephrine, inhaled bronchodilators, colloidal fluid replacement, diphenhydramine, corticosteroids

20. a. Dobutamine (Dobutrex) increases myocardial contractility and causes mild vasodilation by α1-adrenergic stimulation.
    b. Milrinone (Primacor) increases cardiac contractility and output and decreases preload and afterload by directly relaxing vascular smooth muscles.
    c. Nitroglycerin (Nitrol, Tridil) primarily dilates veins, reducing preload.
    d. Nitroprusside (Nipride) acts as a potent vasodilator of veins and arteries and may

increase or decrease CO, depending on the extent of preload and afterload reduction. Others: diuretics, ACE inhibitors, β-adrenergic blockers

21. c. Rationale: Prevention of shock necessitates identification of persons who are at risk and a thorough baseline nursing assessment with frequent ongoing assessments to monitor and detect changes in clients at risk. Frequent monitoring of all clients' vital signs is not necessary. Aseptic technique for all invasive procedures should always be implemented but will not prevent all types of shock. Health promotion activities that reduce the risk for precipitating conditions, such as coronary artery disease or anaphylaxis, may help prevent shock in some selected cases.

22. Vital signs, level of consciousness, skin, urine output, peripheral pulses with capillary refill

23. a. 3;  b. 2;  c. 3;  d. 5;  e. 2;  f. 1;  g. 3;  h. 1; i. 2;  j. 5

24. c. Rationale: If the metabolic acidosis is compensated, the pH will be within the normal range, and if the client is hyperventilating to blow off carbon dioxide to reduce the acid load of the blood, $PaCO_2$ will be decreased.

25. d. Rationale: Although some clients in shock may be treated with anti-anxiety and sedative drugs to control anxiety and apprehension, the nurse should always acknowledge the client's feelings and explain procedures before they are carried out and inform the client of the plan of care and its rationale. Members of the clergy should be called only if the client requests or agrees to a visit, and while visits by family may have a therapeutic effect on some clients, family visits may increase stress in others.

26. a. T; b. F, results; c. F, SIRS; d. T; e. T; f. F, lungs

27. a. 4;  b. 2;  c. 4;  d. 2;  e. 1;  f. 3;  g. 1;  h. 3; i. 5;  j. 5;  k. 6

28. d. Rationale: A respiratory rate above 20/min and a WBC count of less than $4 \times 10^9$/L ($4 \times 10^3$/μL) or more than $12 \times 10^9$/L ($12 \times 10^3$/μL) meet the clinical manifestation and laboratory finding criteria for determining the presence of SIRS. Other criteria include $PaCO_2$ less than 32 mm Hg, heart rate greater than 90/min, and temperature greater than 38°C (101.4°F) or less than 36°C (97°F).

29. a. Rationale: It is believed that early enteral feedings in the client in shock increase the blood supply to the GI tract and help prevent translocation of GI bacteria and endotoxins into the blood, preventing initial or additional infection in clients in shock. Surgical removal of necrotic tissue, especially from burns, eliminates a source of infection in critically ill clients, as does the use of strict aseptic technique in all client procedures.

Known infections are treated with specific agents, and broad-spectrum agents are used only until organisms are identified.

30. d. Rationale: The presence of MODS is confirmed when there is defined clinical evidence of failure of more than one organ. Elevated serum lipase and amylase levels indicate pancreatic failure, a serum creatinine of 200 μmol/L (2.3 mg/dL) indicates kidney failure, and a platelet count of $15 \times 10^9$/L ($15 \times 10^3$/μL) indicates hematological failure. Other criteria include urine output less than 0.5 mL/kg/hr, BUN 12 mmol/L (33.6 mg/dL) or greater, WBC count $1 \times 10^9$/L ($1 \times 10^3$/μL), upper or lower GI bleeding, Glasgow Coma Scale score 6 or less, and hematocrit 0.20 (20%) or less. A respiratory rate of 45/min, $PaCO_2$ of 60, and a chest x-ray with bilateral diffuse, patchy infiltrates indicate respiratory failure but not other organ damage.

**Case Study**

1. Indwelling catheter leading to urinary tract infection; compromised client—elderly, chronic illnesses of diabetes and heart failure

2. Aseptic technique in catheter placement; increased fluid intake to flush catheter; consult with physician regarding prophylactic antimicrobials; early detection of changes in urine, temperature

3. Release of endotoxins by Gram-negative bacteria that cause inflammatory responses is the initial insult. The endotoxins bind to monocytes and lymphocytes, stimulating the release of tumour necrosis factor and interleukin 1 (IL-1), which in turn cause release or activation of platelet-activating factor, prostaglandins, leukotrienes, thromboxane A-2, kinins, and complement. The result is widespread vasodilation and increased capillary permeability. Histamine also is released, which causes increased capillary permeability. The end result is decreased systemic vascular resistance (SVR) and normal or increased cardiac output (CO) as a result of the decreased SVR. Myocardial function is also suppressed by myocardial depressant factor. Death is associated with persistent increase in heart rate and CO, with low SVR and refractory hypotension with progression to MODS.

4. The widespread vasodilation caused by the inflammatory processes and increased capillary permeability causing fluid loss to the interstitium cause hypotension.

5. Decreased LOC—decreased tissue perfusion to the brain and hypoxia of brain cells

Warm, dry, and flushed skin—massive vasodilation

Tachycardia—activation of sympathetic nervous system with β-adrenergic stimulation increasing heart rate

Tachypnea—compensation for tissue hypoxia and metabolic acidosis

Fever—bacterial infection

Decreased SVR—profound vasodilation

Increased cardiac output—occurs as a result of decreased vascular resistance

Oliguria—inadequate renal perfusion and possible renal failure

Hyperglycemia—sympathetic nervous system stimulation causes glycogenolysis by the liver

6. To monitor fluid replacement and cardiac function because of multiple system involvement
7. Blood gases:
   * pH—indicates an acidosis, typical of the metabolic acidosis of anaerobic metabolism of shock
   * $PaO_2$—very low, indicating a marked hypoxemia
   * $PaCO_2$—also low as a result of hyperventilation to compensate for the metabolic acidosis
   * $HCO_3^-$—the bicarbonate is low because it is used to neutralize the acids of anaerobic metabolism.
   * $SaO_2$—a very low oxygen saturation. Normal should be 96%–100%, and the client's level indicates severe hypoxemia.
8. Hemodynamic pressures:
   * Right atrial pressure (RAP)—normal is 2 to 8 mm Hg. Marked vasodilation would decrease venous return to the heart, and it would be expected to be decreased.
   * Pulmonary artery pressure (PAP)—normal is 10 to 20 mm Hg and is an indicator of afterload or systemic vascular resistance. The client's PAP would be expected to be decreased in septic shock, where there is profound vasodilation.
   * Pulmonary artery wedge pressure (PAWP)—normal is 6 to 12 mm Hg and is an indicator of afterload or systemic vascular resistance. The client's PAWP would be expected to be low.
   * Cardiac output (CO)—normal is 4 to 8 L/min. The client's CO would be expected to be elevated, illustrating the high cardiac output typical of septic shock.
   * Systemic vascular resistance (SVR)—normal is 900 to 1400 dynes/sec/cm$^{-5}$. Vasodilation would produce a decreased SVR.
9. Fluid therapy is used to increase vascular volume and blood pressure to increase tissue perfusion. Dopamine is used to increase vasoconstriction and strengthen myocardial contractions to elevate systemic vascular resistance.
10. *Nursing diagnoses:*
    * Altered tissue perfusion related to deficit in capillary blood supply
    * Altered protection related to neurosensory alterations
    * Hyperthermia related to inflammatory process
    * Risk for disuse syndrome related to perceptual-cognitive impairment
    *Collaborative problems:*
    Potential complications: heart failure; ARDS; DIC; organ ischemia—neurological, renal, GI; MODS

# CHAPTER 66

1. c. Rationale: Respiratory failure results when the transfer of oxygen or carbon dioxide functions of the respiratory system are impaired, and although the definition is determined by $PaO_2$ and $PaCO_2$ levels, the major factor in respiratory failure is inadequate gas exchange to meet tissue $O_2$ needs. Absence of ventilation is respiratory arrest, and partial airway obstruction may not necessarily cause respiratory failure. Acute hypoxemia may be caused by factors other than pulmonary dysfunction.
2. a. HO; b. HO; c. HC; d. HO; e. HO; f. HC; g. HC; h. HO; i. HC
3. a. T; b. F, 1 or less; c. T; d. F, air in the lung from passing into the blood; e. F, V/Q mismatch; f. F, diffusion limitation
4. a. 3; b. 4; c. 2; d. 5; e. 1
5. a. 3; b. 1; c. 2; d. 4
6. b. Rationale: Hypercapnic respiratory failure is associated with alveolar hypoventilation with increases in alveolar and arterial $CO_2$ and often is caused by problems outside the lungs. A client with slow, shallow respirations is not exchanging enough gas volume to eliminate $CO_2$. Deep, rapid respirations reflect hyperventilation and often accompany lung problems that cause hypoxemic respiratory failure. Pulmonary edema and large airway resistance cause obstruction of oxygenation and result in a V/Q mismatch or shunt typical of hypoxemic respiratory failure.
7. d. Rationale: In a client with normal lung function, respiratory failure is commonly defined as a $PaO_2 \leq 60$ mm Hg or a $PaCO_2 > 45$ mm Hg or both, but because the client with chronic pulmonary disease normally maintains low $PaO_2$ and high $PaCO_2$, acute respiratory failure in these clients can be defined as an acute decrease in $PaO_2$ or increase in $PaCO_2$ from the client's baseline parameters, accompanied by an acid pH. The

pH of 7.28 reflects an acidemia and a loss of compensation in the client with chronic lung disease.

8. a. HO; b. HC; c. HC; d. HO; e. HO; f. HC; g. HC

9. a. Rationale: Because the brain is very sensitive to a decrease in oxygen delivery, restlessness, agitation, disorientation, and confusion are early signs of hypoxemia, for which the nurse should be alert. Mild hypertension is also an early sign, accompanied by tachycardia. Central cyanosis is an unreliable, late sign of hypoxemia, and cardiac arrhythmias also occur later.

10. d. Rationale: The increase in respiratory rate required to blow off accumulated $CO_2$ predisposes to respiratory muscle fatigue, and the slowing of a rapid rate in a client in acute distress indicates tiring and the possibility of respiratory arrest unless ventilatory assistance is provided. A decreased I/E ratio, orthopnea, and accessory muscle use are common findings in respiratory distress but do not necessarily signal respiratory fatigue or arrest.

11. a. Rationale: Clients with a shunt are usually more hypoxemic than are clients with a V/Q mismatch because the alveoli are filled with fluid, which prevents gas exchange. Hypoxemia secondary to an intrapulmonary shunt is usually not responsive to high $O_2$ concentrations, and the client will usually require positive pressure ventilation. Hypoxemia associated with a V/Q mismatch usually responds favourably to oxygen administration at 1 to 3 L/min by nasal cannula. Removal of secretions with coughing and suctioning is not generally effective in reversing an acute hypoxemia secondary to a shunt.

12. a. Rationale: When there is impaired function of the one lung, the client should be positioned with the unaffected lung in the dependent position to promote perfusion to the functioning tissue. If the diseased lung is positioned dependently, more V/Q mismatch would occur. The head of the bed may be elevated, or a reclining chair may be used, with the client positioned on the unaffected side, to maximize thoracic expansion if the client has increased work of breathing.

13. b. Rationale: Augmented coughing by applying pressure on the thorax or abdominal muscles at the beginning of expiration helps produce muscle movement, increases pleural pressure and expiratory flows, and assists the cough to remove secretions in the client who is exhausted. An oral airway is used only if there is a possibility that the tongue will obstruct the airway. Huff coughing is indicated for clients with problems with endotracheal tubes in place, which prevent glottal closure, and slow, pursed-lip breathing is used to prevent air trapping and give the client a sense of control over breathing.

14. c. Rationale: Hemodynamic monitoring with a pulmonary artery catheter is instituted in severe respiratory failure to determine the amount of blood flow to tissues and the response of the lung and heart to hypoxemia. Continuous blood pressure monitoring may be performed, but blood pressure is a reflection of cardiac activity, which can be determined by the pulmonary artery catheter findings. Arterial blood gas values are important to evaluate oxygenation and ventilation status and V/Q mismatches.

15. d. Rationale: Drug therapy indicated for acute respiratory failure depends on the symptoms that are present and the underlying cause of the respiratory failure. Bronchodilators and IV corticosteroids are used if bronchospasm and inflammation are present; antibiotics are used if infection is present; diuretics are used if pulmonary congestion is caused by heart failure; and sedatives may be used if anxiety and agitation increase the degree of hypoxemia.

16. d. Rationale: NIPPV involves the application of a face mask and delivery of a volume of air under inspiratory pressure. Because the device is worn externally, the client must be able to cooperate in its use, and frequent access to the airway for suctioning or inhaled medications must not be necessary. It is not indicated when high levels of oxygen are needed or respirations are absent.

17. a. Rationale: Although ARDS may occur in the client who has virtually any severe illness or trauma and may be both a cause and result of SIRS; the most common precipitating insults of ARDS are septic shock and gastric aspiration.

18. a. Interstitial and alveolar edema from damage to vascular endothelium and increased capillary permeability
    b. Atelectasis from destruction of type II cells, resulting in inactivation of surfactant
    c. Hyaline membrane formation from exudation of high molecular weight substances in the edema fluid

19. c. Rationale: In the fibrotic phase of ARDS, diffuse scarring and fibrosis of the lungs occur, resulting in decreased surface area for gas exchange and continued hypoxemia due to diffusion limitation. Although edema is resolved, lung compliance is decreased because of interstitial fibrosis, and long-term mechanical ventilation is required with a poor prognosis for survival.

20. a. Rationale: Hypoxemia that does not respond to oxygenation by any route is a hallmark of ARDS and is always present. $PaCO_2$ levels may be normal until the client is no longer able to compen-

sate in response to the hypoxemia. Bronchial breath sounds may be associated with the progression of ARDS. Pulmonary capillary wedge pressures, which are normally elevated in cardiogenic pulmonary edema, are normal in the pulmonary edema of ARDS.

21. c. Rationale: Early signs of ARDS are insidious and difficult to detect, but the nurse should be alert for any early signs of hypoxemia, such as restlessness, dyspnea, and decreased mentation, in clients at risk for ARDS. Abnormal findings on physical examination or diagnostic studies, such as adventitious lung sounds, signs of respiratory distress, respiratory alkalosis, or decreasing $PaO_2$, are usually indications that ARDS has progressed beyond the initial stages.

22. b. Rationale: Nosocomial pneumonia is one of the most common complications of ARDS, and early detection requires frequent monitoring of sputum smears and cultures and assessment of the quality, quantity, and consistency of sputum. Blood in gastric aspirate may indicate a stress ulcer, and subcutaneous emphysema of the face, neck, and chest occurs with barotrauma during mechanical ventilation. Oral infections may result from prophylactic antibiotics and impaired host defenses but are not common.

23. a. Rationale: Because ARDS is precipitated by a physiological insult, a critical factor in its prevention and early management is treatment of the underlying condition. Prophylactic antibiotics, treatment with diuretics and fluid restriction, and mechanical ventilation are also used as ARDS progresses.

24. a. Rationale: PEEP used with mechanical ventilation applies positive pressure to the airway and lungs at the end of exhalation, keeping the lung partially expanded and preventing collapse of the alveoli and helping to open up collapsed alveoli. Permissive hypercapnia is allowed when the client with ARDS is ventilated with smaller tidal volumes to prevent barotrauma. Extracorporeal membrane oxygenation and extracorporeal $CO_2$ removal involve passing blood across a gas-exchanging membrane outside the body and then returning oxygenated blood back to the body.

25. c. Rationale: PEEP increases intrathoracic and intrapulmonic pressures, compresses the pulmonary capillary bed, and reduces blood return to both the right and left side of the heart. Preload (CVP) and cardiac output are decreased, often with a dramatic decrease in blood pressure.

26. d. Rationale: When a client with ARDS is supine, alveoli in the posterior areas of the lung are dependent and fluid-filled, and the heart and mediastinal contents place more pressure on the lungs, predisposing to atelectasis. If the client is turned prone, air-filled, non-atelectic alveoli in the anterior portion of the lung receive more blood, and perfusion may be better matched to ventilation, causing less V/Q mismatch. Lateral rotation therapy is used to stimulate postural drainage and help mobilize pulmonary secretions.

**Case Study**

1. The client is experiencing hypercapnic respiratory failure, reflected by the elevated $PaCO_2$ and pH of 7.3. In this case severe COPD, with destruction of alveoli and terminal respiratory units, has led to hypoventilation, with less removal of $CO_2$ and less space for $O_2$ in the alveoli. The client with severe COPD always has some degree of decompensation resulting in chronic respiratory failure, but an acute exacerbation or infection may cause an acute decompensation, thus producing an acute or chronic respiratory failure.

2. The primary contributing factor to the onset of the acute failure is the pneumonia, but other factors include the presence of chronic lung disease, her age, and immunosuppression with steroids.

3. The primary pathophysiological effects of hypercapnia are a respiratory acidosis resulting from retained $CO_2$ and a hypoxemia resulting from alveolar retention of $CO_2$. Clinical manifestations of hypercapnic respiratory failure that Mrs. C. is experiencing include the dyspnea, shortness of breath, sitting in a tripod position, and using pursed-lip breathing, in addition to her ABG values. Other manifestations of hypercapnia that the nurse should assess Mrs. C. for include morning headache, somnolence, confusion, arrhythmias, and muscle weakness. Because she is also hypoxemic, she should be assessed for mild hypertension, tachycardia, prolonged expiration, and accessory respiratory muscle use.

4. The tripod position helps decrease the work of breathing, because propping the arms up increases the antero-posterior diameter of the chest and changes pressures in the thorax. Pursed-lip breathing causes an increase in $SaO_2$ because it slows respiration, allows more time for expiration, and prevents the small bronchioles from collapsing.

5. Non-invasive positive pressure ventilation (NIPPV) is delivered by placing a mask over the client's nose or nose and mouth; and the client breathes spontaneously while positive pressure is delivered. It may be used as a treatment for clients with acute or chronic respiratory failure and helps decrease the work of breathing, without the need for endotracheal intubation. It is not

appropriate for the client who has absent respirations, excessive secretions, a decreased level of consciousness, high $O_2$ requirements, facial trauma, or hemodynamic instability.

6. Treatment of acute respiratory failure is directed toward reversing the disease process that resulted in the failure. Mrs. C.'s COPD is chronic and irreversible, but the IV antibiotics are critical in treating the pneumonia that precipitated the acute on chronic respiratory failure. The bronchodilators and corticosteroids will help with airway inflammation and spasm, but it cannot be expected that she will recover without treatment of the infection.

7. *Nursing diagnoses:*
   - Ineffective breathing pattern related to expiratory obstruction to airflow
   - Ineffective airway clearance related to increased airway resistance
   - Impaired gas exchange related to alveolar hypoventilation
   - Risk for impaired skin integrity related to NIPPV mask

   *Collaborative problems:*
   Potential complications: hypoxia; hypercapnia; respiratory and metabolic acidosis; arrhythmias

## CHAPTER 67

1. a. Level II; b. Level II; c. Level IV; d. Level V; e. Level I; f. Level II; g. Level III

2. b. Rationale: During the primary survey of emergency care, assessment and immediate interventions for life-threatening problems affecting airway, breathing, circulation, and disability are performed. The triage system is used initially to determine the priority of care for clients, and history of the illness or accident is part of the secondary survey. Any emergency department should be able to stabilize and initially treat a client if the client requires specialized care unavailable at the admitting facility.

3. a. Inhalation injury, airway obstruction, upper airway wounds or trauma
      Interventions: Jaw-thrust, artificial airway, suctioning
   b. Anaphylaxis, flail chest, hemothorax, open or tension pneumothorax
      Interventions: Ventilate with bag-valve mask at 100% oxygen, chest tube insertion or needle thoracostomy, endotracheal intubation
   c. Cardiac injury, pericardial tamponade, shock, uncontrolled external hemorrhage
      Interventions: CPR and ALS if no pulse, two large-bore IVs with infusions of fluids or

blood, pneumatic antishock garment for pelvic fracture, direct pressure to bleeding
   d. Head injury, stroke
      Interventions: Monitor LOC, consider hyperventilation if signs of herniation, elevate head of bed 30 degrees

4. a. Rationale: Specific injuries are associated with specific types of accidents and events surrounding an incident, and details of the incident and the trajectory of penetrating injuries are important in identifying and treating injury. Alcohol use is assessed with blood testing, and although information may be used for regulatory agencies, the primary use of the information is for treatment of the client.

5. a. Cardiac monitoring; b. Pulse oximetry monitoring; c. Indwelling urinary catheter; d. Oro- or nasogastric tube; e. Laboratory studies

6. b. Rationale: A nasally placed tube is contraindicated if the client has facial fractures or a possible basilar skull fracture, because the tube could enter the brain. It would not be contraindicated in the other conditions.

7. a. Allergies; b. Medications; c. Past health history, pregnancy status; d. Last meal; e. Events of the illness or injury

8. b. Rationale: Tetanus immunoglobulin provides passive immunity for tetanus and is used in treatment of a tetanus-prone wound if the client has not had at least three doses of active tetanus toxoid. The client would also receive tetanus toxoid to initiate active immunity in the case of tetanus-prone wounds. If the client has fewer than three doses of tetanus toxoid and a non–tetanus-prone wound, only tetanus toxoid would be administered to initiate active immunity. In the actively immunized client, tetanus toxoid is administered for tetanus-prone wounds if it has been more than five years since the last dose, and it is also administered for non–tetanus-prone wounds if it has been more than 10 years since the last dose.

9. a. Rationale: Before organ donor coordinators are notified, the family members should be made aware of the possibility of organ donation and have a chance to discuss the issue. The best way is just to question them about the possibility without influencing them to make a decision they would later question. If there is interest, the organ donor coordinator can be notified to assist in screening, counselling, and obtaining consent.

10. a. 4; b. 5; c. 2; d. 5; e. 4; f. 5; g. 3; h. 5; i. 4; j. 1

11. c. Rationale: Rewarming of frostbitten tissue is extremely painful, and analgesia should be administered during the process. The affected part is submerged in a warm water bath at approxi-

mately 37°C to 40°C (98.6°F to 104°F), and massage or scrubbing of the tissue should be avoided because of the potential for tissue damage. Blisters form in hours to days following the injury and are not an immediate concern.

12. a. Rationale: Unconsciousness, bradycardia, and slowed respiratory rate are signs of moderate hypothermia, and movement of the client should be avoided to prevent ventricular fibrillation, a common complication of hypothermia and rewarming. Active core rewarming is indicated for moderate to severe hypothermia. Axillary temperatures are inadequate to monitor core temperature, so esophageal, rectal, or indwelling urinary catheter thermometers are used. The client should be assessed for other injuries but should not be exposed, in order to prevent further loss of heat.

13. b. Rationale: Clients with severe hypothermia appear dead on presentation and exhibit fixed, dilated pupils, respirations so slow that they may not be detected, unconsciousness, and absent reflexes. Shivering is seen in mild hypothermia, and moderate hypothermia is characterized by slowed respirations, blood pressure obtainable only by Doppler, and rigidity.

14. a. F; b. B; c. S; d. B; e. S; f. B

15. a. Rationale: The most important life-threatening consequence of near-drowning of any type is hypoxia from fluid-filled and poorly ventilated alveoli, and airway and oxygenation are first priorities. Correction of metabolic (anaerobic) acidosis occurs with effective ventilation and oxygenation; lactated Ringer's or normal saline solution is started to manage fluid balance; and mannitol or furosemide may be used to treat free-water and cerebral edema.

16. d. Rationale: As edema increases with the response to snake or insect bites, watches, rings, or constrictive clothing on an affected part may cause circulatory obstruction and should be removed before the onset of edema. Ice and tourniquets are not recommended because both may cause tissue necrosis, and elevation of the extremity causes increased absorption and circulation of venom.

17. a. Rationale: Wood ticks or dog ticks release a neurotoxin as long as the tick head is attached to the body, and tick removal is essential for effective treatment. Tick removal leads to return of muscle movement, usually within 48 to 72 hours. There is no antidote, and hemodialysis is not known to remove the neurotoxin. Antibiotics are used to treat Lyme disease and Rocky Mountain spotted fever, infections spread by tick bites.

18. a. F, human; b. T; c. F, washing with large amounts of water; d. F, water or milk; e. T

19. b, e, f

20. a. 3; b. 1; c. 4; d. 2

21.

| Agent | Bacterial | Viral | Person-to-Person Spread | Antibiotic Treatment | Active Vaccine | Passive Vaccine/ Antitoxin |
|---|---|---|---|---|---|---|
| Botulism | x | | | | | x |
| Anthrax | x | | | x | x | |
| Plague | x | | x | x (if early) | | |
| Hemorrhagic fever | | x | x | | | |
| Tularemia | x | | | x | | |
| Small pox | | x | x | | x | x |

22. a. 6;  b. 4;  c. 2;  d. 1;  e. 4;  f. 6;  g. 3;  h. 2; i. 6;  j. 5;  k. 3; l. 1
23. b. Rationale: Ionizing radiation exposure in a sublethal dose will cause nausea and vomiting within two to four hours of exposure, hair loss in two days to two weeks, and coagulopathies in two days to two weeks.

## Case Study

1. Advanced age and prolonged exposure to heat over several days are risk factors for Mr. M.'s development of heat stroke.
2. ABGs—decreased $PaO_2$; electrolytes—decreased serum sodium, chloride, potassium; CBC—hemoconcentration with elevated hemoglobin and hematocrit; BUN and creatinine—elevated; serum glucose—decreased; coagulation studies—decreased prothrombin time, decreased bleeding times; liver function tests—elevated enzymes; UA—elevated specific gravity, protein, possible microscopic hematuria
3. Clothing would be removed, and fans and tepid water mist may be used, as well as ice water baths. If the temperature is not reduced by these methods, ice water lavage or cold water peritoneal dialysis may be used.
4. 100% oxygen to compensate for the hypermetabolic state, with intubation and mechanical ventilation if necessary; IV crystalloid salt solution with CVC or PA catheter to monitor fluid status; cooling methods with monitoring of core temperature; indwelling catheter and I&O; administration of chlorpromazine (Thorazine) to control shivering during cooling process
5. Mrs. M. should be told that Mr. M. is very seriously ill and that there is a chance he might not recover because heat stroke has a very high morbidity and mortality rate. She should be kept informed of the treatment he is receiving and his response to treatment, and she should be provided with emotional support.
6. *Nursing diagnoses:*
   - Hyperthermia related to environmental exposure
   - Decreased cardiac output related to hypermetabolic process
   - Deficient fluid volume related to fluid loss excessive of intake
   - Altered protection related to altered mental state
   - Risk for injury related to seizure activity
   - Risk for impaired skin integrity related to immobility
   *Collaborative problems:*
   Potential complications: hypovolemic shock; cerebral edema; seizures; hypoxia; electrolyte imbalance; renal failure